Gastrointestinal Tract and Liver Diseases: Mechanisms, Diagnosis and Treatment

Gastrointestinal Tract and Liver Diseases: Mechanisms, Diagnosis and Treatment

Editor: Adan Bowler

AMERICAN
MEDICAL PUBLISHERS
www.americanmedicalpublishers.com

AMERICAN
MEDICAL PUBLISHERS
www.americanmedicalpublishers.com

Cataloging-in-Publication Data

Gastrointestinal tract and liver diseases : mechanisms, diagnosis and treatment / edited by Adan Bowler.
p. cm.
Includes bibliographical references and index.
ISBN 979-8-88740-130-0
1. Gastrointestinal system--Diseases. 2. Liver--Diseases. 3. Gastrointestinal system--Diseases--Diagnosis.
4. Liver--Diseases--Diagnosis. 5. Gastrointestinal system--Diseases--Treatment. 6. Liver--Diseases--Treatment.
7. Gastrointestinal system. 8. Gastro I. Bowler, Adan.
RC816 .G37 2023
616.33--dc23

American Medical Publishers,
41 Flatbush Avenue,
1st Floor, New York,
NY 11217, USA

ISBN 979-8-88740-130-0 (Hardback)

Contents

Preface

The gastrointestinal tract is a passage way containing major organs of the digestive system from mouth to anus. The digestive system in humans comprises the gastrointestinal tract along with the accessory organs including the gallbladder, pancreas, salivary glands, liver and tongue. One of the significant diseases associated with gastrointestinal tract is the liver disease. Upset stomach and nausea are signs of liver disease. As the ability of the liver to take out the toxins decreases; it increases the digestive distress. Liver disorders can be genetic or caused due to viral infections, alcohol use and even obesity. Primary cancers of the gastrointestinal tract can eventually metastasize and cause secondary lesions or liver malignancies. One of the significant mechanisms that cause liver diseases is DNA damage. Diagnostic tests like liver function test, which are a group of blood tests, can be used to examine the proper functioning of liver. This book unravels the recent studies on gastrointestinal tract and liver diseases. Also included herein is a detailed explanation of the diagnosis, mechanisms and treatment of these diseases. This book is a resource guide for experts as well as students.

This book unites the global concepts and researches in an organized manner for a comprehensive understanding of the subject. It is a ripe text for all researchers, students, scientists or anyone else who is interested in acquiring a better knowledge of this dynamic field.

I extend my sincere thanks to the contributors for such eloquent research chapters. Finally, I thank my family for being a source of support and help.

Editor

1

Targeting Certain Interleukins as Novel Treatment Options for Liver Fibrosis

Su Yeon An[1], *Anca D. Petrescu*[1] *and Sharon DeMorrow*[1,2,3]*

[1]Division of Pharmacology and Toxicology, College of Pharmacy, The University of Texas at Austin, Austin, TX, United States, [2]Department of Internal Medicine, Dell Medical School, The University of Texas at Austin, Austin, TX, United States, [3]Research Division, Central Texas Veterans Healthcare System, Temple, TX, United States

***Correspondence:** Sharon DeMorrow sharon.demorrow@austin.utexas.edu

The liver is a major metabolic organ and an immunologically complex organ. It produces and uses many substances such as acute phase proteins, cytokines, chemokines, and complementary components to maintain the balance between immunity and tolerance. Interleukins are important immune control cytokines, that are produced by many body cells. In liver injury, interleukins are produced in large amount by various cell types, and act as pro-inflammatory (e.g. interleukin (IL)-6, IL-13, IL-17, and IL-33) as well as anti-inflammatory (e.g. IL-10) functions in hepatic cells. Recently, interleukins are regarded as interesting therapeutic targets for the treatment of liver fibrosis patients. Hepatic cells such as hepatocytes, hepatic stellate cells, and hepatic macrophages are involved to the initiation, perpetuation, and resolution of fibrosis. The understanding of the role of interleukins in such cells provides opportunity for the development of therapeutic target drugs. This paper aims to understand the functional roles of interleukins in hepatic and immune cells when the liver is damaged, and suggests the possibility of interleukins as a new treatment target in liver fibrosis.

Keywords: interleukins, hepatocytes, macrophages, hepatic stellate cells, $CD4^+$ T helper cells, liver fibrosis

INTRODUCTION

Fibrosis is the pathological feature and the end result of chronic inflammatory reaction induced by various types of injuries in several organs including skin, kidney, lung, heart, intestine, and liver. Therefore chronic fibroproliferative diseases is a major public health problem (Nanchahal and Hinz, 2016). In the liver, progressive fibrosis caused by injury, inflammation, and extracellular matrix (ECM) accumulation ultimately results in cirrhosis or hepatocellular carcinoma. The only effective treatment for these terminal liver disorders is liver transplantation (Bataller and Brenner, 2005; Bansal et al., 2016). For this reason, treatment at the liver fibrosis stage that prevents the progression of the disease, and that leads to resolution is very important.

Abbreviations: α-SMA, α-smooth muscle actin; CCl4, Carbon tetrachloride; CD4 T cells; CD4+ T helper cells; DAMP, Danger associated molecular patterns; ECM, Extracellular matrix; ERK, Extracellular signal regulated kinase; HSCs, Hepatic stellate cells; IL, Interleukin; IL-10R, IL-10 receptor; ILC2, Innate lymphoid cells; JAK, Janus kinase; MAPK; Mitogen-activated protein kinase; MCs, Mast cells; MoMFs, Monocytes-derived macrophages; MyD88, Myeloid differentiation primary response gene 88; NF-κB; Nuclear factor-κB, PDGF, Platelet-derived growth factor; STAT, Signal transducer and activator of transcription; TGF-β, Transforming growth factor-β; Th, T helper; TRAF6, Tumor necrosis factor receptor-associated factor 6; Tregs, Regulatory T cells; TYK, Tyrosine kinase.

The initiation, perpetuation and resolution of liver fibrosis is a complex process of communication between cells receiving a multitude of signals consisting of various growth factors, chemokines and cytokines (Kubes and Jenne, 2018). Interleukins, a cytokine family that include chemokines, interferons, lymphokines, and tumor necrosis factors, were first thought to be expressed in leukocytes alone, but it was later found that about 40 types of interleukins were produced by many other body cells. Interleukins play an essential role in the activation and differentiation of immune cells as well as proliferation, maturity, migration, and adhesion. They can also have pro-inflammatory or anti-inflammatory or both properties (Hammerich and Tacke, 2014).

IL-6 and IL-1 are representative keystone cytokines in liver disease and have both pro and anti-inflammatory properties. IL-6 is a main regulatory factor in processes of wound healing and tissue regeneration related to various liver injures. It was concluded that IL-6/STAT3 signaling prevents cholestasis and liver fibrosis and has role in regulation of hepatocyte and cholangiocyte functions in the model of sclerosing cholangitis (Mair et al., 2010). However, more recent publications reveal negative effects of IL-6 which can directly induce transition of HSCs to myofibroblast-like cells, in hepatic fibrosis (Kagan et al., 2017). Very recent studies on the role of JAK-STAT signaling in hepatocellular carcinoma (HCC) emphasized that members of IL-6 family of cytokines have emerged as important regulatory factors and are considered to be targets for therapeutic intervention (Lokau et al., 2019). IL-1 family consists of 11 cytokines of the innate immune system. These cytokines trigger various immune responses to liver injuries, i.e. IL-1α, β and IL-33 are proinflammatory cytokines; in contrast, IL-1Ra, IL-36Ra, IL-37, and IL-38 have anti-inflammatory responses, while IL-18 was found to be pro- and anti-inflammatory under different circumstances (Barbier et al., 2019; Chan and Schroder, 2020). Additionally, IL-1 cytokines activate mast cells (MCs) to secrete inflammatory mediators (chemokines and cytokines including IL-1, IL-33 and TNF), and this effect can be counteracted by IL-37 (Gallenga et al., 2019). Thus, it has been determined that IL-37 is an anti-inflammatory cytokine that interacts with IL-18Ra chain and decreases the inflammatory effects of IL-1 cytokines (Toniato et al., 2017; Caraffa et al., 2019; Gugliandolo et al., 2019). Cytokines from IL-36 subfamily of IL-1 are produced by activated MCs and have strong pro-inflammatory effects which can be balanced by IL-38 which binds to IL-36R inducing anti-inflammatory activity (Varvara et al., 2018; Gallenga et al., 2019). Numerous studies have investigated the role of each cytokine and receptor from this family in various types of liver injuries, and have been reviewed in detail recently (He et al., 2021).

This review presents and emphasizes certain interleukins as potential therapeutic targets for liver fibrosis. We specifically focused on the pro-inflammatory interleukins: interleukin (IL)-13, IL-17, and IL-33, anti-inflammatory interleukin: IL-10 based on the numerous studies published in recent years that clearly showed their functions and effects. Furthermore, this review summarizes the origin, function, and signal pathway of these selected interleukins and, also shows the functions of these specific interleukins in hepatocytes, hepatic stellate cells (HSCs), and hepatic macrophages which are main players in liver fibrosis.

CD4$^+$ T HELPER CELLS

The innate and adaptive immune responses occurring simultaneously or sequentially in time, are initiated by Kupffer cells that recognize liver damage. Following liver injury, inflammatory lymphocytes infiltrate the damaged hepatic parenchyma (Dong et al., 2019; Li et al., 2019). T lymphocytes, which are activated through antigen-specific manner of dendritic cells, help the B lymphocytes to create antigen-specific antibodies, or to remove infected cells. Specially, CD4$^+$ T helper cells (CD4 T cells) serve as the total commander of immunity. CD4 T cells can be classified into at least four subsets, referred to as T helper (Th) cells type 1, Th2, Th17, and induced regulatory T cells (Tregs). These cells play a major role in mediating immune response through the secretion of specific cytokines (Luckheeram et al., 2012).

Th1 cells play a particularly important role in mediating immune responses against intracellular pathogens, resistance to mycobacterial infections, and induction of some autoimmune diseases. Their principal cytokine products are interferon gamma, lymphotoxin α, and IL-2 (Paul and Seder, 1994). Th2 cells mediate immune response to extracellular parasites, including helminths, and play an important role in induction and persistence of asthma and other allergic diseases. Th2 cells produce IL-4, IL-5, IL-9, IL-13, IL-10, IL-25, and amphiregulin (Luckheeram et al., 2012). Th17 cells are responsible for mediating immune responses against extracellular fungi and bacteria, and for inducing the many organ-specific autoimmune diseases. Th17 cells produce IL-17, IL-17f, IL-21, and IL-22 (Zhu and Paul, 2008). IL-17 leads to the induction of pro-inflammatory cytokines, including IL-6, IL-1, tumor necrosis factor-α (TNF-α), and thus has an important role in inducing inflammatory responses (Luckheeram et al., 2012). Tregs play a critical role in the maintenance of self-tolerance to self and foreign antigen. Increasing Tregs numbers and/or enhancing their suppressive function may be beneficial for preventing allograft rejection and treating autoimmune diseases. The main effector cytokines of Tregs include IL-10, transforming growth factor-β (TGF-β), and IL-35 (Zhu and Paul, 2008; Luckheeram et al., 2012).

CD4 T cells release a wide range of inflammatory intermediates, particularly interleukins, which can act as the pro-inflammatory, anti-inflammatory, or two functions in liver fibrosis (Hammerich and Tacke, 2014; Sziksz et al., 2020). However, selecting interleukins with conflicting functions depending on the stage of liver disease as a therapeutic target requires more attention in the treatment process. In the case of IL-6 or IL-22, it prevents fibrogenesis but promotes hepatocellular carcinoma, so the risk of tumor occurrence should be considered in the treatment of patients with hepatic fibrosis (Schmidt-Arras and Rose-John, 2016; Wu et al., 2020). Therefore, it is very important to select and study targets capable of blocking pro-inflammatory (IL-13, IL-17, and IL-33) or inducing anti-inflammatory interleukin (IL-10) in the complex process of liver fibrosis.

TARGET INTERLEUKINS

Interleukin-10

IL-10, one of the major anti-inflammatory cytokines, controls neutrophil infiltration and suppresses various pro-inflammatory mediators (Louis et al., 1998; Sziksz et al., 2020). IL-10 can be produced by Th2 cells but also by Th1, Th17, Tregs, $CD8^+$ T, and B lymphocytes. In the liver, IL-10 is expressed in various cell types, including hepatocytes, Kupffer cells, sinusoidal endothelial cells, HSCs, and lymphocytes (Hammerich and Tacke, 2014; Sziksz et al., 2020). Functional IL-10 receptor (IL-10R) complexes are tetramers consisting of two IL-10R1 and two IL-10R2 chains. IL-10 homodimer binding to its receptor activate Janus kinase (JAK) 1 and Tyrosine kinase (TYK) 2. Signal transducer and activator of transcription (STAT) 3 binds to IL-10R1 and phosphorylates, and then phosphorylated STAT3 translocate to the nucleus (**Figure 1**) (Verma et al., 2016).

Interleukin-13

IL-13 is an immunoregulatory cytokine secreted by predominantly Th2 cells. IL-13 has multiple effects on the differentiation and function of monocytes and macrophages. Although IL-13 plays an important role in the induction of allergic responses and inflammation as anti-inflammatory cytokine, it is a critical pro-fibrotic factor in liver fibrosis associated with Schistosoma and non-Schistosoma infection (De Vries, 1998; Liu et al., 2012). Additionally, IL-13 has been implicated in inflammatory bowel disease, asthma, and parasitic nematode expulsion (Grunig et al., 1998; Hershey, 2003). IL-13 induces many of the same responses and functional properties as IL-4 and shares a receptor subunit, the α subunit of the IL-4 receptor. IL-13 binds to the complex receptor system comprised of IL-4 receptor and two IL-13 binding proteins, IL-13Rα1 and IL-13Rα2. Signaling through the type II receptor (IL-4 receptor and IL13Rα1) leads to activation of JAK1 or JAK2/TYK2, STAT6, STAT3, and STAT1. Then, STAT dimerization and nuclear translocation occurs, followed by activation of gene transcription (**Figure 1**) (McCormick and Heller, 2015). IL-13 receptor is expressed on human B cells, basophils, eosinophils, mast cells, endothelial cells, fibroblasts, monocytes, macrophages, respiratory epithelial cells, and smooth muscle cells (Hershey, 2003).

Interleukin-17

IL-17 (now IL-17A) is an ancient pro-inflammatory cytokine with important roles in defense against bacteria and fungi. IL-17 are produced primarily by a T-cell subset termed Th17 cells, but can also be produced by neutrophils and other lymphocytes (Onishi and Gaffen, 2010). IL-17 signals through the IL-17RA-RC complex, and the IL-17 receptor recruits Act1 for downstream signaling. The Act1 with the IL-17 receptor complex contributes to the recruitment of Tumor necrosis factor receptor associated factor 6 (TRAF6). Then, these kinases promote the production of pro-inflammatory cytokines, chemokines, and-microbial peptides, through the pathway such as nuclear factor-κB (NF-κB), activator protein, and CCAAT/enhancer binding protein pathways (**Figure 1**) (Onishi and Gaffen, 2010; Meng et al., 2012).

Interleukin-33

IL-33 is the most recently identified member of IL-1 family of cytokines and is mainly expressed by stromal cells. IL-33 has been shown to induce the Th2 phenotype in Th cell, and therefore promotes progression of Th2-related diseases like several acute and chronic inflammatory diseases, including asthma, atopic dermatitis, rheumatoid arthritis, and ulcerative colitis among others (Schmitz et al., 2005; Sanada et al., 2007). The activity of IL-33 is mediated by binding to the heterodimeric ST2/IL-1 receptor associated protein receptor. Afterward, the complex recruits intracellular signaling molecules, including myeloid differentiation primary response 88 (MyD88)/IL-1 receptor-associated kinase/TRAF6, activating NF-κB, as well as extracellular signal regulated kinase (ERK) 1/2, c-Jun N-terminal kinase, p38 and phosphatidylinositol 3-kinase/protein kinase B (**Figure 1**) (Pinto et al., 2018; Barbier et al., 2019). Recently, IL-33 has gained attention as a new target or as an early alarm of liver fibrogenesis, as Th2 cells are strongly associated with fibrosis progression (Hammerich and Tacke, 2014; Weiskirchen and Tacke, 2016).

CONTRIBUTION OF THESE TARGET INTERLEUKINS IN THE HEPATIC CELLS

Interleukins in Hepatocytes

Hepatocytes are the major parenchymal cells that are important for liver function in metabolism, detoxification, and alcohol processing, and protein synthesis. Hepatocytes also activate innate and adaptive immunity when they are damaged by hepatotropic virus, an intracellular bacterium, or repeated or continuous injury (Crispe, 2016; Zhou et al., 2016). The initial reaction of hepatocytes injury by multiple factors is cell stress and cell death. The stressed and dying hepatocytes release damage-associated molecular patterns (DAMPs), reactive oxygen species, pro-inflammatory signals, and proliferation-associated cytokines through cross-talk with surrounding cells such as HSCs, endothelial cells, and immune cells (Tu et al., 2015; Yan et al., 2018). The reaction of hepatocytes indicate that hepatocytes contribute to the progress and resolution of liver fibrosis as active participants, not victims or bystanders (Tu et al., 2015).

McHedlidze et al. showed that damaged hepatocytes secreted IL-33 and that extracellular IL-33 leads to accumulation and activation of innate lymphoid cells (ILC2) (McHedlidze et al., 2013). Activated ILC2 by IL-33 produce IL-13, which induced the activation and trans-differentiation of HSCs through type-II IL-4 receptor-dependent signaling and STAT6. Further studies have identified IL-33 as key mediator of hepatic fibrosis by demonstrating that IL-33 deficiency ameliorates liver fibrosis

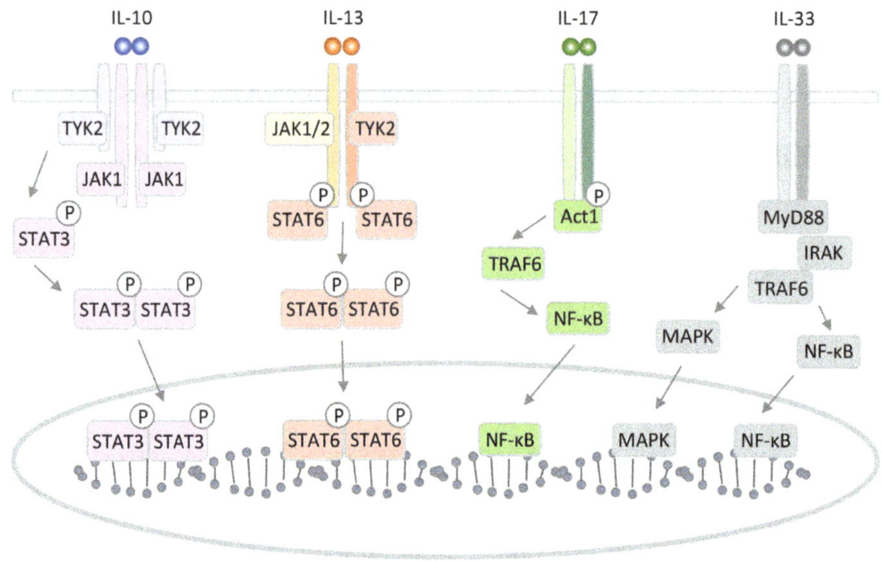

FIGURE 1 | Schematic representation of IL-10, 13, 17, and 33 interaction mechanism with their specific receptors. IL-10 can form a homodimer that binds to the tetrameric heterodimer IL-10 receptor and initiates an intracellular signaling pathway involving STAT3 as key translocation nuclear factor. IL-13 binding to type II receptor complex leads to activation of JAK and phosphorylation of members of the STAT family. The IL-17 receptor complex, which consists of IL-17RA and IL-17RC, activates downstream signaling pathways by recruiting an adaptor molecule named Act1. IL-33 triggers MAPK and NF-κB leading to inflammatory response.

induced by bile duct ligation and carbon tetrachloride (CCl_4) (McHedlidze et al., 2013).

Hepatocytes produce IL-10 which downregulates pro-inflammatory responses and has a potential modulatory effect on liver fibrosis (Sziksz et al., 2020). IL-10 gene therapy attenuated hepatic fibrosis and prevented cell apoptosis in a thioacetamide-treated liver. IL-10 gene transfer reduced not only mRNA level of liver TGF-β1, TNF-α, collagen α1, and cell adhesion molecule, but also decreased the activation of α-smooth muscle actin (α-SMA) and cyclooxygenase-2 (Hung et al., 2005). Other studies have shown that the modification with the IL-10 gene on the buffalo rat liver cells, a rat hepatocytes line, decreased a marked ability to stimulate the primary HSCs proliferation and their expression of α-SMA and procollagen type I, and an accelerated apoptosis of the HSCs was induced (Chen et al., 2012). These results suggest that IL-10 gene therapy might be an effective therapeutic reagent for liver fibrosis.

Interleukins in HSCs

HSCs play a pivotal role in the initiation, perpetuation, and resolution of liver fibrosis. In response to liver injury, quiescent HSCs trans-differentiate into myofibroblasts, and activated HSCs secrete pro-fibrogenic cytokines, growth factors, and ECM molecules (Higashi et al., 2017). Action of HSCs is also regulated by several soluble factors such as TGFβ, platelet-derived growth factor (PDGF), IL-1β, and interleukins. These soluble factors are derived from hepatocytes, macrophages, and other immune cells. In the case of interleukins, IL-17, IL-13, and IL-33 promote hepatic fibrogenesis through activation of hepatic stellate cells. In contrast, IL-10 and IL-22 protect from development of fibrosis by suppressing pro-fibrogenic function of HSCs (Hammerich and Tacke, 2014).

Many studies demonstrated that IL-13 is the pre-dominant profibrotic Th2 cytokine in Schistosomiasis infection which leads to granuloma formation and subsequent fibrosis development in the liver. Also, they show that blockade of IL-13 prevented liver fibrogenesis (Chiaramonte et al., 1999; Fallon et al., 2000; Chiaramonte et al., 2001). In the liver, IL-13 directly induces expression of collagen I and other critical fibrosis-associated genes such as α-SMA and connective tissue growth factor (CTGF) in HSCs (Liu et al., 2012). In HSCs, IL-13 induced CTGF by activating TGF-β-independent activin receptor-like kinase/Smad signaling via the Erk-mitogen-activated protein kinase (MAPK) pathway (Liu et al., 2011). A different study by Sui et al. showed that IL-13 stimulated proliferation of HSCs and secretion of TGF-β and PDGF by activation protein kinase C in LX-2, a cell line of human HSCs (Sui et al., 2018).

Numerous studies show that levels of IL-17 and its receptor increased in response to liver injury. Specially, the pro-inflammatory signaling of IL-17 has been widely studied in HSCs and Kupffer cells (Meng et al., 2012; Tan et al., 2013). Meng et al. demonstrated that IL-17 induced production of collagen type 1 in HSCs through activation of STAT3 signaling pathway. In addition, the author has demonstrated that the activation of fibrin in IL-17-induced HSCs required STAT3 by showing failure to induce collagen-a1 expression in STAT3-deficient HSCs (Meng et al., 2012). A different study showed that pharmacologic inhibition of IL-17-induced ERK1/2 or p38 significantly attenuated HSCs activation and collagen expression (Tan et al., 2013). *In vivo* experiments demonstrated that blocking IL-17 with anti-IL-17A mAb significantly improved liver function and decreased hepatocellular necrosis, pro-inflammatory cytokines, neutrophils and macrophages influx in bile duct ligation-induced liver fibrosis mice (Zhang et al., 2016).

Previous studies have shown that soluble IL-33 increases the secretion of Th2 cytokines such as IL-6, IL-4 and IL-13, which promote HSCs proliferation, TGF-β synthesis and fibrogenesis (Wynn, 2004; Schmitz et al., 2005). Meanwhile, another study showed that activated HSCs with recombinant IL-33 released IL-6, TGF-β, α-SMA, and collagen via MAPK pathways mediated by ERK, c-Jun N-terminal kinase, and p38 protein kinases. Furthermore, the activation of HSCs, liver injury, and inflammatory cell infiltration were reduced in ST2 (IL-33 receptor)-deficient mice (Tan et al., 2017). Marvie et al. identified that IL-33 is upregulated in human and murine fibrosis, and is expressed by HSCs. Activated HSCs was a source of IL-33 that is strongly associated with fibrosis in chronic liver injury (Marvie et al., 2009). These results suggest that IL-33 can play an important role in the cross-talk between HSCs and Th2 cells in liver fibrosis.

The profibrogenic function of HSCs is suppresses by IL-10 which is one of the major anti-inflammatory cytokines. The increase of α-SMA and NF-κB in HSCs was attenuated by ectogenic IL-10 in CCl4-induced liver fibrosis (Zhang et al., 2006). Recently, studies demonstrated that IL-10 induced senescence of activated HSCs via STAT3-p53 pathway to attenuate liver fibrosis (Huang et al., 2020). The therapeutic effects of IL-10 were shown in experiments *in vivo* in which IL-10 gene therapy reduced the expression of fibrosis-related genes including TGF-β, TNF-α, and collagen α1, and also decreased the activation of α-SMA in thioacetamide-induced liver fibrosis (Hung et al., 2005).

Interleukins in Hepatic Macrophages

Hepatic macrophages consist of Kupffer cells, the largest population of liver resident macrophages, and inflammatory monocytes-derived macrophages (MoMFs) recruited from blood circulation and originated from bone marrow, spleen, and peritoneum. Recruited MoMFs undergo a process of differentiation into M1 (classically activated) or M2 (alternatively activated) species depending on the micro-environment (Van der Heide et al., 2019). Generally, following liver injury by many different factors, the resident Kupffer cells are activated and produce cytokines and chemokines to recruit monocytes and neutrophils. The recruited Ly6C+ MoMFs release pro-fibrotic molecules like TGF-β, TNF-α, IL-1β, PDGF and CC chemokine ligand 2, and these cytokines activate HSCs and promote liver fibrosis (Dong et al., 2019; Van der Heide et al., 2019). Recently, novel methods on targeting liver macrophages in fibrosis focus on regulating the activation of Kupffer cells, MoMFs recruitment, and macrophage polarization and differentiation (Tacke, 2017).

Kupffer cells not only express the receptor of IL-17, but also produce IL-17 which is mainly produced by Th17 cells (Ge and You, 2008). Meng et al. demonstrated that Kupffer cells, stimulated by IL-17, expressed inflammatory cytokines IL-6, IL-1β, TNF-α, and TGF-β1, which in turn, induced trans-differentiation of HSCs into fibrogenic myofibroblasts, and further facilitated differentiation of IL-17 producing cells (Meng et al., 2012). A very recent study showed that IL-17 is a cytokine that promotes tumors, critically controlling the inflammatory response in macrophages and the cholesterol synthesis in steatotic hepatocytes in the experimental model of alcohol-induced hepatocellular carcinoma. Therefore, the authors suggested the possibility of IL-17 as a potential treatment target for patients with alcohol-induced hepatocellular carcinoma as well as fibrosis (Ma et al., 2020).

Kupffer cells provide an anti-inflammatory microenvironment by secreting the anti-inflammatory cytokines IL-10 (Heymann et al., 2015; Van der Heide et al., 2019). Antigen presentation to Kupffer cells induces the arrest of CD4 T cells and the secretion of IL-10, an immunosuppressive cytokine, which results in promoting the immune tolerance (Van der Heide et al., 2019). Alternatively, activated M2 macrophages inhibit inflammatory reactions and secrete IL-10, IL-4/IL-13, TGF-β, and vascular endothelial growth factor-α to facilitate tissue repair. In contrast to the M2, M1 is pro-inflammatory, microbicidal, and tumoricidal. M1 also releases numerous inflammatory cytokines e.g., TNF-α, IL-1, IL-6, IL-12, IL-15, and IL-18 (Roszer, 2015; Wang et al., 2018). IL-10 mRNA was upregulated from both Kupffer cells *in vitro* and in whole liver after treatment with lipopolysaccharide or CCl4. Also, IL-10 inhibited production of superoxide and TNF-α in rat Kupffer cells following lipopolysaccharide treatment. Furthermore, IL-10−/− mice showed significantly more severe fibrosis than wild type controls after 70 days of injection with CCl4. The authors concluded that synthesized IL-10 may modulate Kupffer cells action during the liver inflammation and fibrosis, and influence subsequent progression of fibrosis (Thompson et al., 1998).

DISCUSSION

In this review, we have shown the main roles of interleukins in a complex and active cross-talk between hepatic cells responses during liver injury, and their potential as therapeutic targets. Fibrosis is characterized by abnormal ECM derived from HSCs, but it is a dynamic process driven by cytokine-mediated signaling pathways, starting with hepatocytes which are directly involved in the initiation and progression of fibrosis, continuing with macrophages that promote inflammation and present antigens to CD4 T cells which then adjust the immune responses. Interleukins are an immunomodulatory cytokine that is deeply involved from the initiation to the resolution of fibrosis. Recently, the development of a targeted therapy related to liver fibrosis using monoclonal antibodies against interleukins has received considerable interest (**Table 1**). This antibody treatment targeting interleukins has shown potential as a therapeutic agent in various liver diseases through animal experiments. Treatment with monoclonal antibody neutralizing IL-1β and IL-1 receptor antagonist have been tested in clinical trials. While the anti-cytokine therapies can prevent the progression of hepatic fibrogenesis in the early stages of liver injury, they are not a cure for advanced liver fibrosis. Therefore, treatment at the liver fibrosis stage that prevents the progression of the disease, and that leads to resolution is very important. In addition, hepatic fibrosis

TABLE 1 | Strategies targeting interleukins for liver disease.

Agent	Condition or disease	Objective or effector function	Trial number	References
		Antibodies		
Monoclonal antibody neutralizing IL-1β (Canakinumab)	Alcoholic hepatitis	Explore the potential benefits of the IL-1β antibody (Canakinumab) in the treatment of alcoholic hepatitis	NCT03775109	Dinarello et al. (2012)
IL-1 receptor antagonist (Anakinra)	Alcoholic hepatitis	Determine the clinical efficacy and safety of IL-1 receptor antagonist (Anakinra, plus zinc) in participants with clinically severe alcoholic hepatitis	NCT04072822	Meier et al. (2019), Dasarathy et al. (2020)
Polymorphism of IL-1β and TNF-α	Hepatitis B, HCC, Chronic liver disease	Find the effects of polymorphism of IL-1β and TNF-α and their interaction on susceptibility and severity of HBV-related HCC	NCT00629486	Dondeti et al. (2016)
Anti-IL-20 or IL-20R1 monoclonal antibody	Short-term and long-term CCl4 -induced liver injury	Attenuated hepatocyte damage, inhibited TGF-β1 production, liver fibrosis, HSC activation, and ECM accumulation	–	Chiu et al. (2014)
Monoclonal antibody neutralizing IL-11 and anti-IL11RA	Non-alcoholic steatohepatitis	Prevents liver inflammation and steatosis, reverses severe hepatocyte damage, reduces hepatic immune cells and TGFβ1 levels	–	Widjaja et al. (2019)
		Fusion protein		
Nanocomplexes with IL-22 gene	Acetaminophen-induced liver injury, Concanavalin A-induced hepatitis. NAFLD	Activated STAT3/Erk signaling, inhibition of reactive oxygen species generation, ameliorate acetaminophen-induced liver injury	–	Chen et al. (2017), Chen et al. (2018), Zai et al. (2019)
Fusion protein of IL-6 and the soluble IL-6 receptor	D-galactosamine induced acute liver injury	Reversed the state of hepatotoxicity, stimulated liver regeneration	–	Galun et al. (2000)
Fusion protein of IL-28B and human serum albumin	Cell culture-derived hepatitis C virus	Inhibited hepatitis C virus infection	–	Fayad et al. (2013)
Fusion protein of IL-13 cytotoxin	Nonalcoholic steatohepatitis	Decline in fibrosis and liver enzymes without organ toxicity, ameliorates pathological features of NASH	–	Shimamura et al. (2008)

CCl4, carbon tetrachloride; ECM, extracellular matrix; HBV, hepatitis B virus; HCC, hepatocellular carcinoma; HSC, hepatic stellate cells; IL, interleukin; NAFLD, nonalcoholic fatty liver disease; STAT3/Erk, signal transducer and activator of transcription 3/extracellular signal regulated kinase; TGF, tumor growth factor; TNF, tumor necrosis factor.

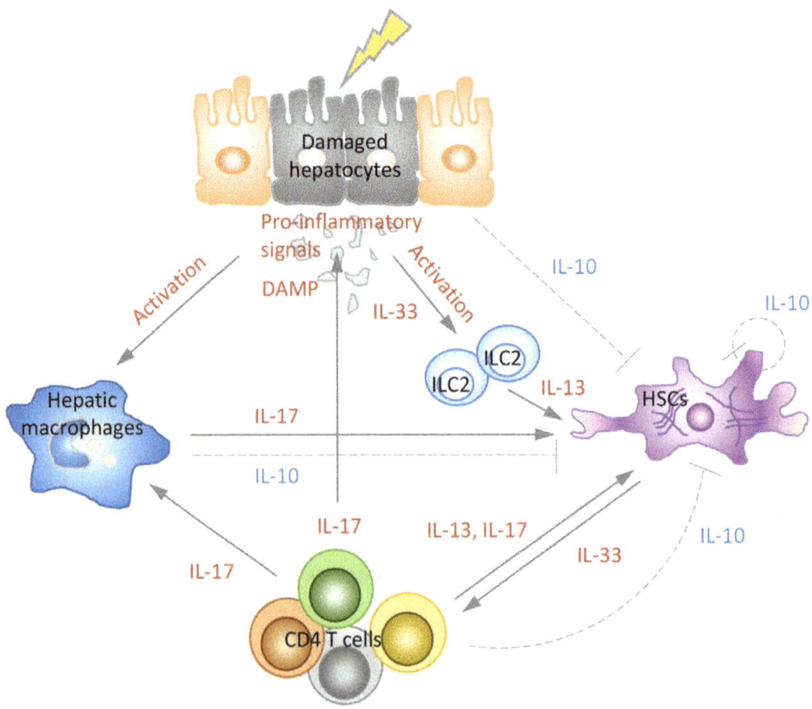

FIGURE 2 | Role of interleukins in development and resolution of liver fibrosis. The combination of signals from inflammatory environment, hepatocytes death, activated macrophages and CD4 T cells stimulates HSCs to proliferate and synthesize collagen and induce fibrosis. IL-33 induces the production of IL-13, and IL-13 and IL-17 directly mediate the activation of HSCs. In the model of fibrosis resolution, hepatocytes, macrophages, HSCs, and CD4 T cells activate the negative feedback loops that reduce immune-mediated fibrosis by secreting IL-10 that prevent activation of HSCs and production of collagen.

TABLE 2 | Roles of IL-10, 13, 17, and 33 in fibrotic disease.

Interleukin	Producing cell	Receptor	Liver	Lung	Heart	Intestine
IL-10	Basophils, B cells, dendritic cells, eosinophils, neutrophils, macrophages Mast cells, Th2 cells	IL-10R1(a), IL-10R2 (b)	IL-10 inhibited HSCs activation Louis et al. (1998) IL-gene therapy reduced the expression of profibrotic genes Hung et al. (2005) IL-10 KO mice showed more severe liver fibrosis Thompson et al. (1998)	IL-10 KO mice increased inflammation after intratracheal instillation of silica Huaux et al. (1998) genetic delivery of IL-10 attenuated the TGF-β production Nakagome et al. (2006)	The lack of IL-10 resulted more severe myocardial fibrosis Verma et al. (2012) the administration of rIL-10 improved cardiac remodeling Krishnamurthy et al. (2009) IL-10 treatment decreased the myocardial inflammation in mice with autoimmune myocarditis Zimmermann et al. (2012)	Loss of function mutations in the gene of IL-10 caused early onset of IBD Kotlarz et al. (2012) IL-10 supplementation did not result clinical improvements in CD patients Marlow et al. (2013)
IL-13	Basophils, B cells, endothelial cells, eosinophils, epithelial cells, fibroblasts, mast cells, macrophages, monocytes, smooth muscle cells, Th2 cells	IL-4Rα, IL13Rα1	Blockade of IL-13 prevented liver fibrogenesis Chiaramonte et al. (2001) IL-13 induced production of collagen, α-SMA Chiaramonte et al. (1999)	IL-13−/− and IL-4/13−/− mice were protected from lung fibrosis development in response to FITC inoculation Kolodsick et al. (2004) IL-13 and IL-4 are elevated in the bronchial alveolar lavage fluid of IPF patients Park et al. (2009)	Il13Rα1-deficient mice develop severe myocardial dysfunction Amit et al. (2017) deficiency of IL-13 leads to increased leukocyte infiltration and reduced M2-like differentiation of the monocytes in the myocardium Hofmann et al. (2014)	IL-13 production by type 2 NKT cells demonstrated to be critical for colitis development Heller et al. (2002) IL-13 is not increased in fibrotic CD muscle layer Vainer et al. (2000)
IL-17	B cells, dendritic cells, macrophages, Th17 cells	IL-17RA, IL-17RC	The increased level of IL-17 activated HSCs and induced collagen production Meng et al. (2012) elevated levels of IL-17 were also found in the fibrotic livers of patients with hepatitis B virus and cirrhosis related liver damage Du et al. (2013)	Anti-IL-17A neutralizing antibody attenuated pulmonary fibrosis and ECM deposition Chen et al. (2014) in humans, elevated levels of IL-17 and IL-1β were seen in the BAL fluid of patients with IPE Wilson et al. (2010)	IL-17 directly induced VA *in vivo* and *in vitro* in a dose-dependent manner Chang et al. (2018) IL-17 induced cardiac fibrosis both *in vitro* and *in vivo* via PKCβ/Erk1/2/NF-κB signaling pathway Liu et al. (2012)	IL-17 induced HSP47 as well as type I collagen in human intestinal myofibroblasts Honzawa et al. (2014) IL-17 contributed significantly for stricture development in CD Yagi et al. (2007) level of fecal IL-17 was elevated in patients with active CD Biancheri et al. (2013)
IL-33	Basophils, B cells, CD8+T cells, dendritic cells, eosinophils, ILC2s, macrophages, mast cells, natural killer cells, Th2 cells, Tregs cells	ST2, IL1RAcP	IL-33−/− mice showed decrease in collagen deposition and ECM-related gene expression McHedlidze et al. (2013) production of IL-13 in Th2 cells Marvie et al. (2009) IL-33 exacerbated liver fibrosis in mice Gao et al. (2016)	Level of IL-33 was elevated in the bronchoalveolar lavage fluids of patients with IPF Lee et al. (2017) treatment with anti-IL-33 antibody markedly reduced airway inflammation and lung fibrosis Luzina et al. (2013)	Recombinant IL-33 reduced aortic atherosclerotic plaque development Miller et al. (2008) ST2−/− mice showed more cardiac fibrosis and impaired survival Sanada et al. (2007) expression levels of IL-33/ST2 in human myocardial tissue were associated with cardiac fibrosis Tseng et al. (2017)	Inhibition of endogenous ST2-mediated signaling by treatment with neutralizing antibody improved DSS-induced colitis Sedhom et al. (2013) IL-33 has extenuating effects in chronic DSS-induced colitis Grobeta et al. (2012)

BAL, bronchoalveolar lavage; CD, crohn's disease; DSS, dextran sulfate sodium; ECM, extracellular matrix; Erk, extracellular signal regulated kinase; HSCs, hepatic stellate cells; HSP, heat shock protein; IBD, inflammatory bowel diseases; IL, interleukin; IPF, idiopathic pulmonary fibrosis; KO, knock-out; NF-κb, nuclear factor-κb; NKT, natural killer T cells; PCK, protein kinase C; r, recombinant; SMA, smooth muscle actin; TGF, tumor growth factor; VA, ventricular arrhythmia.

treatment strategies using various fusion proteins are detailed in **Table 1**. Targeting IL-22 is particularly promising as an alternative strategy to directly break the cycle of inflammatory cytokine and chemokine signaling, and the fusion protein using the IL-22 gene and nanocomplex is considered a new strategy to improve liver disease (Chen et al., 2017; Chen et al., 2018; Chen et al., 2020).

Damaged hepatocytes activate hepatic macrophages, and release DAMPs and IL-33. ILC2, which is activated by IL-33 released by hepatocytes, secretes IL-13, that can induce the activity of HSCs. Stimulated macrophages modulate antigen-presentation of CD4 T cells and produce IL-17 together with CD4 T cells, directly affecting the activity of HSCs and collagen production. Additionally, CD4 cells can promote fibrosis by stimulating macrophages and HSCs with IL-17 or IL-13. The quiescent HSCs receiving various pro-inflammatory signals not only transdifferentiate into myofibroblasts to produce collagen, but secrete pro-fibrogenic cytokines such as IL-33 to play pivotal role in fibrosis. On the other hand, during fibrosis resolution, these cells reverse myofibroblast activation with IL-10 and regulate the restoration of homeostasis (**Figure 2**). This suggests that strategies using prevention of pro-inflammatory interleukins or induction of anti-inflammatory interleukins for the treatment of liver fibrosis may be effective.

IL-3, IL-17 and IL-33 induce liver fibrosis through various mechanisms, therefore an approach targeting them as a major participant in the "fibrosis pathway" is expected to be worthwhile. The blockade of IL-13 can be reversed to reduce liver pathology even when fibrosis is already established. IL-17 signals contribute to the pathogenesis of liver damage and IL-17 inhibition can potentially be an effective treatment for liver disease. Furthermore, IL-17 may be a treatment target for alcohol-induced liver damage and hepatocellular carcinoma. An approach aimed at the IL-33/ST2 path could be a potential therapeutic target for human patients suffering from chronic hepatitis and liver fibrosis (Hammerich and Tacke, 2014; Weiskirchen and Tacke, 2016; Zhang et al., 2016; Ma et al., 2020). IL-10 is a typical anti-inflammatory cytokine that shows signals of conservation mechanism in multiple organs. Specially in the fibrous liver, IL-10 has been proven to induce resolution of fibrosis, therefore it is suggested as a potential therapeutic target (Steen et al., 2020). However, the half-life of recombinant IL-10 *in vivo* is relatively short, and non-targeted administration can cause systemic side effects (Chen et al., 2012). Therefore, increasing numbers of studies have aimed to use IL-10 gene transfer and IL-10 gene therapy might be an effective treatment for liver fibrosis.

Fibrosis can occur in almost any organ or tissue, including lung, heart, and intestine, and is associated with a variety of diseases. Although liver fibrosis has been addressed in this review, treatment with specific interleukins can be applied to several tissue fibrosis. **Table 2** shows studies using interleukin 10, 13, 17, and 33 in various fibrotic tissues (Ng et al., 2018; Wijsenbeek et al., 2018; Sziksz et al., 2020). However, there are some practical problems such as the relevant doses of recombinant interleukins, the route of administration, and the costs of production of the cytokine itself, that need to be addressed to move from the experimental stage to the clinical stage. If these hurdles are overcome, a new treatment strategy targeting specific interleukins will be able to deliver expected therapeutic effects not only in the liver, but also in other tissues as well.

AUTHOR CONTRIBUTIONS

SA and SD developed the outline for this review, SA wrote the first draft with the assistance of AP, SD edited and approved the final version.

ACKNOWLEDGMENTS

This work was completed with support from the Veterans Health Administration and with resources and the use of facilities at the Central Texas Veterans Health Care System, Temple, Texas. The contents do not represent the views of the U.S. Department of Veterans Affairs or the United States Government.

REFERENCES

Amit, U., Kain, D., Wagner, A., Sahu, A., Nevo-Caspi, Y., Gonen, N., et al. (2017). New role for interleukin-13 receptor α1 in myocardial homeostasis and heart failure. *J. Am. Heart Assoc.* 6 (5), e005108. doi:10.1161/JAHA.116.005108

Bansal, R., Nagórniewicz, B., and Prakash, J. (2016). Clinical advancements in the targeted therapies against liver fibrosis. *Mediators Inflamm.* 2016, 7629724. doi:10.1155/2016/7629724

Barbier, L., Ferhat, M., Salamé, E., Robin, A., Herbelin, A., Gombert, J. M., et al. (2019). Interleukin-1 family cytokines: keystones in liver inflammatory diseases. *Front. Immunol.* 10, 2014. doi:10.3389/fimmu.2019.02014

Bataller, R., and Brenner, D. A. (2005). Liver fibrosis. *J. Clin. Invest.* 115, 209–218. doi:10.1172/JCI24282

Biancheri, P., Pender, S. L., Ammoscato, F., Giuffrida, P., Sampietro, G., Ardizzone, S., et al. (2013). The role of interleukin 17 in Crohn's disease-associated intestinal fibrosis. *Fibrogenesis Tissue Repair* 6, 13. doi:10.1186/1755-1536-6-13

Caraffa, A., Gallenga, C. E., Kritas, S. K., Ronconi, G., Di Emidio, P., and Conti, P. (2019). CAR-T cell therapy causes inflammation by IL-1 which activates inflammatory cytokine mast cells: anti-inflammatory role of IL-37. *J. Biol. Regul. Homeost Agents* 33, 1981–1985. doi:10.23812/EditorialCaraffa

Chan, A. H., and Schroder, K. (2020). Inflammasome signaling and regulation of interleukin-1 family cytokines. *J. Exp. Med.* 217, e20190314. doi:10.1084/jem.20190314

Chang, S. L., Hsiao, Y. W., Tsai, Y. N., Lin, S. F., Liu, S. H., Lin, Y. J., et al. (2018). Interleukin-17 enhances cardiac ventricular remodeling via activating MAPK pathway in ischemic heart failure. *J. Mol. Cell. Cardiol.* 122, 69–79. doi:10.1016/j.yjmcc.2018.08.005

Chen, W., Zai, W., Fan, J., Zhang, X., Zeng, X., Luan, J., et al. (2020). Interleukin-22 drives a metabolic adaptive reprogramming to maintain mitochondrial fitness and treat liver injury. *Theranostics* 10, 5879–5894. doi:10.7150/thno.43894

Chen, W., Zhang, X., Fan, J., Zai, W., Luan, J., Li, Y., et al. (2017). Tethering interleukin-22 to apolipoprotein A-I ameliorates mice from acetaminophen-induced liver injury. *Theranostics* 7, 4135–4148. doi:10.7150/thno.20955

Chen, W., Luan, J., Wei, G., Zhang, X., Fan, J., Zai, W., et al. (2018). Vivo hepatocellular expression of interleukin-22 using penetratin-based hybrid nanoparticles as potential anti-hepatitis therapeutics. *Biomaterials*, 187, 66–80. doi:10.1016/j.biomaterials.2018.09.046

Chen, Y., Li, C., Weng, D., Song, L., Tang, W., Dai, W., et al. (2014). Neutralization of interleukin-17A delays progression of silica-induced lung inflammation and fibrosis in C57BL/6 mice. *Toxicol. Appl. Pharmacol.* 275, 62–72. doi:10.1016/j.taap.2013.11.012

Chen, Y. X., Huang, Y. H., Zheng, W. D., Chen, Z. X., Zhang, L. J., and Wang, X. Z. (2012). Interleukin-10 gene modification attenuates hepatocyte activation of rat hepatic stellate cells *in vitro*. *Mol. Med. Rep.* 7, 371–378. doi:10.3892/mmr.2012.1228

Chiaramonte, M. G., Cheever, A. W., Malley, J. D., Donaldson, D. D., and Wynn, T. A. (2001). Studies of murine schistosomiasis reveal interleukin-13 blockade as a treatment for established and progressive liver fibrosis. *Hepatology* 34, 273–282. doi:10.1053/jhep.2001.26376

Chiaramonte, M. G., Donaldson, D. D., Cheever, A. W., and Wynn, T. A. (1999). An IL-13 inhibitor blocks the development of hepatic fibrosis during a T-helper type 2-dominated inflammatory response. *J. Clin. Invest.* 104, 777–785. doi:10.1172/JCI7325

Chiu, Y. S., Wei, C. C., Lin, Y. J., Hsu, Y. H., and Chang, M. S. (2014). IL-20 and IL-20R1 antibodies protect against liver fibrosis. *Hepatology* 60, 1003–1014. doi:10.1002/hep.27189

Crispe, I. N. (2016). Hepatocytes as immunological agents. *J. Immunol.* 196, 17–21. doi:10.4049/jimmunol.1501668

Dasarathy, S., Mitchell, M. C., Barton, B., Mcclain, C. J., Szabo, G., Nagy, L. E., et al. (2020). Design and rationale of a multicenter defeat alcoholic steatohepatitis trial: (DASH) randomized clinical trial to treat alcohol-associated hepatitis. *Contemp. Clin. Trials* 96, 106094. doi:10.1016/j.cct.2020.106094

De Vries, J. E. (1998). The role of IL-13 and its receptor in allergy and inflammatory responses. *J. Allergy Clin. Immunol.* 102, 165–169. doi:10.1016/s0091-6749(98)70080-6

Dinarello, C. A., Simon, A., and Van Der Meer, J. W. (2012). Treating inflammation by blocking interleukin-1 in a broad spectrum of diseases. *Nat. Rev. Drug Discov.* 11, 633–652. doi:10.1038/nrd3800

Dondeti, M. F., El-Maadawy, E. A., and Talaat, R. M. (2016). Hepatitis-related hepatocellular carcinoma: insights into cytokine gene polymorphisms. *World J. Gastroenterol.* 22, 6800–6816. doi:10.3748/wjg.v22.i30.6800

Dong, X., Liu, J., Xu, Y., and Cao, H. (2019). Role of macrophages in experimental liver injury and repair in mice. *Exp. Ther. Med.* 17, 3835–3847. doi:10.3892/etm.2019.7450

Du, W. J., Zhen, J. H., Zeng, Z. Q., Zheng, Z. M., Xu, Y., Qin, L. Y., et al. (2013). Expression of interleukin-17 associated with disease progression and liver fibrosis with hepatitis B virus infection: IL-17 in HBV infection. *Diagn. Pathol.* 8, 40. doi:10.1186/1746-1596-8-40

Fallon, P. G., Richardson, E. J., Mckenzie, G. J., and Mckenzie, A. N. (2000). Schistosome infection of transgenic mice defines distinct and contrasting pathogenic roles for IL-4 and IL-13: IL-13 is a profibrotic agent. *J. Immunol.* 164, 2585–2591. doi:10.4049/jimmunol.164.5.2585

Fayad, H. J., Lamare, F., Le Rest, C. C., Bettinardi, V., and Visvikis, D. (2013). Generation of 4-dimensional CT images based on 4-dimensional PET-derived motion fields. *J. Nucl. Med.* 54, 631–638. doi:10.2967/jnumed.112.110809

Gallenga, C. E., Pandolfi, F., Caraffa, A., Kritas, S. K., Ronconi, G., Toniato, E., et al. (2019). Interleukin-1 family cytokines and mast cells: activation and inhibition. *J. Biol. Regul. Homeost Agents* 33, 1–6.

Galun, E., Zeira, E., Pappo, O., Peters, M., and Rose-John, S. (2000). Liver regeneration induced by a designer human IL-6/sIL-6R fusion protein reverses severe hepatocellular injury. *FASEB J.* 14, 1979–1987. doi:10.1096/fj.99-0913com

Gao, Y., Liu, Y., Yang, M., Guo, X., Zhang, M., Li, H., et al. (2016). IL-33 treatment attenuated diet-induced hepatic steatosis but aggravated hepatic fibrosis. *Oncotarget* 7, 33649–33661. doi:10.18632/oncotarget.9259

Ge, D., and You, Z. (2008). Expression of interleukin-17RC protein in normal human tissues. *Int. Arch. Med.* 1, 19. doi:10.1186/1755-7682-1-19

Groβ, P., Doser, K., Falk, W., Obermeier, F., and Hofmann, C. (2012). IL-33 attenuates development and perpetuation of chronic intestinal inflammation. *Inflamm. Bowel Dis.* 18, 1900–1909. doi:10.1002/ibd.22900

Grünig, G., Warnock, M., Wakil, A. E., Venkayya, R., Brombacher, F., Rennick, D. M., et al. (1998). Requirement for IL-13 independently of IL-4 in experimental asthma. *Science* 282, 2261–2263. doi:10.1126/science.282.5397.2261

Gugliandolo, A., Caraffa, A. L., Gallenga, C. E., Kritas, S. K., Ronconi, G., Trubiani, O., et al. (2019). Mesenchymal stem cells and IL-37: a powerful combination. *J. Biol. Regul. Homeost Agents* 33, 1019–1022.

Hammerich, L., and Tacke, F. (2014). Interleukins in chronic liver disease: lessons learned from experimental mouse models. *Clin. Exp. Gastroenterol.* 7, 297–306. doi:10.2147/CEG.S43737

He, Y., Hwang, S., Ahmed, Y. A., Feng, D., Li, N., Ribeiro, M., et al. (2021). Immunopathobiology and therapeutic targets related to cytokines in liver diseases. *Cell. Mol. Immunol.* 18, 18–37. doi:10.1038/s41423-020-00580-w

Heller, F., Fuss, I. J., Nieuwenhuis, E. E., Blumberg, R. S., and Strober, W. (2002). Oxazolone colitis, a Th2 colitis model resembling ulcerative colitis, is mediated by IL-13-producing NK-T cells. *Immunity* 17, 629–638. doi:10.1016/s1074-7613(02)00453-3

Hershey, G. K. (2003). IL-13 receptors and signaling pathways: an evolving web. *J. Allergy Clin. Immunol.* 111, 677–691. doi:10.1067/mai.2003.1333

Heymann, F., Peusquens, J., Ludwig-Portugall, I., Kohlhepp, M., Ergen, C., Niemietz, P., et al. (2015). Liver inflammation abrogates immunological tolerance induced by Kupffer cells. *Hepatology* 62, 279–291. doi:10.1002/hep.27793

Higashi, T., Friedman, S. L., and Hoshida, Y. (2017). Hepatic stellate cells as key target in liver fibrosis. *Adv. Drug Deliv. Rev.* 121, 27–42. doi:10.1016/j.addr.2017.05.007

Hofmann, U., Knorr, S., Vogel, B., Weirather, J., Frey, A., Ertl, G., et al. (2014). Interleukin-13 deficiency aggravates healing and remodeling in male mice after experimental myocardial infarction. *Circ. Heart Fail.* 7, 822–830. doi:10.1161/CIRCHEARTFAILURE.113.001020

Honzawa, Y., Nakase, H., Shiokawa, M., Yoshino, T., Imaeda, H., Matsuura, M., et al. (2014). Involvement of interleukin-17A-induced expression of heat shock protein 47 in intestinal fibrosis in Crohn's disease. *Gut* 63, 1902–1912. doi:10.1136/gutjnl-2013-305632

Huang, Y. H., Chen, M. H., Guo, Q. L., Chen, Z. X., Chen, Q. D., and Wang, X. Z. (2020). Interleukin-10 induces senescence of activated hepatic stellate cells via STAT3-p53 pathway to attenuate liver fibrosis. *Cell. Signal.* 66, 109445. doi:10.1016/j.cellsig.2019.109445

Huaux, F., Louahed, J., Hudspith, B., Meredith, C., Delos, M., Renauld, J. C., et al. (1998). Role of interleukin-10 in the lung response to silica in mice. *Am. J. Respir. Cell Mol. Biol.* 18, 51–59. doi:10.1165/ajrcmb.18.1.2911

Hung, K. S., Lee, T. H., Chou, W. Y., Wu, C. L., Cho, C. L., Lu, C. N., et al. (2005). Interleukin-10 gene therapy reverses thioacetamide-induced liver fibrosis in mice. *Biochem. Biophys. Res. Commun.* 336, 324–331. doi:10.1016/j.bbrc.2005.08.085

Kagan, P., Sultan, M., Tachlytski, I., Safran, M., and Ben-Ari, Z. (2017). Both MAPK and STAT3 signal transduction pathways are necessary for IL-6-dependent hepatic stellate cells activation. *PLoS One* 12, e0176173. doi:10.1371/journal.pone.0176173

Kolodsick, J. E., Toews, G. B., Jakubzick, C., Hogaboam, C., Moore, T. A., Mckenzie, A., et al. (2004). Protection from fluorescein isothiocyanate-induced fibrosis in IL-13-deficient, but not IL-4-deficient, mice results from impaired collagen synthesis by fibroblasts. *J. Immunol.* 172, 4068–4076. doi:10.4049/jimmunol.172.7.4068

Kotlarz, D., Beier, R., Murugan, D., Diestelhorst, J., Jensen, O., Boztug, K., et al. (2012). Loss of interleukin-10 signaling and infantile inflammatory bowel disease: implications for diagnosis and therapy. *Gastroenterology* 143, 347–355. doi:10.1053/j.gastro.2012.04.045

Krishnamurthy, P., Rajasingh, J., Lambers, E., Qin, G., Losordo, D. W., and Kishore, R. (2009). IL-10 inhibits inflammation and attenuates left ventricular remodeling after myocardial infarction via activation of STAT3 and suppression of HuR. *Circ. Res.* 104, e9–18. doi:10.1161/CIRCRESAHA.108.188243

Kubes, P., and Jenne, C. (2018). Immune responses in the liver. *Annu. Rev. Immunol.* 36, 247–277. doi:10.1146/annurev-immunol-051116-052415

Lee, J. U., Chang, H. S., Lee, H. J., Jung, C. A., Bae, D. J., Song, H. J., et al. (2017). Upregulation of interleukin-33 and thymic stromal lymphopoietin levels in the lungs of idiopathic pulmonary fibrosis. *BMC Pulm. Med.* 17, 39. doi:10.1186/s12890-017-0380-z

Li, S., Tan, H. Y., Wang, N., Feng, Y., Wang, X., and Feng, Y. (2019). Recent insights into the role of immune cells in alcoholic liver disease. *Front. Immunol.* 10, 1328. doi:10.3389/fimmu.2019.01328

Liu, Y., Meyer, C., Müller, A., Herweck, F., Li, Q., Müllenbach, R., et al. (2011). IL-13 induces connective tissue growth factor in rat hepatic stellate cells via TGF-β-independent Smad signaling. *J. Immunol.* 187, 2814–2823. doi:10.4049/jimmunol.1003260

Liu, Y., Munker, S., Müllenbach, R., and Weng, H. L. (2012). IL-13 signaling in liver fibrogenesis. *Front. Immunol.* 3, 116. doi:10.3389/fimmu.2012.00116

Lokau, J., Schoeder, V., Haybaeck, J., and Garbers, C. (2019). Jak-stat signaling induced by interleukin-6 family cytokines in hepatocellular carcinoma. *Cancers (Basel)* 11, 1704. doi:10.3390/cancers11111704

Louis, H., Van Laethem, J. L., Wu, W., Quertinmont, E., Degraef, C., Van Den Berg, K., et al. (1998). Interleukin-10 controls neutrophilic infiltration, hepatocyte proliferation, and liver fibrosis induced by carbon tetrachloride in mice. *Hepatology* 28, 1607–1615. doi:10.1002/hep.510280621

Luckheeram, R. V., Zhou, R., Verma, A. D., and Xia, B. (2012). $CD4^{+}$T cells: differentiation and functions. *Clin. Dev. Immunol.* 2012, 925135. doi:10.1155/2012/925135

Luzina, I. G., Kopach, P., Lockatell, V., Kang, P. H., Nagarsekar, A., Burke, A. P., et al. (2013). Interleukin-33 potentiates bleomycin-induced lung injury. *Am. J. Respir. Cell Mol. Biol.* 49, 999–1008. doi:10.1165/rcmb.2013-0093OC

Ma, H. Y., Yamamoto, G., Xu, J., Liu, X., Karin, D., Kim, J. Y., et al. (2020). IL-17 signaling in steatotic hepatocytes and macrophages promotes hepatocellular carcinoma in alcohol-related liver disease. *J. Hepatol.* 72, 946–959. doi:10.1016/j.jhep.2019.12.016

Mair, M., Zollner, G., Schneller, D., Musteanu, M., Fickert, P., Gumhold, J., et al. (2010). Signal transducer and activator of transcription 3 protects from liver injury and fibrosis in a mouse model of sclerosing cholangitis. *Gastroenterology* 138, 2499–2508. doi:10.1053/j.gastro.2010.02.049

Marlow, G. J., Van Gent, D., and Ferguson, L. R. (2013). Why interleukin-10 supplementation does not work in Crohn's disease patients. *World J. Gastroenterol.* 19, 3931–3941. doi:10.3748/wjg.v19.i25.3931

Marvie, P., Lisbonne, M., L'helgoualc'h, A., Rauch, M., Turlin, B., Preisser, L., et al. (2009). Interleukin-33 overexpression is associated with liver fibrosis in mice and humans. *J. Cell Mol. Med.* 14, 1726–1739. doi:10.1111/j.1582-4934.2009.00801.x

McCormick, S. M., and Heller, N. M. (2015). Commentary: IL-4 and IL-13 receptors and signaling. *Cytokine* 75, 38–50. doi:10.1016/j.cyto.2015.05.023

McHedlidze, T., Waldner, M., Zopf, S., Walker, J., Rankin, A. L., Schuchmann, M., et al. (2013). Interleukin-33-dependent innate lymphoid cells mediate hepatic fibrosis. *Immunity* 39, 357–371. doi:10.1016/j.immuni.2013.07.018

Meier, R. P. H., Meyer, J., Montanari, E., Lacotte, S., Balaphas, A., Muller, Y. D., et al. (2019). Interleukin-1 receptor antagonist modulates liver inflammation and fibrosis in mice in a model-dependent manner. *Int. J. Mol. Sci.* 20 (6), 1295. doi:10.3390/ijms20061295

Meng, F., Wang, K., Aoyama, T., Grivennikov, S. I., Paik, Y., Scholten, D., et al. (2012). Interleukin-17 signaling in inflammatory, Kupffer cells, and hepatic stellate cells exacerbates liver fibrosis in mice. *Gastroenterology* 143, 765–776.e3. doi:10.1053/j.gastro.2012.05.049

Miller, A. M., Xu, D., Asquith, D. L., Denby, L., Li, Y., Sattar, N., et al. (2008). IL-33 reduces the development of atherosclerosis. *J. Exp. Med.* 205, 339–346. doi:10.1084/jem.20071868

Nakagome, K., Dohi, M., Okunishi, K., Tanaka, R., Miyazaki, J., and Yamamoto, K. (2006). *In vivo* IL-10 gene delivery attenuates bleomycin induced pulmonary fibrosis by inhibiting the production and activation of TGF-beta in the lung. *Thorax* 61, 886–894. doi:10.1136/thx.2005.056317

Nanchahal, J., and Hinz, B. (2016). Strategies to overcome the hurdles to treat fibrosis, a major unmet clinical need. *Proc. Natl. Acad. Sci. U.S.A.* 113, 7291–7293. doi:10.1073/pnas.1607896113

Ng, B., Dong, J., D'agostino, G., Viswanathan, S., Widjaja, A. A., Lim, W. W., et al. (2018). Interleukin-11 is a therapeutic target in idiopathic pulmonary fibrosis. *Sci. Transl Med.* 11, eaaw1237. doi:10.1126/scitranslmed.aaw1237

Onishi, R. M., and Gaffen, S. L. (2010). Interleukin-17 and its target genes: mechanisms of interleukin-17 function in disease. *Immunology* 129, 311–321. doi:10.1111/j.1365-2567.2009.03240.x

Park, S. W., Ahn, M. H., Jang, H. K., Jang, A. S., Kim, D. J., Koh, E. S., et al. (2009). Interleukin-13 and its receptors in idiopathic interstitial pneumonia: clinical implications for lung function. *J. Korean Med. Sci.* 24, 614–620. doi:10.3346/jkms.2009.24.4.614

Paul, W. E., and Seder, R. A. (1994). Lymphocyte responses and cytokines. *Cell* 76, 241–251. doi:10.1016/0092-8674(94)90332-8

Pinto, S. M., Subbannayya, Y., Rex, D. A. B., Raju, R., Chatterjee, O., Advani, J., et al. (2018). A network map of IL-33 signaling pathway. *J. Cell Commun. Signal.* 12, 615–624. doi:10.1007/s12079-018-0464-4

Roszer, T. (2015). Understanding the mysterious M2 macrophage through activation markers and effector mechanisms. *Mediators Inflamm.* 2015, 816460. doi:10.1155/2015/816460

Sanada, S., Hakuno, D., Higgins, L. J., Schreiter, E. R., Mckenzie, A. N., and Lee, R. T. (2007). IL-33 and ST2 comprise a critical biomechanically induced and cardioprotective signaling system. *J. Clin. Invest.* 117, 1538–1549. doi:10.1172/JCI30634

Schmidt-Arras, D., and Rose-John, S. (2016). IL-6 pathway in the liver: from physiopathology to therapy. *J. Hepatol.* 64, 1403–1415. doi:10.1016/j.jhep.2016.02.004

Schmitz, J., Owyang, A., Oldham, E., Song, Y., Murphy, E., Mcclanahan, T. K., et al. (2005). IL-33, an interleukin-1-like cytokine that signals via the IL-1 receptor-related protein ST2 and induces T helper type 2-associated cytokines. *Immunity* 23, 479–490. doi:10.1016/j.immuni.2005.09.015

Sedhom, M. A., Pichery, M., Murdoch, J. R., Foligné, B., Ortega, N., Normand, S., et al. (2013). Neutralisation of the interleukin-33/ST2 pathway ameliorates experimental colitis through enhancement of mucosal healing in mice. *Gut* 62, 1714–1723. doi:10.1136/gutjnl-2011-301785

Shimamura, T., Fujisawa, T., Husain, S. R., Kioi, M., Nakajima, A., and Puri, R. K. (2008). Novel role of IL-13 in fibrosis induced by nonalcoholic steatohepatitis and its amelioration by IL-13R-directed cytotoxin in a rat model. *J. Immunol.* 181, 4656–4665. doi:10.4049/jimmunol.181.7.4656

Steen, E. H., Wang, X., Balaji, S., Butte, M. J., Bollyky, P. L., and Keswani, S. G. (2020). The role of the anti-inflammatory cytokine interleukin-10 in tissue fibrosis. *Adv. Wound Care (New Rochelle)* 9, 184–198. doi:10.1089/wound.2019.1032

Sui, G., Cheng, G., Yuan, J., Hou, X., Kong, X., and Niu, H. (2018). Interleukin (IL)-13, prostaglandin E2 (PGE2), and prostacyclin 2 (PGI2) activate hepatic stellate cells via protein kinase C (PKC) pathway in hepatic fibrosis. *Med. Sci. Monit.* 24, 2134–2141. doi:10.12659/msm.906442

Sziksz, E., Pap, D., Lippai, R., Béres, N. J., Fekete, A., Szabó, A. J., et al. (2020). Fibrosis related inflammatory mediators: role of the IL-10 cytokine family. *Mediators Inflamm.* 2015, 764641. doi:10.1155/2015/764641

Tacke, F. (2017). Targeting hepatic macrophages to treat liver diseases. *J. Hepatol.* 66, 1300–1312. doi:10.1016/j.jhep.2017.02.026

Tan, Z., Liu, Q., Jiang, R., Lv, L., Shoto, S. S., Maillet, I., et al. (2017). Interleukin-33 drives hepatic fibrosis through activation of hepatic stellate cells. *Cell. Mol. Immunol.* 15, 388–398. doi:10.1038/cmi.2016.63

Tan, Z., Qian, X., Jiang, R., Liu, Q., Wang, Y., Chen, C., et al. (2013). IL-17A plays a critical role in the pathogenesis of liver fibrosis through hepatic stellate cell activation. *J. Immunol.* 191, 1835–1844. doi:10.4049/jimmunol.1203013

Thompson, K., Maltby, J., Fallowfield, J., Mcaulay, M., Millward-Sadler, H., and Sheron, N. (1998). Interleukin-10 expression and function in experimental murine liver inflammation and fibrosis. *Hepatology* 28, 1597–1606. doi:10.1002/hep.510280620

Toniato, E., Frydas, I., Robuffo, I., Ronconi, G., Caraffa, A., Kritas, S. K., et al. (2017). Activation and inhibition of adaptive immune response mediated by mast cells. *J. Biol. Regul. Homeost Agents* 31, 543–548.

Tseng, C. C. S., Huibers, M. M. H., Van Kuik, J., De Weger, R. A., Vink, A., and De Jonge, N. (2018). The interleukin-33/ST2 pathway is expressed in the failing human heart and associated with pro-fibrotic remodeling of the myocardium. *J. Cardiovasc. Transl Res.* 11, 15–21. doi:10.1007/s12265-017-9775-8

Tu, T., Calabro, S. R., Lee, A., Maczurek, A. E., Budzinska, M. A., Warner, F. J., et al. (2015). Hepatocytes in liver injury: victim, bystander, or accomplice in progressive fibrosis? *J. Gastroenterol. Hepatol.* 30, 1696–1704. doi:10.1111/jgh.13065

Vainer, B., Nielsen, O. H., Hendel, J., Horn, T., and Kirman, I. (2000). Colonic expression and synthesis of interleukin 13 and interleukin 15 in inflammatory bowel disease. *Cytokine* 12, 1531–1536. doi:10.1006/cyto.2000.0744

Van der Heide, D., Weiskirchen, R., and Bansal, R. (2019). Therapeutic targeting of hepatic macrophages for the treatment of liver diseases. *Front. Immunol.* 10, 2852. doi:10.3389/fimmu.2019.02852

Varvara, G., Tettamanti, L., Gallenga, C. E., Caraffa, A., D'ovidio, C., Mastrangelo, F., et al. (2018). Stimulated mast cells release inflammatory cytokines: potential suppression and therapeutical aspects. *J. Biol. Regul. Homeost Agents* 32, 1355–1360.

Verma, R., Balakrishnan, L., Sharma, K., Khan, A. A., Advani, J., Gowda, H., et al. (2016). A network map of Interleukin-10 signaling pathway. *J. Cell Commun. Signal.* 10, 61–67. doi:10.1007/s12079-015-0302-x

Verma, S. K., Krishnamurthy, P., Barefield, D., Singh, N., Gupta, R., Lambers, E., et al. (2012). Interleukin-10 treatment attenuates pressure overload-induced hypertrophic remodeling and improves heart function via signal transducers and activators of transcription 3-dependent inhibition of nuclear factor-κB. *Circulation* 126, 418–429. doi:10.1161/CIRCULATIONAHA.112.112185

Wang, L. X., Zhang, S. X., Wu, H. J., Rong, X. L., and Guo, J. (2019). M2b macrophage polarization and its roles in diseases. *J. Leukoc. Biol.* 106, 345–358. doi:10.1002/JLB.3RU1018-378RR

Weiskirchen, R., and Tacke, F. (2016). Interleukin-33 in the pathogenesis of liver fibrosis: alarming ILC2 and hepatic stellate cells. *Cell Mol. Immunol.* 14, 143–145. doi:10.1038/cmi.2016.62

Widjaja, A. A., Singh, B. K., Adami, E., Viswanathan, S., Dong, J., D'agostino, G. A., et al. (2019). Inhibiting interleukin 11 signaling reduces hepatocyte death and liver fibrosis, inflammation, and steatosis in mouse models of nonalcoholic steatohepatitis. *Gastroenterology* 157, 777–792. doi:10.1053/j.gastro.2019.05.002

Wijsenbeek, M. S., Kool, M., and Cottin, V. (2018). Targeting interleukin-13 in idiopathic pulmonary fibrosis: from promising path to dead end. *Eur. Respir. J.* 52, 1802111. doi:10.1183/13993003.02111-2018

Wilson, M. S., Madala, S. K., Ramalingam, T. R., Gochuico, B. R., Rosas, I. O., Cheever, A. W., et al. (2010). Bleomycin and IL-1beta-mediated pulmonary fibrosis is IL-17A dependent. *J. Exp. Med.* 207, 535–552. doi:10.1084/jem.20092121

Wu, Y., Min, J., Ge, C., Shu, J., Tian, D., Yuan, Y., et al. (2020). Interleukin 22 in liver injury, inflammation and cancer. *Int. J. Biol. Sci.* 16, 2405–2413. doi:10.7150/ijbs.38925

Wynn, T. A. (2004). Fibrotic disease and the T(H)1/T(H)2 paradigm. *Nat. Rev. Immunol.* 4, 583–594. doi:10.1038/nri1412

Yagi, Y., Andoh, A., Inatomi, O., Tsujikawa, T., and Fujiyama, Y. (2007). Inflammatory responses induced by interleukin-17 family members in human colonic subepithelial myofibroblasts. *J. Gastroenterol.* 42, 746–753. doi:10.1007/s00535-007-2091-3

Yan, Y. Y., Lin, S., and Zhu, Y. Y. (2018). Damage-associated molecular patterns and liver failure. *Zhonghua Gan Zang Bing Za Zhi* 24, 636–640. doi:10.3760/cma.j.issn.1007-3418.2016.08.017

Zai, W., Chen, W., Wu, Z., Jin, X., Fan, J., Zhang, X., et al. (2019). Targeted interleukin-22 gene delivery in the liver by polymetformin and penetratin-based hybrid nanoparticles to treat nonalcoholic fatty liver disease. *ACS Appl. Mater. Inter.* 11, 4842–4857. doi:10.1021/acsami.8b19717

Zhang, L. J., Zheng, W. D., Shi, M. N., and Wang, X. Z. (2006). Effects of interleukin-10 on activation and apoptosis of hepatic stellate cells in fibrotic rat liver. *World J. Gastroenterol.* 12, 1918–1923. doi:10.3748/wjg.v12.i12.1918

Zhang, S., Huang, D., Weng, J., Huang, Y., Liu, S., Zhang, Q., et al. (2016). Neutralization of interleukin-17 attenuates cholestatic liver fibrosis in mice. *Scand. J. Immunol.* 83, 102–108. doi:10.1111/sji.12395

Zhou, Z., Xu, M. J., and Gao, B. (2016). Hepatocytes: a key cell type for innate immunity. *Cell Mol. Immunol.* 13, 301–315. doi:10.1038/cmi.2015.97

Zhu, J., and Paul, W. E. (2008). CD4 T cells: fates, functions, and faults. *Blood* 112, 1557–1569. doi:10.1182/blood-2008-05-078154

Zimmermann, O., Homann, J. M., Bangert, A., Müller, A. M., Hristov, G., Goeser, S., et al. (2012). Successful use of mRNA-nucleofection for overexpression of interleukin-10 in murine monocytes/macrophages for anti-inflammatory therapy in a murine model of autoimmune myocarditis. *J. Am. Heart Assoc.* 1, e003293. doi:10.1161/JAHA.112.003293

2

Salidroside Inhibits CCl_4-Induced Liver Fibrosis in Mice by Reducing Activation and Migration of HSC Induced by Liver Sinusoidal Endothelial Cell-Derived Exosomal SphK1

Qiannan Ye[1,2], Yang Zhou[3], Changqing Zhao[1,2], Lieming Xu[1,2,4,5] and Jian Ping[1,5]**

[1]Shuguang Hospital Affiliated to Shanghai University of Traditional Chinese Medicine, Shanghai, China, [2]Institute of Liver Diseases, Shanghai University of Traditional Chinese Medicine, Shanghai, China, [3]Yueyang Hospital Affiliated to Shanghai University of Traditional Chinese Medicine, Shanghai, China, [4]Shanghai Key Laboratory of Traditional Chinese Medicine, Shanghai, China, [5]Key Laboratory of Liver and Kidney Diseases, Ministry of Education, Shanghai, China

***Correspondence:**
Lieming Xu
xulieming@shutcm.edu.cn
Jian Ping
pingjian@aliyun.com

Sphingosine kinase 1 (SphK1)/Sphingosine-1-phosphate (S1P)/S1PRs signaling pathway is known to involve the advancement of liver fibrosis. Exosomal SphK1 promotes hepatic stellate cells (HSC) migration. Salidroside (Sal) inhibits liver fibrosis, but its mechanism is yet to be elucidated. This study was to explore the influences of Sal on the SphK/S1P/S1PRs signaling pathway in liver fibrosis induced by carbon tetrachloride (CCl_4) *in vivo*, and investigated the mechanism of Sal affecting the migration and activation of HSC triggered by exosomal SphK1 *in vitro*. Our data showed that Sal reduced the activities of alanine transaminase (ALT), aspartate aminotransferase (AST) in serum, and hydroxyproline (Hyp) content in the liver tissue. Sal subdued the expression of α-smooth muscle actin (α-SMA), fibronectin (FN) and type I collagen (Col I) of the liver. Sal also reduced mitochondria-induced hepatocyte apoptosis and to inhibit JNK activation. Furthermore, Sal remarkably eradicated the influence of SphK1, SphK2, S1P, and S1PRs triggered by CCl_4, whether stimulating or hindering. Compared with serum-derived exosomes from model group mice, serum-derived exosomes from Sal group mice expressed lower SphK1 and reduced JS 1 (mouse HSC cell line) migration. In addition, Sal was also observed to subdue Col I expression, AKT activation, and LX-2 migration induced by exosomal SphK1 from SK-HEP-1 (a kind of liver sinusoidal endothelial cells (LSEC) cell line). In conclusion, Sal could effectively alleviate liver injury, hepatocyte apoptosis, and liver fibrosis *in vivo*, providing supports that the protective effects of Sal might be realized by suppressing JNK activation and modulating the SphK/S1P/S1PRs axis. *In vitro*, it was observed that Sal might alleviate LX-2 migration and activation induced by exosomal SphK1 by inhibiting the AKT activation.

Keywords: salidroside, liver fibrosis, SphK/S1P/S1PRs, exosomes, liver sinusoidal endothelial cells, hepatic stellate cell

INTRODUCTION

Liver fibrosis involves excessive accumulation of collagen and extracellular matrix (ECM). It is a reversible over-repair process of liver tissue damage due to various chronic liver injuries (Hernandez-Gea and Friedman, 2011). Hepatic stellate cell (HSC) activation is supposedly the critical event that initiates and develops liver fibrosis (Tsuchida and Friedman, 2017), though the exact pathogenesis is yet to be understood. Current effective treatment for liver fibrosis involves etiological treatment, such as antiviral therapy, the use of immunosuppressive agents, and others. This calls for researching effective therapies for alleviating liver fibrosis.

Exosomes are small vesicles released by various cells and distributed in several body fluids. Exosomes can mediate information exchange among cells and are a part of numerous physiological and pathological activities, including cell growth, proliferation, differentiation, and apoptosis (van Niel et al., 2018). Hepatocytes and liver sinusoidal endothelial cells (LSECs) have been shown in recent investigations to interact with HSCs via exosomes, in turn regulating the biological activity of HSCs (Sung et al., 2018). For instance, the miR-192 content in exosomes from palmitic acid-stimulated hepatocytes was found to be considerably increased, and these exosomes stimulated the activation of HSCs (Lee et al., 2017). LSECs secrete exosomes that express high amounts of Sphingosine kinase 1 (SphK1), which promote HSC migration by triggering AKT phosphorylation (Wang et al., 2015).

SphK/Sphingosine-1-phosphate (S1P)/S1PRs signaling pathway participates in tissue fibrosis progression, including liver fibrosis (Kono et al., 2007; Sato et al., 2016; Wang et al., 2019). The renal tissues of mice with unilateral ureteral ligation-caused renal interstitial fibrosis, the SphK1 levels, and autophagy-related proteins were found to have remarkably amplified as fibrosis advanced. The SphK1 protein expression was also detected to be upregulated in the lung tissue of bleomycin-induced pulmonary fibrosis model mice. In addition, when the SphK1 expression was blocked by SphK inhibitors or siRNA, the high expression of α-smooth muscle actin (α-SMA) and fibronectin (FN) induced by transforming growth factor β1 (TGF-β1) was observed to be lowered (Kono et al., 2007). Likewise, the SphK1 expression and its product S1P were recorded to increase progressively as the liver fibrosis advanced in the bile duct ligation (BDL) and carbon tetrachloride (CCl_4)-induced liver fibrosis, mouse model. Furthermore, S1P promoted liver fibrosis angiogenesis via binding to its ligands. Nevertheless, obstructing the binding of S1P to ligands perhaps inhibits angiogenesis in fibrotic liver tissue, in turn lowering the degree of liver fibrosis (Yang et al., 2013). These findings indicate that SphK/S1P/S1PRs signaling pathway plays an essential role in organ fibrosis.

A phenolic compound, Salidroside (Sal), occurs in plants of *Rhodiola rosea* L. Sal has been reported in recent researches to possess several pharmacological properties, such as anti-inflammatory (Xu et al., 2019), antioxidative (Jiansheng and Ying, 2012), and anticancerous (Ren et al., 2019). Earlier researches evidenced Sal to exhibit curative effects on numerous liver diseases. For instance, Sal reduces drug-induced liver injury (Yuan et al., 2019), guards the liver against ischemia/reperfusion injury (Cai et al., 2017), and eases nonalcoholic fatty liver disease (NAFLD) by AMPK-dependent TXNIP/NLRP3 pathway (Zheng et al., 2018). Another study reported Sal obstructing HSC activation and autophagy by downregulating NF-κB and TGF-β1/Smad3 signaling pathway (Feng et al., 2018), though it is unclear whether the effect of Sal on liver fibrosis is correlated to the SphK/S1P/S1PRs signal pathway. In one of our earlier investigations, Sal was observed to hinder the HSCs migration by obstructing AKT phosphorylation (Zhang et al., 2012). Based on literature reports evidencing exosomes to overexpress SphK1 derived from LSEC promoted LX-2-migration by upregulating the AKT activation, Sal was theorized to subdue HSC migration and activation by regulating exosome-mediated communication between LSEC and HSC.

The effects of Sal on SphK/S1P/S1PRs signal pathway in mouse with liver fibrosis caused by CCl_4 and how it regulates the migration and activation of LX-2 induced by exosomal SphK1 from LSECs were explored in this study *in vivo* and *in vitro*, respectively. The outcomes support the efficacy of Sal as an antifibrotic drug and back the SphK/S1P/S1PRs efficiency as a therapeutic target for liver fibrosis.

MATERIALS AND METHODS

Materials

Sal was procured from Shanghai Tauto Biotechnology (Shanghai, China), the alanine transaminase (ALT), aspartate aminotransferase (AST), and hydroxyproline (Hyp) detection kits were acquired from Nanjing Jiancheng Bioengineering Institute (Nanjing, China). FN, type I collagen (Col I), Bax and Bcl-2 antibodies were obtained from Abcam (Cambridge, United Kingdom). JNK, p-JNK, PARP, and cleaved caspase 3 antibodies were purchased from Cell Signaling Technology (Massachusetts, United States). SphK1, SphK2, S1PR1, S1PR2, S1PR3, CD9, and tumor susceptibility gene 101 (TSG101) antibodies were procured from ImmunoWay Biotechnology Company (Suzhou, China). Antibody against GAPDH was provided by Proteintech (Wuhan, China). TdT-mediated dUTP nick end labeling (TUNEL) Apoptosis Assay Kit, 2-(4-Amidinophenyl)-6-indolecarbamidine dihydrochloride (DPAI), and Cy3-labeled goat anti-rabbit IgG were all bought from Beyotime Institute of Biotechnology (Shanghai, China). The S1P Assay Kit (S1P-ELISA) was delivered by Echelon Biosciences (Salt Lake City, United States).

Animals

Male C57BL/6J, SPF grade mice weighing 20 ± 2 g, were supplied by Shanghai Sippr-BK laboratory animal Co. Ltd. (Shanghai, China). They were placed in the experimental animal center of Shanghai University of Traditional Chinese Medicine, China. The Committee on the Care and Use of Live Animals for Teaching and Research of the Shanghai University of Traditional Chinese Medicine sanctioned the animal experiments.

Animal Treatments

Following a week-long adaptive feeding, 45 male mice were divided into the control group included 15 mice, while the modeling group had 30. The modeling group animals were intraperitoneally injected with 15% CCl_4 (diluted with olive oil) at 2 ml/kg thrice a week, whereas those in the control group were administered an equal dosage of olive oil intraperitoneally. After a week of modeling, the modeling group was segregated into Model and Sal groups. The Model and Sal groups were continued to model with CCl_4 for 5 weeks, while the Control group was injected intraperitoneally with equal dose of olive oil. The Sal group animals were administered Sal (20 mg/kg) through gavage for 5 weeks. Simultaneously, those in the Control and Model groups were both treated with equal doses of ddH_2O. At the end of five weeks, the mice were sacrificed on anesthetizing with pentobarbital sodium, and the serum and liver tissue samples were preserved for subsequent experiments.

Serum Biochemical Test

The instructions provided along with the kit were followed to detect ALT and AST levels in the mice serum.

Pathological Evaluation of Liver

Fixation of the liver tissues was carried out in 10% neutral formalin for 48 h. They were then dehydrated stepwise with ethanol, followed by xylene permeation, and finally paraffin-embedded. Sections of 4 μm thickness were prepared for HE and Sirius red staining.

Determination of Hyp Content

Following the kit directions, the Hyp contents in liver tissues were determined.

Human Samples

Healthy volunteers and cirrhosis patients were selected for collecting human liver tissue and serum samples from the Department of Hepatobiliary Surgery, Renji Hospital, Affiliated to Shanghai Jiao Tong University. The Ethics Committee of Shuguang Hospital, Affiliated to Shanghai University of Traditional Chinese Medicine, sanctioned this study.

Isolation of Primary Liver Sinusoidal Endothelial Cells From Mice

Wild and Model groups of five male mice each were formed. The Model group mice were injected with CCl4 intraperitoneally to create a liver fibrosis model. They were then used to isolate primary LSECs. Using density gradient centrifugation in combination with CD146 magnetic bead (Miltenyi Biotec, Germany) separation, the primary LSEC of mice was isolated as the earlier reports (Liu et al., 2011; Meyer et al., 2016). Mouse liver tissue was perfused *in situ* and digested using an enzyme solution of collagenase D and DNase (Roche, Germany). Density gradient centrifugation was performed using OptiPrep solution (Axis-Shield, Norway) and incubation with CD146 magnetic bead for 30 min at 4°C. Thus isolated LSECs were cultured in Col I-coated dishes along with ECM medium, comprising 5% FBS, 2% endothelial cell growth supplement, and maintained with 5% CO_2 at 37°C in a humidified incubator.

Cell Culture

Propagation of human immortalized HSCs (LX-2) and mouse immortalized HSCs (JS 1) was carried out in DMEM, supplemented with 10% FBS, 100 U/ml penicillin, and 0.1 mg/ml streptomycin. The SK-HEP-1 cells, obtained from the Chinese Academy of Sciences, were grown in MEM, containing 10% FBS, 100 U/ml penicillin, and 0.1 mg/ml streptomycin. All cell lines were maintained with 5% CO_2 in a humidified incubator at 37°C.

Cell Transfection

The lentiviral vectors containing human SphK1 (LV-SphK1) or empty plasmid (LV-Cr) were procured from HANBIO Biotech (Shanghai, China). A 24-well plate was used to culture SK-HEP-1 to a confluence of 30–50%. They were then cultured in a fresh medium containing lentiviral vectors (MOI = 30) and polybrene (5 μg/ml) for 24 h, and then in a fresh medium for further culturing, followed by incubation for 48 h. The transfection efficiency of cells was studied using an inverted microscope and were incubated with a medium containing puromycin (1 μg/ml) to eliminate the untransfected cells. The transfected cells were cultured further, and the culture medium was used to isolate exosomes.

Isolation of Exosomes

SK-HEP-1 cells were cultured in 150 mm dishes to a confluence of 80–90%. They were then cultured in MEM with 10% exosome-free serum for 24 h. The supernatant was ultracentrifuged to obtain the exosomes. The supernatant was first centrifuged at 4°C, 300 ×g, for 10 min to eliminate cells. The supernatant was centrifuged again at 4°C, 2,000 ×g, for 10 min to eradicate dead cells. The supernatant was centrifuged at 4°C, 10,000 ×g, for another 30 min to eliminate cell debris. Eventually, the supernatant was ultracentrifuged at 4°C, 100,000 ×g for 70 min, and the precipitate collected was the exosomes. The thus isolated exosomes were resuspended in PBS or DMEM medium for subsequent *in vitro* studies.

Identification of Exosomes

A transmission electron microscope was utilized to study the morphology of isolated exosomes (van Niel et al., 2018). This was followed by detecting typical exosomal marker proteins, CD9 and TSG101, by Western blot (WB) analysis.

Cell Treatment

LX-2 and JS 1 were cultured in 60 mm dishes to a confluence of 80–90%. LX-2 cells were allocated to Cr-exo and Cirrhosis-exo groups and incubated with serum exosomes (30 μg/ml) from healthy volunteers and cirrhosis patients, respectively, to study the migration of LX-2 cells. Also, JS 1 cells were distributed into Cr-exo, M-exo, and Sal-exo groups and incubated with serum exosomes (30 μg/ml) from corresponding mice to detect JS 1 cells' migration. The LX-2 cells were then divided into Cr-exo, SphK1$^+$-exo, Cr-exo + Sal, and SphK1$^+$-exo + Sal groups and incubated with 30 μg/ml exosomes of transfected SK-HEP-1 cell culture media and/or Sal (10^{-5} M) to study the LX-2 cells migration and activation.

Transwell Migration Assays

LX-2 or JS 1 cells were cultured in Col I-coated migration cups to a confluence of 80–90%. Then, exosomes and/or Sal were added to the lower chamber, and with the same medium being added to the upper chamber as well. Incubation was carried out for 24 h, and the migration cups were then taken out and air-dried. Fixation of the cells on the lower surface of the migration cup was done using 4% paraformaldehyde and staining with crystal violet. The total number of cells that migrated to the bottom was recorded with an inverted microscope (Olympus, Tokyo, Japan) and evaluated using ImageJ software (NIH, United States).

Di-Acetylated-Low-Density Lipoprotein Assays

The adhered LSECs were incubated in ECM medium comprising DiI-Ac-LDL (Yiyuan Biotech, Guangzhou, China) for 4 h in the dark. The cells were then rinsed thrice with PBS, fixed with 4% paraformaldehyde for 15 min, and rinsed again with PBS. The endocytosis of DiI-Ac-LDL by LSECs was studied using an inverted fluorescence microscope (Olympus, Tokyo, Japan).

TUNEL Assay

According to the manufacturer's instructions, sections of frozen liver tissue of 8 μm thickness were prepared and incubated with TUNEL.

Immunofluorescence Staining

The LSECs were collected following 3 days of culturing, rinsed with PBS, and fixed using 4% paraformaldehyde for 30 min at room temperature. The frozen sections of mice liver tissue were fixed with precooled acetone for 15 min. Once fixed, the cells and frozen sections were rinsed again with PBS and incubated using 0.1% X-Triton-100 for 15 min at room temperature to disrupt the membrane. They were permeabilized and blocked using 5% BSA at room temperature for 1 h and then incubated with respective primary antibodies at 4°C overnight. The following day, they were incubated with anti-rabbit IgG (Cy3-labeled) in the dark at room temperature for 1 h and rinsed again with PBS. The cells were then stained using DAPI and rinsed using PBS. The sample was sealed, and their fluorescence was studied with the help of an inverted fluorescence microscope.

Protein Isolation and Western Blotting Analysis

RIPA lysate comprising complete Mini, PMSF, and phosphatase inhibitors was utilized to isolate liver tissues and cells' total protein. Protein quantification was performed with the BCA protein assay kit (Beyotime Institute of Biotechnology, Shanghai, China). An equivalent amount (30 μg) of proteins was electrophoresed by SDS-PAGE and transferred to PVDF membranes (Millipore, United States). The membranes were then incubated with blocking buffer (Beyotime Institute of Biotechnology, Shanghai, China) at room temperature for 1 h and incubated with respective primary antibodies overnight at 4°C. The membranes were rinsed using PBS-T for 20 min and treated with anti-rabbit IgG or anti-mouse IgG for 1 h. The membranes were rinsed with PBS-T again, and the images were recorded by means of Odyssey imaging system (LI-COR, United Kingdom) and analyzed with the ImageJ software. A part of the membranes was also stained with ponceau after incubating with antibodies.

RNA Isolation and RT-PCR Analysis

TRIzol total RNA preparation kit (Shanghai Sangon Biotech, Shanghai, China) was utilized to isolate the total RNA of cells and synthesized to cDNA with a ReverAid First Strand cDNA Synthesis Kit (Thermo, United States) following the manufacturer's procedures. The cDNA was mixed with primers and SYBR Green Real-time PCR Master Mix (TOYOBO, Japan) in a certain ratio; the relative expressions of mRNA were measured utilizing the ViiA 7 Real-Time PCR System (ABI, Carlsbad, CA, United States). Primer sequences used for detection of Sphk1, SphK2, S1PR1,2,3 were shown in **Table 1**.

Statistical Analysis

The outcomes have been recorded in terms of mean ± standard error of the mean. The differences among groups were evaluated via *t*-test or One-way ANOVA using SPSS 21.0 software. Values of $p < 0.05$ were considered statistically significant.

RESULTS

Sal Alleviated CCl_4-Induced Liver Fibrosis in Mice

Serum ATL and AST were detected to be considerably higher in the Model group than those in the Control group ($p < 0.01$) (**Figure 1A**), indicating obvious liver function damage due to CCl_4. Nevertheless, these changes were observed to be reversed by Sal ($p < 0.05$ or $p < 0.01$) (**Figure 1A**). HE staining revealed that CCl_4 resulted in collagen deposition, structural destruction, and inflammatory cell infiltration in liver lobules and portal areas. Sal treatment was found to remarkably alleviate these histopathological lesions (**Figure 1B**).

Besides, Sirius red staining revealed excessive collagen deposition in the Model group than that in the control group, and Sal was noted to lower the collagen deposition (**Figures 1C,D**) substantially. Then, the effect of Sal on liver fibrosis was further examined by identifying the Hyp content in liver tissue and the characteristic indicators of liver fibrosis, including FN, Col I, and α-SMA. The Hyp content in liver tissues of the Model group was found to be remarkably higher as compared with that of the control group. Sal treatment

TABLE 1 | Primer sequences for PCR.

Gene	Forward (5′-3′)	Reverse (5′-3′)
SphK1[a]	TGACTTGGAAAGAAAGGCTCT	GCAATGGGGAGTGTCTTCTAT
SphK2[a]	GCACGGCGAGTTTGGTTC	GAGACCTCATCCAGAGAGACTAG
S1PR1[a]	TGAGCGAGGCTGCTGTTTC	AGAGGGCGAGGTTGAGTGAG
S1PR2[a]	CCT TGA CTG GCT TGA ACT TTC	ACCCTCAGAACACAGACAGGT
S1PR3[a]	ACCAAGAAAATGTCACCGTGT	ACTCCCCTACACACTGCTCTG
SphK1[b]	CGACGAGGACTTTGTGCTAGT	AAACATCTCACTGCCCAGGT
GAPDH[b]	AGCCACATCGCTCAGACACC	GTACTCAGCGCCAGCATCG

[a]Mouse
[b]human.

reduced the Hyp level ($p < 0.01$) (**Figure 1E**). Moreover, higher quantities of FN, Col I, and α-SMA proteins were expressed in the Model group, which were considerably subdued by Sal administration ($p < 0.05$ or $p < 0.01$) (**Figure 1F**), signifying Sal reduced CCl_4-induced liver fibrosis.

Sal Alleviated CCl_4-Induced Apoptosis of Hepatocytes in Mice via Regulating JNK Activation

Considering the defensive effect of Sal on liver injury and fibrosis, Sal's influence on hepatocyte apoptosis was further studied by TUNEL staining. As indicated in **Figure 2A**, the apoptotic hepatocytes in the Model group were significantly amplified compared with those in the control group. Apoptotic cells in the Sal group as compared with the Model group were observed to be considerably reduced, indicating Sal's efficacy in alleviating CCl_4-induced hepatocyte apoptosis.

Sal's efficiency in expressing classic proteins in the mitochondrial apoptosis pathway and the role of the JNK signaling pathway in CCl_4-induced liver fibrosis were also investigated. Higher levels of cleaved caspase 3, cleaved PARP and Bax were expressed in the Model group, while Bcl-2 was lowered. Sal therapy was detected to reverse these changes and upregulate the ratio of Bcl-2 to Bax ($p < 0.05$ or $p < 0.01$) (**Figure 2B**). As displayed in **Figure 2B**, CCl_4 supported JNK phosphorylation in liver tissues. Sal therapy was recorded to downregulate the enhanced expression of p-JNK in model mice ($p < 0.05$) (**Figure 2B**). These findings indicate Sal considerably reduced mitochondria-mediated hepatocytes apoptosis by inhibiting JNK phosphorylation.

Sal Regulated the SphK/S1P/S1PR Signaling Pathway in the Liver of Mice

Sal's antifibrosis efficacy in relation to the regulation of SphK/S1P/S1PR signaling pathway was studied by examining the expression levels of SphK, S1P, and S1PRs. The protein and mRNA levels of SphK1 were detected to be upregulated, and SphK2 protein and mRNA expression downregulated in the liver tissues of the Model group as compared with those in the control group ($p < 0.05$ or $p < 0.01$) (**Figures 3A,C**). Sal was found to inhibit these effects ($p < 0.01$) (**Figures 3A,C**). Moreover, a high S1P level was observed in the model group ($p < 0.01$) (**Figure 3B**), and Sal was found to lower its level.

In addition, CCl_4 was also detected to regulate S1PRs, the receptors of S1P. Notably, it also amplified the expression of S1PR1 and S1PR3 but subdued that of S1PR2. Sal substantially eradicated the effects of S1PRs triggered by CCl_4, whether stimulating or hindering (**Figure 3C**).

Sal Inhibited the Expression of SphK1 in Serum Exosomes and the Migration of HSC Induced by Serum Exosomes

Serum exosomes from mice and humans were successfully isolated in this research, and their characteristics were analyzed by electron microscopy (**Figure 4A**), while the expression of markers of exosomes, TSG101 and CD9, was identified by Western blot (**Figure 4B**). SphK1 was noted to be highly expressed in serum exosomes from liver cirrhosis patients, which encouraged the migration of LX-2 ($p < 0.01$) (**Figures 4C,D**). A similar remarkably high expression of SphK1 in the serum exosomes derived from mice with liver fibrosis was recorded ($p < 0.01$) (**Figure 4E**). Moreover, Sal treatment was detected to downregulate the expression of SphK1 in serum exosomes ($p < 0.05$) (**Figure 4E**). As theorized, the serum exosomes in the mice with liver fibrosis were also found to encourage the migration of JS 1, and the serum exosomes of the Sal group to subdue the migration of JS 1 ($p < 0.01$) (**Figure 4F**).

SphK1 was Highly Expressed in Primary LSEC of Mice With Liver Fibrosis Induced by CCl_4

Serum-derived exosomes contain too many contents, not limited to a certain organ or even a certain type of cell. Therefore, it is very difficult to trace whether the components in serum exosomes originate from a certain cell. Considering the special anatomical position of LSEC and HSC and the essential role of the interaction between LSECs and HSC in the process of liver fibrosis (Deleve, 2015), we cultured the primary LSEC and detected its expression of SphK1, trying to prove the source of SphK1. The freshly isolated LSECs were

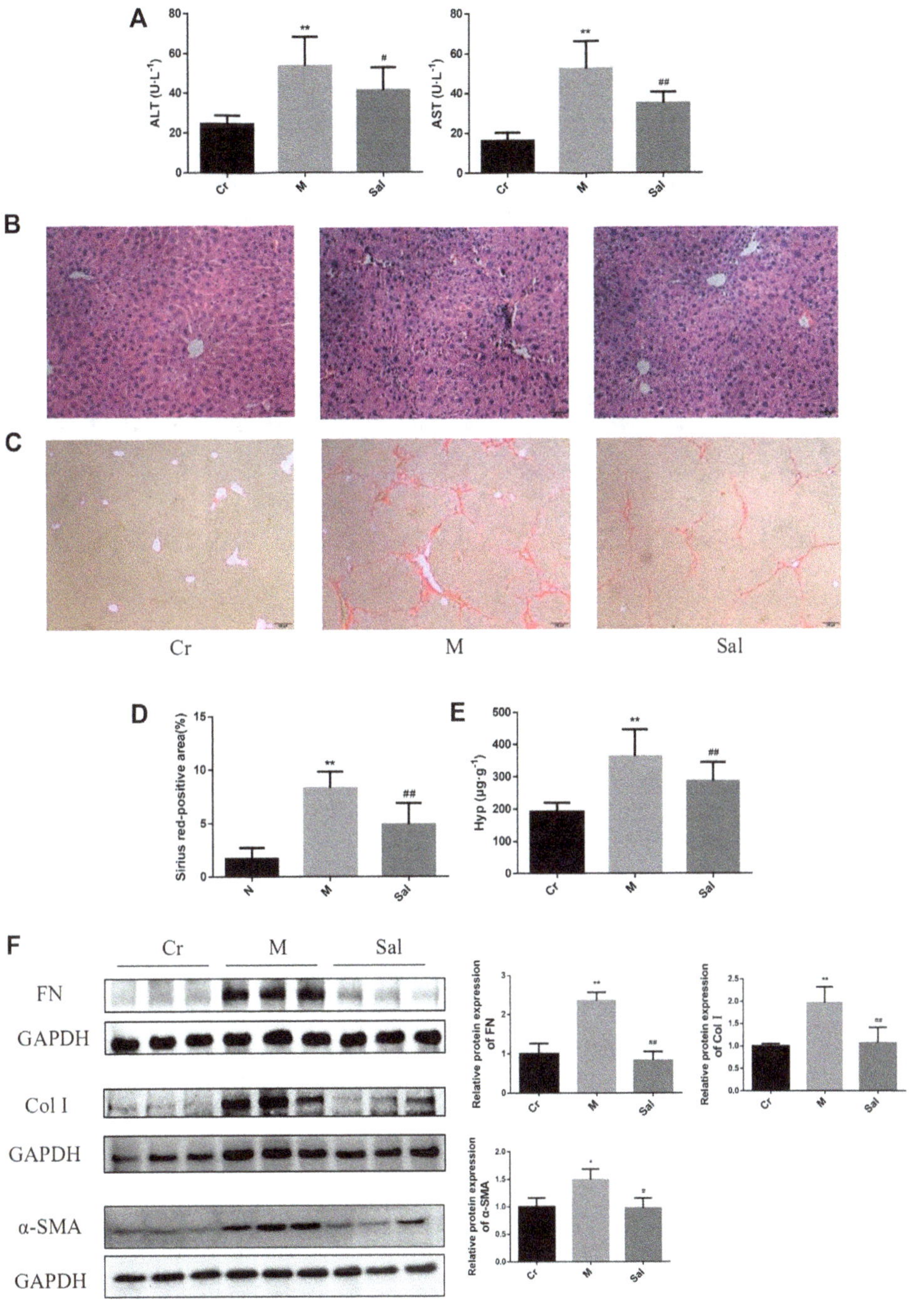

FIGURE 1 | Effects of Sal on liver injury and fibrosis induced by CCl_4. **(A)**: Levels of serum ATL and AST in different groups. **(B)**: HE staining of liver tissues in each group (×100). **(C)**: Sirius red staining of liver tissue sections (×100). **(D)**: Sirius red-positive area. **(E)**: Contents of Hyp in liver tissue. $^{**}p < 0.01$, vs. Cr; $^{\#\#}p < 0.01$, vs. M. **(F)**: Expressions of FN, Col I, and α-SMA in mice liver tissue were detected by WB. ($n = 15$, $^{*}p < 0.05$, $^{**}p < 0.01$, vs Cr; $^{\#}p < 0.05$, $^{\#\#}p < 0.01$, vs M.) ALT: alanine transaminase; AST: aspartate aminotransferase; Hyp: hydroxyproline; Cr: control group; M: model group; Sal: salidroside group. α-SMA: α-smooth muscle actin; FN: fibronectin; Col I: type I collagen; Cr: control group; M: model group; Sal: salidroside group.

small and spherical. During the *in vitro* culture, the LSECs were observed to gradually stretch out and adopt a long spindle shape (**Figure 5A**). **Figures 5B,C** present isolated LSECs phagocytosed Dil-Ac-LDL and expressed CD31, both of which are features of LSECs. Primary LSECs were also isolated from liver fibrosis model mice prompted by CCl_4, which expressed considerably higher SphK1 than that in the Wild mice ($p < 0.01$) (**Figure 5D**).

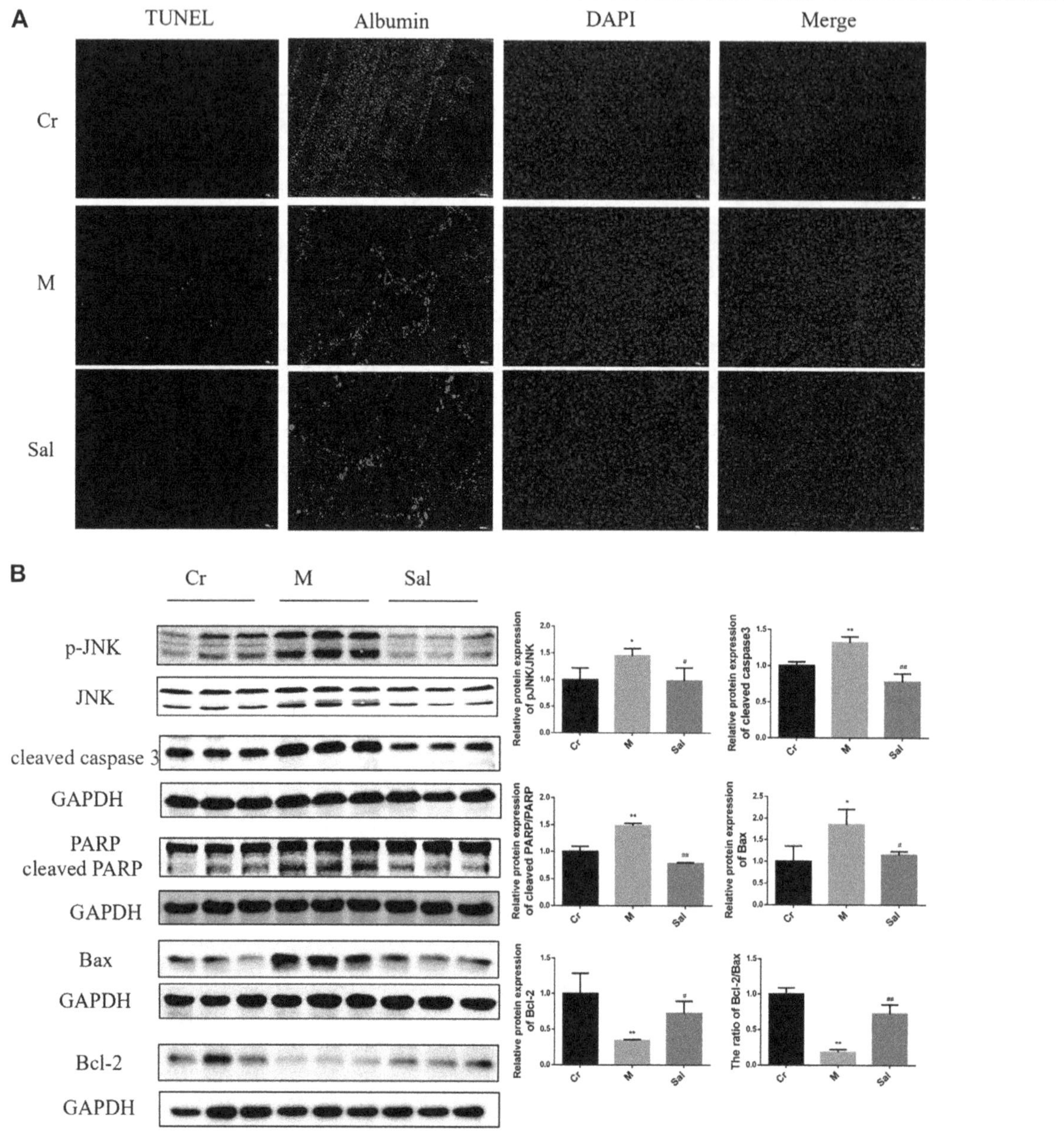

FIGURE 2 | Effect of Sal on apoptosis of hepatocytes in mice with liver fibrosis induced by CCl_4. **(A)**: Immunofluorescence staining of TUNEL and Albumin (×100). **(B)**: Effects of Sal on the expression of p-JNK, cleaved caspase3, cleaved RARP, Bax, and Bcl-2 in mice liver induced by CCl_4. ($n = 15$, $^*p < 0.05$, $^{**}p < 0.01$, vs. Cr; $^{\#}p < 0.05$, $^{\#\#}p < 0.01$, vs. M.). DAPI: 4′,6-diamidino-2-phenylindole; TUNEL: TdT-mediated dUTP nick end labeling.

Sal Alleviated Exosomal SphK1-Induced LX-2 Migration and Activation by Inhibiting AKT Activation

High levels of SphK1 were detected in primary mouse LSECs of liver fibrosis mice. Although the effect of exosomal SphK1 was tried to be studied on LSECs and HSC, the exosomes could not be derived owing to the inadequate number of primary LSECs. Thus, SK-HEP-1 cell lines that function similarly to LSECs were used (Cogger et al., 2008). Overexpression SphK1, SK-HEP-1, was established, and exosomes were isolated from the culture medium to study how exosomal SphK1 influenced the function of LX-2. As displayed in **Figures 6A,B**, substantially protein and mRNA expression of SphK1 was detected in SK-HEP-1 cells transfected with the lentivirus carrying SphK1 as compared with empty vector-transfected SK-HEP-1 cells ($p < 0.05$ or $p < 0.01$) (**Figures 6A,B**).

As predicted, the exosomes from the culture medium of SphK$^+$-SK-HEP-1 cells released significant quantities of SphK1. Moreover, upregulation of FN was recorded in the exosomes of SphK$^+$-SK-HEP-1 cells ($p < 0.05$ or $p < 0.01$) (**Figures 6D,E**). LX-2 cells were incubated with exosomes to

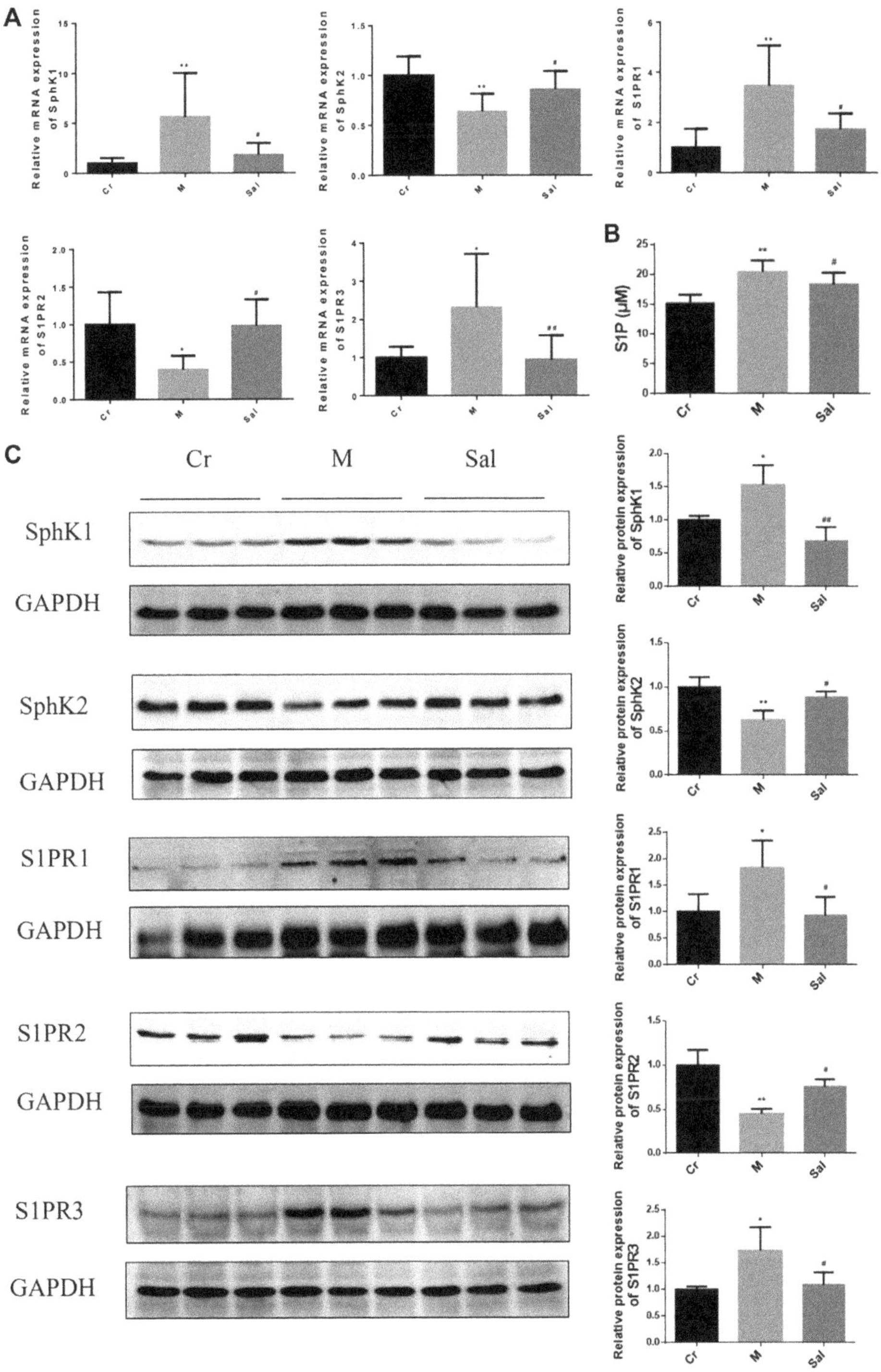

FIGURE 3 | Effects of Sal on the expressions of SphK/S1P/S1PRs signaling pathway in mice liver induced by CCl_4. **(A)**: The mRNA expressions of SphK1, SphK2, SPPR1, S1PR2 and S1PR3 in mice liver tissue. **(B)**: Level of S1P in serum from mice. **(C)**: The protein expressions of SphK1, SphK2, of S1PR1, S1PR2, and S1PR3 in mice liver tissue (n = 15, $^{*}p < 0.05$, $^{**}p < 0.01$, vs Cr; $^{\#}p < 0.05$, $^{\#\#}p < 0.01$, vs. M.) SphK1: Sphingosine kinase 1; S1P: Sphingosine-1-phosphate; S1PR1: Sphingosine 1-phosphate receptor 1; S1PR2: Sphingosine 1-phosphate receptor 2; S1PR3: Sphingosine 1-phosphate receptor 3.

explore the influence of exosomal SphK1 on the function of LX-2. As displayed in Figure 8F and G, the exosomal SphK1 caused the migration of LX-2 and the Col I level in LX-2, which could be reversed by Sal ($p < 0.05$ or $p < 0.01$) (**Figures 6F,G**). Earlier studies have evidenced AKT phosphorylation to support HSC activation, while exosomal SphK1 was found to encourage AKT

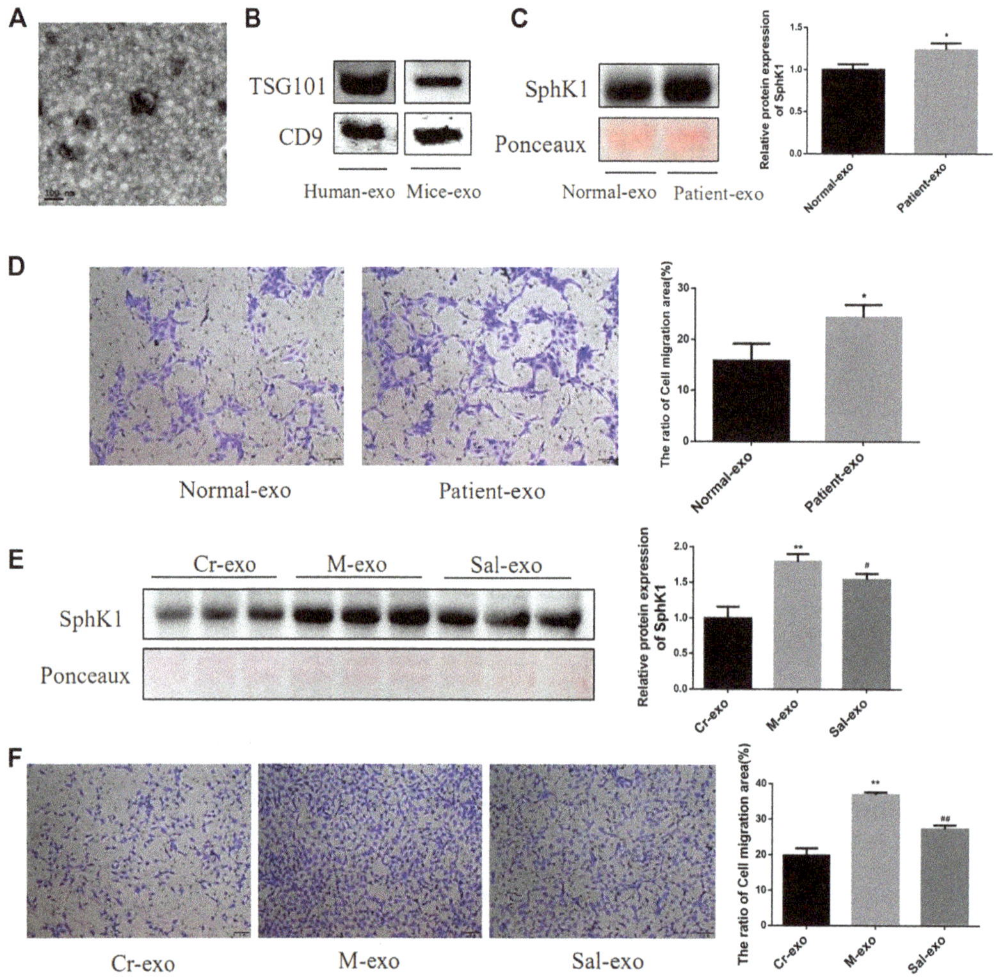

FIGURE 4 | Characteristics of serum exosomes and their effect on migration of HSC. **(A)**: Serum exosomes had a double-layer membrane structure. **(B)**: Expression of TSG101 and CD9 in serum exosomes from human and mice. **(C)**: Expression of SphK1 in serum exosomes from human ($n = 6$, $^{*}p < 0.05$, vs. Normal-exo.) **(D)**: Effects of serum exosomes from different populations on LX-2 migration ($n = 6$, $^{*}p < 0.05$, vs Normal-exo.) **(E)**: Expression of SphK1 in serum exosomes from different groups of mice ($n = 15$, $^{**}p < 0.01$, vs. Cr-exo, $^{\#}p < 0.05$, vs. M-exo,) **(F)**: Effects of serum exosomes from different groups of mice on JS 1 migration ($n = 15$, $^{**}p < 0.01$, vs Cr-exo, $^{\#\#}p < 0.01$, vs. M-exo.) TSG101: tumor susceptibility gene 101.

activation, and Sal reduces this effect in this research ($p < 0.05$ or $p < 0.01$) (**Figure 6G**). Thus, Sal was theorized to lessen LX-2 migration and activation induced by exosomal SphK1 by hindering AKT activation.

DISCUSSION

According to the complex pathological mechanism of fibrosis, multiple targets and pathways are the traits of traditional Chinese medicine. Traditional Chinese herbal medicine has been increasingly substantiated to treat liver fibrosis (Li, 2020), as it has effectively established the protective influence of Sal on liver fibrosis (Wu et al., 2003; Feng et al., 2018). Sal has already been proved to inhibit the migration of HSC in one of our earlier researches (Zhang et al., 2012). Exosomes have been explored extensively in recent years for their vital function as carriers for drug delivery. Earlier studies have revealed curcumin-encapsulated exosomes to possess anti-inflammatory, antioxidant, and anticancerous properties (Oskouie et al., 2018). In this study, a mouse model of liver fibrosis triggered by CCl_4 was replicated further to investigate Sal's potential influence on liver fibrosis. Exosomes carrying SphK1 secreted by SK-HEP-1, a cell line with endothelial cell function, were also isolated, and their effect on HSC function and the effect of Sal treatment *in vitro* was analyzed.

Inflammation is a significant feature of fibrosis; constraining hepatic inflammation is essential in treating liver fibrosis. Previous studies have reported that Sal reduces liver fibrosis through anti-inflammatory (Feng et al., 2018). In this study, Sal was not just found to efficiently reduce the serum concentrations of ALT and AST in CCl_4-induced liver fibrosis mice but also to hinder the infiltration of inflammatory cells into the liver tissue, evidencing that Sal could ease the damage caused by inflammation in the process of liver fibrosis. Unfortunately, in

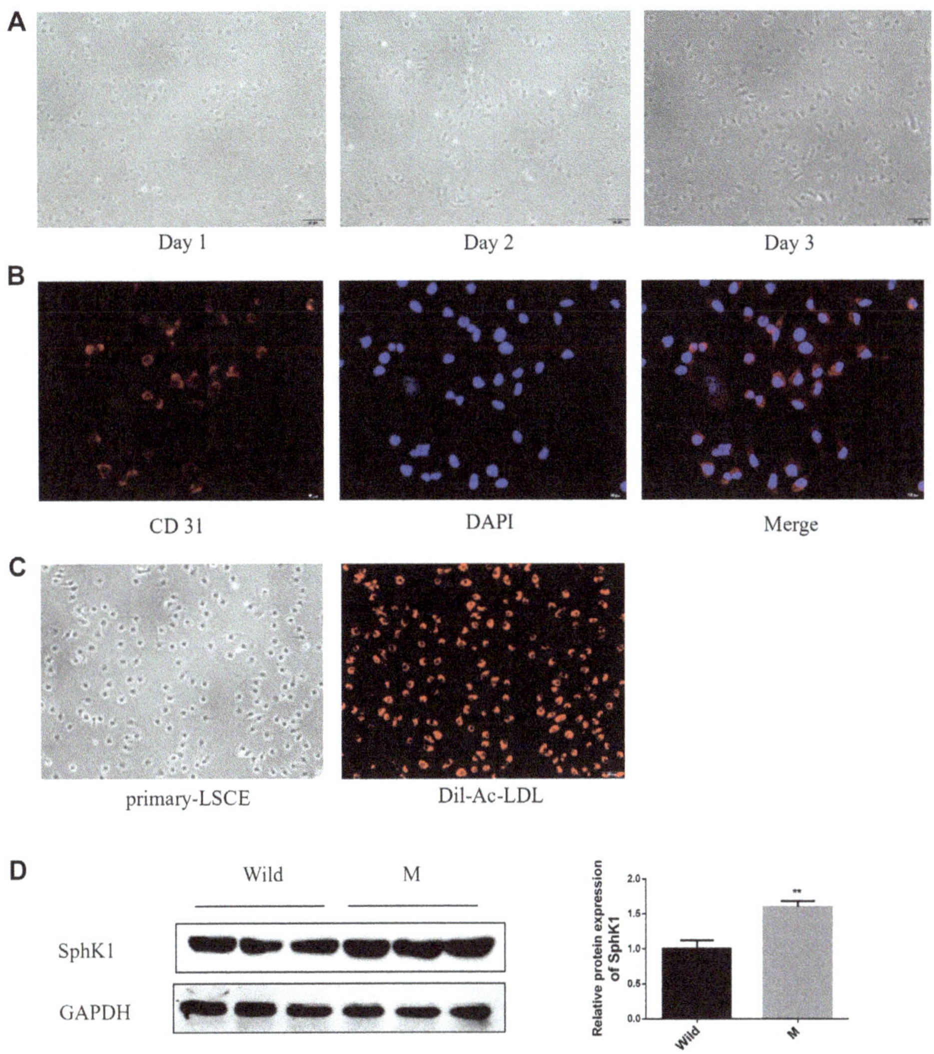

FIGURE 5 | Expression of SphK1 in LSECs isolated from mice with liver fibrosis induced by CCl_4. **(A)**: Morphology of isolated mouse primary LSECs. **(B)**: Isolated mouse primary LSEC could phagocytosis Dil-Ac-LDL. **(C)**: Isolated mouse primary LSECs expressed CD31. **(D)**: LSEC of mice with liver fibrosis upregulated the expression of SphK1 ($n = 5$, $^{**}p < 0.01$, vs. Wild.)

order to reserve as much serum as possible for the extraction of exosomes, this study did not detect IL1, IL6, TNF-α and other inflammatory factors in mouse serum, and failed to explain the anti-inflammatory effect of Sal more intuitively.

Cell apoptosis is known to have an essential role in embryonic development and tissue homeostasis (Tuzlak et al., 2016), but apoptotic cells can activate a series of pathological events under certain circumstances (Schwabe and Luedde, 2018). Apoptosis of damaged hepatocytes amplified inflammation, HSC activation, and liver fibrosis (Kisseleva and Brenner, 2020). Cell apoptosis primarily includes extrinsic and intrinsic pathways. The intrinsic or the mitochondrial-mediated apoptosis pathway is essentially regulated by the Bcl-2 family (Bock and Tait, 2020). Bcl-2 family is divided into 3 categories on the basis of function and structure: BH3, the apoptosis initiator; the antiapoptotic guardians, such as Bcl-2; and the proapoptotic proteins, such as Bax and Bak (Czabotar et al., 2014). Various cytotoxic stimuli activate BH3 pathologically, subduing the expression of antiapoptotic proteins and activating proapoptotic proteins, thus destroying the permeability of the mitochondrial inner membrane. Mitochondrial apoptosis is known to be co-regulated by the Bcl-2 family; the ratio of Bcl-2 to Bax is the key determining factor of apoptosis (Yu et al., 2021). Damaged mitochondria secrete cytochrome C that in turn is known to activate the caspase family, which is a group of cysteine protease that participates in cell apoptosis (Van Opdenbosch and Lamkanfi, 2019). Of these, caspase-3 is the central link and an essential initiator of the apoptosis process (Galluzzi et al., 2016). Caspase-3 physiologically exists as an inactive zymogen. Caspase-3 is rapidly cleaved and activated to trigger cell death signals in case of various injuries (Lim et al., 2021). In the present study, the hepatocyte apoptosis was observed in the Model group, the

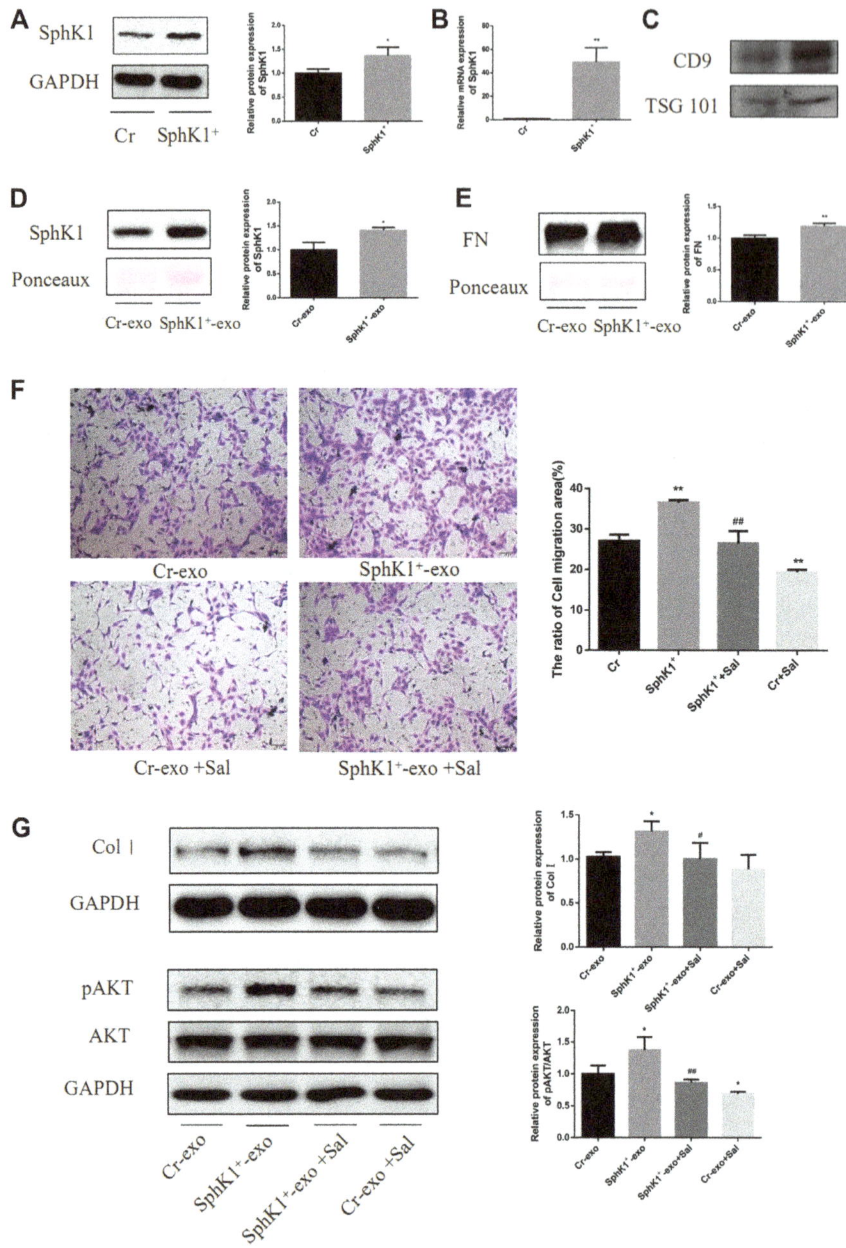

FIGURE 6 | Effects of Sal on exosomal SphK1-induced LX-2 migration and activation. **(A)**: Expression of SphK1 in transfected cells was detected by WB. **(B)**: Expression of SphK1 in transfected cells was detected by PCR. **(C)**: Expression of TSG101 and CD9 in exosomes from culture mediums. **(D,E)**: Expression of SphK1 and FN in exosomes from culture mediums of transfected cells. ($n = 3$, $^{**}p < 0.01$, vs Cr-exo.) **(F)**: Sal inhibited exosomal SphK1-induced LX-2 migration and activation. **(G)**: Sal inhibited exosomal SphK1-induced AKT phosphorylation in LX-2. ($n = 3$, $^{*}p < 0.05$, $^{**}p < 0.01$, vs. Cr-exo; $^{\#}p < 0.05$, $^{\#\#}p < 0.01$, vs. SphK1^{+}-exo.).

expression of cleaved caspase 3, cleaved PARP and Bax were upregulated, while Bcl-2 was downregulated. Sal was observed to reverse the high expression of Bax and low expression of Bcl-2 induced by CCl_4 and upregulate the ratio of Bcl-2 to Bax. Sal was also observed to inhibit the activation of caspase-3 and PRAP, the substrate of caspase-3, thereby hindering cell apoptosis.

SphK1 has been shown to be involved in the regulation of mitochondrial permeability transition by several studies. Besides, SphK1 deficiency hinders JNK activation and defends acetaminophen-induced hepatocyte death (Li et al., 2019), whereas SphK1 overexpression was found to aggravate cell apoptosis (Lu et al., 2018). In this study, Sal was detected to alleviate hepatocytes apoptosis as well as JNK activation. The effect of Sal on the SphK/S1P/S1PRs signaling pathway in CCl_4-induced hepatic fibrosis mice was also explored. S1P, bioactive sphingomyelin, is released by Sphingosine kinases (SphKs) catalyzing Sphingosine, which participates in regulating various biological activities such as cell proliferation and migration. Two subtypes of SphK are SphK1 and SphK2 (Ogretmen, 2018). SphK1 can migrate from the cytoplasm to the plasma membrane and promote S1P formation on the cell membrane under the influence of growth factors, hormones, or cytokines. Furthermore, SphK1 occurs chiefly in the cytoplasm, whereas SphK2 in the nucleus and mitochondrial inner membrane, which can likely upsurge the S1P concentration in the nucleus (Spiegel and Milstien, 2011). High quantities of SphK1 expression have been shown recently to aid in the progression of liver fibrosis (Sato et al., 2016), whereas SphK1 inhibition substantially reduces the degree of liver fibrosis (Yang et al., 2013). Another study found compared with that in healthy volunteers, the level of SphK2 was reduced in the liver of patients with alcoholic cirrhosis and hepatocellular carcinoma, and SphK2 deficiency could aggravate liver injury induced by alcohol (Kwong et al., 2019). Our date suggested that the expression of SphK1 in the fibrotic liver was remarkably upregulated, and the SphK2 level was obviously reduced, in agreement with the findings of earlier researches. While Sal could reverse these changes, whether these changes were stimulating or hindering. Moreover, there are growing researches regarding of the expression level of S1P and its ligands and their roles in liver fibrosis. For instance, Yang et al. (Yang et al., 2013) reported the expression of S1P increased progressively with the aggravation of liver fibrosis in mice induced by CCl_4 or BDL. Besides, their study displayed these changes of S1P are not only manifested in fibrotic animals but also upregulated in liver tissues from hepatitis B, C, and alcoholic cirrhosis patients (Yang et al., 2013). In this study, high concentrations of S1P were also found in the mice serum with liver fibrosis and Sal reversed the change of S1P. Earlier studies have established that S1PR1, S1PR2, and S1PR3 can be expressed in human liver fibroblasts (hepatic myofibroblast, hMFs). Remarkably, S1PR1 and S1PR3 occurred in high concentrations in fibrotic liver tissues, whereas S1PR2 expression was downregulated (Li et al., 2011), the findings being in agreement with those of our experiments. Essentially, Sal reversed the increase in S1PR1 and S1PR3 and the decrease in S1PR2 induced by CCl_4. Based on published research, the differences in the SphK/S1P/S1PRs signaling pathway among humans, rats, and mice samples may be owing to the species differences and diverse fibrogenesis mechanisms. Additional studies are indispensable to investigate the role of the SphK/S1P/S1PRs signaling pathway in regulating liver fibrosis and its therapeutic significance.

After observing the effects of Sal on SphK1 and S1PRs *in vivo*, we tried to clarify whether the influence of Sal on SphK1 and S1PRs in liver tissue could be localized on certain cells. Considering the key role of HSC in liver fibrosis, LX-2 was treated with PMA (an agonist of SphK1) and/or Sal. The results showed that Sal could inhibit HSC migration induced by PMA, but did not affect the expressions of SphK1 and S1PRs in LX-2 (Data not shown). Combined with previous studies reported that exosomal SphK1 derived by LSEC could induce HSC migration (Wang et al., 2015). Therefore, we tried to illustrate effect of Sal on HSC based on regulation of LSEC exosomes on HSC.

Exosomes are extracellular vesicles of diameters ranging from 50 to 150 nm (van Niel et al., 2018). They possess the same characteristics containing "exosome marker" proteins related to exosome biogenesis and secretion, such as the Rab family, GTPase, ALG-2-interacting protein X (ALIX), and TSG101. Exosomes are also rich in heat shock proteins, such as HSP60, HSP70, and HSP90; integrins; and tetraspanins, viz, CD9, CD63, CD81, and CD82. However, the inclusions of exosomes are highly heterogeneous based on the state and type of cells (Sung et al., 2018). For instance, the expression of CD81 in serum exosomes of patients with chronic hepatitis C was significantly higher than that in the healthy volunteers and patients in the virus response phase (Martin-Walter et al., 2012). The exosomes of lipid-induced hepatocyte secreted high amounts of miR-128-3p, which stimulated HSC migration after being taken up by HSC(Povero et al., 2015). In this study, serum exosomes derived from liver cirrhosis patients or mice with liver fibrosis released high concentrations of SphK1 and promoted HSC migration. Simultaneously, compared with serum-derived exosomes from Model group mice, serum-derived exosomes from Sal group mice expressed lower SphK1 and reduced JS 1 migration. In addition, exosome-mediated intercellular communication has been shown to require docking on the plasma membrane in an earlier study (Teng and Fussenegger, 2021). Also, integrins, lipids, heparan sulfate proteoglycans, and ECM components (especially FN and laminin) can function as mediators in the intercellular interaction (van Niel et al., 2018). In this study, the expression of FN was upregulated in exosomes of $SphK^{+}$-SK-HEP-1 cells, signifying that the FN on the surface of exosomes mediated interactions between exosomes and cells thus influencing the function of the recipient cells. The concentration of SphK1 was amplified in primary LSECs of liver fibrosis mice. Also, exosomal SphK1 derived from SK-HEP-1, a cell line with a similar function to that of LSECs, promoted the migration, activation, and AKT phosphorylation of LX-2. Sal relieved these effects. These outcomes indicated that Sal likely alleviated the migration and activation of LX-2 induced by exosomal SphK1 by inhibiting the activation of AKT.

To conclude, our study evidenced that Sal could effectively reduce liver injury, hepatocyte apoptosis, and liver fibrosis *in vivo*. In addition, the protective efficacy of Sal might be comprehended by regulating JNK activation and controlling the SphK/S1P/S1PRs axis. Moreover, Sal was observed to reduce the migration and activation of LX-2 induced by exosomal SphK1 by subduing the activation of AKT *in vitro*. In summary, the present study explained the anti-fibrosis mechanism of Sal based on the perspective of regulating the biological activity of HSC by LSEC-derived exosomes. More experiments are needed to further explain the role of Sal on liver fibrosis.

ETHICS STATEMENT

The studies were approved by The Ethics Committee of Shuguang Hospital, Affiliated to Shanghai University of Traditional Chinese Medicine and The Committee on the Care and Use of Live Animals for Teaching and Research of the Shanghai University of Traditional Chinese Medicine. All participants provided written informed consent.

AUTHOR CONTRIBUTIONS

QY carried out the experiment and wrote the manuscript. YZ, CZ, LX, and JP guided the experiments and reviewed the manuscript.

REFERENCES

Bock, F. J., and Tait, S. W. G. (2020). Mitochondria as Multifaceted Regulators of Cell Death. *Nat. Rev. Mol. Cel Biol* 21 (2), 85–100. doi:10.1038/s41580-019-0173-8

Cai, L., Li, Y., Zhang, Q., Sun, H., Yan, X., Hua, T., et al. (2017). Salidroside Protects Rat Liver against Ischemia/reperfusion Injury by Regulating the GSK-3β/Nrf2-dependent Antioxidant Response and Mitochondrial Permeability Transition. *Eur. J. Pharmacol.* 806, 32–42. doi:10.1016/j.ejphar.2017.04.011

Cogger, V. C., Arias, I. M., Warren, A., Mcmahon, A. C., Kiss, D. L., Avery, V. M., et al. (2008). The Response of Fenestrations, Actin, and Caveolin-1 to Vascular Endothelial Growth Factor in SK Hep1 Cells. *Am. J. Physiology-Gastrointestinal Liver Physiol.* 295 (1), G137–G145. doi:10.1152/ajpgi.00069.2008

Czabotar, P. E., Lessene, G., Strasser, A., and Adams, J. M. (2014). Control of Apoptosis by the BCL-2 Protein Family: Implications for Physiology and Therapy. *Nat. Rev. Mol. Cel Biol* 15 (1), 49–63. doi:10.1038/nrm3722

Deleve, L. D. (2015). Liver Sinusoidal Endothelial Cells in Hepatic Fibrosis. *Hepatology* 61 (5), 1740–1746. doi:10.1002/hep.27376

Feng, J., Chen, K., Xia, Y., Wu, L., Li, J., Li, S., et al. (2018). Salidroside Ameliorates Autophagy and Activation of Hepatic Stellate Cells in Mice via NF-Kb and TGF-β1/Smad3 Pathways. *Dddt* 12, 1837–1853. doi:10.2147/DDDT.S162950

Galluzzi, L., López-Soto, A., Kumar, S., and Kroemer, G. (2016). Caspases Connect Cell-Death Signaling to Organismal Homeostasis. *Immunity* 44 (2), 221–231. doi:10.1016/j.immuni.2016.01.020

Hernandez-Gea, V., and Friedman, S. L. (2011). Pathogenesis of Liver Fibrosis. *Annu. Rev. Pathol. Mech. Dis.* 6 (6), 425–456. doi:10.1146/annurev-pathol-011110-130246

Jiansheng, X., and Ying, L. (2012). Effects of Salidroside on Exhaustive Exercise-Induced Oxidative Stress in Rats. *Mol. Med. Rep.* 6 (5), 1195–1198. doi:10.3892/mmr.2012.1060

Kisseleva, T., and Brenner, D. (2020). Molecular and Cellular Mechanisms of Liver Fibrosis and its Regression. *Nat. Rev. Gastroenterol. Hepatol.* 18 (3), 151–166. doi:10.1038/s41575-020-00372-7

Kono, Y., Nishiuma, T., Nishimura, Y., Kotani, Y., Okada, T., Nakamura, S.-i., et al. (2007). Sphingosine Kinase 1 Regulates Differentiation of Human and Mouse Lung Fibroblasts Mediated by TGF-B1. *Am. J. Respir. Cel Mol Biol* 37 (4), 395–404. doi:10.1165/rcmb.2007-0065OC

Kwong, E. K., Liu, R., Zhao, D., Li, X., Zhu, W., Wang, X., et al. (2019). The Role of Sphingosine Kinase 2 in Alcoholic Liver Disease. *Dig. Liver Dis.* 51 (8), 1154–1163. doi:10.1016/j.dld.2019.03.020

Lee, Y.-S., Kim, S. Y., Ko, E., Lee, J.-H., Yi, H.-S., Yoo, Y. J., et al. (2017). Exosomes Derived from Palmitic Acid-Treated Hepatocytes Induce Fibrotic Activation of Hepatic Stellate Cells. *Sci. Rep.* 7 (1). doi:10.1038/s41598-017-03389-2

Li, C., Zheng, S., You, H., Liu, X., Lin, M., Yang, L., et al. (2011). Sphingosine 1-phosphate (S1P)/S1P Receptors Are Involved in Human Liver Fibrosis by Action on Hepatic Myofibroblasts Motility. *J. Hepatol.* 54 (6), 1205–1213. doi:10.1016/j.jhep.2010.08.028

Li, H. (2020). Advances in Anti Hepatic Fibrotic Therapy with Traditional Chinese Medicine Herbal Formula. *J. Ethnopharmacology* 251, 112442. doi:10.1016/j.jep.2019.112442

Li, L., Wang, H., Zhang, J., Sha, Y., Wu, F., Wen, S., et al. (2019). SPHK1 Deficiency Protects Mice from Acetaminophen-Induced ER Stress and Mitochondrial Permeability Transition. *Cell Death Differ* 27, 1924–1937. doi:10.1038/s41418-019-0471-x

Lim, J.-Y., Lee, J.-H., Yun, D.-H., Lee, Y.-M., and Kim, D.-K. (2021). Inhibitory Effects of Nodakenin on Inflammation and Cell Death in Lipopolysaccharide-Induced Liver Injury Mice. *Phytomedicine* 81, 153411. doi:10.1016/j.phymed.2020.153411

Liu, W., Hou, Y., Chen, H., Wei, H., Lin, W., Li, J., et al. (2011). Sample Preparation Method for Isolation of Single-Cell Types from Mouse Liver for Proteomic Studies. *Proteomics* 11 (17), 3556–3564. doi:10.1002/pmic.201100157

Lu, J., Yi, Y., Pan, R., Zhang, C., Han, H., Chen, J., et al. (2018). Berberine Protects HK-2 Cells from Hypoxia/reoxygenation Induced Apoptosis via Inhibiting SPHK1 Expression. *J. Nat. Med.* 72 (2), 390–398. doi:10.1007/s11418-017-1152-z

Meyer, J., Lacotte, S., Morel, P., Gonelle-Gispert, C., and Bühler, L. (2016). An Optimized Method for Mouse Liver Sinusoidal Endothelial Cell Isolation. *Exp. Cel Res.* 349 (2), 291–301. doi:10.1016/j.yexcr.2016.10.024

Ogretmen, B. (2018). Sphingolipid Metabolism in Cancer Signalling and Therapy. *Nat. Rev. Cancer* 18 (1), 33–50. doi:10.1038/nrc.2017.96

Oskouie, M. N., Aghili Moghaddam, N. S., Butler, A. E., Zamani, P., and Sahebkar, A. (2018). Therapeutic Use of Curcumin-encapsulated and Curcumin-primed Exosomes. *J. Cel. Physiol.* 234 (6), 8182–8191. doi:10.1002/jcp.27615

Povero, D., Panera, N., Eguchi, A., Johnson, C. D., Papouchado, B. G., de Araujo Horcel, L., et al. (2015). Lipid-Induced Hepatocyte-Derived Extracellular Vesicles Regulate Hepatic Stellate Cells via MicroRNA Targeting Peroxisome Proliferator-Activated Receptor-γ. *Cell Mol. Gastroenterol. Hepatol.* 1 (6), 646–663. doi:10.1016/j.jcmgh.2015.07.007

Ren, M., Xu, W., and Xu, T. (2019). Salidroside Represses Proliferation, Migration and Invasion of Human Lung Cancer Cells through AKT and MEK/ERK Signal Pathway. *Artif. Cell Nanomedicine, Biotechnol.* 47 (1), 1014–1021. doi:10.1080/21691401.2019.1584566

Sato, M., Ikeda, H., Uranbileg, B., Kurano, M., Saigusa, D., Aoki, J., et al. (2016). Sphingosine Kinase-1, S1P Transporter Spinster Homolog 2 and S1P2 mRNA Expressions Are Increased in Liver with Advanced Fibrosis in Human. *Sci. Rep.* 6 (1), 32119. doi:10.1038/srep32119

Schwabe, R. F., and Luedde, T. (2018). Apoptosis and Necroptosis in the Liver: a Matter of Life and Death. *Nat. Rev. Gastroenterol. Hepatol.* 15 (12), 738–752. doi:10.1038/s41575-018-0065-y

Spiegel, S., and Milstien, S. (2011). The Outs and the Ins of Sphingosine-1-Phosphate in Immunity. *Nat. Rev. Immunol.* 11 (6), 403–415. doi:10.1038/nri2974

Sung, S., Kim, J., and Jung, Y. (2018). Liver-Derived Exosomes and Their Implications in Liver Pathobiology. *Ijms* 19 (12), 3715. doi:10.3390/ijms19123715

Teng, F., and Fussenegger, M. (2021). Shedding Light on Extracellular Vesicle Biogenesis and Bioengineering. *Adv. Sci.* 8 (1), 2003505. doi:10.1002/advs.202003505

Tsuchida, T., and Friedman, S. L. (2017). Mechanisms of Hepatic Stellate Cell Activation. *Nat. Rev. Gastroenterol. Hepatol.* 14 (7), 397–411. doi:10.1038/nrgastro.2017.38

Tuzlak, S., Kaufmann, T., and Villunger, A. (2016). Interrogating the Relevance of Mitochondrial Apoptosis for Vertebrate Development and Postnatal Tissue Homeostasis. *Genes Dev.* 30 (19), 2133–2151. doi:10.1101/gad.28929810.1101/gad.289298.116

van Niel, G., D'Angelo, G., and Raposo, G. (2018). Shedding Light on the Cell Biology of Extracellular Vesicles. *Nat. Rev. Mol. Cel Biol* 19 (4), 213–228. doi:10.1038/nrm.2017.125

Van Opdenbosch, N., and Lamkanfi, M. (2019). Caspases in Cell Death, Inflammation, and Disease. *Immunity* 50 (6), 1352–1364. doi:10.1016/j.immuni.2019.05.020

Wang, E., He, X., and Zeng, M. (2019). The Role of S1P and the Related Signaling Pathway in the Development of Tissue Fibrosis. *Front. Pharmacol.* 9, 1504. doi:10.3389/fphar.2018.01504

Wang, R., Ding, Q., Yaqoob, U., de Assuncao, T. M., Verma, V. K., Hirsova, P., et al. (2015). Exosome Adherence and Internalization by Hepatic Stellate Cells Triggers Sphingosine 1-phosphate-dependent Migration. *J. Biol. Chem.* 290 (52), 30684–30696. doi:10.1074/jbc.M115.671735

Welker, M. W., Reichert, D., Susser, S., Sarrazin, C., Martinez, Y., Herrmann, E., et al. (2012). Soluble Serum CD81 Is Elevated in Patients with Chronic Hepatitis C and Correlates with Alanine Aminotransferase Serum Activity. *PLoS One* 7 (2), e30796. doi:10.1371/journal.pone.0030796

Wu, X.-L., Zeng, W. Z., Wang, P. L., Lei, C. T., Jiang, M. D., Chen, X. B., et al. (2003). Effect of Compound Rhodiola Sachalinensis A Bor on CCl4-Induced Liver Fibrosis in Rats and its Probable Molecular Mechanisms. *Wjg* 9 (7), 1559–1562. doi:10.3748/wjg.v9.i7.1559

Xu, N., Huang, F., Jian, C., Qin, L., Lu, F., Wang, Y., et al. (2019). Neuroprotective Effect of Salidroside against Central Nervous System Inflammation-induced Cognitive Deficits: A Pivotal Role of Sirtuin 1-dependent N Rf-2/HO -1/NF -κ B Pathway. *Phytotherapy Res.* 33 (5), 1438–1447. doi:10.1002/ptr.6335

Yang, L., Yue, S., Yang, L., Liu, X., Han, Z., Zhang, Y., et al. (2013). Sphingosine Kinase/sphingosine 1-phosphate (S1P)/S1P Receptor axis Is Involved in Liver Fibrosis-Associated Angiogenesis. *J. Hepatol.* 59 (1), 114–123. doi:10.1016/j.jhep.2013.02.021

Yu, H.-h., Qiu, Y.-x., Li, B., Peng, C.-y., Zeng, R., and Wang, W. (2021). Kadsura Heteroclita Stem Ethanol Extract Protects against Carbon Tetrachloride-Induced Liver Injury in Mice via Suppression of Oxidative Stress, Inflammation, and Apoptosis. *J. Ethnopharmacology* 267, 113496. doi:10.1016/j.jep.2020.113496

Yuan, Y., Wu, X., Zhang, X., Hong, Y., and Yan, H. (2019). Ameliorative Effect of Salidroside from Rhodiola Rosea L. On the Gut Microbiota Subject to Furan-Induced Liver Injury in a Mouse Model. *Food Chem. Toxicol.* 125, 333–340. doi:10.1016/j.fct.2019.01.007

Zhang, Z., Ping, J., and Xu, L. (2012). Screening Chinese Medicine Components for Inhibition of Human Hepatic Stellate Cell Migration. *J. Clin. Hepatol.* 28 (3), 183–188. doi:10.3969/j.issn.1001-5256.2012.03.00

Zheng, T., Yang, X., Li, W., Wang, Q., Chen, L., Wu, D., et al. (2018). Salidroside Attenuates High-Fat Diet-Induced Nonalcoholic Fatty Liver Disease via AMPK-dependent TXNIP/NLRP3 Pathway. *Oxidative Med. Cell Longevity* 2018, 1–17. doi:10.1155/2018/8597897

3

Exosomes in Intestinal Inflammation

Kanchana K. Ayyar and Alan C. Moss*

Division of Gastroenterology, Department of Medicine, Boston Medical Center, Boston, MA, United States

***Correspondence:**
Kanchana K. Ayyar
kanchana.ayyar@bmc.org

Exosomes are 30–150 nm sized vesicles released by a variety of cells, and are found in most physiological compartments (feces, blood, urine, saliva, breast milk). They can contain different cargo, including nucleic acids, proteins and lipids. In Inflammatory Bowel Disease (IBD), a distinct exosome profile can be detected in blood and fecal samples. In addition, circulating exosomes can carry targets on their surface for monoclonal antibodies used as IBD therapy. This review aims to understand the exosome profile in humans and other mammals, the cargo contained in them, the effect of exosomes on the gut, and the application of exosomes in IBD therapy.

Keywords: IBD, colitis, extracellular vesicles, exosomes, inflammation

INTRODUCTION

Exosomes are biological nanovesicles (30–150 nm) that are made by most cell types (Gross et al., 2012). They fuse with the plasma membrane of the cell and are released outside, they can be detected in almost all biological fluids (Edgar, 2016). The exosomal membrane is made of lipids and proteins (Mathivanan et al., 2010). The cargo contained within the exosomes can be proteins, nucleic acids and lipids which may or may not be similar to those of the parent cell (Valadi et al., 2007). Neighboring and/or distant cells can benefit from the cargo of circulating exosomes. They function as signaling molecules and can bring about regulation. The knowledge of their autocrine, paracrine, juxtacrine, and endocrine regulation has aroused the curiosity of many researchers. Studies indicate that exosomes play a role in extracellular matrix remodeling and signal transmission (Beshbishy et al., 2020). They also play vital roles in many disease conditions like cancer, neurodegenerative disorders, cardiovascular diseases, diabetes and others like Inflammatory Bowel Disease (IBD) by regulating immunity, inflammation, and tissue homeostasis.

Inflammatory Bowel Disease (IBD) has been widely thought to be a western disease; however, the global prevalence of IBD has been increasing since 2000. One in 200 individuals in Western countries suffers from IBD (Ng et al., 2017). Crohn's disease (CD) and ulcerative colitis (UC) are the two distinct disorders of IBD. CD and UC differ in the symptoms, complications, part of the gastrointestinal (GI) tract they affect, pathophysiology, disease course and management. UC affects the colon and is characterized by continuous lesions and superficial inflammation, which can lead to erosions, ulcers and bloody diarrhea. CD is progressive and destructive—many patients have systemic, extra intestinal manifestations, which strongly affects their quality of life due to risk of hospitalization, complications and surgery (Torres et al., 2017).

The pathogenesis of IBD is still ambiguous, the process is linked to genetic, environmental, gut microbiota and immune response factors (Ocansey et al., 2019). Some individuals with IBD have a genetic predisposition due to which there is a failure in maintaining intestinal homeostasis (Console et al., 2019). Intestinal Epithelial Cells (IECs) are constantly exposed to numerous bacteria and dietary-derived antigens. In order to defend itself, the human body needs to mount a robust immune response against invading pathogens, however if this response is prolonged it can be deleterious to the host leading to acute and chronic inflammatory disorder. Thus, the cells of the body employ intricate signaling network to control inflammation (Ayyar and Reddy, 2018). This system includes many small extra cellular components such as extra-cellular vesicles (EV), non-coding RNAs (ncRNA) like miRNA (microRNA), snRNA (small nucleolar RNA), siRNA (small interfering RNA), lncRNA (long non-coding RNA), and others (Ayyar et al., 2014). The immune system of the intestinal mucosa employs the use of such extra-cellular factors such as exosomes to maintain a balance between exhibiting tolerance toward normal microbiota and food proteins and eliciting an immune response toward enteric pathogens. Exosomes regulate cells of the immune system, gut microbes and factors maintaining the gut barrier within the IBD microenvironment. This helps repair damage and restore intestinal mucosal functions. IBD therapy is directed at improving immune regulation and easing intestinal mucosal inflammation. Exosome based therapy can help achieve these goals. In this article, we review the contents of exosomes and their effects in IBD; focusing on their effect on immune cells and gut microbiota. We also examine the potential applications of exosomes and exosomal cargo as biomarkers of IBD and in IBD therapy.

EXOSOMES

Exosomes, prostasomes, ectosomes, microvesicles, microparticles, tolerosomes, and nanovesicles are collectively referred as EVs. Currently, exosomes cannot be easily separated from other EVs (Beshbishy et al., 2020). Thus, exosomes separated from biological fluids and cell culture supernatants that are used for research are regarded as EVs, as stated in the guidelines developed by the International Society of Extracellular Vesicles (ISEV) (Théry et al., 2018). Existence of EVs was documented for the first time in 1946 (Chargaff and West, 1946). By 1977, the release of membrane fragments was considered a ubiquitous feature of viable cells. Till 1980, they were commonly considered as cellular debris (P. Wolf, 1967). The discovery of exosomes occurred in 1983. Pan and Johnstone reported that during maturation of reticulocytes in sheep, small vesicles were engaged in the release of transferrin receptors into the extracellular milieu (Pan and Johnstone, 1983). These vesicles were termed exosomes in 1989 (Johnstone et al., 1989). Subsequent studies demonstrated that exosomes originate from endosomal vesicles.

Biogenesis of Exosomes

Exosomes have a lipid bilayer membrane and are incapable of replicating. The process by which exosomes are synthesized differs from other EVs. These vesicles are forged from a novel multi-step "exosome biogenesis" pathway. The plasma membrane of the cell buds inwards to form membrane enclosed compartments called early endosomes (Pant et al., 2012). Early endosomes mature into late endosomes, these are also called multivesicular bodies (MVB). MVBs acquire intraluminal vesicles (ILVs) in their lumen. Inward budding of early endosomal membrane results in generation of ILVs. ILVs contain biologically active molecules like lipids (Subra et al., 2010), proteins (André et al., 2004) and nucleic acids (Valadi et al., 2007). These components may be selectively enriched by the endosomal sorting complexes required for transport (ESCRTs) (Tamai et al., 2010). The process may also be orchestrated by ESCRT-independent mechanisms which involve tetraspanins or lipids (Colombo et al., 2013). Depending on the molecules used, the mechanism is considered ESCRT dependent or ESCRT independent (Stuffers et al., 2009). The resultant MVBs can have two fates: survive as exosomes or perish. Fusion of MVBs with plasma membrane leads to their release in extracellular space as exosomes (Gruenberg and Goot, 2006). Alternatively, MVBs may fuse with lysosomes which leads to degradation of their content (Palmulli and Van Niel, 2018). Exosomes are released by exocytosis pathway in the course of cellular crosstalk or during receptor removal mechanisms. Growth factor receptors on the plasma membrane play a pivotal role in the exocytosis pathway (Stoorvogel et al., 2002). It is not yet fully understood as to how exosomes are released. Even though considerable progress has been made in this field, substantial gap exists in our knowledge of cargo sorting mechanisms in exosomes and other vesicular bodies.

Characterization of Exosomes

A few minimal requirements have been made mandatory by ISEV to establish the existence of exosome in a study. Experimental methods like electron microscopy, concentration monitoring techniques, and western blotting are needed to identify the presence of exosomes (Théry et al., 2018). Also, physical properties like particle size are calculated during isolation via ultracentrifugation, density gradient separation, and polymer-based precipitation methods. (Chang et al., 2020). Under TEM (Transmission Electron Microscopy), exosomes resemble cup-shaped lipoidal vesicles (Théry et al., 2009). Most exosomes bear tetraspanin proteins and this superfamily of proteins was considered to be a definitive marker of exosomes. Recent research indicates that micro-vesicles (MVs) also bear CD63, CD9, and CD81 tetraspanin proteins (Simons and Raposo, 2009). Many studies on exosomes have shown Alix and TSG101 (Tumor Susceptibility Gene 101 protein) and heat shock proteins HSC70 and HSP90 to be associated with these vesicles (Maas et al., 2017). The main difference between endosomes and MVs is that MVs are derived from outward blebbing of the plasma membrane (Agrahari et al., 2019).

Trafficking of Exosomes

The cell to cell communication by exosomes can occur via three mechanisms. The first mechanism involves receptor-ligand interaction. Signaling receptors of target cell interact directly with exosomal transmembrane proteins (Munich et al., 2012). In the second mechanism, the plasma membrane of target cell fuses with exosome, the contents of the exosome is directly delivered into the cytosol (Mulcahy et al., 2014). In the third mechanism, the exosomes get internalized by target cells. The internalized exosomes may either merge with endosomes, undergo transcytosis and be released for uptake by neighboring cells or the exosomes mature into lysosome in the target cells and are degraded (Tian et al., 2013). Some of the factors that influence internalization of exosomes have been studied. Exosomal lipid rafts and annexins are essential for exosomal internalization (Koumangoye et al., 2011). This is not to say that all factors responsible for internalization of exosomes are present only on exosomes. The proteins mediating internalization of exosomes are present on both target cells and exosomes (Escrevente et al., 2011). Apart from proteins, alteration of cholesterol content leading to disruption of lipid rafts also impairs exosomal internalization (Gonda et al., 2019). We still lack knowledge of how a mechanism is preferred over another by the exosome and/or the cell; is it condition, cell type or exosome specific?

Exosomal Cargo

Cell-to-cell communication is essential and exosomes help in facilitating this cellular crosstalk (Carrière et al., 2016). The lumen of the exosome contains the cargo-which could be lipids, proteins, nucleic acid like mRNAs, microRNAs, and other non-coding RNAs (ncRNA) (Sato-Kuwabara et al., 2015). The cargo can be same or different from that of the parent cell. Exosomes contain proteins primarily present in endosomes, plasma membrane and cytosol. They rarely enclose factors originating from the nucleus, mitochondria, endoplasmic reticulum or golgi. Also, formation and secretion of exosomes is a cost intensive process for the cell requiring enzymes and ATP (adenosine triphosphate) (J. Zhang et al., 2015). We believe there is mechanism in the cell for actively selecting exosomes and their cargos.

Proteins

Exosomal research data from different sources reveal that they share common exosomal constituents. As of 2016, 41,860 exosomal proteins, >7,540 exosomal RNA, and 1,116 exosomal lipid molecules have been cataloged from more than 286 exosome-based studies defined as per ISEV guidelines (Keerthikumar et al., 2016). Exosomes have two different kinds of protein content. The first kind depends on the cell and tissue from which it originates, while the other kind of protein constitutively occurs in exosomes and can be used as exosomal markers (Console et al., 2019). TSG101, Charged Multivesicular Body Protein 2a (CHMP2A), Ras-related protein Rab-11B (RAB11B), CD9, CD63, and CD81 are currently used as exosomal protein markers (Gross et al., 2012). Other common proteins documented in exosomes include adhesion molecules, heat shock proteins (such as HSC73, HSC90), annexins I, II, V, and VI, cytoskeletal proteins (synenin, actin, moesin, albumin) and GTPases (Samanta et al., 2018). Interestingly, some cytoskeletal proteins, glycolytic enzymes, and argonaute 1–4 (required for miRNA stability) are not detected in exosomes (Jeppesen et al., 2019).

Lipids

The current knowledge regarding the lipid content of exosomes is limited. Exosomes may contain cholesterol, sphingomyelin, ceramide, and phosphatidylserine. Cholesterol was found in the membrane of internal vesicles of MVB (Möbius et al., 2003). This is relevant as many membrane transporters are sensitive to cholesterol (Dickens et al., 2017). The structure of exosomal membrane is analogus to that of the plasma membrane; it also contains detergent resistant subdomains (Colombo et al., 2014).

Nucleic Acids

The other cargo contained within exosomes is nucleic acids (DNA, mRNA, miRNA, lncRNA, and ncRNA). The delivery of nucleic acids to cells can alter expression of genes and regulate the immune status in neighboring tissue. miRNAs can modulate immune responses by production and release of cytokines and chemokines resulting in a feedback regulation of immune homeostasis (Ayyar and Reddy, 2017). The nucleic acid content within exosomes differ. Identifying them will help us understand the role they may play in many processes. As exosomes are produced by almost all cells, they can be harvested from physiological fluids and their contents may indicate health of the tissues (healthy vs. diseased). They have the potential to be used as biomarkers: a diagnostic tool. A recent study suggests that the DNA found in small EVs are of extracellular origin that are released via an autophagy and multivesicular-endosome-dependent but exosome independent mechanism (Jeppesen et al., 2019). The source of different EV components and their functions is listed in **Table 1**.

Exosomes in Inflammatory Bowel Disease

The role of exosomes in IBD has garnered interest among researchers. Exosomal proteins, RNAs and lipids regulate factors of IBD like immune cells, gut microbiota and the mucosal barrier (Chang et al., 2020). Many studies have used exosomes from a variety of starting materials to study the process of IBD alleviation and related factors of interest. Translational studies are being conducted to tap into the possible use of exosomes as diagnostic markers and drug delivery systems, and also on the utility of modified exosomes in IBD therapy (Ocansey et al., 2020). Many of the studies cited in this review do not differentiate between the different types of EVs like exosomes, endosomes and MVBs, hence for the sake of convenience we have used the general term EVs while describing study findings.

Exosomal Profile in Intestinal Mucosa

Epithelial cells, Paneth cells, macrophages, and lymphocytes are cells in the intestinal tract that are directly exposed to digested food, microbes, and foreign antigens making immune homeostasis a challenging and complex process (Peterson and Artis, 2014). While maintaining immune homeostasis, the intestinal barrier strikes a perfect balance by clearing pathogenic bacteria and maintaining immune tolerance with the commensals. Evidence indicates that dysregulation of intestinal homeostasis leads to IBD pathogenesis. Intestinal homeostasis depends on effective crosstalk between extracellular factors, EVs and the host's intestinal immune defense (comprised of the mucus membrane, intestinal epithelial cells (IECs) and the immune cells) (Avila-Calderón et al., 2015). EVs act not only as communicator between cells but also between cells and organisms (Chang et al., 2020). This is important as the mammalian intestine encounters 10 trillion (10^{13}) microbes (10X the number of total cells in a mammalian body) (Sartor, 2008). EVs from micro-organisms and the host body communicate and help maintain a peaceful coexistence, maintaining intestinal immune homeostasis which is a major determinant of health (Sommer et al., 2017). Physiological fluids also contain EVs which affect the intestinal microbiota.

Exosomes From Intestinal Epithelial Cells

IECs play a major role in immune modulation in the gut that even though they are not professional antigen presenting cells (APC), they bear major histocompatibility complex (MHC) I, II, and HLA-DM (Lin et al., 2005). The knowledge of IEC releasing EVs has been known for a while now (Van Niel et al., 2001). IEC EVs like parent cells, contain immunomodulatory molecules. They also express MHC I and II, expression of which is elevated during inflammation as compared to basal

TABLE 1 | Source and function of different extracellular vesicle components in IBD.

Exosomal component	Source	Role	References
A33 antigen	Intestinal epithelial cells	Cell-cell recognition and signaling	Van Niel et al. (2001)
Annexin A1	Intestinal epithelial cells	Promotes wound healing	Leoni et al. (2015)
CCL20 and prostaglandin E2	Intestinal epithelial cells	Recruit Th17 cells through MyD88 mediated pathway	Deng et al. (2015)
CD63 and EpCAM	Intestinal epithelial cells	Induces DC apoptosis Suppresses DC maturation inhibits antigen presentation by DCs in rats	Kojima et al. (2018)
GELNs lipids	Grapes	Induces Lgr5+ stem cells Enhances *in vivo* targeting of intestinal stem cells Remodels and protects intestinal tissue against DSS-induced colitis	Ju et al. (2013)
Integrin αvβ6	Intestinal epithelial cells	Promotes production of active TGF-β in DCs and Tregs	Chen et al. (2011)
Metallothionein-2	Bone marrow-derived MSCs	Maintenance of intestinal barrier integrity Polarization of M2b macrophages Induction of IL-10 from macrophages	(Liu et al. (2019)
MHC I and II	Intestinal epithelial cells	Initiating immune response	Van Niel et al. (2001)
miR-223	Mice colonic epithelial cells	Modulates communication between IL-23 signal pathway and claudin-8 in IBD development Modulates intestinal barrier integrity	Wang et al. (2016)
miR-23a and miR-155	Neutrophils	Induces replication fork collapse Inhibits homologous recombination Induces accumulation of double strand breaks	Butin-Israeli et al. (2019)
miR-34c and PlncRNA1	Intestinal epithelial cell line Caco-2	Modulates ZO-1, MAZ, and occludin expression Modulates intestinal barrier integrity	Chen et al. (2017)
miR-4334, miR-219 and miR-338	Porcine milk	Prevents LPS-induced intestinal inflammation, apoptosis and damage via inhibiting TLR4/NF-κB and p53 pathways	Xie et al. (2019)
Mdo-miR7267–3p	Ginger	Shapes gut microbiota Improves barrier function Ameliorates colitis via IL-22-dependent mechanisms	Teng et al. (2019)
Myeloperoxidase (MPO)	Intestinal epithelial cells	Contributes to oxidative stress against microbes	Zhang et al. (2018)
Myeloperoxidase (MPO)	Neutrophils	Damages intestinal barrier by production of oxidative radicals, inhibiting wound closure and healing	Slater et al. (2017)
NEAT1	Mouse intestinal mucosa and serum	Down-regulation of NEAT1 Suppresses inflammatory response by modulating intestinal epithelial barrier and via exosome-mediated polarization of macrophages in IBD	Liu et al. (2018)
PSMA7	Oral mucosal cells	Responsible for degradation of proteins Controls autoimmune disorders and immune tolerance	Zheng et al. (2017)
Sphingosine-1-phosphate	Intestinal epithelial cells	Promotes tumorigenesis	(Patmanathan et al. (2017)
Tetraspanin 14–3-3 protein, enolase and heat shock proteins	Hookworm	Protection against colitis by significantly suppressing IFNγ, IL-6,IL-1β, and IL-17a and upregulating anti-inflammatory cytokine IL-10	(Eichenberger et al. (2018)
TGF-β	Intestinal epithelial cells	Inhibit $CD4^+$ T cell proliferation	Jiang et al. (2016)

condition (Van Niel et al., 2001). EVs released from these cells can be released apically or basolaterally. They carry A33 antigen, whose expression is confined to the intestinal epithelium (Van Niel et al., 2001). A33 is now considered a marker for IEC exosomes (Van Niel et al., 2003; Lin et al., 2005; Mallegol et al., 2007).

IEC EVs are known to interact with Dendritic cells (DC) (Mallegol et al., 2007). They stimulate DC, Treg and macrophage maturation with tolerogenic properties through immunoregulatory signals (Jeffrey et al., 2018). Also, tolerogenic DCs are essential for maintaining intestinal homeostasis (Peterson and Artis, 2014). The cytokine, TGF-β is produced in tolerogenic DCs and Tregs in its latent form as LTGF-β. IEC EVs carrying integrin αvβ6 are internalized by intestinal tolerogenic DCs, wherein they help activate TGF-β, induce Treg cells and initiate tolerogenic responses in the gut (Chen et al., 2011). $CD4^+$ T cell proliferation is inhibited by TGF-β containing IEC EVs (Jiang et al., 2016). IEC EVs have a wide spectrum immuno modulatory effect. EVs expressing CD63 and EpCAM (Epithelial cell adhesion molecule) suppress DC maturation and inhibit antigen presentation by DCs and also induce DC apoptosis in post-trauma immune dysfunction in rats (Kojima et al., 2018). EpCAM plays a unique role in immuno-modulation by facilitating a physical interaction between intraepithelial lymphocytes and IECs (Jiang et al., 2016). Annexin 1 (ANXA1) is crucial for maintaining the intestinal barrier during inflammatory response; it is found in exosomes released from IECs (Leoni et al., 2015). These ANXA 1 containing EVs help in resolving inflammation in murine colitis, their number increases during wound healing (Leoni et al., 2013; Perretti and D'Acquisto, 2009). These EVs bind to formyl peptide receptors (FPRs) and may be employed to activate wound repair in epithelial cells (Leoni et al., 2015). In IBD patients, mucosal-luminal interface EVs express MPO (myeloperoxidase). MPO is a defense protein which creates oxidative stress against microbes in the intestines (X. Zhang et al., 2018). At the same time, intestinal fluid EVs from IBD patients have a pro-inflammatory effect on IECs *in-vitro* (Mitsuhashi et al., 2017).

This disparity can be attributed to the source of EVs. EVs secreted by *Bacteroides fragilis* induce secretion of host mucosal EVs containing sphingosine-1-phosphate, CCL20, and prostaglandin E2 (Deng et al., 2015). Th17 cells are sequestered by Prostaglandin E2 and CCL20 via MyD88-mediated pathway (Deng et al., 2015), while sphingosine-1-phosphate plays a role in tumorigenesis (Kunkel et al., 2013; Hait and Maiti, 2017; Patmanathan et al., 2017). Conversely, it is possible that CCL20 and other pro-inflammatory cytokines are inhibited by EVs derived from healthy intestinal mucosa (Deng et al., 2015). **Figure 1** summarizes exosomal effects of IEC derived exosomes on intestinal barrier functions and immunity.

Exosomes From Immune Cells

The mucosal barrier maintains immune homeostasis in the gut by spatially separating the gut microbiota from the host immune system. In IBD, there is dysfunction of the barrier, immune dysregulation and dysbiosis. Both the innate and the adaptive immune system signals lead to IBD pathogenesis. The innate immune response is quicker; it involves phagocytosis, antigen presentation and provides stimulus for initiation of the adaptive immune response. The process involves macrophages, DCs, neutrophils, and monocytes (Ayyar et al., 2014). Many APCs have been reported to secrete exosomes, these exosomes may also bear MHC molecules (Morelli et al., 2004).

DCs are professional APCs of the immune system and can initiate an immune response upon sensing antigens. Based on the stage and maturation of parent DCs, DC derived exosomes may have immune stimulatory/suppressive effects (Lindenbergh and Stoorvogel, 2018; H.; Zhang et al., 2019). EVs from DCs can inhibit T-cell proliferation, this could play a key role in modulating inflammation in IBD (Kim et al., 2007; Tkach et al., 2017). Mature DC-derived exosomes that contain tumor antigens potentially could induce anti-tumor immunity in *in-vitro* trials, while immature exosomes could induce peripheral tolerance by T-cell immunosuppression (Yang et al., 2010). TGF-β1-modified bone marrow derived DCs (BMDC) produce exosomes that induce $CD4^{+}Foxp3^{+}$Tregs and attenuate Th17 population in lymphocytes from mesenteric lymph nodes of inflammatory site in DSS induced mice (Cai et al., 2012). Similarly, IL-10 treated DC exosomes inhibit 2,4,6-trinitrobenzenesulfonic acid (TNBS) induced colitis in rats by stimulating $CD4^{+}CD25^{+}$Tregs (Yang et al., 2010). In a similar study, EVs from *Schistosoma japonicum*-soluble antigen-treated DCs provided protection during acute IBD development (Tkach et al., 2017; L. Wang et al., 2017). Immune tolerance can be achieved through regulation of activated T cells, by harnessing the immunosuppressive activity of exosomes. APC derived exosomes can activate $CD4^{+}$ and/or $CD8^{+}$ T lymphocytes, their antigen presentation capacity relies on DC, indicating that APCs take up DC derived exosomes to promote T cell activation. Exosomes may quickly transfer immune information via APCs (Van Niel et al., 2003).

IBD progression is affected in myriad ways by other immune cell derived EVs. Neutrophil infiltration occurs in IBD and is accompanied by liberating MPO into the extracellular space. MPO results in production of oxidative radicals which damage the gut barrier. It was found that MPO was delivered to IEC via EVs and inflammatory response was enhanced, inhibiting wound closure and healing (Slater et al., 2017). EVs also contain miRNAs as cargo; miRNAs are excellent regulators of immune response (Ayyar et al., 2014). EVs containing proinflammatory miRNAs can promote doublestrand breaks (DSBs) in affected colonic epithelia (Butin-Israeli et al., 2019). Neutrophil derived EVs can contain miR-23a and miR-155. These EVs promote lamin B1- dependent replication fork collapse and also suppress homologous recombination (HR) by repressing RAD51 (Bui and Sumagin, 2019; Butin-Israeli et al., 2019). During transepithelial migration of granulocytes, granulocyte EVs accumulate on IECs. This promotes the recruitment of granulocytes accompanied by a loss of epithelial cadherins (Butin-Israeli et al., 2016). On the other hand, granulocytic myeloid-derived suppressor cells-derived EVs diminish number of Th1 cells and a resultant surge is observed in Treg population in colitis induced mice (Y. Wang et al., 2016). WNT signaling is essential for intestinal epithelium and homeostasis (Kuhnert et al., 2004; Gregorieff et al., 2005). Intestinal stem cells can be rescued by macrophage-derived EVs. They can also improve enterocyte survival post radiation via modulation of WNT signaling pathway (Saha et al., 2016). **Figure 2** shows the general modulatory features of immune-cell-derived exosomes on the immune system.

Exosomal Profile in Animals

Many studies have been conducted in rats and mice to study the effects exosomes in IBD. A radical difference was observed in the proportion of gut-bacteria derived EVs in feces of DSS (dextran sulfate sodium) induced colitis mice in comparison with those from healthy mice (Kang et al., 2013). The fecal EVs can be IEC-derived, microbiome-derived or may come from the diet. When healthy exosomes from mice were transferred to IBD-induced mice, it was observed that the disease severity markedly reduced in recipient mice (Jiang et al., 2016). This shows that exosomes have therapeutic potential. Another study showed that the protein load of exosomes in healthy and acute-colitis induced mice was different. A total of 56 acute phase proteins and immunoglobulins were found to be differentially expressed between the two groups (Wong et al., 2016). *Lactobacillus* and Bifidobacterium are known probiotics which are administered to IBD patients. DCs and EV isolated from TLR2 (toll-like-receptor 2) knockout mice and healthy mice were co-cultured with these bacteria. It was observed that TLR2/6 activity in DCs was reduced significantly (van Bergenhenegouwen et al., 2014). The effect was reversed upon EV depletion suggesting an immunosuppressive role of these EVs. Fecal OMVs (outer membrane vesicles) from colitis induced rats (DSS) reduced the expression of enzyme UDP-glucuronosyltransferase 1A1 (UGT1A1) in human Caco-2 cells while OMVs from healthy rats upregulated the enzyme expression (X. J. Gao et al., 2018). UGT1A1 helps in maintaining the Intestinal epithelial barrier. This study shows that rat OMVs can modulate mucosal immunity. EVs isolated from mesenteric lymph modulated the immune response through DC suppression in post-trauma immune dysfunction in rats (Kojima et al., 2018). When exosomes are introduced in naïve rats from IBD induced rats, antigen specific tolerance is detected; these exosomes were briefly called tolerosomes (Karlsson et al., 2001).

Exosomal Profile in Blood

Diseases like Cancer, inflammatory diseases and infections result in change in exosome composition of patients as compared to

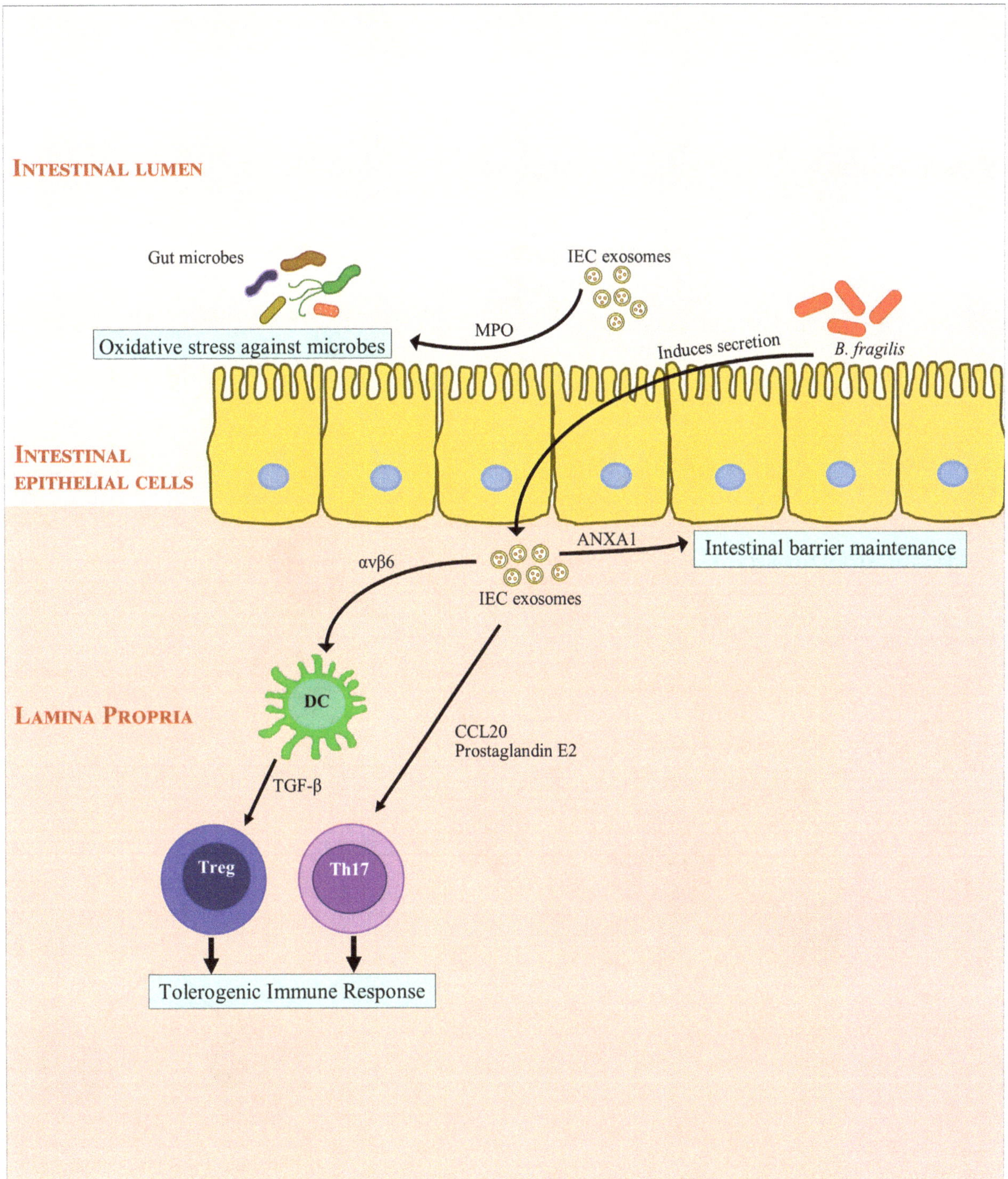

FIGURE 1 | Modulation of intestinal inflammation by intestinal epithelial cell derived exosomes. Intestinal epithelial cell derived exosomes help maintain gut immune homeostasis through secretion of Annexin A1. They induce a tolerogenic immune response by secretion of integrin, cytokines and chemokines. They also protect the gut immune barrier from bacterial invasion by secreting myeloperoxidase which creates oxidative stress against bacteria. ANXA1, Annexin A1; αvβ6, Integrin αvβ6; *B. fragilis*, *Bacteroides fragilis*; CCL20, C-C Motif Chemokine Ligand 20; DC, dendritic cell; IEC, Intestinal epithelial cells; MPO: myeloperoxidase; Th17, TGF-β, transforming growth factor β; T helper 17; Treg, regulatory T cell.

healthy controls. These changes can be observed in biological fluids like blood and blood components, saliva, stool, urine. These fluids represent an excellent tool for identification of biomarkers (Barile and Vassalli, 2017). Unfortunately, there are not many reports of EVs or exosomes in blood/serum. In 2015, Leoni et al. looked at serum exosome levels in IBD patients. They found that

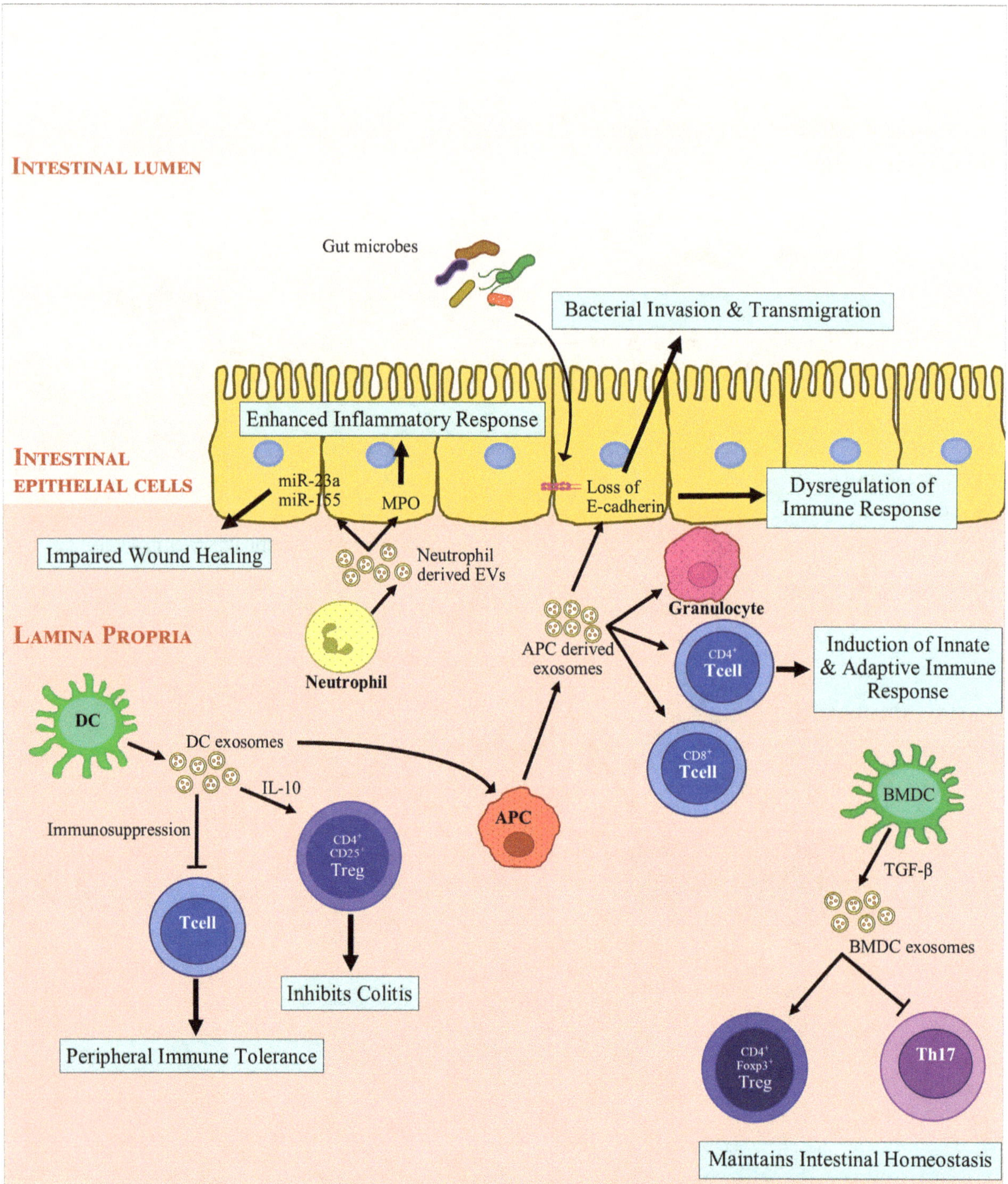

FIGURE 2 | Modulation of intestinal inflammation by immune cell derived extracellular vesicles. Exosomes derived from immune cells promote anti-inflammatory responses by inducing immune tolerance and triggering regulatory T cells (Treg) activation while inhibiting T helper cells. Exosome-treated immune cells further express exosomes that encourage anti-inflammatory responses. Mature APC derived exosomes promote loss of E-cadherin, which leads to breach of barrier integrity and facilitates bacterial invasion and transmigration. These exosomes also recruit immune cells and drive a pro-inflammatory immune response. Neutrophil derived exosomes secrete myeloperoxidase and miRNAs which are taken up by intestinal epithelial cells. miR-23a and miR-155 can introduce double strand breaks and impair wound healing in degenerated colonic epithelium. In summary, depending on the parent cells, exosomes derived from immune cells can drive toward a pro-inflammatory or an anti-inflammatory response. APC, antigen presenting cell; BMDC, Bone marrow derived dendritic cell; CD, cluster of differentiation; DC, dendritic cell; EV, extracellular vesicles; FOXP3, Forkhead box protein 3; IL-10, Interleukin 10; miR, microRNA; MPO: myeloperoxidase; TGF-β, transforming growth factor β; Th17, T helper 17; Treg, regulatory T cell.

exosomes released from IECs, entered circulation and expressed ANXA 1, which is crucial for maintaining the intestinal barrier during inflammatory response. Serum of IBD patients contain good number of such vesicles (Leoni et al., 2015). Additional research on the serum exosomal content in IBD patients will help better our understanding.

Role of Dietary EVs in Inflammatory Bowel Disease

The source of exosome existing in human body could be produced by human cells such as immune cells, IECs, tumor cells or by plant cells which are introduced through dietary food. As almost all biological cells produce exosomes; many of the edible foods that we consume contain exosomes.

Plant Derived Exosomes

Some studies have been conducted on exosomes derived from edible plants. *Curcuma longa* and grapes contain exosomes that helps in alleviating IBD. *Curcuma longa* is a medical herb, the exosomes derived from this plant may inactivate NF-κB to alleviate colitis and improve intestinal wound repair (H. Zhang et al., 2019). Exosome-like nanoparticles (ELN) from grape juice play a protective role in DSS-induced colitis mice when administered via the oral route (Ju et al., 2013). ELNs from ginger rhizome strongly inhibit NLRP3 (nucleotide-binding domain and leucine-rich repeat-containing family, pyrin domain-containing 3) inflammasome activation. Events occurring downstream of inflammasome activation like secretion of cytokines IL-1β and IL-18, auto cleavage of caspase-1 and pyroptotic cell death can also be impeded by these ELNs (Chen et al., 2019). Broccoli derived ELNs inhibit induced colitis in mice. These ELNs help in the activation of AMPK (AMP [adenosine monophosphate]-activated protein kinase) in DCs, which promotes DC tolerance and prevents DC activation, leading to inhibition of DSS induced colitis in mice (Deng et al., 2017).

Milk Derived Exosomes

Breast milk not only provides nutrition but also helps shape the neonate gut immune system (Turfkruyer and Verhasselt, 2015). Breast milk has immunoglobulin which help in responding precisely to encountered antigens (Walker and Iyengar, 2015; Doare et al., 2018). Recent studies have shown EVs contained in milk can affect intestinal homeostasis (Admyre et al., 2007). Bioactive milk exosomes are known to carry miRNAs, mRNAs, lncRNAs, TGF-β and a variety of other proteins and lipids (Reinhardt et al., 2012; Reinhardt et al., 2013; Pieters et al., 2015; Tomé-Carneiro et al., 2018). Exosomes are resistant to the harsh conditions in the gastrointestinal tract (Benmoussa et al., 2016; Liao et al., 2017; Kahn et al., 2018) but are actively captured by intestinal epithelial cells (T. Wolf et al., 2015). It has been observed that a considerable portion of milk exosomes (from consumed milk) enter circulation in rodents and humans (Baier et al., 2014; Manca et al., 2018; Betker et al., 2019). The fate of unabsorbed exosomes is not yet known. There is strong evidence that milk exosomes are crucial for maturation and intestinal function (Gao H. N. et al., 2019; Gao R. et al., 2019; Hock et al., 2017; Li et al., 2019; Miyake et al., 2020; Reif et al., 2019; Xie et al., 2020). Strong evidence indicates that human, porcine and bovine milk exosomes aid intestinal cell growth in mice (Gao H. N. et al., 2019; Hock et al., 2017; Reif et al., 2019). Milk exosomes can also attenuate LPS-induced apoptosis (Xie et al., 2019), and prevent intestinal endothelial cell damage (R. Gao et al., 2019b; Miyake et al., 2020). They also enhance goblet cell numbers and mucin production (Li et al., 2019). They can also modify bacterial growth, and promote intestinal microbiota (Doare et al., 2018; Zhou et al., 2019). Interestingly, pasteurized fresh milk contains more bioactive milk exosomes as compared to fermented milk products like yoghurt (Yu et al., 2017). **Figure 3** describes the role of microbiome derived OMVs and dietary exosomes in modulating intestinal inflammation.

Role of Microbiota Derived Outer Membrane Vesicles in Inflammatory Bowel Disease

All biological life forms are capable of producing EVs. These include micro-organisms encountered in the intestinal tract like protozoa, archaea, bacteria and fungi (Brown et al., 2015). It has been reported that commensal microbes can modulate IECs and immune cells in the intestine by affecting maturation and other related functions. As alterations in intestinal microbiota affect the pathogenesis and development of IBD, the EVs secreted by the commensal microbes may help maintain gut immune homeostasis (Geveres et al., 2014). The involvement of extracellular factors from microbes in modulating immune response has been observed as early as 1967 (S. Chatterjee and Das, 1967). In 1967, Chatterjee and Das showed that the bacteria, *Neisseria meningitides* secreted endotoxins as cell wall blebs *in-vivo* (S. Chatterjee and Das, 1967). However, the mechanism has not yet been understood thoroughly.

Pathogenic bacteria exist in the intestines and their EVs can negatively influence gut homeostasis. They breach the intestinal barrier and facilitate mucosal invasion leading to IBD pathogenesis. *Helicobacter pylori* infection in the gut leads to gastritis, ulceration and malignancy. In 2003, a study found that it was not necessary for the bacterium to associate with the epithelial cell to cause disease, the OMVs released by the bacteria could interact with the host epithelial cell and bring about an adverse reaction (Ismail et al., 2003). Enterohemorrhagic *Escherichia coli* (EHEC) O157 EVs promote IL-8 secretion in IECs through TLR5 and TLR4/MD-2 pathway (Bielaszewska et al., 2018). They also induce apoptosis by delivering hemolysin from EHEC to endothelial cells and mitochondria (Bielaszewska et al., 2013). UGT1A1 is an important part of intestinal epithelial barrier. Fecal OMVs isolated from colitis induced rats (DSS) reduced the expression of UGT1A1 in human Caco-2 cells while, OMVs from healthy rats upregulated UGT1A1 (X. J. Gao et al., 2018). This shows that gut microbiota can regulate intestinal UGT1A1 expression. *Vibrio cholera* secretes two proteases, hemagglutinin protease (HAP) and calcium-dependent trypsin-like serine protease (VesC) in association with OMVs, these are transported to human IECs in an active form. Studies show that HAP induces apoptosis and VesC induces necrosis and increases IL-8 secretion in host cells. Data also suggests that VesC promotes intestinal colonization of *V. cholerae* in mice (Mondal et al., 2016).

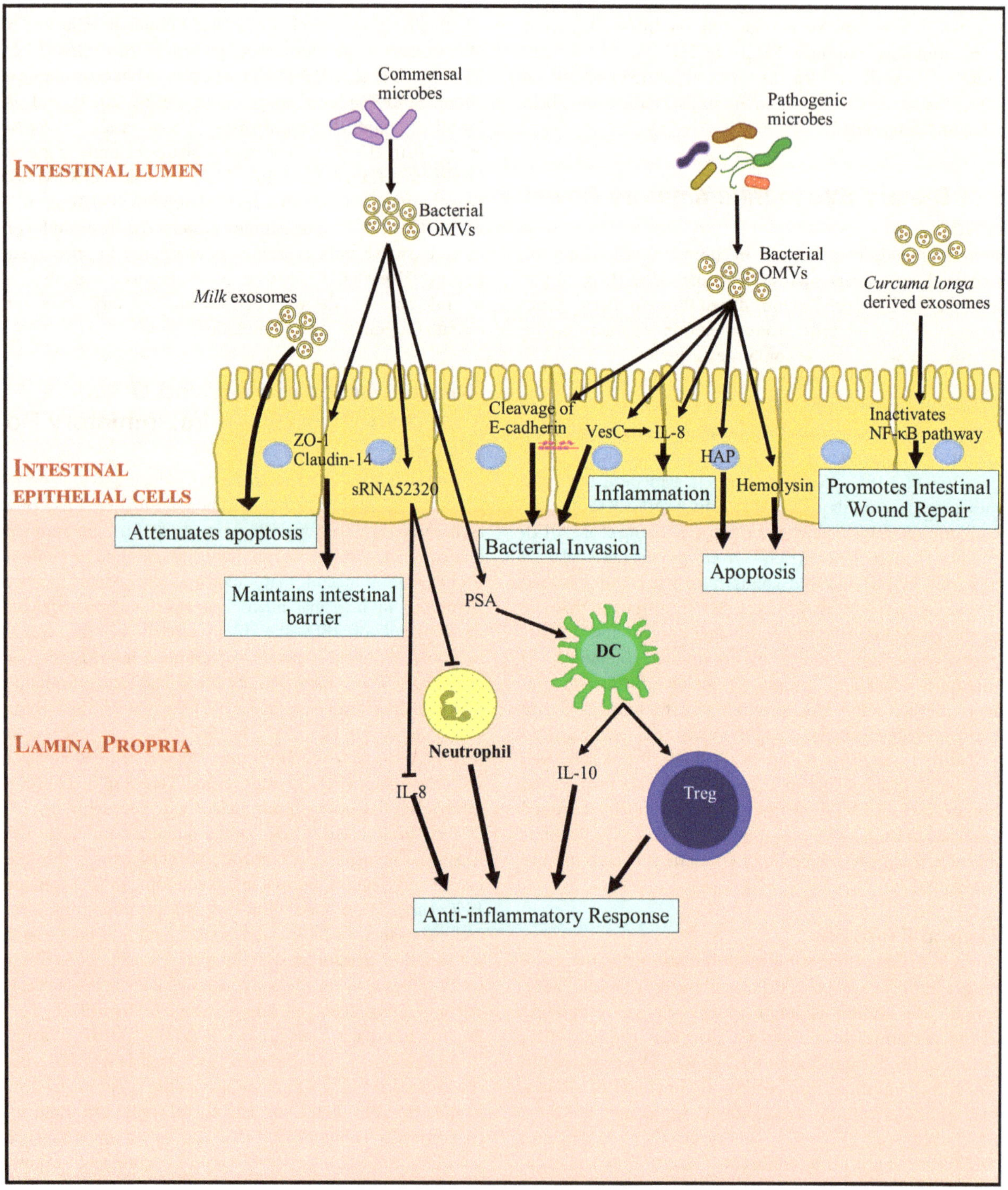

FIGURE 3 | Modulation of intestinal inflammation by microbiome derived outer membrane vesicles and dietary exosomes. Exosomes and OMVs (outer membrane vesicles) through their functional components, directly or indirectly interact with gut intestinal epithelial cells (IECs). Dietary exosomes attenuate apoptosis and promote intestinal wound repair. OMVs from commensal bacteria induce the proliferation of IECs and development of the intestinal tract, and indirectly enhance barrier functions by inhibiting components of the inflammatory environment that negatively impact tight junction molecules and IECs. They also interact with immune cells and promote an anti-inflammatory immune response. On the other hand, pathogenic bacteria, though their OMVs can induce inflammation and apoptosis. They can also cause a breach in the epithelial barrier by cleaving E-cadherin. This facilitates bacterial invasion and transmigration into the intestinal tissue. DC, dendritic cell; HAP, hemagglutinin protease; IL, Interleukin; NF-κB, nuclear factor kappa light chain enhancer of activated B cells; OMV, outer membrane vesicle, PSA: capsular polysaccharide; sRNA52320, shortRNA 52320; Treg, regulatory T cell; VesC, calcium-dependent trypsin-like serine protease; ZO-1, Zonula occludens 1.

Also, IECs take up these EVs and stimulate the MAPK and NF-κB pathways in a nucleotide-binding oligomerization domain-containing 1 (NOD1)-dependent manner. This causes a change in the expression of IL-8, GM-CSF, CCL2, CCL20, and thymic stromal lymphopoietin (D. Chatterjee and Chaudhuri, 2013). Epithelial cadherin is essential for maintaining epithelial integrity, EVs from *Campylobacter jejuni* cleaved epithelial cadherin and facilitated the infiltration of pathogenic bacteria into IECs (Elmi et al., 2016; Boehm et al., 2018). Evidence suggests that immune responses mounted against commensal like *Bacteroides thetaiotaomicron* could trigger colitis in genetically vulnerable hosts (Hickey et al., 2015).

Microbiome derived EVs present in the host can also help maintain gut immune homeostasis. The innate immune defense of the gut relies heavily on the integrity of the epithelial layer which acts as a barrier. Apart from IECs that reinforce this barrier, probiotic bacteria can also influence barrier integrity by regulating the pro-inflammatory signals, reinforcing tight junctions between IECs and by facilitating cross-talk between commensals, gut epithelia and the mucosal immunity. *Escherichia coli* C25, is a commensal organism present in the human gut, the OMVs released by this bacterium elicits a moderate pro-inflammatory response via secretion of IL-8 *in vitro* (Patten et al., 2017). This response is beneficial to the host as healthy human intestine has a low-level inflammatory environment. OMVs from *E. coli* C25 have also shown to regulate the translocation of parent bacteria across the intestinal epithelium. This aids in maintaining a favorable symbiotic relationship with the host (Patten et al., 2017). Another probiotic bacteria, *E. coli* Nissle 1917 (EcN) helps in maintaining tight junctions by secreting OMVs and soluble factors which induce ZO-1 and claudin-14 expression, and inhibit claudin-2 expression (Alvarez et al., 2016). The pro-inflammatory effect of *E. coli* OMVs can be ameliorated by *Akkermansia muciniphila* EVs. Also, *A. muciniphila* EVs are depleted in colitis induced mice as compared to healthy mice, indicating that they play a protective role in IBD. Indeed, IBD indicators like loss of body weight, length of colon, infiltration of colon wall are maintained when *A. muciniphila* EVs are delivered orally (Kang et al., 2013). *B. fragilis* OMVs containing PSA (capsular polysaccharide) can protect against inflammation in TNBS colitis mice model. This is achieved by production of anti-inflammatory cytokines by DCs, enhancing the Treg response (Shen et al., 2012). *Pseudomonas aeruginosa* releases EVs which contains shortRNAs (sRNA), this sRNA was shown to reduce IL-8 secretion from LPS (lipopolysaccharide) induced IECs. This sRNA termed as sRNA52320 can also attenuate cytokine secretion and neutrophil infiltration (Koeppen et al., 2016). *B. thetaiotaomicron* produces a phosphatase, BTMinpp which is packaged inside OMVs, thus protecting its catalytic activity. This enzyme promotes intracellular Ca^{2+} signaling in IECs and thereby the physiological responses of the digestive system are sustained (Stentz et al., 2014). Additionally, *E. coli* OMVs (probiotic and commensal strains) induce more anti-inflammatory cytokines in explanted colonic tissue, although a modest expression of proinflammatory cytokines, such as IL-6 and IL-8 is also observed (Fábrega et al., 2016).

The host can also combat EVs from pathogenic microbes. OMVs secreted from bacteria contain cargo and this cargo is recognized by pattern recognition receptors (PRR) of the host immune system which mount an inflammatory response. The OMV released from *E. coli* contains peptidoglycan which is recognized by NOD1 receptor. This triggers the NOD1 signaling cascade, inducing the expression of pro-inflammatory molecules like NF-κB, IL-6, and IL-8 (Cañas et al., 2018). However, the OMVs may escape immune surveillance and enter IECs via clathrin-dependent endocytosis resulting in host cell DNA damage (Cañas et al., 2016). It's not just the EVs from bacteria that regulate host cells but EVs present in the host's physiological fluid can also interact with bacteria and promote bacterial aggregation (van Bergenhenegouwen et al., 2014). Pathogenic bacteria and commensals derived EVs regulate inter-species communication in the gut which leads to immunoregulation of signaling pathways. The source and functions of different OMV components and their function in IBD is listed in **Table 2**.

EXOSOMAL COMPONENTS AS BIOMARKERS FOR INFLAMMATORY BOWEL DISEASE

Micro-environmental changes take place at the site of intestinal mucosal inflammation: nutrient shortage, dysregulated oxygen supply in tissue and production of reactive nitrogen and oxygen

TABLE 2 | Source and function of different bacterial outer membrane vesicle components in IBD.

Component	Source	Role	References
BTMinpp	*Bacteroides thetaiotaomicron*	Promotes intracellular CA^{++} signaling in IECs	Stentz et al. (2014)
Calcium-dependent trypsin-like serine protease (VesC)	*Vibrio cholera*	Plays a role in intestinal colonization of bacteria Induces necrosis Increase IL-8 secretion in host cells	Mondal et al. (2016)
Capsular polysaccharide (PSA)	*Bacteroides fragilis*	Induces anti-inflammatory cytokine production in DCs Enhances Treg response	Shen et al. (2012)
Hemagglutinin protease (HAP)	*Vibrio cholera*	Induces apoptosis in intestinal epithelial cells	Mondal et al. (2016)
Hemolysin	Enterohemorrhagic *E.coli*	Apoptosis of endothelial cells	Bielaszewska et al. (2013)
Peptidoglycan	*Escherichia coli*	Triggers NOD1 signaling cascade Induces expression of IL-6, IL-8 and NF-κB	Cañas et al. (2018)
sRNA52320	*Pseudomonas aeruginosa*	Reduces IL-8 secretion from LPS induced IECs Attenuates neutrophil infiltration	Koeppen et al. (2016)

species. Mucosal barrier, cell fate, immune regulation, and gut microbiota are affected by the consequent oxidative and hypoxia derived stress (Taylor and Colgan, 2007; Cao, 2018). An inflammatory cascade is triggered within this microenvironment through intricate crosstalk between different cell types (Marafini et al., 2019). Inflammatory cells such as granulocytes, macrophages and monocytes, and also cells of the adaptive immune system like B and T cells are sequestered within the site of active inflammation, by cytokines like IL-8 (Marafini et al., 2019). When the intestinal barrier is intact, it is very difficult for luminal antigens to approach the lamina propria. When immune cells are within the lamina propria, a tolerance system is set in place which limits induction of an immune response. On the other hand, when barrier integrity is compromised, antigens trespass the barrier and the tolerance system is invalidated. This culminates in secretion of chemokines, recruitment and infiltration of immune cells, further aggravating inflammation (Neurath, 2019). The current diagnosis of IBD involves invasive procedures like endoscopy and colonoscopy. They are also expensive, time-consuming and inconvenient for the patients. There is a need to develop a less-invasive, faster, reliable detection method for IBD.

The origin of exosomes present in the intestinal tract can be host cells, diet or microbial organisms (Chang et al., 2020). The EV content in bile samples of individuals suffering from malignant common bile stenosis was significantly higher than those seen in the bile samples of healthy controls, suggesting that the nature of EVs differs with respect to health condition of the body (Severino et al., 2017). ANXA1 is crucial for maintaining the intestinal barrier during inflammatory response; it is found in exosomes released from intestinal epithelial cells (IEC). Serum of IBD patients contain good number of such vesicles, making it a promising biomarker for intestinal inflammation (Leoni et al., 2015). Proteasome Subunit Alpha type 7 (PSMA7) is found in oral exosomes secreted by the oral mucosal cells of IBD patients. The expression of PSMA7 isolated from saliva in IBD patients is remarkably different than those in healthy controls and is a good biomarker candidate (Zheng et al., 2017). More exosomal characterization studies on biological fluids from IBD patients would help in identifying novel biomarkers that could help in early diagnosis of IBD.

EFFECT OF EXOSOMES ON CURRENT INFLAMMATORY BOWEL DISEASE TREATMENT

IBD treatment involves anti-inflammatory drugs, immune system suppressors, and biologics supplemented with antibiotics and dietary supplements. Biologics are the newest category of drugs in IBD treatment. Most of them are monoclonal antibodies which neutralize inflammation causing proteins in the body. The most common form of biologics administered to IBD patients are TNF blocking agents e.g.,: Infliximab, Adalimumab, Golimumab, and Certolizumab. Other biologics used in IBD treatment are Vedolizumab, which is a $\alpha_4\beta_7$ blocker and Ustekinumab, which blocks the IL12-IL23 pathway.

A recent study detected $\alpha_4\beta_7$ integrin expression on the surface of circulating exosomes from serum of IBD patients being treated with Vedolizumab (VDZ) (Domenis et al., 2020). These $\alpha_4\beta_7$ expressing exosomes were able to bind to VDZ competitively *in-vitro*. In IBD treatment, VDZ acts by binding to the $\alpha_4\beta_7$ integrin found on a subset of T cells and prevents their trafficking into the gut. This data suggests that exosomes could be involved in mediating VDZ resistance in IBD patients by sequestration of therapeutic molecules into vesicles. Most IBD patients on treatment with a biologic drug respond poorly to a second biologic drug (Gisbert ad Chaparro, 2020). The study by Domenis et al. (2020) reports that the serum exosomal concentration and vesicle surface expression of $\alpha_4\beta_7$ integrin was greater in the serum of patients on TNF blocking drugs compared to TNF naïve patients. The resultant exosomal sequestration of VDZ also increased in patients on TNF blocking drugs suggesting that previous treatment with a biologic drug alters the expression of α4β7 integrin and binding capacity of circulating exosomes. This potentially explains the reduced efficacy of VDZ in IBD patients who were previously treated with TNF blocking agents.

To date this is the only study correlating the effect of exosomes on IBD treatment modalities. Further studies in this direction would help design better treatment strategies that could increase drug bioavailability.

ROLE OF EXOSOMES IN INFLAMMATORY BOWEL DISEASE THERAPY

Exosomes are natural carriers of functional RNAs, proteins and have the characteristics to be employed for transporting drugs or biologicals. They can also be employed for tissue repair and regeneration. Modification of exosomes either biologically or chemically will boost their therapeutic potential (Ocansey et al., 2020). IBD is characterized by disruption of the immune system and abnormal stimulation of immune cells. As mentioned in this review, DC derived EVs through immune excitation or repression mitigate IBD progression. Hence, it is plausible that immune cells derived EVs may be the new therapeutic intervention for IBD.

The interest in EV research also propels the exploration of artificial nanoparticles as tool for disease treatment. Studies have looked at EV-like nanoparticles as treatment for IBD. Bioadhesive chitosan has been developed, which can be delivered by oral route to accumulate in a safe and specific way to affected areas in the GI tract (Han et al., 2019). Intestinal organoids containing 5-ASA-loaded nanoparticles have been used to relieve IBD (Davoudi et al., 2018). Mannosylated bioreducible cationic polymers have been used to synthesize RNAi (RNA interference) nanoparticles to lower cell-death and improve treatment efficacy in IBD (Xiao et al., 2013). EVs are bio-compatible and stable than artificial nanoparticles as they are innate in nature, being derived from cells and microbes. EVs can also be engineered, enhancing their role in treatment and therapy in IBD (Hood and Wickline, 2012; Hood, 2016). Promising results have been observed with Rifaximin loaded EVs (Kumar and Newton, 2017; García-

Manrique et al., 2018). These studies demonstrate that EVs have a potential use in drug delivery.

Breast milk is known to have immunoglobulins, approximately 15 years ago it was discovered that it contains immune-modulatory EVs (Admyre et al., 2007). Since then milk EVs have received considerable attention and a lot of studies have been conducted to understand the process of drug delivery in the intestinal tract. EVs are resilient to gastric/pancreatic digestion (Hata et al., 2010), indicating that breast milk EVs are delivered to intestines of infants (Kahn et al., 2018). Milk derived EVs were also observed in human intestinal crypt-like cells, indicating a possible role in neonatal mucosal immunity (Liao et al., 2017). Several studies recommend that IEC viability, stem-cell activity and proliferation capacity increase when treated with milk derived EVs (T. Chen et al., 2016; Gao H. N. et al., 2019; Hock et al., 2017). Breast milk EVs can prevent cell death in IECs and decrease necrotizing enterocolitis (NEC) (Lucas and Cole, 1990; Martin et al., 2018). They also offer the possibility of delivering drugs in milk (Schanler et al., 1992; Zamrik et al., 2018). Small molecules such as siRNA are ideal candidate for therapy but they are unstable during delivery. A 2017 study showed that AF488 could be encapsulated in milk whey and EVs would ensure their delivery to Caco-2 cells (Shandilya et al., 2017).

Protein cargo content of EVs have also been researched. Intestinal EVs contain high levels of the cytokine, TGF-β1 which induces Treg cells and immunosuppressive DCs in IBD mice (Jiang et al., 2016). Meanwhile, ANXA1 containing exosomes stimulates epithelial cell repair in a colitis mice-model. Increased amount of ANXA1 is also observed in sera of IBD patients, the increase is directly proportionate to disease severity (Leoni et al., 2015). This provides strong evidence to use EV components as biomarkers for disease severity and IBD progression but may also have a role in therapy. Anti-tumor immunity can be induced by mature DC-derived exosomes carrying tumor antigens in *in-vitro* trials (Yang et al., 2010). Most translational EV studies are still in the pre-clinical stages with data available from animal and cellular models. Additional research would help in exploring the application of EVs in diagnostics and therapeutics in a clinical setting.

DISCUSSION

Evidence from recent studies on exosomes in particular and EVs in general indicate that these extracellular vesicles are capable of modulation of genes and cellular function and can thereby regulate inflammation and immune response. Based on our review of published studies, it is evident that exosomal cargo is strongly associated with the nature of the cells which produces them. Exosomal components are optimal for use as biomarkers as they can be extracted with minimal invasive techniques from most biological fluids like blood, urine, saliva, and feces. Existing data in IBD is limited to initial characterizations of exosomes in blood and fecal samples. Further studies are required to identify sensitive and specific markers of mucosal inflammation, and ideally inflammatory pathways. This could guide treatment decisions when several mechanisms of drug action are available to clinicians. As researchers we need to make efforts to develop robust methodologies for isolation of exosomes from fecal samples to ensure results are reliable and reproducible.

AUTHOR CONTRIBUTIONS

KKA and ACM conceptualized the review. KKA wrote the manuscript. ACM edited the manuscript.

REFERENCES

Admyre, C., Johansson, S. M., Qazi, K. R., Filén, J.-J., Lahesmaa, R., Norman, M., et al. (2007). Exosomes with Immune Modulatory Features Are Present in Human Breast Milk. *J. Immunol.* 179 (3), 1969–1978. doi:10.4049/jimmunol.179.3.1969

Agrahari, V., Agrahari, V., Burnouf, P.-A., Chew, C. H., and Burnouf, T. (2019). Extracellular Microvesicles as New Industrial Therapeutic Frontiers. *Trends Biotechnol.* 37 (7), 707–729. doi:10.1016/j.tibtech.2018.11.012

Alvarez, C.-S., Badia, J., Bosch, M., Giménez, R., and Baldomà, L. (2016). Outer Membrane Vesicles and Soluble Factors Released by Probiotic escherichia Coli Nissle 1917 and Commensal ECOR63 Enhance Barrier Function by Regulating Expression of Tight junction Proteins in Intestinal Epithelial Cells. *Front. Microbiol.* 7 (DEC), 1–14. doi:10.3389/fmicb.2016.01981

André, F., Chaput, N., Schartz, N. E. C., Flament, C., Aubert, N., Bernard, J., et al. (2004). Exosomes as Potent Cell-free Peptide-Based Vaccine. I. Dendritic Cell-Derived Exosomes Transfer Functional MHC Class I/Peptide Complexes to Dendritic Cells. *J. Immunol.* 172 (4), 2126–2136. doi:10.4049/jimmunol.172.4.2126

Avila-Calderón, E. D., Araiza-Villanueva, M. G., Cancino-Diaz, J. C., López-Villegas, E. O., Sriranganathan, N., Boyle, S. M., et al. (2015). Roles of Bacterial Membrane Vesicles. *Arch. Microbiol.* 197 (Issue 1), 1–10. doi:10.1007/s00203-014-1042-7

Ayyar, K. K., and Reddy, K. V. R. (2018). MAPK and NF-κB Signalling Pathways Regulate the Expression of miRNA, Let-7f in Human Endocervical Epithelial Cells. *J. Cel. Biochem.* 119 (January), 4751–4759. doi:10.1002/jcb.26665

Ayyar, K. K., Saha, D., Shroff, A., and Kvr, R. (2014). *MicroRNAs: the Key Regulators of PRR Signaling* 2 (3), 116–121.

Ayyar, K., and Reddy, K. V. R. (2017). Transcription Factor CCAAT/enhancer-binding Protein-β Upregulates microRNA,let-7f-1 in Human Endocervical Cells. *Am. J. Reprod. Immunol.* 78 (6), e12759. doi:10.1111/aji.12759

Baier, S. R., Nguyen, C., Xie, F., Wood, J. R., and Zempleni, J. (2014). MicroRNAs Are Absorbed in Biologically Meaningful Amounts from Nutritionally Relevant Doses of Cow Milk and Affect Gene Expression in Peripheral Blood Mononuclear Cells, HEK-293 Kidney Cell Cultures, and Mouse Livers. *J. Nutr.* 144 (10), 1495–1500. doi:10.3945/jn.114.196436

Barile, L., and Vassalli, G. (2017). Exosomes: Therapy Delivery Tools and Biomarkers of Diseases. *Pharmacol. Ther.* 174, 63–78. doi:10.1016/j.pharmthera.2017.02.020

Benmoussa, A., Lee, C. H. C., Laffont, B., Savard, P., Laugier, J., Boilard, E., et al. (2016). Commercial Dairy Cow Milk Micrornas Resist Digestion under Simulated Gastrointestinal Tract Conditions. *J. Nutr.* 146 (11), 2206–2215. doi:10.3945/jn.116.237651

Beshbishy, A. M., Alghamdi, S., Onyiche, T. G. E., Zahoor, M., Rivero-Perez, N., Zaragoza-Bastida, A., et al. (2020). Biogenesis, Biologic Function and Clinical Potential of Exosomes in Different Diseases. *Appl. Sci. (Switzerland)MDPI AG* 10 (13), 4428. doi:10.3390/app10134428

Betker, J. L., Angle, B. M., Graner, M. W., and Anchordoquy, T. J. (2019). The Potential of Exosomes from Cow Milk for Oral Delivery. *J. Pharm. Sci.* 108 (4), 1496–1505. doi:10.1016/j.xphs.2018.11.022

Bielaszewska, M., Marejková, M., Bauwens, A., Kunsmann-Prokscha, L., Mellmann, A., and Karch, H. (2018). Enterohemorrhagic *Escherichia coli* O157 Outer Membrane Vesicles Induce Interleukin 8 Production in Human Intestinal Epithelial Cells by Signaling via Toll-like Receptors TLR4 and TLR5 and Activation of the Nuclear Factor NF-κB. *Int. J. Med. Microbiol.* 308 (7), 882–889. doi:10.1016/j.ijmm.2018.06.004

Bielaszewska, M., Rüter, C., Kunsmann, L., Greune, L., Bauwens, A., Zhang, W., et al. (2013). Enterohemorrhagic *Escherichia coli* Hemolysin Employs Outer Membrane Vesicles to Target Mitochondria and Cause Endothelial and Epithelial Apoptosis. *Plos Pathog.* 9 (12), e1003797–30. doi:10.1371/journal.ppat.1003797

Boehm, M., Simson, D., Escher, U., Schmidt, A.-M., Bereswill, S., Tegtmeyer, N., et al. (2018). Function of Serine Protease HtrA in the Lifecycle of the Foodborne Pathogen Campylobacter Jejuni. *Eur. J. Microbiol. Immunol.* 2 (July), 1–8. doi:10.1556/1886.2018.00011

Brown, L., Wolf, J. M., Prados-Rosales, R., and Casadevall, A. (2015). Through the wall: Extracellular Vesicles in Gram-Positive Bacteria, Mycobacteria and Fungi. *Nat. Rev. Microbiol.* 13 (10), 620–630. doi:10.1038/nrmicro3480

Bui, T. M., and Sumagin, R. (2019). Progressing from Recurring Tissue Injury to Genomic Instability: A New Mechanism of Neutrophil Pathogenesis. *DNA Cel Biol.* 38 (8), 747–753. doi:10.1089/dna.2019.4842

Butin-Israeli, V., Houser, M. C., Feng, M., Thorp, E. B., Nusrat, A., Parkos, C. A., et al. (2016). Deposition of Microparticles by Neutrophils onto Inflamed Epithelium: a New Mechanism to Disrupt Epithelial Intercellular Adhesions and Promote Transepithelial Migration. *FASEB J.* 30 (12), 4007–4020. doi:10.1096/fj.201600734R

Butin-Israeli, V., Bui, T. M., Wiesolek, H. L., Mascarenhas, L., Lee, J. J., Mehl, L. C., et al. (2019). Neutrophil-induced Genomic Instability Impedes Resolution of Inflammation and Wound Healing. *J. Clin. Invest.* 129 (2), 712–726. doi:10.1172/JCI122085

Cai, Z., Zhang, W., Yang, F., Yu, L., Yu, Z., Pan, J., et al. (2012). Immunosuppressive Exosomes from TGF-β1 Gene-Modified Dendritic Cells Attenuate Th17-Mediated Inflammatory Autoimmune Disease by Inducing Regulatory T Cells. *Cell Res* 22 (3), 607–610. doi:10.1038/cr.2011.196

Cañas, M.-A., Fábrega, M.-J., Giménez, R., Badia, J., and Baldomà, L. (2018). Outer Membrane Vesicles from Probiotic and Commensal escherichia Coli Activate NOD1-Mediated Immune Responses in Intestinal Epithelial Cells. *Front. Microbiol.* 9 (MAR), 1–13. doi:10.3389/fmicb.2018.00498

Cañas, M.-A., Giménez, R., Fábrega, M.-J., Toloza, L., Baldomà, L., and Badia, J. (2016). Outer Membrane Vesicles from the Probiotic *Escherichia coli* Nissle 1917 and the Commensal ECOR12 Enter Intestinal Epithelial Cells via Clathrin-dependent Endocytosis and Elicit Differential Effects on DNA Damage. *PLoS ONE* 11 (8), e0160374–22. doi:10.1371/journal.pone.0160374

Cao, S. S. (2018). Cellular Stress Responses and Gut Microbiota in Inflammatory Bowel Disease. *Gastroenterol. Res. Pract.* 2018, 1–13. doi:10.1155/2018/7192646

Carrière, J., Barnich, N., and Nguyen, H. T. T. (2016). Exosomes: From Functions in Host-Pathogen Interactions and Immunity to Diagnostic and Therapeutic Opportunities. *Rev. Physiol. Biochem. Pharmacol.* 172, 39–75. doi:10.1007/112_2016_7

Chang, X., Wang, S.-L., Zhao, S.-B., Shi, Y.-H., Pan, P., Gu, L., et al. (2020). Extracellular Vesicles with Possible Roles in Gut Intestinal Tract Homeostasis and IBD. *Mediators Inflamm.* 2020, 1–14. doi:10.1155/2020/1945832

Chargaff, E., and West, R. (1946). The Biological Significance of the Thromboplastic Protein of Blood. *J. Biol. Chem.* 166, 189–197. doi:10.1016/s0021-9258(17)34997-9

Chatterjee, D., and Chaudhuri, K. (2013). *Vibrio cholerae* O395 Outer Membrane Vesicles Modulate Intestinal Epithelial Cells in a NOD1 Protein-dependent Manner and Induce Dendritic Cell-Mediated Th2/Th17 Cell Responses. *J. Biol. Chem.* 288 (6), 4299–4309. doi:10.1074/jbc.M112.408302

Chatterjee, S. N., and Das, J. (1967). Electron Microscopic Observations on the Excretion of Cell-wall Material by *Vibrio cholerae*. *J. Gen. Microbiol.* 49 (1), 1–11. doi:10.1099/00221287-49-1-1

Chen, T., Xie, M.-Y., Sun, J.-J., Ye, R.-S., Cheng, X., Sun, R.-P., et al. (2016). Porcine Milk-Derived Exosomes Promote Proliferation of Intestinal Epithelial Cells. *Sci. Rep.* 6 (September), 1–12. doi:10.1038/srep33862

Chen, T., Xue, H., Lin, R., Huang, Z., et al. (2017). MiR-34c and PlncRNA1 Mediated the Function of intestinal Epithelial Barrier by regulating Tight Junction Proteins in Inflammatory Bowel Disease. *Biochem. Biophys. Res. Commun.* 486 (1), 6–13. doi:10.1016/j.bbrc.2017.01.115

Chen, X., Song, C.-H., Feng, B.-S., Li, T.-L., Li, P., Zheng, P.-Y., et al. (2011). Intestinal Epithelial Cell-Derived Integrin αβ6 Plays an Important Role in the Induction of Regulatory T Cells and Inhibits an Antigen-specific Th2 Response. *J. Leukoc. Biol.* 90 (4), 751–759. doi:10.1189/jlb.1210696

Chen, X., Zhou, Y., and Yu, J. (2019). Exosome-like Nanoparticles from Ginger Rhizomes Inhibited NLRP3 Inflammasome Activation. *Mol. Pharmaceutics* 16 (6), 2690–2699. doi:10.1021/acs.molpharmaceut.9b00246

Colombo, M., Moita, C., Van Niel, G., Kowal, J., Vigneron, J., Benaroch, P., et al. (2013). Analysis of ESCRT Functions in Exosome Biogenesis, Composition and Secretion Highlights the Heterogeneity of Extracellular Vesicles. *J. Cel Sci.* 126 (24), 5553–5565. doi:10.1242/jcs.128868

Colombo, M., Raposo, G., and Théry, C. (2014). Biogenesis, Secretion, and Intercellular Interactions of Exosomes and Other Extracellular Vesicles. *Annu. Rev. Cel Dev. Biol.* 30 (1), 255–289. doi:10.1146/annurev-cellbio-101512-122326

Console, L., Scalise, M., and Indiveri, C. (2019). Exosomes in Inflammation and Role as Biomarkers. *Clinica Chim. Acta* 488 (July 2018), 165–171. doi:10.1016/j.cca.2018.11.009

Davoudi, Z., Peroutka-Bigus, N., Bellaire, B., Wannemuehler, M., Barrett, T. A., Narasimhan, B., et al. (2018). Intestinal Organoids Containing Poly(lactic-Co -glycolic Acid) Nanoparticles for the Treatment of Inflammatory Bowel Diseases. *J. Biomed. Mater. Res.* 106 (4), 876–886. doi:10.1002/jbm.a.36305

Deng, Z., Mu, J., Tseng, M., Wattenberg, B., Zhuang, X., Egilmez, N. K., et al. (2015). Enterobacteria-secreted Particles Induce Production of Exosome-like S1P-Containing Particles by Intestinal Epithelium to Drive Th17-Mediated Tumorigenesis. *Nat. Commun.* 6 (1), 1–15. doi:10.1038/ncomms7956

Deng, Z., Rong, Y., Teng, Y., Mu, J., Zhuang, X., Tseng, M., et al. (2017). Broccoli-Derived Nanoparticle Inhibits Mouse Colitis by Activating Dendritic Cell AMP-Activated Protein Kinase. *Mol. Ther.* 25 (7), 1641–1654. doi:10.1016/j.ymthe.2017.01.025

Dickens, D., Chiduza, G. N., Wright, G. S. A., Pirmohamed, M., Antonyuk, S. V., and Hasnain, S. S. (2017). Modulation of LAT1 (SLC7A5) Transporter Activity and Stability by Membrane Cholesterol. *Sci. Rep.* 7 (1), 1–13. doi:10.1038/srep43580

Doare, K. Le., Holder, B., Bassett, A., and Pannaraj, P. S. (2018). Mother's Milk: A Purposeful Contribution to the Development of the Infant Microbiota and Immunity. *Front. Immunol.* Vol. 9, 1. doi:10.3389/fimmu.2018.00361

Domenis, R., Marino, M., Cifù, A., Scardino, G., Curcio, F., and Fabris, M. (2020). Circulating Exosomes Express α4β7 Integrin and Compete with CD4+ T Cells for the Binding to Vedolizumab. *PLOS ONE* 15 (11), e0242342. doi:10.1371/journal.pone.0242342

Edgar, J. R. (2016). Q&A: What Are Exosomes, Exactly? *BMC Biol.* 14 (1), 1–7. doi:10.1186/s12915-016-0268-z

Eichenberger, R. M., Ryan, S., Jones, L., Buitrago, G., Polster, R., Montes de Oca, M , et al. (2018). Hookworm Secreted Extracellular Vesicles Interact With Host Cells and Prevent Inducible Colitis in Mice. *Front. Immunol.* 9, 850.

Elmi, A., Nasher, F., Jagatia, H., Gundogdu, O., Bajaj-Elliott, M., Wren, B., et al. (2016). Campylobacter Jejuniouter Membrane Vesicle-Associated Proteolytic Activity Promotes Bacterial Invasion by Mediating Cleavage of Intestinal Epithelial Cell E-Cadherin and Occludin. *Cell Microbiol.* 18 (4), 561–572. doi:10.1111/cmi.12534

Escrevente, C., Keller, S., Altevogt, P., and Costa, J. (2011). Interaction and Uptake of Exosomes by Ovarian Cancer Cells. *BMC Cancer* 11 (1), 108. doi:10.1186/1471-2407-11-108

Fábrega, M. J., Aguilera, L., Giménez, R., Varela, E., Cañas, M. A., Antolín, M., et al. (2016). Activation of Immune and Defense Responses in the Intestinal Mucosa by Outer Membrane Vesicles of Commensal and Probiotic *Escherichia coli* Strains. *Front. Microbiol.* 7 (MAY). doi:10.3389/fmicb.2016.00705

Gao, H. N., Guo, H. Y., Zhang, H., Xie, X. L., Wen, P. C., and Ren, F. Z. (2019a). Yak-milk-derived Exosomes Promote Proliferation of Intestinal Epithelial Cells in an Hypoxic Environment. *J. Dairy Sci.* 102 (2), 985–996. doi:10.3168/jds.2018-14946

Gao, R., Zhang, R., Qian, T., Peng, X., He, W., Zheng, S., et al. (2019b). A Comparison of Exosomes Derived from Different Periods Breast Milk on Protecting against Intestinal Organoid Injury. *Pediatr. Surg. Int.* 35 (12), 1363–1368. doi:10.1007/s00383-019-04562-6

Gao, X.-J., Li, T., Wei, B., Yan, Z.-X., Hu, N., Huang, Y.-J., et al. (2018). Bacterial Outer Membrane Vesicles from Dextran Sulfate Sodium-Induced Colitis Differentially Regulate Intestinal UDP-Glucuronosyltransferase 1A1 Partially through Toll-like Receptor 4/Mitogen-Activated Protein Kinase/ Phosphatidylinositol 3-Kinase Pathway. *Drug Metab. Dispos* 46 (3), 292–302. doi:10.1124/dmd.117.079046

Liu, R., Tang, A., Wang, X., Chen, X., Zhao, L., Xiao, Z., et al.(2018). Inhibition of lncRNA NEAT1 Suppresses the Inflammatory Response in IBD by Modulating the intestinal Epithelial Barrier and by exosome-Mediated Polarization of Macrophages. *Int. J. Mol. Med.* 42, 2903–2913. doi:10.3892/ijmm.2018.3829

García-Manrique, P., Gutiérrez, G., and Blanco-López, M. C. (2018). Fully Artificial Exosomes: Towards New Theranostic Biomaterials. *Trends Biotechnol.* 36 (Issue 1), 10–14. doi:10.1016/j.tibtech.2017.10.005

Geveres, D., Kugathasan, S., Denson, L. A., Vazquez-Baeza, Y., Van Treuren, W., Ren, B., et al. (2014). The Treatment-Naïve Microbiome in New-Onset Crohn ' S Disease. *Cell Host Microbe* 15(3), 382–392. doi:10.1016/j.chom.2014.02.005

Gisbert, J. P., and Chaparro, M. (2020). Predictors of Primary Response to Biologic Treatment [Anti-TNF, Vedolizumab, and Ustekinumab] in Patients with Inflammatory Bowel Disease: From Basic Science to Clinical Practice. *J. Crohn's Colitis* 14 (5), 694–709. doi:10.1093/ecco-jcc/jjz195

Gonda, A., Kabagwira, J., Senthil, G. N., and Wall, N. R. (2019). Internalization of Exosomes through Receptor-Mediated Endocytosis. *Mol. Cancer Res.* 17 (Issue 2), 337–347. doi:10.1158/1541-7786.MCR-18-0891

Gregorieff, A., Pinto, D., Begthel, H., Destrée, O., Kielman, M., and Clevers, H. (2005). Expression Pattern of Wnt Signaling Components in the Adult Intestine. *Gastroenterology* 129 (2), 626–638. doi:10.1016/j.gastro.2005.06.007

Gross, J. C., Chaudhary, V., Bartscherer, K., and Boutros, M. (2012). Active Wnt Proteins Are Secreted on Exosomes. *Nat. Cel Biol* 14 (10), 1036–1045. doi:10.1038/ncb2574

Gruenberg, J., and van der Goot, F. G. (2006). Mechanisms of Pathogen Entry through the Endosomal Compartments. *Nat. Rev. Mol. Cel Biol* 7, 495–504. doi:10.1038/nrm1959

Hait, N. C., and Maiti, A. (2017).The Role of Sphingosine-1-Phosphate and Ceramide-1-Phosphate in Inflammation and Cancer. *Mediators Inflamm.*, 2017. 1–17. doi:10.1155/2017/4806541

Han, W., Xie, B., Li, Y., Shi, L., Wan, J., Chen, X., et al. (2019). Orally Deliverable Nanotherapeutics for the Synergistic Treatment of Colitis-Associated Colorectal Cancer. *Theranostics* 9 (24), 7458–7473. doi:10.7150/thno.38081

Hata, T., Murakami, K., Nakatani, H., Yamamoto, Y., Matsuda, T., and Aoki, N. (2010). Isolation of Bovine Milk-Derived Microvesicles Carrying mRNAs and microRNAs. *Biochem. Biophysical Res. Commun.* 396 (2), 528–533. doi:10.1016/j.bbrc.2010.04.135

Hickey, C. A., Kuhn, K. A., Donermeyer, D. L., Porter, N. T., Jin, C., Cameron, E. A., et al. (2015). Colitogenic Bacteroides Thetaiotaomicron Antigens Access Host Immune Cells in a Sulfatase-dependent Manner via Outer Membrane Vesicles. *Cell Host & Microbe* 17 (5), 672–680. doi:10.1016/j.chom.2015.04.002

Hock, A., Miyake, H., Li, B., Lee, C., Ermini, L., Koike, Y., et al. (2017). Breast Milk-Derived Exosomes Promote Intestinal Epithelial Cell Growth. *J. Pediatr. Surg.* 52 (5), 755–759. doi:10.1016/j.jpedsurg.2017.01.032

Hood, J. L. (2016). Post Isolation Modification of Exosomes for Nanomedicine Applications. *Nanomedicine* 11 (13), 1745–1756. doi:10.2217/nnm-2016-0102

Hood, J. L., and Wickline, S. A. (2012). A Systematic Approach to Exosome-Based Translational Nanomedicine. *WIREs Nanomed Nanobiotechnol* 4 (4), 458–467. doi:10.1002/wnan.1174

Ismail, S., Hampton, M. B., and Keenan, J. I. (2003). *Helicobacter pylori* Outer Membrane Vesicles Modulate Proliferation and Interleukin-8 Production by Gastric Epithelial Cells. *Iai* 71 (10), 5670–5675. doi:10.1128/IAI.71.10.5670-5675.2003

Jeffrey, M. P., Strap, J. L., Jones Taggart, H., and Green-Johnson, J. M. (2018). Suppression of Intestinal Epithelial Cell Chemokine Production by Lactobacillus Rhamnosus R0011 and Lactobacillus Helveticus R0389 Is Mediated by Secreted Bioactive Molecules. *Front. Immunol.* 9 (NOV), 1–13. doi:10.3389/fimmu.2018.02639

Jeppesen, D. K., Fenix, A. M., Franklin, J. L., Higginbotham, J. N., Zhang, Q., Zimmerman, L. J., et al. (2019). Reassessment of Exosome Composition. *Cell* 177 (2), 428–445. doi:10.1016/j.cell.2019.02.029

Jiang, L., Shen, Y., Guo, D., Yang, D., Liu, J., Fei, X., et al. (2016). EpCAM-dependent Extracellular Vesicles from Intestinal Epithelial Cells Maintain Intestinal Tract Immune Balance. *Nat. Commun.* 7, 1–15. doi:10.1038/ncomms13045

Johnstone, R., Bianchini, A., and Teng, K. (1989). Reticulocyte Maturation and Exosome Release: Transferrin Receptor Containing Exosomes Shows Multiple Plasma Membrane Functions. *Blood* 74 (5), 1844–1851. doi:10.1182/blood.v74.5.1844.1844

Ju, S., Mu, J., Dokland, T., Zhuang, X., Wang, Q., Jiang, H., et al. (2013). Grape Exosome-like Nanoparticles Induce Intestinal Stem Cells and Protect Mice from DSS-Induced Colitis. *Mol. Ther.* 21 (7), 1345–1357. doi:10.1038/mt.2013.64

Kahn, S., Liao, Y., Du, X., Xu, W., Li, J., and Lönnerdal, B. (2018). Exosomal MicroRNAs in Milk from Mothers Delivering Preterm Infants Survive *In Vitro* Digestion and Are Taken up by Human Intestinal Cells. *Mol. Nutr. Food Res.* 62 (11), 1701050. doi:10.1002/mnfr.201701050

Kang, C.-S., Ban, M., Choi, E.-J., Moon, H.-G., Jeon, J.-S., Kim, D.-K., et al. (2013). Extracellular Vesicles Derived from Gut Microbiota, Especially Akkermansia Muciniphila, Protect the Progression of Dextran Sulfate Sodium-Induced Colitis. *PLoS ONE* 8 (10), e76520. doi:10.1371/journal.pone.0076520

Karlsson, M., Lundin, S., Dahlgren, U., Kahu, H., Pettersson, I., and Telemo, E. (2001). "Tolerosomes" Are Produced by Intestinal Epithelial Cells. *Eur. J. Immunol.* 31 (10), 2892–2900. doi:10.1002/1521-4141(2001010)31:10<2892::AID-IMMU2892>3.0.CO;2-I

Keerthikumar, S., Chisanga, D., Ariyaratne, D., Al Saffar, H., Anand, S., Zhao, K., et al. (2016). ExoCarta: A Web-Based Compendium of Exosomal Cargo. *J. Mol. Biol.* 428 (4), 688–692. doi:10.1016/j.jmb.2015.09.019

Kim, S. H., Bianco, N. R., Shufesky, W. J., Morelli, A. E., and Robbins, P. D. (2007). Effective Treatment of Inflammatory Disease Models with Exosomes Derived from Dendritic Cells Genetically Modified to Express IL-4. *J. Immunol.* 179 (4), 2242–2249. doi:10.4049/jimmunol.179.4.2242

Koeppen, K., Hampton, T. H., Jarek, M., Scharfe, M., Gerber, S. A., Mielcarz, D. W., et al. (2016). A Novel Mechanism of Host-Pathogen Interaction through sRNA in Bacterial Outer Membrane Vesicles. *Plos Pathog.* 12 (6), e1005672. doi:10.1371/journal.ppat.1005672

Kojima, M., Costantini, T. W., Eliceiri, B. P., Chan, T. W., Baird, A., and Coimbra, R. (2018). Gut Epithelial Cell-Derived Exosomes Trigger Posttrauma Immune Dysfunction. *J. Trauma Acute Care Surg.* 84 (2), 257–264. doi:10.1097/TA.0000000000001748

Koumangoye, R. B., Sakwe, A. M., Goodwin, J. S., Patel, T., and Ochieng, J. (2011). Detachment of Breast Tumor Cells Induces Rapid Secretion of Exosomes Which Subsequently Mediate Cellular Adhesion and Spreading. *PLoS ONE* 6 (9), e24234. doi:10.1371/journal.pone.0024234

Kuhnert, F., Davis, C. R., Wang, H.-T., Chu, P., Lee, M., Yuan, J., et al. (2004). Essential Requirement for Wnt Signaling in Proliferation of Adult Small Intestine and colon Revealed by Adenoviral Expression of Dickkopf-1. *Proc. Natl. Acad. Sci.* 101 (1), 266–271. doi:10.1073/pnas.2536800100

Kumar, J., and Newton, A. M. J. (2017). Rifaximin - Chitosan Nanoparticles for Inflammatory Bowel Disease (IBD). *Iad* 11 (1). doi:10.2174/1872213x10666161230111226

Kunkel, G. T., MacEyka, M., Milstien, S., and Spiegel, S. (2013). Targeting the Sphingosine-1-Phosphate axis in Cancer, Inflammation and beyond. *Nat. Rev. Drug Discov.* 12 (Issue 9), 688–702. doi:10.1038/nrd4099

Leoni, G., Alam, A., Neumann, P.-A., Lambeth, J. D., Cheng, G., McCoy, J., et al. (2013). Annexin A1, Formyl Peptide Receptor, and NOX1 Orchestrate Epithelial Repair. *J. Clin. Invest.* 123 (1), 443–454. doi:10.1172/JCI65831

Leoni, G., Neumann, P.-A., Kamaly, N., Quiros, M., Nishio, H., Jones, H. R., et al. (2015). Annexin A1-Containing Extracellular Vesicles and Polymeric Nanoparticles Promote Epithelial Wound Repair. *J. Clin. Invest.* 125 (3), 1215–1227. doi:10.1172/JCI76693

Li, B., Hock, A., Wu, R. Y., Minich, A., Botts, S. R., Lee, C., et al. (2019). Bovine Milk-Derived Exosomes Enhance Goblet Cell Activity and Prevent the Development of Experimental Necrotizing Enterocolitis. *PLoS ONE* 14 (1), e0211431–12. doi:10.1371/journal.pone.0211431

Liao, Y., Du, X., Li, J., and Lönnerdal, B. (2017). Human Milk Exosomes and Their microRNAs Survive Digestion *In Vitro* and Are Taken up by Human Intestinal Cells. *Mol. Nutr. Food Res.* 61 (11), 1700082. doi:10.1002/mnfr.201700082

Lin, X. P., Almqvist, N., and Telemo, E. (2005). Human Small Intestinal Epithelial Cells Constitutively Express the Key Elements for Antigen Processing and the Production of Exosomes. *Blood Cell Mol. Dis.* 35 (2), 122–128. doi:10.1016/j.bcmd.2005.05.011

Lindenbergh, M. F. S., and Stoorvogel, W. (2018). Antigen Presentation by Extracellular Vesicles from Professional Antigen-Presenting Cells. *Annu. Rev. Immunol.* 36, 435–459. doi:10.1146/annurev-immunol-041015-055700

Liu, H., Liang, Z., Wang, F., et al. (2019). Exosomes From Mesenchymal Stromal Cells Reduce Murine Colonic Inflammation Via A Macrophage-Dependent Mechanism. *JCI Insight* 4(24), e131273. doi:10.1172/jci.insight.131273

Liu, R., Tang, A., Wang, X., Chen, X., Zhao, L., Xiao, Z., and Shen, S. (2018). Inhibition of lncRNA NEAT1 suppresses the inflammatory response in IBD by modulating the intestinal epithelial barrier and by exosome-mediated polarization of macrophages. *International Journal of Molecular Medicine.* 42, 2903–2913. doi:10.3892/ijmm.2018.3829

Lucas, A., and Cole, T. J. (1990). Breast Milk and Neonatal Necrotising Enterocolitis. *The Lancet* 336 (8730-8731), 1519–1523. doi:10.1016/0140-6736(90)93304-8

Maas, S. L. N., Breakefield, X. O., and Weaver, A. M. (2017). Extracellular Vesicles: Unique Intercellular Delivery Vehicles. *Trends Cel Biol.* 27 (3), 172–188. doi:10.1016/j.tcb.2016.11.003

Mallegol, J., Van Niel, G., Lebreton, C., Lepelletier, Y., Candalh, C., Dugave, C., et al. (2007). T84-Intestinal Epithelial Exosomes Bear MHC Class II/Peptide Complexes Potentiating Antigen Presentation by Dendritic Cells. *Gastroenterology* 132 (5), 1866–1876. doi:10.1053/j.gastro.2007.02.043

Manca, S., Upadhyaya, B., Mutai, E., Desaulniers, A. T., Cederberg, R. A., White, B. R., et al. (2018). Milk Exosomes Are Bioavailable and Distinct microRNA Cargos Have Unique Tissue Distribution Patterns. *Sci. Rep.* 8 (1), 1–11. doi:10.1038/s41598-018-29780-1

Marafini, I., Sedda, S., Dinallo, V., and Monteleone, G. (2019). Inflammatory Cytokines: from Discoveries to Therapies in IBD. *Expert Opin. Biol. Ther.* 19 (Issue 11), 1207–1217. doi:10.1080/14712598.2019.1652267

Martin, C., Patel, M., Williams, S., Arora, H., and Sims, B. (2018). Human Breast Milk-Derived Exosomes Attenuate Cell Death in Intestinal Epithelial Cells. *Innate Immun.* 24 (5), 278–284. doi:10.1177/1753425918785715

Mathivanan, S., Ji, H., and Simpson, R. J. (2010). Exosomes: Extracellular Organelles Important in Intercellular Communication. *J. Proteomics* 73 (10), 1907–1920. doi:10.1016/j.jprot.2010.06.006

Mitsuhashi, S., Feldbrügge, L., Csizmadia, E., Mitsuhashi, M., Robson, S. C., Moss, A. C., et al. (2016). Luminal Extracellular Vesicles (EVs) in Inflammatory Bowel Disease (IBD) Exhibit Proinflammatory Effects on Epithelial Cells and Macrophages. *Inflamm. Bowel Dis.* 22 (7), 1587–1595. doi:10.1097/MIB.0000000000000840

Miyake, H., Lee, C., Chusilp, S., Bhalla, M., Li, B., Pitino, M., et al. (2020). Human Breast Milk Exosomes Attenuate Intestinal Damage. *Pediatr. Surg. Int.* 36 (2), 155–163. doi:10.1007/s00383-019-04599-7

Möbius, W., van Donselaar, E., Ohno-Iwashita, Y., Shimada, Y., Heijnen, H. F. G., Slot, J. W., et al. (2003). Recycling Compartments and the Internal Vesicles of Multivesicular Bodies Harbor Most of the Cholesterol Found in the Endocytic Pathway. *Traffic* 4 (4), 222–231. doi:10.1034/j.1600-0854.2003.00072.x

Mondal, A., Tapader, R., Chatterjee, N. S., Ghosh, A., Sinha, R., Koley, H., et al. (2016). Cytotoxic and Inflammatory Responses Induced by Outer Membrane Vesicle-Associated Biologically Active Proteases from *Vibrio cholerae*. *Infect. Immun.* 84 (5), 1478–1490. doi:10.1128/IAI.01365-15

Morelli, A. E., Larregina, A. T., Shufesky, W. J., Sullivan, M. L. G., Stolz, D. B., Papworth, G. D., et al. (2004). Endocytosis, Intracellular Sorting, and Processing of Exosomes by Dendritic Cells. *Blood* 104 (10), 3257–3266. doi:10.1182/blood-2004-03-0824

Mulcahy, L. A., Pink, R. C., and Carter, D. R. F. (2014). Routes and Mechanisms of Extracellular Vesicle Uptake. *J. Extracellular Vesicles* 3 (1), 24641. doi:10.3402/jev.v3.24641

Munich, S., Sobo-Vujanovic, A., Buchser, W. J., Beer-Stolz, D., and Vujanovic, N. L. (2012). Dendritic Cell Exosomes Directly Kill Tumor Cells and Activate Natural Killer Cells via TNF Superfamily Ligands. *OncoImmunology* 1 (7), 1074–1083. doi:10.4161/onci.20897

Neurath, M. F. (2019). Targeting Immune Cell Circuits and Trafficking in Inflammatory Bowel Disease. *Nat. Immunol.* 20 (8), 970–979. doi:10.1038/s41590-019-0415-0

Ng, S. C., Shi, H. Y., Hamidi, N., Underwood, F. E., Tang, W., Benchimol, E. I., et al. (2017). Worldwide Incidence and Prevalence of Inflammatory Bowel Disease in the 21st century: a Systematic Review of Population-Based Studies. *The Lancet* 390 (10114), 2769–2778. doi:10.1016/S0140-6736(17)32448-0

Ocansey, D. K. W., Wang, L., Wang, J., Yan, Y., Qian, H., Zhang, X., et al. (2019). Mesenchymal Stem Cell-Gut Microbiota Interaction in the Repair of Inflammatory Bowel Disease: an Enhanced Therapeutic Effect. *Clin. Translational Med.* 8 (1). doi:10.1186/s40169-019-0251-8

Ocansey, D. K. W., Zhang, L., Wang, Y., Yan, Y., Qian, H., Zhang, X., et al. (2020). Exosome-mediated Effects and Applications in Inflammatory Bowel Disease. *Biol. Rev.* 95 (5), 1287–1307. doi:10.1111/brv.12608

Palmulli, R., and Van Niel, G. (2018). To Be or Not to be... Secreted as Exosomes, a Balance Finely Tuned by the Mechanisms of Biogenesis. *Essays Biochem.* 62 (2), 177–191. doi:10.1042/EBC20170076

Pan, B.-T., and Johnstone, R. M. (1983). Fate of the Transferrin Receptor during Maturation of Sheep Reticulocytes *In Vitro*: Selective Externalization of the Receptor. *Cell* 33 (3), 967–978. doi:10.1016/0092-8674(83)90040-5

Pant, S., Hilton, H., and Burczynski, M. E. (2012). The Multifaceted Exosome: Biogenesis, Role in normal and Aberrant Cellular Function, and Frontiers for Pharmacological and Biomarker Opportunities. *Biochem. Pharmacol.* 83 (11), 1484–1494. doi:10.1016/j.bcp.2011.12.037

Patmanathan, S. N., Wang, W., Yap, L. F., Herr, D. R., and Paterson, I. C. (2017). Mechanisms of Sphingosine 1-phosphate Receptor Signalling in Cancer. *Cell Signal.* 34, 66–75. doi:10.1016/j.cellsig.2017.03.002

Patten, D. A., Hussein, E., Davies, S. P., Humphreys, P. N., and Collett, A. (2017). Commensal-derived OMVs Elicit a Mild Proinflammatory Response in Intestinal Epithelial Cells. *Microbiology (United Kingdom)* 163 (5), 702–711. doi:10.1099/mic.0.000468

Perretti, M., and D'Acquisto, F. (2009). Annexin A1 and Glucocorticoids as Effectors of the Resolution of Inflammation62–70). *Nat. Rev. ImmunologyNat Rev Immunol* 9 (Issue 1), 62–70. doi:10.1038/nri2470

Peterson, L. W., and Artis, D. (2014). Intestinal Epithelial Cells: Regulators of Barrier Function and Immune Homeostasis. *Nat. Rev. Immunol.* 14 (Issue 3), 141–153. doi:10.1038/nri3608

Pieters, B. C. H., Arntz, O. J., Broeren, M. G. A., van Caam, A. P. M., Koenders, M. I., et al. (2015). Commercial Cow Milk Contains Physically Stable Extracellular Vesicles Expressing Immunoregulatory TGF-β. *PLoS ONE* 10 (3), e0121123. doi:10.1371/journal.pone.0121123

Reif, S., Elbaum Shiff, Y., and Golan-Gerstl, R. (2019). Milk-derived Exosomes (MDEs) Have a Different Biological Effect on normal Fetal colon Epithelial Cells Compared to colon Tumor Cells in a miRNA-dependent Manner. *J. Transl Med.* 17 (1), 1–10. doi:10.1186/s12967-019-2072-3

Reinhardt, T. A., Lippolis, J. D., Nonnecke, B. J., and Sacco, R. E. (2012). Bovine Milk Exosome Proteome. *J. Proteomics* 75 (5), 1486–1492. doi:10.1016/j.jprot.2011.11.017

Reinhardt, T. A., Sacco, R. E., Nonnecke, B. J., and Lippolis, J. D. (2013). Bovine Milk Proteome: Quantitative Changes in normal Milk Exosomes, Milk Fat Globule Membranes and Whey Proteomes Resulting from *Staphylococcus aureus* Mastitis. *J. Proteomics* 82, 141–154. doi:10.1016/j.jprot.2013.02.013

Saha, S., Aranda, E., Hayakawa, Y., Bhanja, P., Atay, S., Brodin, N. P., et al. (2016). Macrophage-derived Extracellular Vesicle-Packaged WNTs rescue Intestinal Stem Cells and Enhance Survival after Radiation Injury. *Nat. Commun.* 7. doi:10.1038/ncomms13096

Samanta, S., Rajasingh, S., Drosos, N., Zhou, Z., Dawn, B., and Rajasingh, J. (2018). Exosomes: New Molecular Targets of Diseases. *Acta Pharmacol. Sin* 39 (4), 501–513. doi:10.1038/aps.2017.162

Sartor, R. B. (2008). Microbial Influences in Inflammatory Bowel Diseases. *Gastroenterology* 134 (2), 577–594. doi:10.1053/j.gastro.2007.11.059

Sato-Kuwabara, Y., Melo, S. A., Soares, F. A., and Calin, G. A. (2015). The Fusion of Two Worlds: Non-coding RNAs and Extracellular Vesicles - Diagnostic and Therapeutic Implications (Review). *Int. J. Oncol.* 46 (1), 17–27. doi:10.3892/ijo.2014.2712

Schanler, R. J., Burns, P. A., Abrams, S. A., and Garza, C. (1992). Bone Mineralization Outcomes in Human Milk-Fed Preterm Infants. *Pediatr. Res.* 31 (6), 583–586. doi:10.1203/00006450-199206000-00009

Shandilya, S., Rani, P., Onteru, S. K., and Singh, D. (2017). Small Interfering RNA in Milk Exosomes Is Resistant to Digestion and Crosses the Intestinal Barrier *In Vitro*. *J. Agric. Food Chem.* 65 (43), 9506–9513. doi:10.1021/acs.jafc.7b03123

Shen, Y., Torchia, M. L. G., Lawson, G. W., Karp, C. L., Ashwell, J. D., and Mazmanian, S. K. (2012). Outer Membrane Vesicles of a Human Commensal Mediate Immune Regulation and Disease protection. *Cell Host & Microbe* 12 (4), 509–520. doi:10.1016/j.chom.2012.08.004

Simons, M., and Raposo, G. (2009). Exosomes - Vesicular Carriers for Intercellular Communication. *Curr. Opin. Cel Biol.* 21 (4), 575–581. doi:10.1016/j.ceb.2009.03.007
Slater, T. W., Finkielsztein, A., Mascarenhas, L. A., Mehl, L. C., Butin-Israeli, V., and Sumagin, R. (2017). Neutrophil Microparticles Deliver Active Myeloperoxidase to Injured Mucosa to Inhibit Epithelial Wound Healing. *J.I.* 198 (7), 2886–2897. doi:10.4049/jimmunol.1601810
Sommer, F., Anderson, J. M., Bharti, R., Raes, J., and Rosenstiel, P. (2017). The Resilience of the Intestinal Microbiota Influences Health and Disease. *Nat. Rev. Microbiol.* 15 (Issue 10), 630–638. doi:10.1038/nrmicro.2017.58
Stentz, R., Osborne, S., Horn, N., Li, A. W. H., Hautefort, I., Bongaerts, R., et al. (2014). A Bacterial Homolog of a Eukaryotic Inositol Phosphate Signaling Enzyme Mediates Cross-Kingdom Dialog in the Mammalian Gut. *Cel Rep.* 6 (4), 646–656. doi:10.1016/j.celrep.2014.01.021
Stoorvogel, W., Kleijmeer, M. J., Geuze, H. J., and Raposo, G. (2002). The Biogenesis and Functions of Exosomes. *Traffic* 3 (5), 321–330. doi:10.1034/j.1600-0854.2002.30502.x
Stuffers, S., Sem Wegner, C., Stenmark, H., and Brech, A. (2009). Multivesicular Endosome Biogenesis in the Absence of ESCRTs. *Traffic* 10 (7), 925–937. doi:10.1111/j.1600-0854.2009.00920.x
Subra, C., Grand, D., Laulagnier, K., Stella, A., Lambeau, G., Paillasse, M., et al. (2010). Exosomes Account for Vesicle-Mediated Transcellular Transport of Activatable Phospholipases and Prostaglandins. *J. Lipid Res.* 51 (8), 2105–2120. doi:10.1194/jlr.M003657
Tamai, K., Tanaka, N., Nakano, T., Kakazu, E., Kondo, Y., Inoue, J., et al. (2010). Exosome Secretion of Dendritic Cells Is Regulated by Hrs, an ESCRT-0 Protein. *Biochem. Biophysical Res. Commun.* 399 (3), 384–390. doi:10.1016/j.bbrc.2010.07.083
Taylor, C. T., and Colgan, S. P. (2007). Hypoxia and Gastrointestinal Disease. *J. Mol. Med.* 85 (12), 1295–1300. doi:10.1007/s00109-007-0277-z
Teng, Y., Ren, Y., Sayed, M., Hu, X., Lei, C., Kumar, A., et al. (2018). Plant-Derived Exosomal MicroRNAs Shape the Gut Microbiota. *Cell Host Microbe* 24 (5), 637–652.e8. doi:10.1016/j.chom.2018.10.001
Théry, C., Ostrowski, M., and Segura, E. (2009). Membrane Vesicles as Conveyors of Immune Responses. *Nat. Rev. Immunol.* 9 (8), 581–593. doi:10.1038/nri2567
Théry, C., Witwer, K. W., Aikawa, E., Alcaraz, M. J., Anderson, J. D., Andriantsitohaina, R., et al. (2018). Minimal Information for Studies of Extracellular Vesicles 2018 (MISEV2018): a Position Statement of the International Society for Extracellular Vesicles and Update of the MISEV2014 Guidelines. *J. Extracellular Vesicles* 7 (1). doi:10.1080/20013078.2018.1535750
Tian, T., Zhu, Y.-L., Hu, F.-H., Wang, Y.-Y., Huang, N.-P., and Xiao, Z.-D. (2013). Dynamics of Exosome Internalization and Trafficking. *J. Cel. Physiol.* 228 (7), 1487–1495. doi:10.1002/jcp.24304
Tkach, M., Kowal, J., Zucchetti, A. E., Enserink, L., Jouve, M., Lankar, D., et al. (2017). Qualitative Differences in T-cell Activation by Dendritic Cell-derived Extracellular Vesicle Subtypes. *Embo J.* 36 (20), 3012–3028. doi:10.15252/embj.201696003
Tomé-Carneiro, J., Fernández-Alonso, N., Tomás-Zapico, C., Visioli, F., Iglesias-Gutierrez, E., and Dávalos, A. (2018). Breast Milk microRNAs Harsh Journey towards Potential Effects in Infant Development and Maturation. Lipid Encapsulation Can Help. *Pharmacol. Res.* 132, 21–32. doi:10.1016/j.phrs.2018.04.003
Torres, J., Mehandru, S., Colombel, J.-F., and Peyrin-Biroulet, L. (2017). Crohn's Disease. *The Lancet* 389 (10080), 1741–1755. doi:10.1016/S0140-6736(16)31711-1
Turfkruyer, M., and Verhasselt, V. (2015). Breast Milk and its Impact on Maturation of the Neonatal Immune System. *Curr. Opin. Infect. Dis.* 28 (Issue 3), 199–206. doi:10.1097/QCO.0000000000000165
Valadi, H., Ekström, K., Bossios, A., Sjöstrand, M., Lee, J. J., and Lötvall, J. O. (2007). Exosome-mediated Transfer of mRNAs and microRNAs Is a Novel Mechanism of Genetic Exchange between Cells. *Nat. Cel Biol* 9 (6), 654–659. doi:10.1038/ncb1596
van Bergenhenegouwen, J., Kraneveld, A. D., Rutten, L., Kettelarij, N., Garssen, J., and Vos, A. P. (2014). Extracellular Vesicles Modulate Host-Microbe Responses by Altering TLR2 Activity and Phagocytosis. *PLoS ONE* 9 (2), e89121. doi:10.1371/journal.pone.0089121
Van Niel, G., Mallegol, J., Bevilacqua, C., Candalh, C., Brugière, S., Tomaskovic-Crook, E., et al. (2003). Intestinal Epithelial Exosomes Carry MHC Class II/ peptides Able to Inform the Immune System in Mice. *Gut* 52 (12), 1690–1697. doi:10.1136/gut.52.12.1690
Van Niel, G., Raposo, G., Candalh, C., Boussac, M., Hershberg, R., Cerf-Bensussan, N., et al. (2001). Intestinal Epithelial Cells Secrete Exosome-like Vesicles. *Gastroenterology* 121 (2), 337–349. doi:10.1053/gast.2001.26263
Walker, W. A., and Iyengar, R. S. (2015). Breast Milk, Microbiota, and Intestinal Immune Homeostasis. *Pediatr. Res.* 77, 220–228. doi:10.1038/pr.2014.160
Wang, L., Yu, Z., Wan, S., Wu, F., Chen, W., Zhang, B., et al. (2017). Exosomes Derived from Dendritic Cells Treated with Schistosoma Japonicum Soluble Egg Antigen Attenuate DSS-Induced Colitis. *Front. Pharmacol.* 8 (SEP), 651. doi:10.3389/fphar.2017.00651
Wang, Y., Tian, J., Tang, X., Rui, K., Tian, X., Ma, J., et al. (2016). Exosomes Released by Granulocytic Myeloid-Derived Suppressor Cells Attenuate DSS-Induced Colitis in Mice. *Oncotarget* 7 (13), 15356–15368. doi:10.18632/oncotarget.7324
Wolf, P. (1967). The Nature and Significance of Platelet Products in Human Plasma. *Br. J. Haematol.* 13 (3), 269–288. doi:10.1111/j.1365-2141.1967.tb08741.x
Wolf, T., Baier, S. R., and Zempleni, J. (2015). The Intestinal Transport of Bovine Milk Exosomes Is Mediated by Endocytosis in Human Colon Carcinoma Caco-2 Cells and Rat Small Intestinal IEC-6 Cells. *J. Nutr.* 145 (10), 2201–2206. doi:10.3945/jn.115.218586
Wong, W.-Y., Lee, M. M.-L., Chan, B. D., Kam, R. K.-T., Zhang, G., Lu, A.-P., et al. (2016). Proteomic Profiling of Dextran Sulfate Sodium Induced Acute Ulcerative Colitis Mice Serum Exosomes and Their Immunomodulatory Impact on Macrophages. *Proteomics* 16 (7), 1131–1145. doi:10.1002/pmic.201500174
Xiao, B., Laroui, H., Ayyadurai, S., Viennois, E., Charania, M. A., Zhang, Y., et al. (2013). Mannosylated Bioreducible Nanoparticle-Mediated Macrophage-specific TNF-α RNA Interference for IBD Therapy. *Biomaterials* 34 (30), 7471–7482. doi:10.1016/j.biomaterials.2013.06.008
Xie, M.-Y., Chen, T., Xi, Q.-Y., Hou, L.-J., Luo, J.-Y., Zeng, B., et al. (2020). Porcine Milk Exosome miRNAs Protect Intestinal Epithelial Cells against Deoxynivalenol-Induced Damage. *Biochem. Pharmacol.* 175 (November 2019), 113898. doi:10.1016/j.bcp.2020.113898
Xie, M.-Y., Hou, L.-J., Sun, J.-J., Zeng, B., Xi, Q.-Y., Luo, J.-Y., et al. (2019). Porcine Milk Exosome MiRNAs Attenuate LPS-Induced Apoptosis through Inhibiting TLR4/NF-κB and P53 Pathways in Intestinal Epithelial Cells. *J. Agric. Food Chem.* 67 (34), 9477–9491. doi:10.1021/acs.jafc.9b02925
Yang, X., Meng, S., Jiang, H., Chen, T., and Wu, W. (2010). Exosomes Derived from Interleukin-10-Treated Dendritic Cells Can Inhibit Trinitrobenzene Sulfonic Acid-Induced Rat Colitis. *Scand. J. Gastroenterol.* 45 (10), 1168–1177. doi:10.3109/00365521.2010.490596
Yu, S., Zhao, Z., Sun, L., and Li, P. (2017). Fermentation Results in Quantitative Changes in Milk-Derived Exosomes and Different Effects on Cell Growth and Survival. *J. Agric. Food Chem.* 65 (6), 1220–1228. doi:10.1021/acs.jafc.6b05002
Zamrik, S., Giachero, F., Heldmann, M., Hensel, K. O., Wirth, S., and Jenke, A. C. (2018). Impact of an In-House Pediatric Surgery Unit and Human Milk Centered Enteral Nutrition on Necrotizing Enterocolitis. *Biomed. Res. Int.* 2018, 1–6. doi:10.1155/2018/5042707
Zhang, H., Wang, L., Li, C., Yu, Y., Yi, Y., Wang, J., et al. (2019). Exosome-induced Regulation in Inflammatory Bowel Disease. *Front. Immunol.* 10 (JUN), 1–9. doi:10.3389/fimmu.2019.01464
Zhang, J., Li, S., Li, L., Li, M., Guo, C., Yao, J., et al. (2015). Exosome and Exosomal microRNA: Trafficking, Sorting, and Function. *Genomics, Proteomics & Bioinformatics* 13 (1), 17–24. doi:10.1016/j.gpb.2015.02.001
Zhang, X., Deeke, S. A., Ning, Z., Starr, A. E., Butcher, J., Li, J., et al. (2018). Metaproteomics Reveals Associations between Microbiome and Intestinal Extracellular Vesicle Proteins in Pediatric Inflammatory Bowel Disease. *Nat. Commun.* 9 (1), 1–14. doi:10.1038/s41467-018-05357-4
Zheng, X., Chen, F., Zhang, Q., Liu, Y., You, P., Sun, S., et al. (2017). Salivary Exosomal PSMA7: a Promising Biomarker of Inflammatory Bowel Disease. *Protein Cell* 8 (9), 686–695. doi:10.1007/s13238-017-0413-7
Zhou, F., Paz, H. A., Sadri, M., Cui, J., Kachman, S. D., Fernando, S. C., et al. (2019). Dietary Bovine Milk Exosomes Elicit Changes in Bacterial Communities in C57BL/6 Mice. *Am. J. Physiology-Gastrointestinal Liver PhysiologyGastrointestinal Liver Physiol.* 317 (5), G618–G624. doi:10.1152/ajpgi.00160.2019

4

Ultrasonographic Evaluation of Intestinal Fibrosis and Inflammation in Crohn's Disease: The State of the Art

Francesca Ferretti[1†], *Rosanna Cannatelli*[1†], *Sandro Ardizzone*[1], *Jeanette A. Maier*[2] and *Giovanni Maconi*[1*]

[1]Gastroenterology Unit—ASST Fatebenefratelli-Sacco, Department of Biomedical and Clinical Sciences (DIBIC) L. Sacco, Università degli Studi di Milano, Milan, Italy, [2]General Pathology—Department of Biomedical and Clinical Sciences (DIBIC) L. Sacco, Università degli Studi di Milano, Milan, Italy

***Correspondence:**
Giovanni Maconi
giovanni.maconi@unimi.it

†These authors have contributed equally to this work

The evaluation of the degree of inflammation and fibrosis, intrinsic elements in intestinal wall damage of Crohn's disease, is essential to individuate the extent of the lesions and the presence of strictures. This information will contribute to the choice of the appropriate therapeutic approach, the prediction of the response to therapy and the course of the disease. The accurate evaluation of the extent and severity of inflammation and/or fibrosis in Crohn's disease currently requires histopathological analysis of the intestinal wall. However, in clinical practice and research, transmural assessment of the intestinal wall with cross sectional imaging is increasingly used for this purpose. The B-mode ultrasonograhic characteristics of the intestinal wall, the assessment of its vascularization by color Doppler and I.V. contrast agents, and the evaluation of the mechanical and elastic properties by sonoelastography, may provide useful and accurate information on the severity and extent of inflammation and intestinal fibrosis in Crohn's disease. The purpose of this review is to provide an update on current sonographic methods to discriminate inflammation and fibrosis in Crohn's disease.

Keywords: Crohn's disease, fibrosis, inflammation, strictures, ultrasound, sonoelastography

INTRODUCTION

Crohn's disease (CD) is characterized by chronic inflammation and progressive fibrosis. In general, the inflammatory pattern is the most frequent at the onset of the disease, while a stricturing or penetrating evolution can be observed later on (Cosnes et al., 2002).

The complicated course of disease occurs in up to 50% of patients within 20 years of diagnosis, requiring a surgical intervention in half of these cases within 10 years (Peyrin-Biroulet et al., 2010).

The evaluation and characterization of inflammation is pivotal in the detection of the disease, in the characterization of newly diagnosed of CD, and in its monitoring, along with the evaluation of complications (Maaser et al., 2019). The definition of disease activity and onset of fibrosis will shape therapeutic decisions, with prognostic impact on the response to therapy and the risk of recurrence.

Histopathology is still the gold standard for the identification of inflammation and fibrosis. However, despite several scoring systems have been proposed, in particular for strictures, a wide heterogeneity in scoring methods exists and none can be considered as a suitable benchmark (Bettenworth et al., 2019; De Voogd et al., 2020; Gordon et al., 2020). In clinical practice and research, cross-sectional imaging techniques have been proposed as reliable non-invasive alternative approaches for transmural assessment of the intestinal wall to detect inflammatory or fibrotic patterns.

Among different imaging techniques, intestinal ultrasound (IUS) is a radiation-free and cost-effective technique which is increasingly adopted both for the diagnosis and the monitoring of CD. The introduction of small intestine contrast ultrasonography (SICUS) and the contrast-enhanced ultrasound (CEUS) as well as elastography expanded the potential applications of this technique.

However, reliability of IUS in detecting inflammation and fibrosis is still under investigation, as well as its applicability and usefulness in clinical practice to drive the most appropriate treatment. Most of these gaps rely on the absence of reproducible gold standards for evaluating inflammation and fibrosis to be used for complicated and not complicated patients. In fact, if the assessment of pathological features is still awaiting valid and reproducible parameters, the discrimination of fibrosis and inflammation in non-operated patients is mainly indirect and relies essentially on clinical parameters such as biochemical tests and the response to steroid or biologic treatment.

In this review we evaluated the reliability of IUS in assessing inflammation and fibrosis, mainly focusing on the available studies that have used pathological features or the response to treatment as direct and indirect reference parameters.

INTESTINAL ULTRASOUND AND INFLAMMATION

Applications

The identification and characterization of inflammatory features in the small bowel and/or colon are pivotal both for the diagnosis and the monitoring of IBD. The gold standard in the assessment of bowel inflammatory involvement is histology, but non-invasive approaches are demanded to limit the risks and the costs of repeated endoscopic procedures, considering also the limitation of histology in case of inadequate or superficial biopsy sampling. Thus, different non-invasive approaches have been introduced with different degrees of reliability.

Biomarkers such as C reactive protein (CRP) and fecal calprotectin (FC) are useful for monitoring IBD (Vos et al., 2013) although with some risk of false positive results (Maaser et al., 2019). Thus, the available imaging techniques including IUS, computed tomography (CT) and magnetic resonance imaging (MRI) have been increasingly applied to IBD. In a systematic review, Panes et al. compared the diagnostic accuracy of different cross sectional imaging techniques showing a high accuracy both for the CD diagnosis and CD monitoring, with good reliability for assessing disease severity and complications (Panés et al., 2011). If multiple options are available with comparable local expertize, IUS can be considered the first choice due to its non-invasiveness, low costs and repeatability (Calabrese et al., 2016).

Identification and Characterization of Disease Activity in Suspect Crohn's Disease

In case of suspect CD, IUS has shown a 80% sensitivity and 97% specificity for the CD diagnosis when compared with reference standards including clinical evaluation, endoscopy, histology and/or radiology (Calabrese et al., 2016).

The accuracy of US depends on the location and severity of CD (Hollerbach et al., 1998; Astegiano et al., 2001; Parente et al., 2003). In comparison with endoscopy, cross-sectional techniques are less accurate to detect mild inflammatory luminal lesions (Panés et al., 2011).

In suspected involvement of small bowel (SB), IUS and SB capsule endoscopy (SBCE) yield similar findings. Indeed, IUS shows 72% of sensitivity and 84% of specificity (Carter et al., 2018), which can be slightly increased using oral contrast agents (e.g., SICUS) (Kopylov et al., 2017), in particular for the assessment of proximal SB lesions (Petruzziello et al., 2010).

Finally, a comparison of the diagnostic accuracy between MRI and IUS in detecting active CD—defined as the presence of ulcerations at endoscopy, CRP >8 mg/L, Calprotectin >250 μg/g, histological evidence of activity—demonstrated a lower sensitivity of IUS vs. MRI in active SB disease (90 vs. 96%, p 0.01) and a comparable sensitivity in case of active colonic disease (66 vs 63%, p 0.7) (Taylor et al., 2018).

Monitoring of Disease Activity in Known Crohn's Disease

The role of IUS in the evaluation of disease activity is still controversial (Calabrese et al., 2016). In a systematic review Rimola et al. investigated the accuracy of different cross-sectional imaging techniques in assessing disease activity, and found that four US-based parameters (wall thickening, Doppler signal, loss of stratification and reduced peristalsis/compressibility) showed good correlation with endoscopic reference standard (Rimola et al., 2012). MRI showed a good or very good agreement with endoscopic or histologic reference standard when limited small bowel tracts were analyzed, while the results about colonic CD assessment were more conflicting, mainly because of the inconstant use of colonic intraluminal contrast (Rimola et al., 2012). All the MRI-based indexes included wall thickness (in mm) and the degree of wall enhancement after intravenous contrast injection. To date, magnetic resonance index of activity (MaRIA) (Rimola et al., 2011) and Clermont score (Buisson et al., 2015; Buisson et al., 2017) are the two main indexes in the assessment and grading of CD severity and mucosal lesions, evaluating the presence of ulcerations, edema, bowel thickness and relative contrast enhancement (MaRIA) or apparent diffusion coefficient (Clermont). Both have been validated compared with endoscopy, both in ileal and colonic CD. Even if data are conflicting about the concordance and degree of accuracy of these scores, a recent study demonstrated a high and equal efficacy in the detection of mucosal healing (Buisson et al., 2017), showing a substantial accuracy in the detection of endoscopic ulcerations with high specificity (81–82%) and high negative predictive value (82% NPV), while sensitivity and positive predictive values were moderate. Likewise, in a recent study by Yuksel et al., IUS showed a comparable accuracy to MRE in detecting endoscopic activity (Yuksel et al., 2019) where in endoscopically active disease, the most frequent IUS signs were increased BWT (>3 mm) and fibrofatty proliferation (not defined in the study). These findings are in keeping with another study by Livne et al., where IUS parameters, and in particular terminal ileum thickness and mesenteric fat hypertrophy, showed a significant correlation with the MaRIA score (Livne et al., 2020).

However, the main limitation and difficulties in obtaining a conclusion regarding IUS assessment of disease activity are the choice of the IUS parameters and/or their combination (e.g., IUS scores) and the choice of the reference standard adopted to assess activity, whether clinical (i.e. elevated CDAI), biochemical (CRP, fecal calprotectin), radiological and/or histological.

Techniques and Parameters

B-Mode Ultrasound and Color Doppler Imaging

The data in the literature agree on the fact that main parameters suggesting inflammation and disease activity in CD are bowel wall thickening (BWT), color Doppler imaging (CDI), and bowel wall stratification (BWS), along with mesenteric fat hypertrophy and regional lymphadenopathy (Livne et al., 2020). However, these evidences come mostly from the changes of these parameters in response to the therapy.

The definition of the main parameters linked to inflammation has been indirectly obtained by assessing the behavior of the same bowel wall parameters, which result mostly affected, after biologic or corticosteroid treatment and by correlating each feature of bowel wall with the clinical (i.e. elevated CDAI, HBI) and biochemical (CRP, calprotectin) parameters (Goodsall et al., 2020). A large German multi-center study showed the improvement of different IUS parameters (BWT, parietal vascularization assessed by color-Doppler grade, lack of bowel stratification and creeping fat and mesenteric lymph nodes) after pharmacological treatment (Kucharzik et al., 2017).

The fact that BWT is one of the main parameters correlated with inflammation has also been suggested by studies showing that transmural healing, namely the normalization of the BWT (e.g., <3 mm), is strongly correlated with mucosa healing, and recent studies have shown a normalization of the thickened wall in up to 25% of patients treated with anti-TNFα drugs (Castiglione et al., 2013). A good concordance of BWT with other diagnostic studies was demonstrated both with ileocolonoscopy and MRI (Castiglione et al., 2013; Castiglione et al., 2017), thus showing the potential role of IUS in monitoring CD patients, even in pediatric age (Civitelli et al., 2016).

The available studies correlating US and histologic features define a hypoechoic echo pattern, namely the absence or disruption of the regular bowel wall stratification, in case of prevalent inflammatory stenosis (Maconi et al., 2003) and color Doppler US abnormalities of bowel wall (Sasaki et al., 2014a; Sasaki et al., 2014b).

A recent study of Bhatnagar et al. evaluates different mural and extramural US features as potential imaging predictors of histologic inflammation by comparing IUS findings with resection specimens and confirms a significant association of bowel wall and mucosal layer thickness with acute inflammation, while mesenteric fat echogenicity correlates with chronic inflammation (Bhatnagar et al., 2021). A retrospective study measured vascularity by means of color Doppler, using the Limberg score to grade the presence of blood flow within and around the bowel wall as an index of activity and inflammation, and compared the findings with the histologic results obtained on ileum biopsies of 32 CD patients. However, the association between the Limberg score and histologic grades of disease activity was poor (κ = 0.4375) (Drews et al., 2009).

More recently, an ultrasensitive ultrasound microvessel imaging (UMI) technique, able to provide a significant higher sensitivity in depicting smaller vessels compared with conventional Doppler, has been developed and compared to CT/MRI, in a pilot study of Gong et al.(Gong et al., 2020). Altered vascularization was demonstrated in case of severe inflammation, while no significant difference was found between quiescent and mild CD.

Taken into account the data of the literature, an expert consensus on inflammatory activity parameters, combined with a blinded agreement study, showed that BWT is the most important predictor of disease activity for ultrasound with a very high inter-rater agreement and correlation with overall assessment of disease activity. CDI, inflammatory mesenteric fat and BWS, which are important parameters, show moderate or nearly moderate agreement (Novak et al., 2020).

Different US activity scoring systems have been developed so far. A recent systematic review identified different available scoring systems created on the basis of endoscopic, radiologic or histologic reference standards. However, a suboptimal methodology was observed in these studies, suggesting the need for further evaluations to identify a more reliable and standardized index (Bots et al., 2018).

Small Intestine Contrast Ultrasonography (SICUS)

SICUS is a sonographic technique where the evaluation of the small bowel is performed before and after the ingestion of an oral contrast solution (approximately 500 ml of polyethylene glycol solution, PEG). It has been used for the detection and characterization of SB lesions and complications (Pallotta et al., 2012), in particular with a better accuracy than transabdominal US and comparable to radiologic examination (Calabrese et al., 2005; Pallotta et al., 2005). However, an adequate validation for activity monitoring compared with endoscopic score is not available. The actual scores (i.e., SLIC: sonographic lesion index for CD) have been compared to clinical activity (CDAI and CRP levels) and used in the evaluation of the response after induction or maintenance with anti-TNFα therapy (Calabrese et al., 2012; Zorzi et al., 2014). According to this small prospective study, a significant improvement of SLIC was observed after the induction period. Moreover, SICUS-responders to anti-TNFα agents have shown a better long-term outcome in terms of need for surgery, hospitalization rate and use for steroids (Zorzi et al., 2020).

Contrast-Enhanced Ultrasound

Unlike Doppler ultrasound, CEUS is able to detect slow-moving blood flow in small vessels, also in deep-lying bowel wall segments, and can provide qualitative and quantitative evaluations of vascularity and perfusion of the bowel walls. CEUS is performed after the injection of microbubbles (average diameter of 2.5 μm) in the blood stream. The US signals reflected by microbubbles can be easily separated from tissue signals by the softwares of the sonographic machines, and be used to discriminate vascular from avascuar tissues (e.g., to separate phlegmon from abscesses) and to quantify vascularity within the specific tissues. The latter can be assessed in a dynamic qualitative or semiqualitiative way, according to pattern of enhacement (e.g. absence/presence of enhancement of different wall layers), contrast quantification of peak intensity, or using parameters of dynamic CEUS intensity changes over time (e.g. time-intensity curves). In this setting, the application of CEUS in the evaluation of inflammation and disease activity is raising great interest. Migaleddu et al. reported a 93.5% sensitivity and 93.7% specificity of CEUS enhancement patterns in detecting inflammatory activity with a strong correlation with CDAI in 47 CD patients. CEUS accuracy was higher than US or Color Doppler US (Migaleddu et al., 2009).

Besides the pattern of enhancement of the bowel wall, defined as the description of the arrangement of the enhanced layer, Serra et al. quantified the perfusion by using a quantitative ratio between the major thickness of the enhanced layer (E) and the thickness of the entire wall section (W) (Serra et al., 2007). According to this study, an altered pattern of enhancement and a E/W ratio ranging between 0.43 and 0.47 identified active patients with a sensitivity 81% and specificity of 55–63% (Serra et al., 2007).

The perfusion analysis with CEUS has demonstrated a prognostic value in pharmacologically treated patients. Quaia et al. identified different CEUS parameters, including the overall vascularization assessed by the area under the time-intensity curve, to discriminate responders from non-responders in newly diagnosed and treated CD patients after 3 months of therapy (Quaia et al., 2013). Moreover, Saevik et al. showed that, in case of acute exacerbation requiring anti-TNFα drugs or steroids, an high relative perfusion and thickened proper muscle layer at 1 month was predictive of treatment failure (Saevik et al., 2014). Ripolles et al.(Ripollés et al., 2009) demonstrated that an increase of 46% as the threshold brightness value has a 96% sensitivity and 73% specificity in predicting a moderate-to-severe inflammation by endoscopy in 53 CD patients. Moreover, the association was confirmed even when compared with histopathology. Indeed, Ripolles et al. showed a significant association between increased contrast enhancement (CE) and histologic inflammatory score in 28 analyzed segments (Ripollés et al., 2013).

However, comparisons among CEUS and histopathology findings are limited. In a small prospective study, Wilkens et al. compared US, CEUS and MRE parameters with histopathology of 25 patients with small bowel CD undergoing elective surgery, confirming the role of bowel wall thickness as a marker of inflammation, but reporting the failure of CEUS in discriminating between inflammatory and fibrotic lesions (Wilkens et al., 2018).

CEUS has been applied also for the post-surgery recurrence. Paredes et al. developed and applied an activity index to identify postoperative recurrence in 60 CD patients. They found that the combination of a 34.5% cut-off of maximum CE with the other US parameters predicted endoscopic recurrence with a 94.4% of accuracy and a good correlation ($\kappa = 0.82$; $p < 0.001$). A cut-off >46% CE predicted a moderate–severe endoscopic recurrence (Paredes et al., 2013). Recently, a score combining the US wall thickness, the color Doppler grade and contrast parameters showed an high degree of accuracy in the prediction of endoscopic CD activity. A similar accuracy was maintained even without considering CE results in a simpler version of the score (Ripollés et al., 2021).

However, CEUS has some intrinsic limitations if compared to traditional IUS. The perfusion quantification cannot be compared among different scanners, and both time and costs are higher. Moreover, reproducibility is affected by multiple confounding factors depending on the imaging settings of the available instrumentations, on the operator technique such as the injection method and the pressure exerted by the probe on inflamed bowel wall, and also on patients' characteristics such as the body habitus, the depth of the region of interest and the gas in gut cavity (Cheng et al., 2016). However, the recent introduction of specific software integrated into US devices such as Qontrast (Bracco, Milan, Italy) and QLAB (Philips, Koninklijke, Belgium) allows a quantitative and semiquantitative analysis of contrast enhancement, limiting the subjective component of the evaluation.

Sonoelastography

Sonoelastography is a relatively new sonographic technique that assesses the stiffness of tissues. It is already used in clinical practice for several applications, in particular for breast and thyroid evaluation, and it has been more recently also proposed for assessing gastrointestinal tract. Sonoelastography is able to estimate tissue elasticity by means of US force that propagates a wave into the tissue. Since the wave velocity depends on tissue mechanical properties and mainly on its elasticity, it has been assumed that it is able to provide information on histological features and more precisely on the presence of fibrosis of the bowel wall.

There are two types of elastography: strain and shear wave elastography. With strain elastography compressive force is applied to tissues with repeated pulses to measure lesion stiffness. This can be expressed on a color scale (e.g., from red, soft to blue, hard) for qualitative assessment and/or expressed as wall-to-mesenteric fat strain ratio (i.e., "strain ratio"), for semi-quantitative assessment. In contrast to strain elastography, shear-wave elastography uses an acoustic radiation force impulse, which allows measurement of the propagation speed of shear waves within the tissue. Shear waves propagate faster in hard than in soft tissue and this allows to locally quantify its stiffness. This can be qualitatively assessed by analyzing a colour-scaled image and/or quantitively by determining the maximum elasticity value in either kilopascals (kPa) or meters per second. To date, a limited role is reserved for sonoelastography in the identification of disease activity and inflammation. Only one study assessed inflammation on UC patients, showing a significant correlation between qualitative images of real-time strain-elastography and the severity of lesions at colonoscopy (Ishikawa et al., 2011). However, in more recent studies, Serra et al. and Dillman et al. did not find any significant relationship between elastography parameters and inflammation

TABLE 1 | Imaging techniques and assessment of inflammation in CD compared with histology (i.e., reference standard: histopathology resection). Adapted from Bettenworth et al. (2019) and Gordon et al. (2020).

Study Year Type	Pts (n)	Imaging technique	Features	Results
Maconi et al. (2003) 2003 Prospective	43	US	Evaluation of echo pattern (hypoechoic, stratified or mixed)	Successful differentiation between inflammatory, mixed and fibrotic strictures. Inflammatory stenoses showed a hypoechoic echo pattern
Ripollés et al. (2013)	25	CDUS	Assessment of:	Successful differentiation in inflammatory and fibrotic strictures
2013		CEUS	-Wall thickness	Transmural complications, color Doppler grade and percentage of increase in contrast enhancement were significantly associated with the pathology inflammatory score ($p = 0.018$, $p = 0.036$ and $p = 0.005$, respectively)
Prospective			-Inflammatory markers: Loss of stratification, transmural complications, lymphadenopathy -US Doppler signal -Quantitative CE -Presence of stenosis or prestenotic dilation	Sonographic and pathology scores showed a good correlation in inflammation (Spearman's, $r = 0.53$)
Wilkens et al. (2018) 2018	25	CEUS (+CE MR enterography)	Peak signal intensity, time to peak, area under the time-intensity curve, wash-in rate, wash-out rate, wash-in perfusion index, area under the curve during wash-in and wash-out, fall time, mean transit time	Unsuccessful differentiation in none, mild/moderate to severe fibrosis and inflammation using CE imaging Successful determination of the degree of inflammation and fibrosis (none, mild/moderate to severe) using US without CE effects
Prospective				Correlation between US wall thickness and histological inflammation ($p = 0.001$) No correlation was found between the severity of inflammation or fibrosis on histopathology and on CEUS
Girlich et al. (2011) 2011	20	CEUS	Description of the perfusion pattern of the inflamed bowel wall Specific quantification software employ for perfusion assessment	Significant correlation with the parameters of the quantitative CEUS analysis Strong negative correlation ($r = -0.677$, $p < 0.01$) between the histopathological score and the time-to-peak (TTP)
Prospective				Strong correlation between TTP and single parameters of the histopathological scoring system (erosion, crypt architecture, crypt, density of eosinophils, excess of intraepithelial neutrophils)
Serra et al. (2017) 2017 Prospective	26	Strain elastography	Strain ratio measurement	Unsuccessful differentiation in fibrosis and inflammation No correlation was found between strain ratio and inflammation ($p = 0.53$)
Dillman et al. (2014)	12	Shear wave elastography	Shear wave speed	No significant difference in mean shear wave speed between high–score and low–inflammation score bowel segments
2014 Prospective				The relationship between bowel wall shear wave speed and inflammation was less correlative and nonsignificant

(**Table 1**) (Dillman et al., 2014; Serra et al., 2017). Thus, this technique is mainly reserved to the assessment of fibrosis and the differentiation between fibrotic and non-fibrotic stenoses.

INTESTINAL ULTRASOUND AND FIBROSIS

Applications

Due to the transmural inflammation in CD patients, endoscopic assessment should be always combined with cross sectional imaging diagnostic techniques, which provide a panoramic evaluation of gut, beyond the evaluation of the mucosal surface. ECCO-ESGAR guidelines suggest using an imaging technique, such as IUS, MRE or CT enterography for the assessment of the small bowel activity, for the response to treatment or in case of relapse, persistent disease activity, new unexplained symptoms, before changing in therapies and in postoperative recurrence. The guidelines underlined the role of both IUS and MRE for the detection of small bowel strictures, but also pointed out their inability in the evaluation of the fibrosis. Moreover, they suggest that the choice of the technique should be taken accordingly to the center experience (Maaser et al., 2019).

In fact, according to an observational study involving 71 CD patients, the overall accuracy of US was similar to MRE for the detection of the mural lesions. However, the specificity of US was superior to MRE for bowel wall thickness, loss of wall stratification and stenosis, while the MRE had higher sensitivity in the detection of loss of wall stratification and stenosis. US had higher sensitivity in the detection of ascites, while other mesenteric parameters were similar for both techniques (Yuksel et al., 2019).

Identification and Characterization of Strictures

CD is a chronic relapsing inflammatory disease, which evolves in a progressive and irreversible damage of the bowel. According to the Montreal Classification (Sturm et al., 2019), the course of the disease could be penetrating, stricturing or non stricturing/non penetrating. However, this classification is not fixed over time, and the clinical history can change or show mixed types, such as fistula and abscess combined with strictures leading to a high risk of surgery (Gionchetti et al., 2017). This is particularly true for ileal CD, which is usually an inflammatory disease at the time of diagnosis but may become stricturing and penetrating, as well as complicated by strictures and then fistulas and abscesses during the following 10–15 years in almost all patients (Cosnes, 2008).

The stricture, with or without penetrating complication, is still the main indication for surgery, and up to 70% of patients during their life undergo a surgical operation for this complication (Bernell et al., 2000). However, strictures in CD are not always an irreversible condition. The CD strictures show different degrees of inflammation and fibrosis. Rarely, a stricture in CD patients is purely either fibrotic or inflammatory (Rieder et al., 2017).

Since the management and treatment of inflammatory strictures is different from fibrotic strictures, it is useful to differentiate which form is predominant. In particular, inflammation can be successfully treated with medical therapy, such as corticosteroids or targeting TNFα, but fibrosis is an irreversible condition that can be treated only mechanically with balloon dilatation or bowel resection (Gomollón et al., 2017).

Therefore, the differentiation between inflammatory and fibrotic stricture is crucial for the management of CD patients. Unfortunately, no biomarkers, endoscopy or histology could identify the proportion of fibrosis within the stenosis. Likewise, no imaging technique is validated for the identification of the proportion of fibrosis. However, new imaging techniques are emerging and could help in the assessment of the fibrosis within the strictures. In particular, CEUS and Doppler US may evaluate hypervascularity correlated with proportion of inflammation, and sonoelastography, which is a technique that measures the stiffness of tissues, could be used for the identification of fibrosis (Maaser et al., 2019).

The sensitivity and specificity of IUS for the diagnosis of strictures in CD patients range between 80–100% and 63–75%, respectively (Bettenworth et al., 2019), but the differentiation of fibrotic strictures from the inflammatory ones is still a challenge.

The gold standard of the diagnosis of fibrosis remains histology through the analysis of surgical specimens. As reported by Chen et al., smooth muscle hypertrophy and hyperplasia is the most prominent histological change in fibrostenosic bowel strictures. In Crohn's strictures we can find also neuronal and adipose hyperplasia along with active and chronic inflammation and fibrosis. In particular, in Crohn's strictures the normal submucosal collagen and adipose tissue are replaced by fibrosis and accompanied by hyperplasia of the muscularis mucosa, the so called muscularization of the submucosa. The muscularis propria is also thickened and expanded by collagen (Chen et al., 2017). All these factors concur to produce the bowel wall thickening detectable by IUS, and in determining the narrowing of the lumen of the bowel. These are inversely correlated, because even only a bit improvement in the thickening suffice to produce a large increase of the luminal area (Yaffe and Korelitz, 1983).

Several studies have been published about the accuracy of imaging techniques to differentiate between fibrotic and inflammatory components of the stricture. However, only few studies compared these techniques with histology (**Table 2**).

Prognostic Value (Treatment Response)

The assessment of fibrosis on treatment response have been investigated only in one study from Orlando et al. (Orlando et al., 2018). 31 patients without strictures were assessed by strain elastography before a biologic treatment and 3 and 12 months later. Bowel wall thickening and strain ratio have been assessed. The study showed that baseline BWT was not different in patients who responded to the pharmacological treatment and those who underwent operation, while the baseline strain ratio (and so the stiffness of the bowel wall) was significantly greater in patients who underwent operation in the following 2 years and in those who did not reach transmural healing. In particular a SR > 2 was able to discriminate the risk of poor outcome after biologics in the following 2 years (Orlando et al., 2018).

Post Operative Recurrence

A large proportion of CD patients, particularly patients with ileal CD, require surgery due to strictures, penetrating disease, or refractoriness to medical treatment. Noteworthy, more than half of them need further surgeries for the same complication (Buisson et al., 2012). To date, the evaluation of the risk of clinical and surgical recurrence for these patients, relies on assessment of presence and severity of endoscopic recurrence by means of Rutgeert's score, performed within one year after surgery (Gionchetti et al., 2017).

ECCO guidelines have recognized that IUS is a useful emerging tool, alternative to ileocolonoscopy, to identify postoperative recurrence (Maaser et al., 2019). A meta-analysis has shown that the detection by IUS of a pre-anastomic BWT ≥3 mm may detect a postoperative recurrence with an overall sensitivity and specificity of 0.94 (95% CI, 0.86–0.97) and 0.84 (95% CI, 0.62–0.94) and that a post-operative BWT ≥5.5 mm may predict a severe postoperative recurrence (Rutgeert's ≥ 3) with a sensitivity of 83.8% (95% CI, 73.6–90.6%) and specificity of 97.7% (95% CI, 93–99%) (Rispo et al., 2018).

However, it should be acknowledged this meta-analysis included some studies with a small number of patients and with a very high pretest probability of recurrence, thus making the sensitivity of IUS likely oversized. In addition the studies that assessed the accuracy of IUS before 6 months (e.g. at 3 or 6 months) provided disappointing results.

Overall, IUS is now considered a promising tool for assessing postoperative recurrence and to predict the long term outcome of patients. However, prospective studies using IUS coupled with new technologies (e.g., CEUS or elastography) and combined

TABLE 2 | Imaging techniques and characterization of the fibrotic stricture compared with histology.

Study	Year	N pts	Imaging technique	Features	Histopathologic index	Results
Maconi et al. (2003)	2003	43	TUS	Stratified echo pattern or hypoechoic pattern	Fazio et al	Sensitivity 100% specificity 63.3%, PPV 72%, NPV 100% of stratified or mixed echo pattern associated with moderate-severe or intermediate degree of fibrosis in muscolaris mucosae and submucosa
Wilkens et al. (2018)	2018	25	TUS	-Wall thickness	Chiorean et al	-Wall thickness was correlated to fibrosis (r = 0.399, *p* = 0.048)
			CEUS	-Peak enhancement, total area under curve, wash-in and wash-out area under curve, wash-in perfusion index, wash-in rate, rise and fall time, mean transit time local		-No correlation was found between CEUS and fibrosis (r = -0.28, *p* = 0.19)
Ripollés et al. (2013)	2013	25	CDUS	-Stenosis, prestenotic dilatation, color Doppler grade 0 or 1, contrast enhancement <46%	Chiorean et al	-Good correlation between US and histopathological score (Spearman's, r = 0.50)
			CEUS	-A formula to calculate the percentage of increase in wall brightness and the "time-to-peak"		-Using a cut-off of 65% of enhancement increase, CEUS had sensitivity 93%, specificity 69%, PPV 78%, NPV 90%, accuracy 82%
Baumgart et al. (2015)	2015	10	US-based real-time elastography	RTE strain mean values	Collagen deposits	RTE strain values were significantly higher in unaffected segments compared with affected (*p* < 0.001)
Serra et al. (2017)	2017	26	TUS CDUS CEUS RTE	-Thickness and stratification score -Color-Doppler score -CEUS score -Mean strain ratio (MSR)	Chiorean et al.	No correlation was found between thickness score (*p* = 0.198), stratification score (*p* = 0.632), Color-Doppler score (*p* = 0.288), CEUS score (*p* = 0.205) and MSR (*p* = 0.877)
Chen et al. (2018)	2018	35	SWE	Shear-wave elastography (SWE)	Semiquantitativscoring system	Cut-off of SWE 22.5 kPa had sensitivity 69.6%, specificity 91.7% and AUROC 0.822 to differentiate between mild/ moderate and severe fibrosis
Lu et al. (2017)	2017	15	-CEUS	-Peak enhancement	Active and chronic inflammation, fibrosis, and muscular hypertrophy	-Peak enhancement was negatively correlated with fibrosis (r 1/4 20.59, *p* 1/4 0.02)
			-SWE	-SWE measures		-No significant correlation between SWE and fibrosis (*p* = 0.05)

with fecal calprotectin are awaited to estimate the postoperative risk of stenosis and new surgeries in CD patients. On this regard, it has been demonstrated that in post-operative patients, independently of the time from the previous surgery, a BWT >3 mm may double the risk of surgical recurrence compare to patients with BWT <3 mm, and that the incidence of new surgical interventions is positively correlated with the degree of BWT (Cammarota et al., 2013). Likewise, also in patients who undergo conservative surgery (e.g. stricturoplasties or minimal bowel resections) (Maconi et al., 2001), the behavior of BWT may be a relevant prognostic factor. In fact, the improvement of BWT >2 mm compared to baseline or the normalization of BWT at 6–12 months after surgery has significant favorable prognostic impact on clinical and surgical recurrence, while the IUS detection of unchanged or worsened BWT after surgery predicts a high risk of clinical and surgical recurrence (Maconi et al., 2001). However, the real long term prognostic value of postoperative IUS findings needs further confirmations, as well as the usefulness of therapy escalation, if any, in these patients.

Techniques and Parameters

IUS can detect strictures as intestinal segments characterized by thickened bowel walls, narrowing of the lumen with proximal bowel dilatation greater than 25 mm (Maconi et al., 1996; Panés et al., 2011; Maconi et al., 2018). In particular, in a recent systematic review, the features used to identify the stricture were at least one among luminal narrowing, wall thickness and prestenotic dilatation. Using only one feature, the sensitivity was 80% and specificity 75%. The SICUS which uses 500–750 ml of PEG oral solution before IUS had sensitivity 88–98% and specificity 88–100% for the diagnosis of the stricture using all three parameters (Bettenworth et al., 2019).

B-Mode Ultrasound and Color-Doppler Ultrasound

Regarding the accuracy of IUS in suggesting fibrosis of CD, it has been shown that the thickening of the muscularis propria (clearly visible with IUS), but not the entire bowel wall thickening, was predictive of treatment response and, in particular, of poor response to anti-TNFα therapy (Saevik et al., 2014).

A prospective study including 43 CD patients operated for a single ileal stricture shows that the stratified or mixed echopattern of the wall of the stricture was associated with a moderate-severe or intermediate degree of fibrosis showing a 100% sensitivity, 63.3% specificity, 72% PPV and 100% NPV. The hypoechoic echopattern was more related to the presence of neutrophil infiltrate (Maconi et al., 2003).

Wall thickness measured by IUS was reported associated to fibrosis in a small cohort of CD patients but without a significant correlation between CEUS and fibrosis (Wilkens et al., 2018).

A recent study assessed the utility of mural and extramural sonographic features of CD as markers of inflammation and fibrosis in comparison to histological sections of the bowel of 12 operated CD patients. It shows that mucosal thickness was mainly associated with fibrosis (Bhatnagar et al., 2021).

Another study evaluated the accuracy of US, by using several parameters - such as wall thickness, transmural complications, color Doppler grade, quantitative analysis of the contrast enhancement at CEUS and the presence and severity of strictures - to characterize intestinal inflammation and fibrosis in CD strictures. When compared to the histopathology findings, a negative association was found between the color Doppler grade and the pathologic fibrostenotic score (Ripollés et al., 2013).

Contrast-Enhanced Ultrasound

International guidelines recommend the use of CEUS to detect hypervascularity and inflammatory activity of CD strictures (Sidhu et al., 2018). Indeed, the intravenous contrast agent enhances the highly vascularized Crohn's stenotic segments, which are more likely inflammatory stenosis, and it does not enhance the non-vascularized ones, which are likely fibrotic (Wilson and Burns, 2010).

However, the quantitative assessment of the blood flow within the wall of strictures, inflammatory or fibrotic, may be difficult and not always reliable. Several parameters have been identified to describe and give an estimation of the flow such as the wash in rate, the time to peak, the peak enhancement and the area under the curve (Quaia et al., 2018). Using some of these parameters, the first studies evaluated the blood flow within the wall of the strictures compared to histologic findings, showing positive and very promising results. A small study, including 8 CD patients who underwent CEUS and surgery in the following year, has shown that three patients with fibrotic strictures had no or low signal echo intensity after contrast administration (Kratzer et al., 2002). These preliminary results have been confirmed by another study showing that a 65% of contrast enhancement within the stricture wall had sensitivity, specificity, PPV, NPV and accuracy of 93, 69, 78, 90, and 82% for discriminating predominant inflammatory from predominant fibrotic stenoses (Ripollés et al., 2013). These promising results have been confirmed by Lu et al. who showed an inverse correlation between the peak enhancement at CEUS and the histological degree of fibrosis (Lu et al., 2017), but not by other studies (Serra et al., 2017; Wilkens et al., 2018). In particular, Wilkens et al. used several CEUS parameters to characterize the stricture but did not find any positive or negative correlation between CEUS parameters and the histological features of the strictures. Interestingly, also MRE parameters did not show any positive or negative correlation with histological fibrosis and inflammation (Wilkens et al., 2018).

Sonoelastography

An interesting sonographic tool that may be used to characterize the strictures and assess fibrosis is elastography, both strain elastography and shear-wave elastography (SWE). The strain elastography investigates the stiffness of the bowel wall by means of repeated pressures with the probe on the abdominal wall. The system informs the operator when the signal is stable and reliable or reproducible and the image is captured and analyzed. Conventionally, the blue or red color means hard or soft tissue, respectively. The system gives either a qualitative and subjective assessment of the stiffness by examining the colors, and a quantitative estimation of the stiffness, by comparing the value within a region of interest in the wall with a similar one outside of the wall, usually taken from the softer tissue around (Stidham et al., 2011; Lu et al., 2019; Vestito et al., 2019). On the contrary, the SWE is a system that directly calculates the elasticity in kPascal thanks to the diffusion of the beam within the tissue in specific regions of interest, without the necessity to pressurize repeatedly the abdomen (Vestito et al., 2019).

A meta-analysis, whose conclusion has some limitations due to high heterogeneity and patient selection between the six studies included, shows that sonoelastography could be useful to detect fibrosis in CD strictures. Three studies used strain elastography and showed that the strain ratio was higher in strictures with fibrosis compared to strictures without fibrosis ($p = 0.05$). Similar results were found by the other three studies that used SWE, where the strain value was statistically higher in fibrotic stenosis ($p = 0.08$) (Vestito et al., 2019).

A few studies have also compared the sonoelastography results with histological evaluation. Fraquelli et al. assessed the ileal strictures in Crohn's patients by strain elastography, comparing the results with the rate of fibrosis assessed by histology. The ileal wall fibrosis percentages in histological sections showed a significant and positive correlation with ileal wall strain ratios obtained by elastography ($p = 0.005$) (Fraquelli et al., 2015).

A small study, including 16 CD patients with either ileocolonic localization or postoperative recurrence, showed that fibrotic strictures had a significantly higher axial-strain sonoelastography scores than inflammatory strictures (Sconfienza et al., 2016). Chen et al. performed SWE in 35 CD patients who underwent surgery within one week and demonstrated that SWE was significantly higher in patients with fibrosis in the stricture than in patients with inflammation. Setting 22.55 kPa as the cut-off value, the sensitivity was 69.6%, the specificity reached 91.7% with the area under the ROC curve (AUROC) of 0.822, thus allowing to differentiate between mild/moderate and severe fibrosis (Chen et al., 2018).

However, not all the studies showed positive and promising results. Lu et al. did not find a significant correlation between SWE and fibrosis ($p = 0.05$) (Lu et al., 2017), but reported a moderate correlation between SWE and muscular hypertrophy (r 1/4 0.59, p 1/4 0.02) in 15 CD patients. Serra et al. reported data from 26 CD patients who underwent IUS, color-Doppler, CEUS and real time elastography, without finding any correlation between any of the previous techniques and fibrosis score at the histological examination (Serra et al., 2017).

CONCLUSION

Despite the high accuracy of US in detecting strictures, and the promising results obtained with the novel sonographic techniques such as CEUS and sonoelastography, several limitations are still present and more studies are needed before using these technique in routine clinical practice and trials.

Ultrasound is a well-known operator and patient dependent technique and, apart from operator experience, there are bowel segments that are difficult to scan by IUS, such as proximal ileum, jejunum and deep pelvic loops due to intestinal gaseous content, which is rather frequent in patients with chronic strictures. In addition, the fine evaluation of long strictures and multiple strictures may be difficult, particularly in case of quantitative assessment with CEUS and elastography because of need of repeated measurements, and the uncertainty on the exact part of the stenotic segment that should be evaluated. On this regard, MRE, which offers a multiparametric more panoramic view, may be more accurate.

Like MRE, the bowel evaluation with IUS currently allows a multiparametric approach where B-mode, Doppler, CEUS and elastography can be applied to simultaneously assess inflammation and fibrosis in the same segment. A preliminary experience on this multiparametric approach has been performed using in combination IUS, CEUS, and sonoelastography by two readers providing an accuracy of 70 and 75% with the area under the ROC curve (AUROC) of 0.953 and 0.921 and both were significantly higher than the single technique in the detection of fibrosis ($p = 0.001$ and $p < 0.05$, respectively) (Quaia et al., 2018).

In the last years, important steps have been done in this direction. First, a valid gold standard for fibrosis and inflammation, which is mandatory to have reliable studies, has been defined. Important systematic reviews and research groups have appropriately addressed this point (Bettenworth et al., 2019; De Voogd et al., 2020). Then, the concept has emerged that the IUS parameters and scores obtained by each technique need a validation and should be reproducible. This has been done in few studies including this review, but the big challenge remains to assess CD activity (Novak et al., 2020), an issue that will be faced for strictures in the near future.

If these criteria will be fulfilled by IUS and MRI, we will have powerful tools to study strictures and fibrosis of CD, we will able to select the most appropriate diagnostic techniques for our patients, reliable to decide if a stricture should be surgically or medically treated and to monitor its outcome after the therapy.

AUTHOR CONTRIBUTIONS

FF and RC contributed equally. FF and RC: made the literature search, wrote the draft of the manuscript and approved the final manuscript as submitted. SA and JM: edited and critically reviewed the manuscript and approved the final manuscript as submitted. GM: conceptualized and designed the study, made the literature search, critically reviewed the manuscript and approved the final manuscript as submitted.

REFERENCES

Astegiano, M., Bresso, F., Cammarota, T., Sarno, A., Robotti, D., Demarchi, B., et al. (2001). Abdominal Pain and Bowel Dysfunction: Diagnostic Role of Intestinal Ultrasound. *Eur. J. Gastroenterol. Hepatol.* 13 (8), 927–931. doi:10.1097/00042737-200108000-00009

Baumgart, D. C., Müller, H. P., Grittner, U., Metzke, D., Fischer, A., Guckelberger, O., et al. (2015). US-based Real-Time Elastography for the Detection of Fibrotic Gut Tissue in Patients with Stricturing Crohn Disease. *Radiology* 275 (3), 889–899. doi:10.1148/radiol.14141929

Bernell, O., Lapidus, A., and Hellers, G. (2000). Risk Factors for Surgery and Postoperative Recurrence in Crohn's Disease. *Ann. Surg.* 231 (1), 38–45. doi:10.1097/00000658-200001000-00006

Bettenworth, D., Bokemeyer, A., Baker, M., Mao, R., Parker, C. E., Nguyen, T., et al. (2019). Assessment of Crohn's Disease-Associated Small Bowel Strictures and Fibrosis on Cross-Sectional Imaging: a Systematic Review. *Gut* 68 (6), 1115–1126. doi:10.1136/gutjnl-2018-318081

Bhatnagar, G., Rodriguez-Justo, M., Higginson, A., Bassett, P., Windsor, A., Cohen, R., et al. (2021). Inflammation and Fibrosis in Crohn's Disease: Location-Matched Histological Correlation of Small Bowel Ultrasound Features. *Abdom. Radiol.* 46 (1), 144–155. doi:10.1007/s00261-020-02603-6

Bots, S., Nylund, K., Löwenberg, M., Gecse, K., Gilja, O. H., and D'Haens, G. (2018). Ultrasound for Assessing Disease Activity in IBD Patients: A Systematic Review of Activity Scores. *J. Crohn's colitis.* 12 (8), 920–929. doi:10.1093/ecco-jcc/jjy048

Buisson, A., Chevaux, J. B., Allen, P. B., Bommelaer, G., and Peyrin-Biroulet, L. (2012). Review Article: the Natural History of Postoperative Crohn's Disease Recurrence. *Lett. Editors* 35, 625–633. doi:10.1111/j.1365-2036.2012.05002.x

Buisson, A., Hordonneau, C., Goutte, M., Boyer, L., Pereira, B., and Bommelaer, G. (2015). Diffusion-weighted Magnetic Resonance Imaging Is Effective to Detect Ileocolonic Ulcerations in Crohn's Disease. *Aliment. Pharmacol. Ther.* 42 (4), 452–460. doi:10.1111/apt.13287

Buisson, A., Pereira, B., Goutte, M., Reymond, M., Allimant, C., Obritin-Guilhen, H., et al. (2017). Magnetic Resonance Index of Activity (MaRIA) and Clermont Score Are Highly and Equally Effective MRI Indices in Detecting Mucosal Healing in Crohn's Disease. *Dig. Liver Dis.* 49 (11), 1211–1217. doi:10.1016/j.dld.2017.08.033

Calabrese, E., La Seta, F., Buccellato, A., Virdone, R., Pallotta, N., Corazziari, E., et al. (2005). Crohn's Disease: A Comparative Prospective Study of Transabdominal Ultrasonography, Small Intestine Contrast Ultrasonography, and Small Bowel Enema. *Inflamm. Bowel Dis.* 11 (2), 139–145. doi:10.1097/00054725-200502000-00007

Calabrese, E., Zorzi, F., Zuzzi, S., Ooka, S., Onali, S., Petruzziello, C., et al. (2012). Development of a Numerical Index Quantitating Small Bowel Damage as Detected by Ultrasonography in Crohn's Disease. *J. Crohn's Colitis* 6 (8), 852–860. doi:10.1016/j.crohns.2012.01.015

Calabrese, E., Maaser, C., Zorzi, F., Kannengiesser, K., Hanauer, S. B., Bruining, D. H., et al. (2016). Bowel Ultrasonography in the Management of Crohn's Disease. A Review with Recommendations of an International Panel of Experts. *Inflamm. Bowel Dis.* 22 (5), 1168–1183. doi:10.1097/mib.0000000000000706

Cammarota, T., Ribaldone, D. G., Resegotti, A., Repici, A., Danese, S., Fiorino, G., et al. (2013). Role of Bowel Ultrasound as a Predictor of Surgical Recurrence of Crohn's Disease. *Scand. J. Gastroenterol.* 48, 552–555. doi:10.3109/00365521.2013.777774

Carter, D., Katz, L. H., Bardan, E., Salomon, E., Goldstein, S., Ben Horin, S., et al. (2018). The Accuracy of Intestinal Ultrasound Compared with Small Bowel

Capsule Endoscopy in Assessment of Suspected Crohn's Disease in Patients with Negative Ileocolonoscopy. *Therap Adv. Gastroenterol.* 11, 1756284818765908. doi:10.1177/1756284818765908

Castiglione, F., Testa, A., Rea, M., De Palma, G. D., Diaferia, M., Musto, D., et al. (2013). Transmural Healing Evaluated by Bowel Sonography in Patients with Crohn's Disease on Maintenance Treatment with Biologics. *Inflamm. Bowel Dis.* 19 (9), 1928–1934. doi:10.1097/mib.0b013e3182802b87

Castiglione, F., Mainenti, P., Testa, A., Imperatore, N., De Palma, G. D., Maurea, S., et al. (2017). Cross-sectional Evaluation of Transmural Healing in Patients with Crohn's Disease on Maintenance Treatment with Anti-TNF Alpha Agents. *Dig. Liver Dis.* 49 (5), 484–489. doi:10.1016/j.dld.2017.02.014

Chen, W., Lu, C., Hirota, C., Iacucci, M., Ghosh, S., and Gui, X. (2017). Smooth Muscle Hyperplasia/Hypertrophy Is the Most Prominent Histological Change in Crohn's Fibrostenosing Bowel Strictures: A Semiquantitative Analysis by Using a Novel Histological Grading Scheme. *J. Crohns. Colitis.* 11 (1), 92–104. doi:10.1093/ecco-jcc/jjw126

Chen, Y. J., Mao, R., Md, X. H. L., Cao, Q. H., Chen, Z. H., Liu, B. X., et al. (2018). Real-Time Shear Wave Ultrasound Elastography Differentiates Fibrotic from Inflammatory Strictures in Patients with Crohn's Disease. *Inflamm. Bowel Dis.* 24 (10), 2183–2190. doi:10.1093/ibd/izy115

Cheng, W., Gao, X., Wang, W., Zhi, M., Tang, J., Wen, Y.-l., et al. (2016). Preliminary Analysis of Clinical Situations Involved in Quantification of Contrast-Enhanced Ultrasound in Crohn's Disease. *Ultrasound Med. Biol.* 42 (8), 1784–1791. doi:10.1016/j.ultrasmedbio.2016.03.001

Civitelli, F., Nuti, F., Oliva, S., Messina, L., La Torre, G., Viola, F., et al. (2016). Looking beyond Mucosal Healing. *Inflamm. Bowel Dis.* 22 (10), 2418–2424. doi:10.1097/mib.0000000000000897

Cosnes, J., Cattan, S., Blain, A., Beaugerie, L., Carbonnel, F., Parc, R., et al. (2002). Long-term Evolution of Disease Behavior of Crohn's Disease. *Inflamm. Bowel Dis.* 8 (4), 244–250. doi:10.1097/00054725-200207000-00002

Cosnes, J. (2008). Crohn's Disease Phenotype, Prognosis, and Long-Term Complications: what to Expect? *Acta Gastroenterol. Belg.* 71 (3), 303–307.

De Voogd, F. A., Mookhoek, A., Gecse, K. B., De Hertogh, G., Bemelman, W. A., Buskens, C. J., et al. (2020). Systematic Review: Histological Scoring of Strictures in Crohn's Disease. *J. Crohns Colitis* 14 (6), 734–742. doi:10.1093/ecco-jcc/jjz177

Dillman, J. R., Stidham, R. W., Higgins, P. D. R., Moons, D. S., Johnson, L. A., Keshavarzi, N. R., et al. (2014). Ultrasound Shear Wave Elastography Helps Discriminate Low-Grade from High-Grade Bowel Wall Fibrosis in Ex Vivo Human Intestinal Specimens. *J. Ultrasound Med.* 33 (12), 2115–2123. doi:10.7863/ultra.33.12.2115

Drews, B. H., Barth, T. F. E., Hänle, M. M., Akinli, A. S., Mason, R. A., Muche, R., et al. (2009). Comparison of Sonographically Measured Bowel Wall Vascularity, Histology, and Disease Activity in Crohn's Disease. *Eur. Radiol.* 19 (6), 1379–1386. doi:10.1007/s00330-008-1290-5

Fraquelli, M., Branchi, F., Cribiù, F. M., Orlando, S., Casazza, G., Magarotto, A., et al. (2015). The Role of Ultrasound Elasticity Imaging in Predicting Ileal Fibrosis in Crohn's Disease Patients. *Inflamm. Bowel Dis.* 21 (11), 2605–2612. doi:10.1097/mib.0000000000000536

Gionchetti, P., Dignass, A., Danese, S., Magro Dias, F. J., Rogler, G., Lakatos, P. L., et al. (2017). 3rd European Evidence-Based Consensus on the Diagnosis and Management of Crohn's Disease 2016: Part 2: Surgical Management and Special Situations. *J. Crohns Colitis* 11 (2), 135–149. doi:10.1093/ecco-jcc/jjw169

Girlich, C., Jung, E. M., Huber, E., Ott, C., Iesalnieks, I., Schreyer, A., et al. (2011). Comparison between Preoperative Quantitative Assessment of Bowel Wall Vascularization by Contrast-Enhanced Ultrasound and Operative Macroscopic Findings and Results of Histopathological Scoring in Crohn's Disease. *Ultraschall Med.* 32 (2), 154–159. doi:10.1055/s-0029-1245398

Gomollón, F., Dignass, A., Annese, V., Tilg, H., Van Assche, G., Lindsay, J. O., et al. (2017). 3rd European Evidence-Based Consensus on the Diagnosis and Management of Crohn's Disease 2016: Part 1: Diagnosis and Medical Management. *J. Crohns Colitis* 11 (1), 3–25. doi:10.1093/ecco-jcc/jjw168

Gong, P., Song, P., Kolbe, A. B., Sheedy, S. P., Huang, C., Ling, W., et al. (2020). Quantitative Inflammation Assessment for Crohn Disease Using Ultrasensitive Ultrasound Microvessel Imaging. *J. Ultrasound Med.* 39 (9), 1819–1827. doi:10.1002/jum.15290

Goodsall, T. M., Nguyen, T. M., Parker, C. E., Ma, C., Andrews, J. M., Jairath, V., et al. (2020). Systematic Review: Gastrointestinal Ultrasound Scoring Indices for Inflammatory Bowel Disease. *J. Crohns Colitis* 15 (1), 125–142. doi:10.1093/ecco-jcc/jjaa129

Gordon, I. O., Bettenworth, D., Bokemeyer, A., Srivastava, A., Rosty, C., de Hertogh, G., et al. (2020). Histopathology Scoring Systems of Stenosis Associated with Small Bowel Crohn's Disease: A Systematic Review. *Gastroenterology* 158 (1), 137–150. doi:10.1053/j.gastro.2019.08.033

Hollerbach, S., Geissler, A., Schiegl, H., Kullmann, F., Lock, G., Schmidt, J., et al. (1998). The Accuracy of Abdominal Ultrasound in the Assessment of Bowel Disorders. *Scand. J. Gastroenterol.* 33 (11), 1201–1208. doi:10.1080/00365529850172575

Ishikawa, D., Ando, T., Watanabe, O., Ishiguro, K., Maeda, O., Miyake, N., et al. (2011). Images of Colonic Real-Time Tissue Sonoelastography Correlate with Those of Colonoscopy and May Predict Response to Therapy in Patients with Ulcerative Colitis. *BMC Gastroenterol.* 11, 29. doi:10.1186/1471-230x-11-29

Kopylov, U., Yung, D. E., Engel, T., Vijayan, S., Har-Noy, O., Katz, L., et al. (2017). Diagnostic Yield of Capsule Endoscopy versus Magnetic Resonance Enterography and Small Bowel Contrast Ultrasound in the Evaluation of Small Bowel Crohn's Disease: Systematic Review and Meta-Analysis. *Dig. Liver Dis.* 49 (8), 854–863. doi:10.1016/j.dld.2017.04.013

Kratzer, W., von Tirpitz, C., Mason, R., Reinshagen, M., Adler, G., Möller, P., et al. (2002). Contrast-enhanced Power Doppler Sonography of the Intestinal Wall in the Differentiation of Hypervascularized and Hypovascularized Intestinal Obstructions in Patients with Crohn's Disease. *J. Ultrasound Med.* 21 (2), 149. doi:10.7863/jum.2002.21.2.149

Kucharzik, T., Wittig, B. M., Helwig, U., Börner, N., Rössler, A., Rath, S., et al. (2017). Use of Intestinal Ultrasound to Monitor Crohn's Disease Activity. *Clin. Gastroenterol. Hepatol.* 15 (4), 535–542. doi:10.1016/j.cgh.2016.10.040

Livne, M., Amitai, M. M., Klang, E., Ben Horin, S., Ungar, B., Levartovsky, A., et al. (2020). Qualitative Sonographic Assessment of Transmural Ileal Inflammation in Crohn's Disease. *Eur. J. Gastroenterol. Hepatol.* [Epub ahead of print]. doi:10.1097/MEG.0000000000002016

Lu, C., Gui, X., Chen, W., Fung, T., Novak, K., and Wilson, S. R. (2017). Ultrasound Shear Wave Elastography and Contrast Enhancement: Effective Biomarkers in Crohn's Disease Strictures. *Inflamm. Bowel Dis.* 23 (3), 421–430. doi:10.1097/mib.0000000000001020

Lu, C., Merrill, C., Medellin, A., Novak, K., and Wilson, S. R. (2019). Bowel Ultrasound State of the Art: Grayscale and Doppler Ultrasound, Contrast Enhancement, and Elastography in Crohn Disease. *J. Ultrasound Med.* 38 (2), 271–288. doi:10.1002/jum.14920

Maaser, C., Sturm, A., Vavricka, S. R., Kucharzik, T., Fiorino, G., Annese, V., et al. (2019). ECCO-ESGAR Guideline for Diagnostic Assessment in IBD Part 1: Initial Diagnosis, Monitoring of Known IBD, Detection of Complications. *J. Crohn's colitis* 13 (2), 144K–164K. doi:10.1093/ecco-jcc/jjy113

Maconi, G., Bollani, S., and Bianchi Porro, G. (1996). Ultrasonographic Detection of Intestinal Complications in Crohn's Disease. *Dig. Dis Sci.* 41 (8), 1643–1648. doi:10.1007/bf02087914

Maconi, G., Sampietro, G. M., Cristaldi, M., Danelli, P., Russo, A., Porro, G. B., et al. (2001). Preoperative Characteristics and Postoperative Behavior of Bowel Wall on Risk of Recurrence after Conservative Surgery in Crohn's Disease: a Prospective Study. *Ann. Surg.* 233, 345–352. doi:10.1097/00000658-200103000-00007

Maconi, G., Carsana, L., Fociani, P., Sampietro, G. M., Ardizzone, S., Cristaldi, M., et al. (2003). Small Bowel Stenosis in Crohn's Disease: Clinical, Biochemical and Ultrasonographic Evaluation of Histological Features. *Aliment. Pharmacol. Ther.* 18 (7), 749–756. doi:10.1046/j.1365-2036.2003.01673.x

Maconi, G., Nylund, K., Ripolles, T., Calabrese, E., Dirks, K., Dietrich, C., et al. (2018). EFSUMB Recommendations and Clinical Guidelines for Intestinal Ultrasound (GIUS) in Inflammatory Bowel Diseases. *Ultraschall Med.* 39 (3), 304–317. doi:10.1055/s-0043-125329

Migaleddu, V., Scanu, A. M., Quaia, E., Rocca, P. C., Dore, M. P., Scanu, D., et al. (2009). Contrast-enhanced Ultrasonographic Evaluation of Inflammatory Activity in Crohn's Disease. *Gastroenterology* 137 (1), 43–52. doi:10.1053/j.gastro.2009.03.062

Novak, K. L., Nylund, K., Maaser, C., Petersen, F., Kucharzik, T., Lu, C., et al. (2020). Expert Consensus on Optimal Acquisition and Development of the International Bowel Ultrasound Segmental Activity Score (IBUS-SAS): a Reliability and Inter-rater Variability Study on Intestinal Ultrasonography in Crohn's Disease. *J. Crohns Colitis* 15 (4), 609–616. doi:10.1093/ecco-jcc/jjaa216

Orlando, S., Fraquelli, M., Coletta, M., Branchi, F., Magarotto, A., Conti, C. B., et al. (2018). Ultrasound Elasticity Imaging Predicts Therapeutic Outcomes of Patients with Crohn's Disease Treated with Anti-tumour Necrosis Factor Antibodies. *J. Crohns Colitis* 12 (1), 63–70. doi:10.1093/ecco-jcc/jjx116

Pallotta, N., Tomei, E., Viscido, A., Calabrese, E., Marcheggiano, A., Caprilli, R., et al. (2005). Small Intestine Contrast Ultrasonography: an Alternative to Radiology in the Assessment of Small Bowel Disease. *Inflamm. Bowel Dis.* 11 (2), 146–153. doi:10.1097/00054725-200502000-00008

Pallotta, N., Vincoli, G., Montesani, C., Chirletti, P., Pronio, A., Caronna, R., et al. (2012). Small Intestine Contrast Ultrasonography (SICUS) for the Detection of Small Bowel Complications in Crohn's Disease: A Prospective Comparative Study versus Intraoperative Findings. *Inflamm. Bowel Dis.* 18 (1), 74–84. doi:10.1002/ibd.21678

Panés, J., Bouzas, R., Chaparro, M., García-Sánchez, V., Gisbert, J. P., Martínez de Guereñu, B., et al. (2011). Systematic Review: the Use of Ultrasonography, Computed Tomography and Magnetic Resonance Imaging for the Diagnosis, Assessment of Activity and Abdominal Complications of Crohn's Disease. *Aliment. Pharmacol. Ther.* 34 (2), 125–145. doi:10.1111/j.1365-2036.2011.04710.x

Paredes, J. M., Ripollés, T., Cortés, X., Moreno, N., Martínez, M. J., Bustamante-Balén, M., et al. (2013). Contrast-enhanced Ultrasonography: Usefulness in the Assessment of Postoperative Recurrence of Crohn's Disease. *J. Crohn's Colitis* 7 (3), 192–201. doi:10.1016/j.crohns.2012.03.017

Parente, F., Greco, S., Molteni, M., Cucino, C., Maconi, G., Sampietro, G. M., et al. (2003). Role of Early Ultrasound in Detecting Inflammatory Intestinal Disorders and Identifying Their Anatomical Location within the Bowel. *Aliment. Pharmacol. Ther.* 18 (10), 1009–1016. doi:10.1046/j.1365-2036.2003.01796.x

Petruzziello, C., Onali, S., Calabrese, E., Zorzi, F., Ascolani, M., Condino, G., et al. (2010). Wireless Capsule Endoscopy and Proximal Small Bowel Lesions in Crohn's Disease. *World. J. Gastroenterol.* 16 (26), 3299–3304. doi:10.3748/wjg.v16.i26.3299

Peyrin-Biroulet, L., Loftus, E. V., Jr., Colombel, J.-F., and Sandborn, W. J. (2010). The Natural History of Adult Crohn's Disease in Population-Based Cohorts. *Am. J. Gastroenterol.* 105 (2), 289–297. doi:10.1038/ajg.2009.579

Quaia, E., Cabibbo, B., De Paoli, L., Toscano, W., Poillucci, G., and Cova, M. A. (2013). The Value of Time-Intensity Curves Obtained after Microbubble Contrast Agent Injection to Discriminate Responders from Non-responders to Anti-inflammatory Medication Among Patients with Crohn's Disease. *Eur. Radiol.* 23 (6), 1650–1659. doi:10.1007/s00330-012-2754-1

Quaia, E., Gennari, A. G., Cova, M. A., and van Beek, E. J. R. (2018). Differentiation of Inflammatory from Fibrotic Ileal Strictures Among Patients with Crohn's Disease Based on Visual Analysis: Feasibility Study Combining Conventional B-Mode Ultrasound, Contrast-Enhanced Ultrasound and Strain Elastography. *Ultrasound Med. Biol.* 44 (4), 762–770. doi:10.1016/j.ultrasmedbio.2017.11.015

Rieder, F., Fiocchi, C., and Rogler, G. (2017). Mechanisms, Management, and Treatment of Fibrosis in Patients with Inflammatory Bowel Diseases. *Gastroenterology* 152 (2), 340–350. doi:10.1053/j.gastro.2016.09.047

Rimola, J., Ordás, I., Rodriguez, S., García-Bosch, O., Aceituno, M., Llach, J., et al. (2011). Magnetic Resonance Imaging for Evaluation of Crohn's Disease: Validation of Parameters of Severity and Quantitative Index of Activity. Inflammatory Bowel Diseases. *Inflamm. Bowel Dis.* 17 (8), 1759–1768. doi:10.1002/ibd.21551

Rimola, J., Ordás, I., Rodríguez, S., Ricart, E., and Panés, J. (2012). Imaging Indexes of Activity and Severity for Crohn's Disease: Current Status and Future Trends. *Abdom. Imaging* 37 (6), 958–966. doi:10.1007/s00261-011-9820-z

Ripollés, T., Martínez, M. J., Paredes, J. M., Blanc, E., Flors, L., and Delgado, F. (2009). Crohn Disease: Correlation of Findings at Contrast-Enhanced US with Severity at Endoscopy. *Radiology* 253 (1), 241–248. doi:10.1148/radiol.2531082269

Ripollés, T., Rausell, N., Paredes, J. M., Grau, E., Martínez, M. J., and Vizuete, J. (2013). Effectiveness of Contrast-Enhanced Ultrasound for Characterisation of Intestinal Inflammation in Crohn's Disease: a Comparison with Surgical Histopathology Analysis. *J. Crohn's Colitis* 7 (2), 120–128. doi:10.1016/j.crohns.2012.03.002

Ripollés, T., Poza, J., Suarez Ferrer, C., Martínez-Pérez, M. J., Martín-Algíbez, A., and de Las Heras Paez, B. (2021). Evaluation of Crohn's Disease Activity: Development of an Ultrasound Score in a Multicenter Study. *Inflamm. Bowel Dis.* 27 (1), 145–154. doi:10.1093/ibd/izaa134

Rispo, A., Imperatore, N., Testa, A., Nardone, O. M., Luglio, G., Caporaso, N., et al. (2018). Diagnostic Accuracy of Ultrasonography in the Detection of Postsurgical Recurrence in Crohn's Disease: A Systematic Review with Meta-Analysis. *Inflamm. Bowel Dis.* 24, 977–988. doi:10.1093/ibd/izy012

Saevik, F., Nylund, K., Hausken, T., Ødegaard, S., and Gilja, O. H. (2014). Bowel Perfusion Measured with Dynamic Contrast-Enhanced Ultrasound Predicts Treatment Outcome in Patients with Crohn's Disease. *Inflamm. Bowel Dis.* 20 (11), 2029–2037. doi:10.1097/mib.0000000000000159

Sasaki, T., Kunisaki, R., Kinoshita, H., Kimura, H., Kodera, T., Nozawa, A., et al. (2014a). Doppler Ultrasound Findings Correlate with Tissue Vascularity and Inflammation in Surgical Pathology Specimens from Patients with Small Intestinal Crohn's Disease. *BMC Res. Notes* 7, 363. doi:10.1186/1756-0500-7-363

Sasaki, T., Kunisaki, R., Kinoshita, H., Yamamoto, H., Kimura, H., Hanzawa, A., et al. (2014b). Use of Color Doppler Ultrasonography for Evaluating Vascularity of Small Intestinal Lesions in Crohn's Disease: Correlation with Endoscopic and Surgical Macroscopic Findings. *Scand. J. Gastroenterol.* 49 (3), 295–301. doi:10.3109/00365521.2013.871744

Sconfienza, L. M., Cavallaro, F., Colombi, V., Pastorelli, L., Tontini, G., Pescatori, L., et al. (2016). *In-vivo* Axial-Strain Sonoelastography Helps Distinguish Acutely-Inflamed from Fibrotic Terminal Ileum Strictures in Patients with Crohn's Disease: Preliminary Results. *Ultrasound Med. Biol.* 42 (4), 855–863. doi:10.1016/j.ultrasmedbio.2015.11.023

Serra, C., Menozzi, G., Labate, A. M. M., Giangregorio, F., Gionchetti, P., Beltrami, M., et al. (2007). Ultrasound Assessment of Vascularization of the Thickened Terminal Ileum Wall in Crohn's Disease Patients Using a Low-Mechanical Index Real-Time Scanning Technique with a Second Generation Ultrasound Contrast Agent. *Eur. J. Radiol.* 62 (1), 114–121. doi:10.1016/j.ejrad.2006.11.027

Serra, C., Rizzello, F., Pratico', C., Felicani, C., Fiorini, E., Brugnera, R., et al. (2017). Real-time Elastography for the Detection of Fibrotic and Inflammatory Tissue in Patients with Stricturing Crohn's Disease. *J. Ultrasound* 20 (4), 273–284. doi:10.1007/s40477-017-0265-2

Sidhu, P., Cantisani, V., Dietrich, C., Gilja, O., Saftoiu, A., Bartels, E., et al. (2018). The EFSUMB Guidelines and Recommendations for the Clinical Practice of Contrast-Enhanced Ultrasound (CEUS) in Non-hepatic Applications: Update 2017 (Long Version). *Ultraschall Med.* 39 (2), e2–e44. doi:10.1055/a-0586-1107

Stidham, R. W., Xu, J., Johnson, L. A., Kim, K., Moons, D. S., McKenna, B. J., et al. (2011). Ultrasound Elasticity Imaging for Detecting Intestinal Fibrosis and Inflammation in Rats and Humans with Crohn's Disease. *Gastroenterology* 141 (3), 819–826. doi:10.1053/j.gastro.2011.07.027

Sturm, A., Maaser, C., Calabrese, E., Annese, V., Fiorino, G., Kucharzik, T., et al. (2019). ECCO-ESGAR Guideline for Diagnostic Assessment in IBD Part 2: IBD Scores and General Principles and Technical Aspects. *J. Crohns Colitis* 13 (3), 273–284. doi:10.1093/ecco-jcc/jjy114

Taylor, S. A., Mallett, S., Bhatnagar, G., Baldwin-Cleland, R., Bloom, S., Gupta, A., et al. (2018). Diagnostic Accuracy of Magnetic Resonance Enterography and Small Bowel Ultrasound for the Extent and Activity of Newly Diagnosed and Relapsed Crohn's Disease (METRIC): a Multicentre Trial. *Lancet Gastroenterol. Hepatol.* 3 (8), 548–558. doi:10.1016/s2468-1253(18)30161-4

Vestito, A., Marasco, G., Maconi, G., Festi, D., Bazzoli, F., and Zagari, R. M. (2019). Role of Ultrasound Elastography in the Detection of Fibrotic Bowel Strictures in Patients with Crohn's Disease: Systematic Review and Meta-Analysis. *Ultraschall Med.* 40 (5), 646–654. doi:10.1055/a-0865-1842

Vos, M. D., Louis, E. J., Jahnsen, J., Vandervoort, J. G. P., Noman, M., Dewit, O., et al. (2013). Consecutive Fecal Calprotectin Measurements to Predict Relapse in Patients with Ulcerative Colitis Receiving Infliximab Maintenance Therapy. *Inflamm. Bowel Dis.* 19 (10), 2111–2117. doi:10.1097/mib.0b013e31829b2a37

Wilkens, R., Hagemann-Madsen, R. H., Peters, D. A., Nielsen, A. H., Nørager, C. B., Glerup, H., et al. (2018). Validity of Contrast-Enhanced Ultrasonography and Dynamic Contrast-Enhanced MR Enterography in the Assessment of Transmural Activity and Fibrosis in Crohn's Disease. *J. Crohns Colitis* 12 (1), 48–56. doi:10.1093/ecco-jcc/jjx111

Wilson, S. R., and Burns, P. N. (2010). Microbubble-enhanced US in Body Imaging: what Role? *Radiology* 257 (1), 24–39. doi:10.1148/radiol.10091210

Yaffe, B. H., and Korelitz, B. I. (1983). Prognosis for Nonoperative Management of Small-Bowel Obstruction in Crohn's Disease. *J. Clin. Gastroenterol.* 5 (3), 211–216. doi:10.1097/00004836-198306000-00003

Yuksel, I., Kilincalp, S., Coskun, Y., Akinci, H., Hamamci, M., and Alkan, A. (2019). Diagnostic Accuracy of Intestinal Ultrasound and Magnetic Resonance Enterography for the Detection of Endoscopy-Based Disease Activity in Ileocolonic Crohn's Disease. *Eur. J. Gastroenterol. Hepatol.* 31 (7), 809–816. doi:10.1097/meg.0000000000001438

Zorzi, F., Stasi, E., Bevivino, G., Scarozza, P., Biancone, L., Zuzzi, S., et al. (2014). A Sonographic Lesion Index for Crohn's Disease Helps Monitor Changes in Transmural Bowel Damage during Therapy. *Clin. Gastroenterol. Hepatol.* 12 (12), 2071–2077. doi:10.1016/j.cgh.2014.04.036

Zorzi, F., Ghosh, S., Chiaramonte, C., Lolli, E., Ventura, M., Onali, S., et al. (2020). Response Assessed by Ultrasonography as Target of Biological Treatment for Crohn's Disease. *Clin. Gastroenterol. Hepatol.* 18 (9), 2030–2037. doi:10.1016/j.cgh.2019.10.042

5

UPLC-Q-TOF/MS-Based Serum and Urine Metabonomics Study on the Ameliorative Effects of Palmatine on *Helicobacter pylori*–Induced Chronic Atrophic Gastritis

Xing Chen[1,2], Jianzhong Zhang[3], Ruilin Wang[4], Honghong Liu[4], Chunmei Bao[5], Shihua Wu[1,2], Jianxia Wen[1,2], Tao Yang[1,2], Ying Wei[1,2], Sichen Ren[1,2], Yuling Tong[1,2] and Yanling Zhao[1]*

[1] Department of Pharmacy, Fifth Medical Center of PLA General Hospital, Beijing, China, [2] College of Pharmacy, Chengdu University of Traditional Chinese Medicine, Chengdu, China, [3] Center of Disease Control and Prevention, National Institute for Communicable Disease Control and Prevention, Beijing, China, [4] Integrative Medical Center, Fifth Medical Center of PLA General Hospital, Beijing, China, [5] Division of Clinical Microbiology, Fifth Medical Center of PLA General Hospital, Beijing, China

***Correspondence:**
Yanling Zhao
zhaoyl2855@126.com

Objective: The main objective of this study was to investigate the ameliorative effects of Palmatine (Pal) on *Helicobacter pylori* (*H. pylori*) induced chronic atrophic gastritis (CAG)

Method: Body function, serum biochemical indicators and histopathology were used to evaluate the pharmacodynamics of Pal on CAG rats. The target genes expression levels were verified and assessed by RT-PCR and immunohistochemistry (IHC). Moreover, UPLC-Q-TOF/MS analysis based on urine and serum was performed to identify the potential metabolites in the pathological process of CAG induced by *H. pylori*. Metabolic pathway analysis was performed to elucidate the metabolic network associated with Pal treatment of CAG.

Results: Pal (10, 20, 40 mg/kg/day) significantly restored the body function of CAG rats, reduced the serum biochemical indicators, and maintained the integrity of the gastric mucosal epithelial barrier while alleviated gastric histological damage. Metabolomics analysis shows that the therapeutic effect of Pal on CAG involves 10 metabolites and 10 metabolic pathways, of which the Taurine and hypotaurine metabolism, Glycerophospholipid metabolism and Pentose and glucuronate interconversions are closely related to the gastrointestinal protection of Pal, and these metabolic pathways crosstalk with each other due to the internet hub of citric acid cycle.

Conclusions: Metabolomics was used for the first time to identify potential biomarkers of CAG and to illuminate the therapeutic mechanism of Pal on CAG induced by *H. pylori*. The results provided a new insight for further research on CAG treatment.

Keywords: palmatine, *Helicobacter pylori*, chronic atrophic gastritis, metabolomics, molecular mechanisms

INTRODUCTION

Chronic atrophic gastritis (CAG) is a common disease of the digestive system which is considered a precursor condition for gastric cancer (GC). The rate of CAG progression to GC was as high as 2% per year during a 16 years of follow-up report (Lahner et al., 2015). It is understood that GC ranks fourth in the global incidence of various cancers worldwide and is the second cause of cancer-related deaths (Topi et al., 2020). *Helicobacter pylori* (*H. pylori*) is an obligate pathogen in the stomach, and the persistent inflammatory response caused by colonization is the strongest single risk factor for GC (Schulz et al., 2019). It has been recognized by the World Health Organization as a "definite carcinogen" since 1994, and the evidence for its role in gastric cancer (GC) development was expanded and updated in 2012 (Crafa et al., 2018). The risk of carcinogenic risk is closely related to the strain-specific bacterial components, host immune responses and effective drug intervention. Therefore, while focusing on the prevention of gastric cancer risk in people with *H. pylori* infection, delineating the drug treatment and mechanisms for gastric inflammation has profound significance for greatly reducing the incidence of CAG and GC.

Palmatine (Pal, **Figure 2A**) is an isoquinoline alkaloid from *Coptidis rhizoma* (Huanglian in Chinese), and is classified as an anti-inflammatory drug in Chinese Pharmacopeia (Tarabasz and Kukula-Koch, 2020). It can be used to relieve bacterial dysentery, gynecological inflammation and urinary tract-related surgical infections on clinic (Yokozawa et al., 2005; Wang et al., 2017). It has been the subject of scientific interest in recent years due to its multiple antibacterial, antiviral, and gastrointestinal protection biological activities (Li et al., 2018; Chen et al., 2020). However, the largely potential anti-gastritis mechanism of Pal remain unknown, and whether Pal can be safely and effectively used in clinical still needs more investigation.

Recently, omics techniques, such as transcriptomics, proteomics, and metabolomics have been widely used to identify potential disease markers and elucidate biologically related mechanisms. Metabolite profiling provides a clearer explanation of the relationship between drug efficacy, pharmacological effects, and metabolic pathways by analyzing specific biomarkers during disease and drug treatment. It has shown great potential in many life science fields, such as toxicology, disease diagnosis, drug mechanism research and natural product discovery (Wang et al., 2011). Previous studies have shown that *H. pylori* infection causes various metabolic alterations at lesional sites associated with disease transformation attribution. (Nishiumi et al., 2017). To the best of our knowledge, although the metabolites of Pal *in vivo* have been analyzed for quality evaluation or pharmacological activity (Wang et al., 2017), the analysis of Pal and its metabolitesmetabolite changes in *H. pylori*-induced gastritis individuals is currently lacking.

All the considerations above prompted the application of metabolomics to comprehensively explore the gastrointestinal toxicity of Pal and its protective effect on *H. pylori*-induced CAG. In this study, serum biochemical indicators and pathological observations were used to evaluate theameliorative effect of Pal on CAG. UPLC-Q-TOF/MS metabolomics research was applied to obtain and analyze the changes of different metabolites in urine and serum during Pal therapy (**Figure 1**). Finally, it systematically clarified the modulatory properties of Pal on *H. pylori*-induced CAG, and further confirmed the feasibility of Pal for treatment of *H. pylori*-induced CAG.

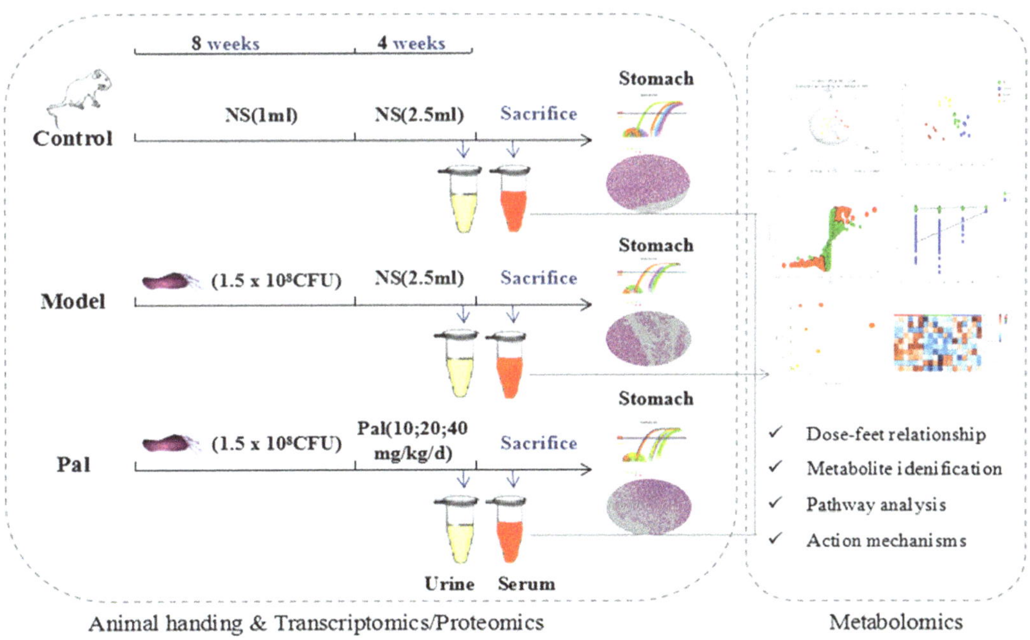

FIGURE 1 | Scheme of the study.

MATERIALS AND METHODS

Chemicals and Reagents

Pal standard ($C_{21}H_{25}NO_4$, purity > 90%, Cat. No.10605-02-4) was purchased from Chroma Biotechnology Co. Ltd (Chengdu, China). Dissolved it into normal saline (NS 0.9%) and diluted to the corresponding concentration for later use.

H. pylori Strains and Growth Condition

H. pylori strain was kindly provided by Prof. Jianzhong which was isolated from CAG patient (No. ZCDC111001). Columbia agar plates (Thermo Fisher Scientific Co., Ltd., Beijing, China) was used for bacterial propagation and shake for 48–72 h under the microaerobic conditions (6% O2, 7.2% CO2, 7.1% H2, 79.7% N2) of Low Oxygen Cell Culture Jar (UNITECH Co., Ltd., Guangzhou, China).

Animals

Male Sprague Dawley (SD) rats (180 ± 20 g) were purchased from Sibeifu Biotechnology Co., Ltd. (Permission No. SCXK (jing) 2016-0002, Beijing, China). Rats were adapted the specific environment (humidity: 55% ± 5%, temperature: 25°C ± 0.5°C and 12-h/12-h light/dark cycle) and given sufficient sterile food and water for 2 weeks. All experimental procedures have been reviewed and approved by the Animal Ethical and Experimental Committee of the Fifth Medical Center of PLA General Hospital (Approval ID: IACUC-2018-010) and strictly implemented in accordance with the "Guide for the Care and Use of Laboratory Animals" (https://grants.nih.gov/grants/olaw/guide-for-the-care-and-use-of-laboratory-animals.pdf).

Induction of CAG

CAG model was induced by *H. pylori* as previously described (Werawatganon, 2014). Live bacteria were collected and adjusted to 1.5×10^8 colony forming units (CFU)/ml with normal saline (NS). Rats were administered with *H. pylori* strains at 1 day intervals to induce CAG model. Hematoxylin and eosin (H & E) staining and a rapid urease kit were used to evaluate the inflammation of stomach tissue at 8 weeks of infection. After CAG model was successfully duplicated, animals were randomly assigned into five groups (n = 6/group): Control group, Model group, Pal group (PalL PalM, PalH = 10, 20, 40 mg/kg/day) respectively. A normal diet was maintained during the 4 weeks of Pal treatment. In this study, the doses of Pal was referenced to previous experiments (Jung et al., 2014).

Sample Collection and Preparation

At the end of the experiment, each rat was put into a metabolic cage (1 per cage) to collect 24-h urine and then sacrificed rats to obtain blood from aorta abdominalis.

Collected the gastric tissue and cut along the large curvature of the stomach, soaked in 10% neutral formalin buffer and embedded in paraffin to observe the pathological changes. The blood was centrifuged at 3.5×10^3 rpm for 12 min to separate the serum and transferred to −8°C for storage before biochemical parameters and metabolomics analysis.

Histopathological Analysis

Cuted 3–5μm thick paraffin slice of stomach tissue. H & E staining was performed for highlighting the pathological damage and inflammation of stomach tissues. The test result was observed with a light microscope (200 ×, 400 × magnifications).

Measurement of Cytokine Concentrations

Serum was stored at −80°C before to cytokine determination. The levels of Pepsinogen I (PG I), Pepsinogen II (PG II), Gastrin17 (G-17) and Ghrelin were quantified by ELISA kits (MLBIO biotechnology Co., Ltd., Shanghai, China) according to the protocols provided by the manufacturer. Synergy H1 Hybrid Reader (Biotek, Winooski, VT, USA) was used to measure the absorbance at 450 nm.

Quantitative RT-PCR

Total RNA was extracted from stomach tissues by using Trizol reagent (Nordic Bioscience, Beijing, China) and then converted into cDNA by reverse transcription kit (Promega, Madison, USA). RT-PCR was selected SYBR Green PCR Master Mix (Nordic Bioscience, Beijing, China) and executed on QuantSTUDIO TM 6 Flex System (Applied Biosystems, Foster City, CA, USA). The level of mRNA was normalized to GAPDH expression based on $2^{-\Delta\Delta CT}$ method. The primers sequences of IFN-γ, Ghrelin, Epithelial cadherin (E-Cadherin), Desmoglein 2 (DSG 2), Zonula occludens-1 (ZO-1) and Mucin 1(Muc1) were listed in **Table 1**.

Immunohistochemistry/ Immunofluorescence

Paraffin sections of stomach tissues were stained with anti-E-Cadherin, anti-DSG 2, anti-ZO-1, anti-Muc1 Ab (**Table 2**) for IHC/immunofluorescence (IF), and lastly examined using NIS Elements Imaging Software Version 4.0 (Olympus, Japan).

TABLE 1 | Primers sequences.

Gene	Forward primer	Reverse primer
Rat IFN-γ	ACAACCCACAGATCCAGCACAAAG	GCTTCCTTAGGCTAGATTCTGGTGAC
Rat Ghrelin	CCAGAAAGCCCAGCAGAGAAAGG	ACATCGAAGGGAGCATTGAACCTG
Rat E-Cadherin	CCTACAATGCTGCCATCGCCTAC	GGGTAACTCTCTCGGTCCAGTCC
Rat Dsg2	CGGAGTGTCTGTGCGGATGC	GGCTGGTCAATGATGGAGAAGGTG
Rat ZO-1	CGCAGCCAGTTCAAACAAAGTTCC	GCAACATCAGCAATCGGTCCAAAG
Rat Muc1	GCCCATCTCTCCCACCATCCC	GGAAGACCGCTGTGCTGTAGTAAG

TABLE 2 | Antibodies and other reagents.

Antibodies	Dilution rate	Manufacturers	Cat.No.
For IHC			
Rabbit anti-Rat Desmoglein2/ DSG2	1/250–1/500	Abcam	ab150372
Rabbit anti-Rat ZO-1 tight junction	1/500	Abcam	ab221547
Rabbit anti-Rat E-Cadherin	1:50–1:200	Cell signaling technology	14472
For IF			
Rabbit anti-Rat Muc1	1/500	Abcam	ab45167

Metabolic Profiling

The serum and urine samples were thawed at room temperature prior to analysis. Added three times methanol to serum or urine and centrifuged at 12,000 rpm for 12 min to precipitate the protein. Collected the supernatant filtrate with nylon filter. Ten microliter of each sample was mixed to prepare quality control (QC), and the remaining samples were used for UPLC-Q-TOF/MS testing.

An Agilent 1290 series UHPLC system (Agilent Technologies, Santa Clara, CA, USA) system was used for serum and urine metabolic profiling analysis. ZORBOX RRHD C18 analytical column (2.1 mm × 100 mm, 1.8 µm., Agilent Technologies, Santa Clara, CA, USA) was used for sample separation at 30°C. The injection volume was 4 µl and flow rate was 0.30ml/min. Solvent A (0.1% formic acid in acetonitrile) and solvent B (0.1% formic acid in water) were mixed into a gradient mobile phase under a 25-min gradient program: 0–1.0 min (95% A); 1.0–9.0 min (95%–60% A); 9.0–19.0 min (60%–10%); 19.0–21.0 min (10%–0% A); 21.0–25.0 min (100% B). Each sample is injected only once, a QC sample and a blank were injected after every 10 samples to ensure the stability and repeatability of the system. Both positive and negative mode electrospray ionization sources (ESI) were used (Electrospray capillary voltage: 4.0kV in ESI+ and 3.5 kV in ESI-; Mass range: 50 to 1,200 m/z; Gas flow:13 L/min; Nebulizer: 20 psi; Sheath gas temperature: 275°C; Sheath gas flow: 12 L/min; Nozzle voltage: 2,000V) in this study.

Data Extraction and Multivariate Analysis

Sample data was extracted by using MassHunter Profinder software (version B.06.00; Agilent, Santa Clara, CA, USA) for analysis and comparison. Data was normalized with MetaboAnalyst 4.0 and then SIMCA-P V14.1 (Umetrics, Umea, Sweden) was used for principal component analysis (PCA) and orthogonal-partial least squares-discriminant analysis (OPLS-DA). The potential biomarkers were identified based on precise molecular weight in the Human Metabolome Database (HMDB) and METLIN (http://metlin.scripps.edu/) database. MetaboAnalyst 4.0 (http://www.metaboanalyst.ca/) was visualized enrichment pathway of potential markers.

Statistical Analysis

Statistical analysis was performed by SPSS 20.0 software program (Chicago, IL, USA) using one-way ANOVA followed by t-test. GraphPad Prism software (version 6.02; Inc., San Diego, USA) was used to visualize the results. $P < 0.05$ was considered statistically significant.

RESULTS

Pal Attenuated Pathological Damage and Inflammation in H. pylori–Induced CAG

During *H. pylori* infection, rats infected with *H. pylori* developed symptoms of inappetence, diarrhea, and the weight gain trend of the model group was markedly slower than control group during the whole experiment (**Figure 2B**). In addition, the positive results of the rapid urease kit proved the reliability of the model (**Figure 2C**). The pathological result showed that the epithelial cells of gastric mucosa in control group were arranged neatly without shedding, and the morphology of submucosal was normal; model group was characterized by thin mucosa and partial mucosa shedding, submucosal edema and eosinophil infiltration in the stomach, atrophy of glands at the junction of the anterior and posterior stomach and reduction of inherent glands (**Figure 2D**). Those changes were similar to CAG patients caused by *H. pylori* in clinic. After 4 weeks of Pal intervention, the body weight of CAG rats gradually recovered, and the pathological gastric mucosal damage was significantly reduced (**Figure 2D**), suggesting that Pal had a significant protective effect on CAG induced by *H. pylori*.

Pal Improved Biomarkers in Serum of H. pylori–Induced CAG

To clarify the activities of several specific markers of *H. pylori*–induced CAG rats, the serum supernatant levels of serum PG I, PG II, and G-17 were estimated. As showed in **Figure 3**, PG I, PG II, PG I/PG II, and G-17 decreased markedly in *H. pylori*–induced model group compared to control group. Conversely, PG I, PG II, and G-17 significantly increased after Pal administration, and the above biomarkers in the PalH group maintained higher levels compared with the PalL group (**Figures 3A–D**). In addition, Pal reversed the decrease in the ratio of PG I/PG II induced by *H. pylori* in the model group, which was more obvious in PalH group (**Figure 3C**). Altogether, these results *in vivo* implied that the activities of several specific markers, including PG I, PG II, and G-17, and the ratio of PG I/PG II, could get dose-dependently improved by Pal intervention.

Pal Relieved the Release Disorder of Ghrelin by Inhibiting IFN-γ

To test whether the CAG rat model induced by *H. pylori* was IFN-γ associated inflammation and would further change the expression of ghrelin, the expression of IFN-γ and ghrelin in stomach and serum were evaluated by RT-PCR and ELISA respectively. Results were presented in **Figure 4**. Evidently, the significant increase of IFN-γ expression in stomach of *H. pylori* infected rats was accompanied by a decrease in the expression of ghrelin, while the concentration of ghrelin in serum was also significantly reduced (**Figures 4A–C**). Accordingly, these

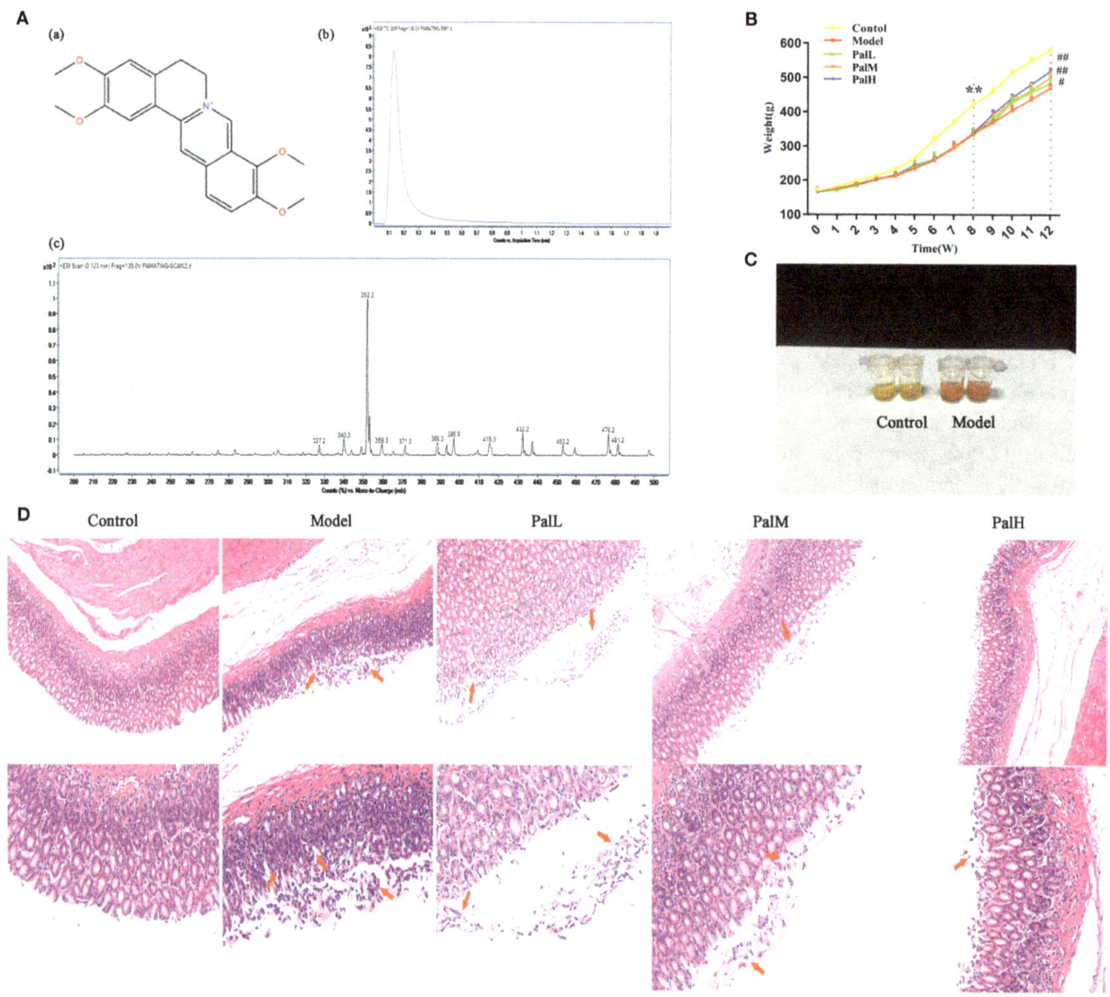

FIGURE 2 | Pal attenuated pathological damage and inflammation in *H. pylori*–induced chronic atrophic gastritis (CAG). **(A)** Chemical structure (a), TIC (b) and Scan (c) chromatogram of Pal. **(B)** Weight of SD rats (n=6). **(C)** Rapid urease test of stomach tissues. **(D)** Morphology and hematoxylin and eosin (H & E) staining of rats stomach (200 × and 400 × magnification). $^{**}P < 0.01$ vs control group. $^{\#}P < 0.05$ and $^{\#\#}P < 0.01$ vs model group. PalL (10 mg/kg); PalM: (20 mg/kg); PalH: (40 mg/kg).

findings indicated that IFN-γ inflammatory response and impaired production of ghrelin in the stomach are associated with CAG induced by *H. pylori*, which ultimately leads to a decrease in the concentration of serum ghrelin (**Figure 4D**). However, Pal could dose-dependently reduced the level of IFN-γ gene and alleviated the release of ghrelin. Consequently, the above results suggested that Pal could restore ghrelin expression by inhibiting IFN-γ and had anti-inflammatory properties in CAG induced by *H. pylori*.

Pal Protected Mucosal Integrity by Modulating Epithelial Junctions and Mucins

To further evaluated the protective effect of Pal on the gastric mucosa of CAG rats induced by *H. pylori*, the mRNA expression of ZO-1, E-cadherin, DSG2, Muc1 were detected using RT-PCR. The results show that the expression of the above mentioned mRNA in the model group was significantly downregulated compared with the control group. However, Pal significantly reversed the inhibitory effect of *H. pylori* (**Figures 5A–D**).

Subsequently, the protein expression of ZO-1, E-cadherin, DSG2, Muc1 were measured to evaluate the integrity on gastric mucosa epithelium. The results showed that all proteins were reduced in model group, indicating that the gastric mucosa epithelium structure was disrupted. In contrast, Pal promoted the expression of ZO-1, E-cadherin, DSG2 and increased the fluorescence intensity of Muc1, and there was a statistically significant difference between the PalH group and the model group (**Figures 5E, F**). Therefore, Pal could protect mucosal integrity by modulating epithelial junctions and mucins, and PalH group was selected for subsequent metabolomics analysis.

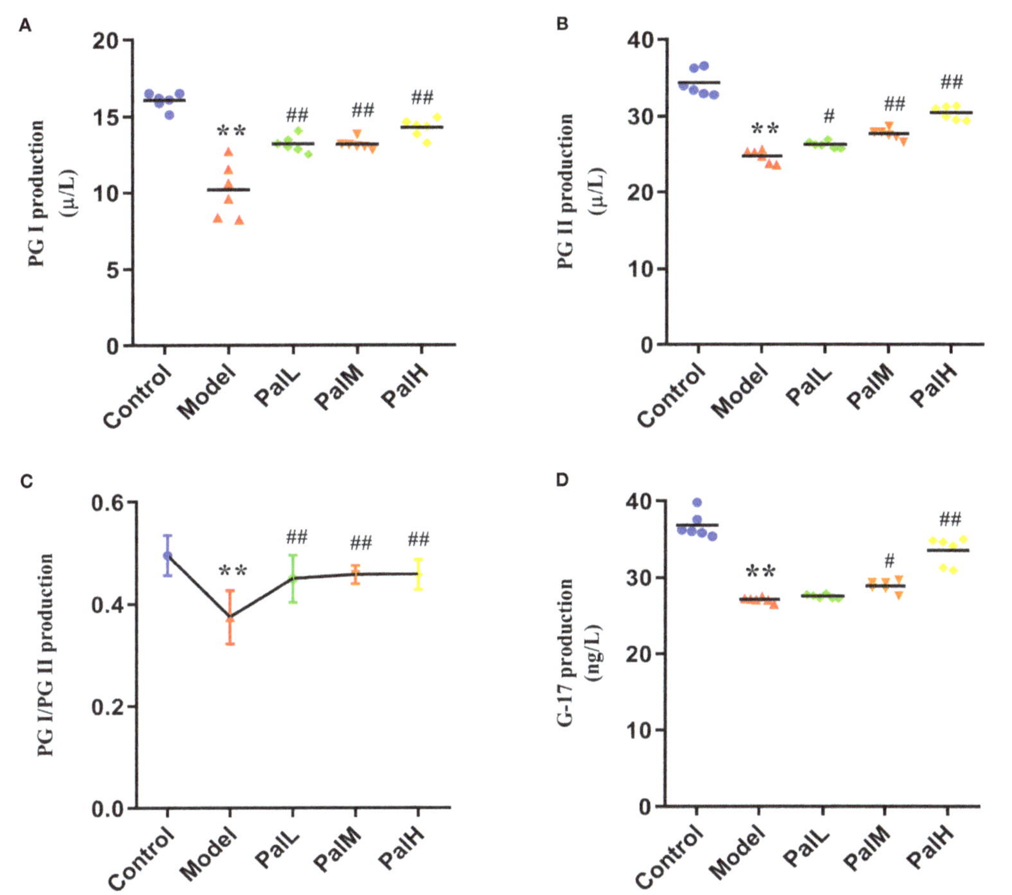

FIGURE 3 | Pal improves biomarkers in serum of *H. pylori*–induced chronic atrophic gastritis (CAG). **(A–D)** PG I **(A)**, PG II **(B)**, PG I/PG II **(C)**, and G-17 **(D)** production in serum was measured by ELISA (n=6). $^{**}P < 0.01$ vs control group. $^{\#}P < 0.05$ and $^{\#\#}P < 0.01$ vs model group. PalL (10 mg/kg); PalM: (20 mg/kg); PalH: (40 mg/kg).

Serum Metabolomics Analysis

PCA is an unsupervised pattern recognition approach used to reduce the dimension of UPLC-MS data and to disclose intrinsic clustering of samples. In this study, PCA was used to summarize and distinguish the metabolic phenotypes and metabolites between control, model, and PalH group in both ESI+ and ESI- models. QC can confirm whether the systematic error of the experiment is within the controllable range. The cluster analysis of QC suggested that the method was stability and repeatability. The PCA score plots showed that clear separations were observed among the clusters of the control, model and PalH group in both ESI+ and ESI– modes (**Figure 6**), which indicated *H. pylori*–induced remarkable changes in serum endogenous metabolites and Pal could restore the metabolic profiling of serum in CAG rats. The R^2X of ESI+ and ESI– PCA models confirmed the credibility of these two models. Thus, the CAG model was successful, and could be used to explore the effects of Pal on CAG induced by *H. pylori*. Subsequently, Summarized the influence of variables on the model according to the corresponding loading scores plots from PCA, multivariate analysis was used to explore specific differential metabolites.

The differential metabolites from control vs model group and model vs PalH group were identified in OPLS-DA mode respectively. The relevant parameter of OPLS-DA model and permutation tests (n=100) demonstrated that the modes had good predictive capabilities. Obvious classifications were observed among control, model and PalH groups in both of ESI+ and ESI- modes. Metabolites that meet a threshold of VIP ≥ 1.0 and | P (corr) | ≥ 0.58 in the corresponding S-plot were considered potential candidates (**Figure 7**). Combined the potential candidates obtained in ESI+ and ESI–. Based on ANOVA analysis ($P < 0.05$), candidates with significant changes were identified as biomarkers in the METLIN and Metaboanalyst databases. Finally, three biomarkers were screened in serum, and relevant information and variation trends between groups were listed in **Table 3** and **Figure 8**.

Urine Metabolomics Analysis

To further explored the overall metabolism in the urine of the CAG, PCA approach was applied to distinguish the metabolic phenotypes and metabolites between control, model, and PalH

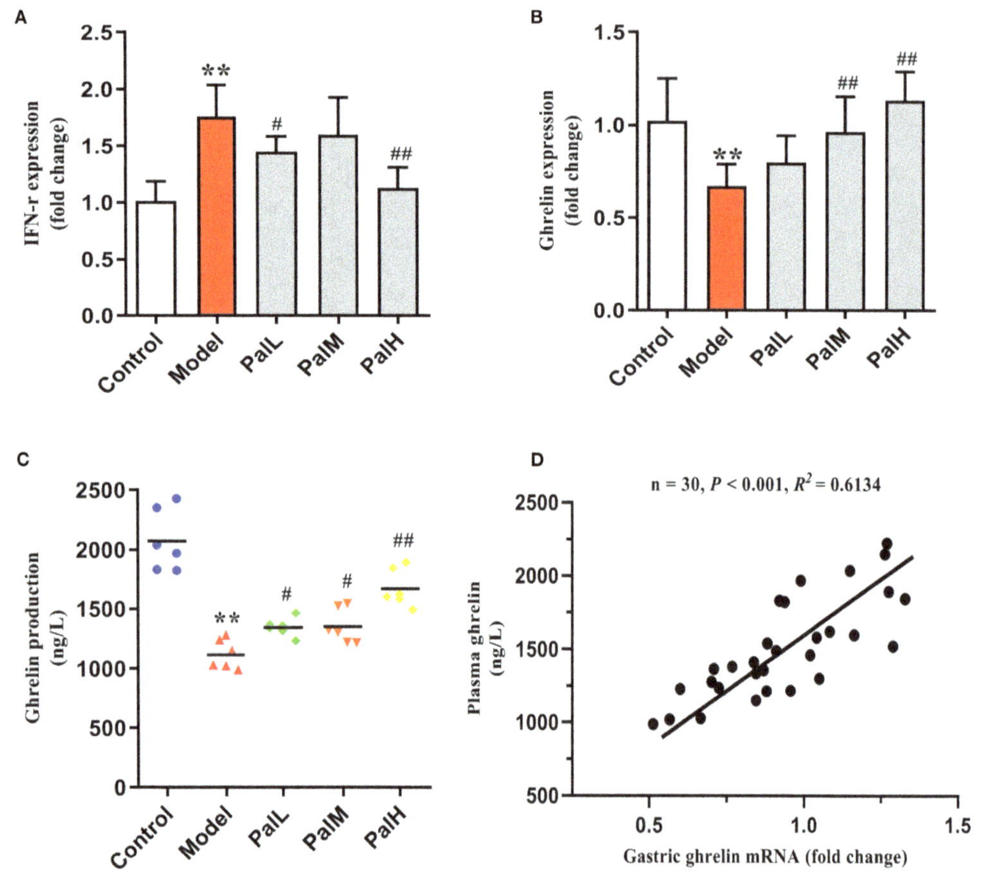

FIGURE 4 | Pal relieved the release disorder of ghrelin by inhibiting IFN-γ. **(A, B)** IFN-γ and ghrelin mRNA in gastric mucosa were analyzed by RT-PCR (n=6). **(C)** ghrelin production in serum was measured by ELISA (n=6). **(D)** Pearson correlation coefficient analysis of ghrelin expression in gastric mucosa and serum. ***P* < 0.01 vs control group. #*P* < 0.05 and ##*P* < 0.01 vs model group. PalL (10 mg/kg); PalM: (20 mg/kg); PalH: (40 mg/kg).

groups. The R^2X of ESI+ and ESI− in PCA models confirmed the reliability of these two models. The PCA score plots indicated remarkable changes of endogenous metabolites in urine induced by *H. pylori* and Pal could restore the metabolic profiling of urine in CAG rats (**Figure 9**).

OPLS-DA score plots showed that the metabolic profile of the model group deviated from control group, and PalH group in both of ESI+ and ESI- modes, suggesting that significant biochemical changes were induced by CAG. The relevant parameter of OPLS-DA mode and permutation tests (n = 100) demonstrated that the modes had good explanatory and predictive capabilities (**Figure 10**). Combined the potential candidates obtained in ESI+ and ESI-, and further determined biomarkers by using ANOVA analysis. Finally, the seven biomarkers in urine were summarized. **Table 3** and **Figure 8** listed the corresponding formulations, quality (m/z), retention time and change trend of each group.

Pathway Analysis of Pal Treatment

The hierarchical cluster analysis heatmap generated according to the relative concentration of metabolic markers in serum and urine can intuitively displayed the differences in metabolic profiles between different samples (**Figure 11A**). Metabo Analyst 4.0 was performed for pathway analysis to visualize the affected metabolic pathways in CAG rats. As shown in **Table 4** and **Figure 11**, Taurine and hypotaurine metabolism, Glycerophospholipid metabolism, Pentose and glucuronate interconversions were considered as the crucial signaling pathways in CAG and Pal treatment. In addition, the related metabolic pathways crosstalk with each other by the citric acid (TCA) cycle. The match status, *P* value, log(P) and impact of each pathway were listed in **Table 4**.

DISCUSSION

Huang Lian has been applied to endocrine system and gastrointestinal diseases in clinic for thousands of years (Zou et al., 2017; Ma et al., 2019). More and more studies regarding the effects of the active ingredients in HuangLian on gastrointestinal diseases is available. Previous studies have shown that Pal and

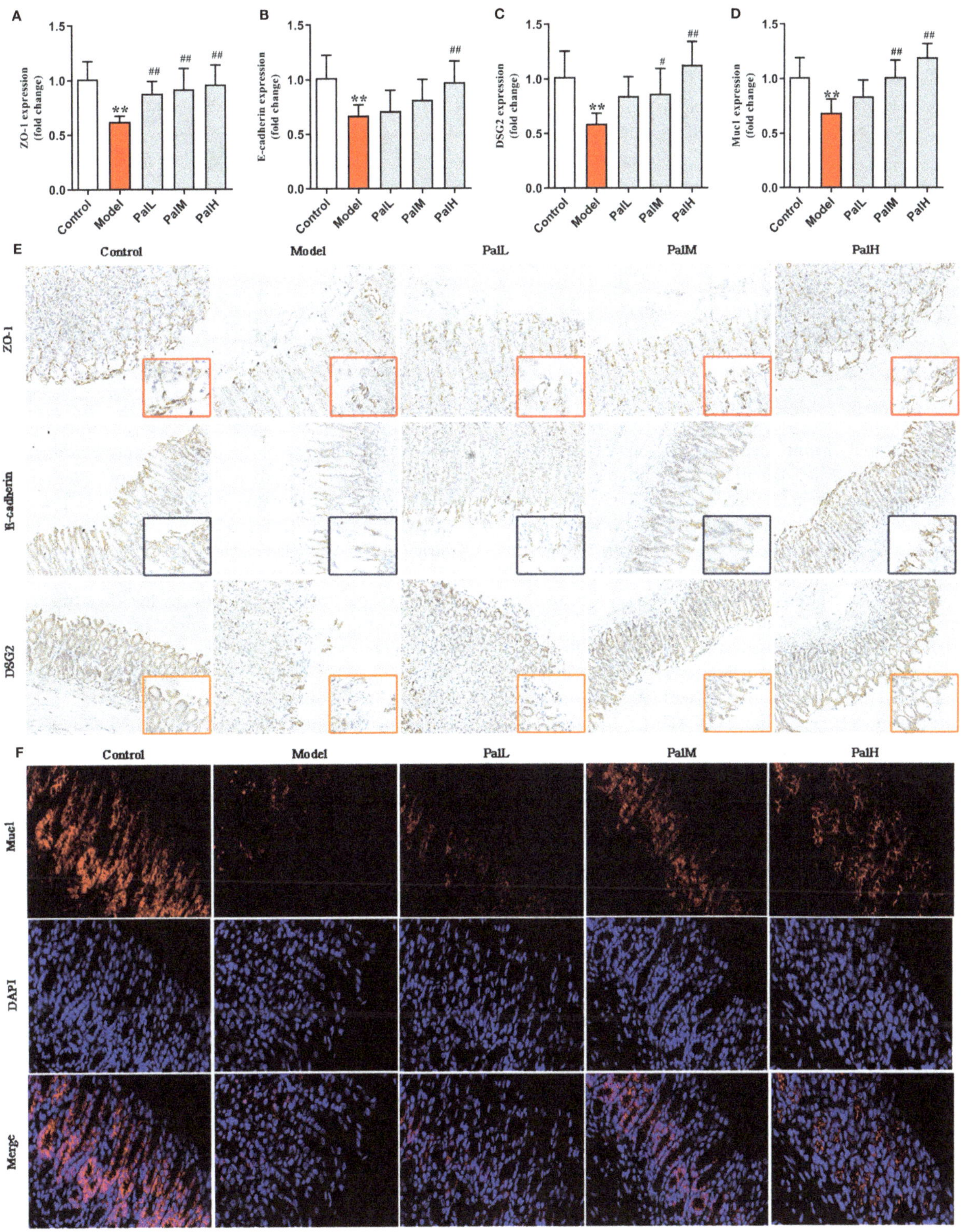

FIGURE 5 | Pal protected mucosal integrity by modulating epithelial junctions and mucins. **(A–D)** ZO-1 **(A)**, E-cadherin **(B)**, Desmoglein 2 (DSG 2) **(C)** and Muc1 **(D)** mRNA in gastric mucosa were analyzed by RT-PCR (n=6). **(E)** Representative immunohistochemical staining images in gastric mucosa showing ZO-1, E-cadherin, DSG2 expressing (200 × and 400 × magnification). **(F)** Representative immunofluorescence staining images in gastric mucosa showing Muc1 expressing (400 × magnification). $^{**}P < 0.01$ vs control group. $^{\#}P < 0.05$ and $^{\#\#}P < 0.01$ vs model group. PalL (10 mg/kg); PalM: (20 mg/kg); PalH: (40 mg/kg).

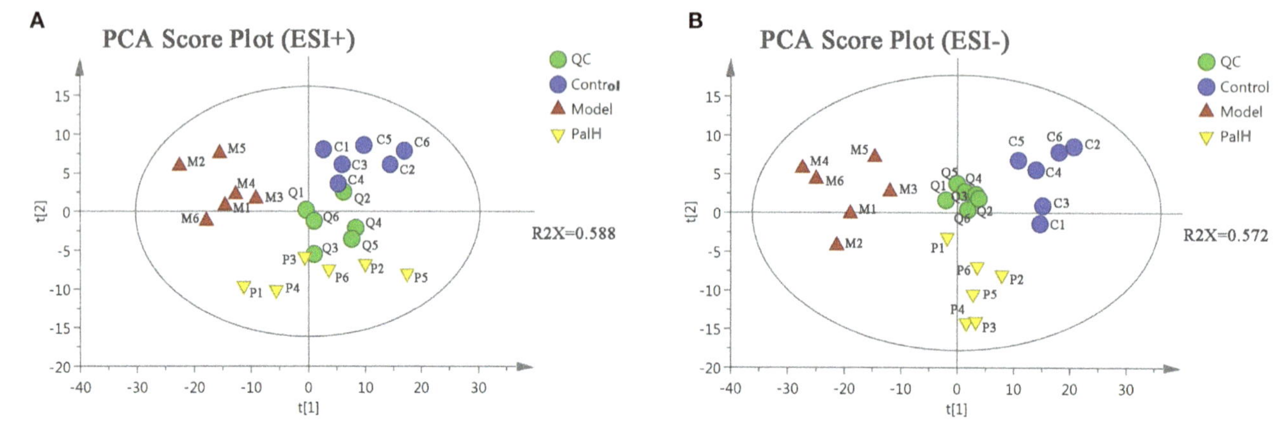

FIGURE 6 | The principal component analysis (PCA) score plot of serum metabolomics analysis. **(A)** ESI+ model. **(B)** ESI- model. PalH: (40 mg/kg).

berberine inhibited the proliferation of gastric cancer cells (MGC803) in a dose-dependent manner and the inhibitory effect more significantly in combination with berberine (Zhao and Zhang, 2011). Jung J et al. demonstrated the antibacterial activity of Pal and its protective effect on gastric injury through the *H. pylori* colony formation experiment and the hydrochloric acid/ ethanol induced gastric ulcer model, and the efficacy is better than berberine (Jung et al., 2014). Moreover, Pal was confirmed to have a clear antibacterial activity against *H. pylori* in a molecular docking simulation experiment (Zhou et al., 2017). Therefore, Pal is considered to be a promising non-antibiotic drug candidate for the treatment of *H. pylori*-induced CAG.

H. pylori-induced gastritis is one of the optimized models used to study CAG. As in humans, weight loss, inappetence, diarrhea, and pathological changes in rats are usually consistent symptoms of CAG (Kishikawa et al., 2020). Given that the intractable characteristic and high morbidity of CAG, UPLC-Q-TOF/MS method based on serum combined with urin metabolomics was firstly investigated in this study to clarify the protective effect of Pal on CAG and attempted to clarify the mechanisms of action.

Gastric infections due to *H. pylori* overgrowth are associated with reduced fundic ghrelin and G-17 expression and increased IFN-γ production (Strickertsson et al., 2011). Ghrelin plays an essential role in the mechanism of gastric mucosal defense, the reduction of ghrelin production in the fundic is the main reason for the decrease of serum ghrelin concentration, and it is closely related to the ratio of PG I/PG II, in which the PG I/PG II < 3 is considered a reliable sign of severe atrophic gastritis. PG I is secreted only by secretory glands of the corpus mucosa, PG II is synthesized by gastric antrum and duodenum, and G-17 is only expressed by G cells of the antral mucosa. Thus the combination of the results of the PG I, PG II, PG I/PG II and G-17 test can more comprehensively and accurately detect the presence of CAG (Osawa et al., 2005; Zagari et al., 2017). In this study, the model group had high levels of pro-inflammatory cytokines IFN-γ, low levels of ghrelin, G-17, PG I, PG II, and PGI/PGII ratios. However, the levels of biomarkers and proinflammatory cytokines was decreased in Pal treatment revealed that Pal could effectively ameliorate CAG triggered by *H. pylori*.

CAG induced by *H. pylori* is triggered by the destruction of gastric mucosal epithelial barrier function, which further leads to excessive response of immune cells to microbiota. The gastrointestinal mucosa can protect the digestive tract from harmful substances and is an important barrier to maintain environmental stability in the digestive tract (Zhang et al., 2014). This mucosal barrier is predominantly composed of apical junctional complex (AJC) and mucins. AJC include tight junctions (TJs), adherens junctions (AJs) and desmosomes. Muc1 is a prototypical member of the membrane bound mucin subfamily. In this study, the expression and distribution of TJ proteins (ZO-1), AJ proteins (E-cadherin), desmosome protein (DSG2), and Muc1 in gastrointestinal epithelial cells infected with *H. pylori* were systematically investigated. The mRNA and protein expression of AJC and Muc1 were significantly downregulated in the model group, suggesting that *H pylori* breached the mucosal layer and increased the permeability of gastric mucosa. However, Pal promoted the mRNA and protein expression of AJC and Muc1, indicating that Pal could protect the gastric mucosal barrier from the *H.pylori* elicited epithelial structural damage by increasing mucin synthesis and improving epithelial AJC.

Subsequently, UPLC-Q-TOF/MS metabolomic analysis was used to determine the fingerprints of serum and urine metabolic characteristics of GCA rats. PCA and OPLS-DA model showed sufficient sensitivity and specificity to distinguish model from control group. The significant difference between the PalH and model group suggested Pal protected CAG by reversing potential metabolites to normal levels. Meanwhile, the biological function and relevant pathway were identified by HMDB and MetaboAnalyst platform to elucidate the underlying mechanism. 10 related endogenous metabolites were selected as potential biomarkers which were associated with Taurine and hypotaurine metabolism,

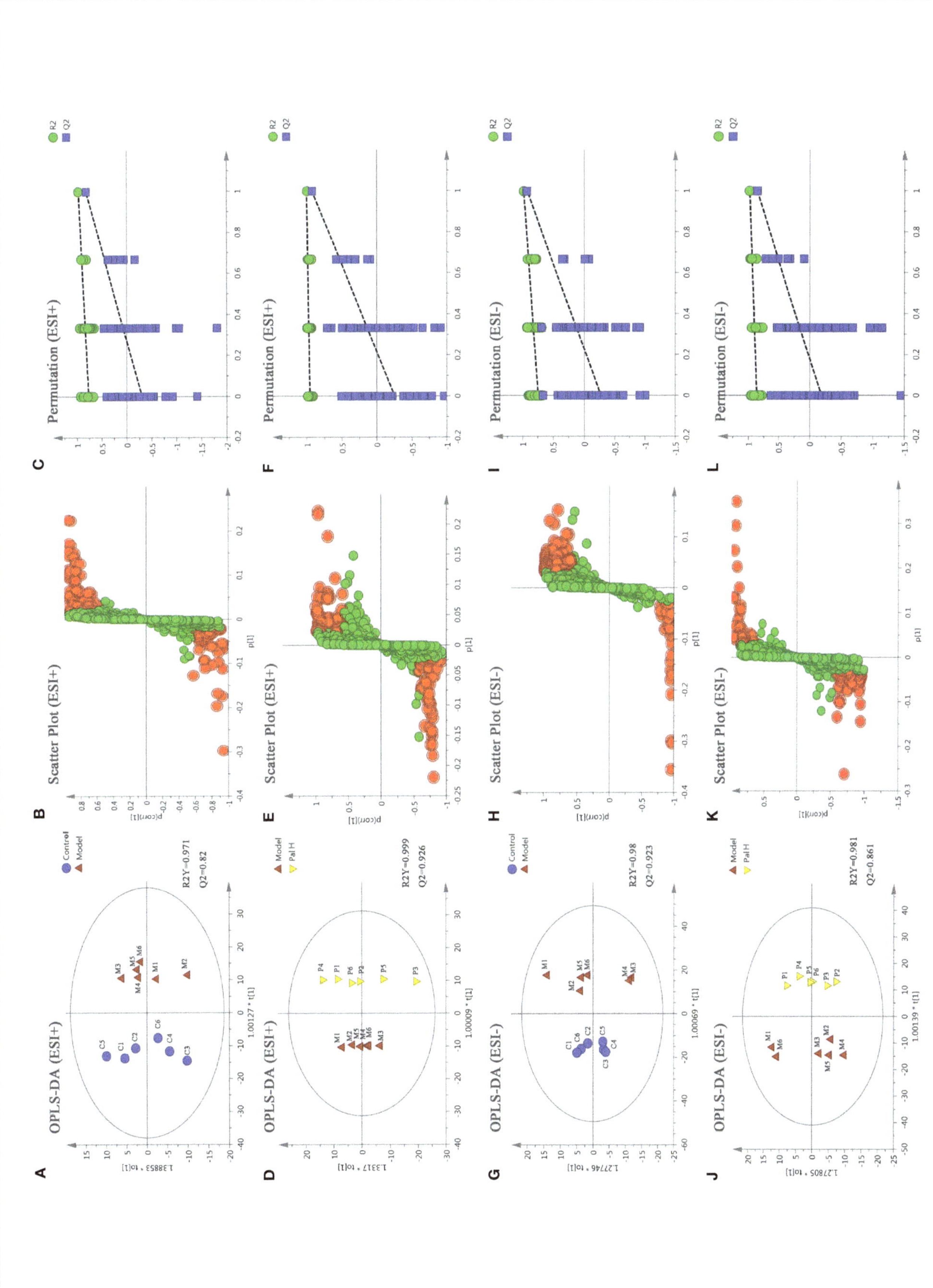

FIGURE 7 | The orthogonal-partial least squares-discriminant analysis (OPLS-DA) score plots, S-plots and 100-permutation test of serum metabolomics analysis. **(A–F)** ESI+ model. **(G–L)** ESI- model. PalH: (40 mg/kg).

TABLE 3 | Identified metabolites of serum and urine.

No	Source	Compound name	Formula	Query mass	Monoisotopic_mass	R.T. (min)	Pathway
1	Serum (ESI+)	Phosphatidylcholine	$C_{46}H_{82}NO_7P$	792.5951	791.5829	7.14	Glycerophospholipid metabolism
2	Serum (ESI-)	LysoPC(16:0/0:0)	$C_{24}H_{50}NO_7P$	496.3396	495.3325	15.35	Glycerophospholipid metabolism
3		Taurine	$C_2H_7NO_3S$	124.0073	125.0147	0.89	Taurine and hypotaurine metabolism; Primary bile acid biosynthesis
4	Urine(ESI +)	Glycerylphosphorylethanolamine	$C_5H_{14}NO_6P$	216.0631	215.0559	5.51	Glycerophospholipid metabolism
5		Pyridoxamine	$C_8H_{12}N_2O_2$	169.0971	168.0898	2.35	Vitamin B6 metabolism
6		Pantetheine	$C_{11}H_{22}N_2O_4S$	279.1318	278.1300	5.39	Pantothenate and CoA biosynthesis
7		Pantothenate	$C_9H_{17}NO_5$	220.1172	219.1107	2.91	Pantothenate and CoA biosynthesis
8		S-Adenosylmethioninamine	$C_{14}H_{23}N_6O_3S$	355.1565	355.1552	0.85	Cysteine and methionine metabolism; Arginine and proline metabolism
9	Urine (ESI-)	β-D-Glucuronoside	$C_{14}H_{18}O_7$	297.0975	298.1053	2.65	Pentose and glucuronate interconversions
10		Oxalosuccinate	$C_6H_6O_7$	189.0038	190.0114	2.72	Citrate cycle (TCA cycle)

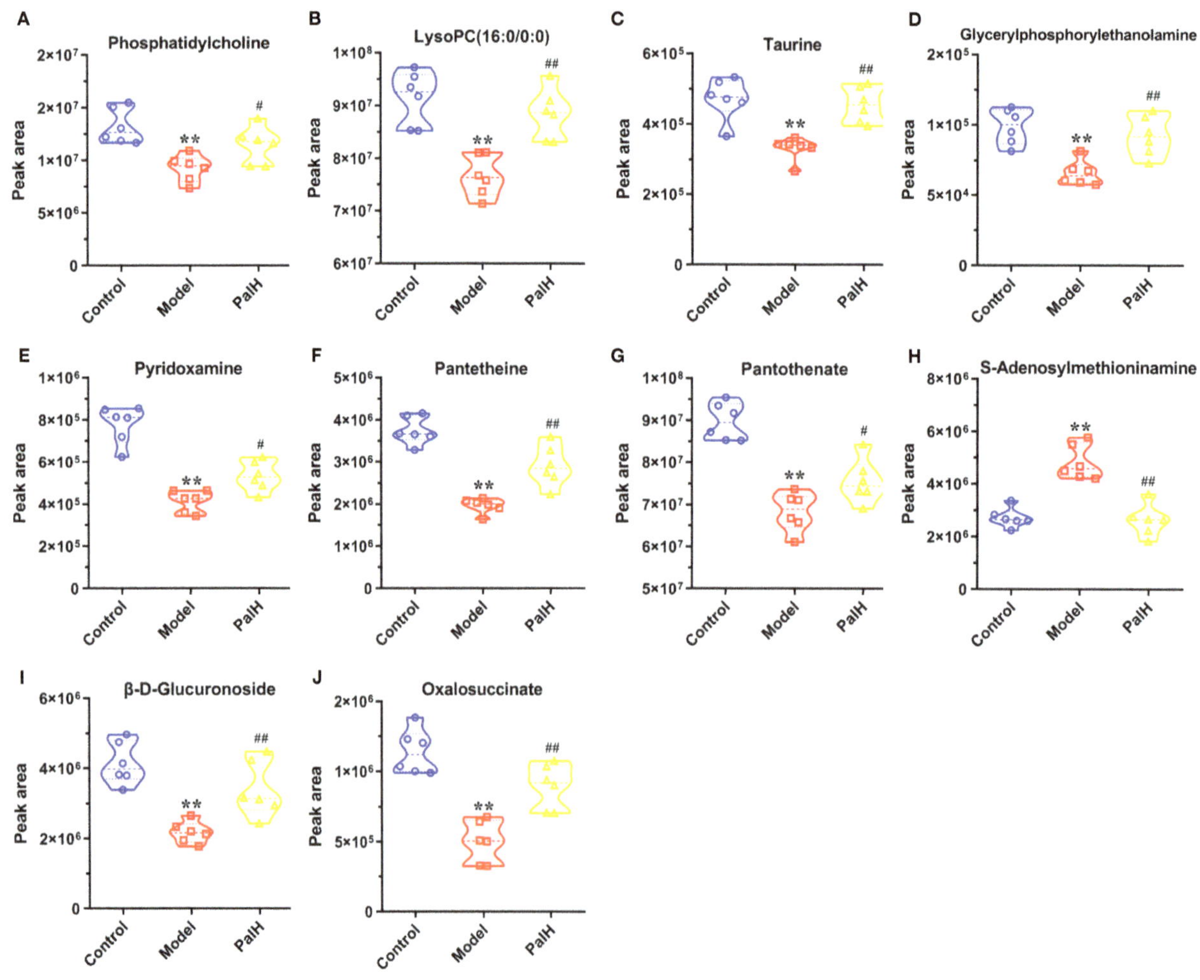

FIGURE 8 | Potential metabolites changes in *H. pylori* - induced CAG with PalH treatment. **(A)** Phosphatidylcholine. **(B)** LysoPC(16:0/0:0). **(C)** Taurine. **(D)** Glycerylphosphorylethanolamine. **(E)** Pyridoxamine. **(F)** Pantetheine. **(G)** Pantothenate. **(H)** S-Adenosylmethioninamine. **(I)** β-D-Glucuronoside. **(J)** Oxalosuccinate. $^{**}P < 0.01$ vs control group. $^{\#}P < 0.05$ and $^{\#\#}P < 0.01$ vs model group. PalH: (40mg / kg).

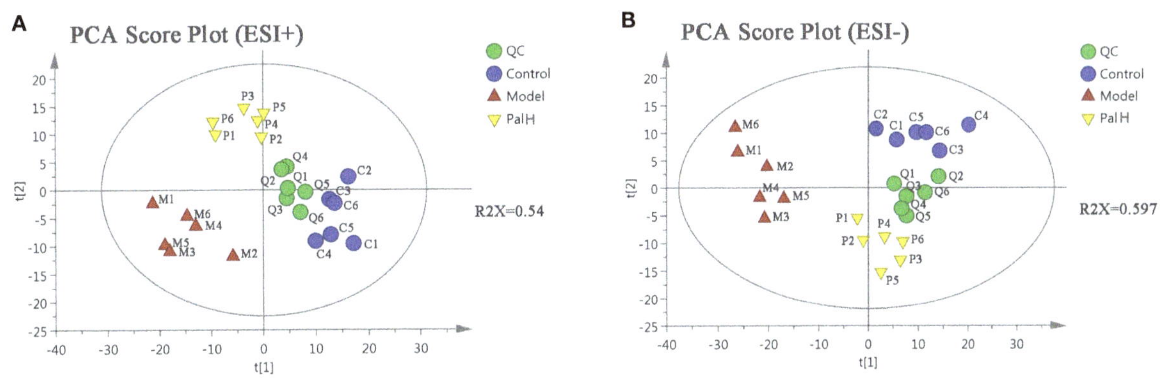

FIGURE 9 | The principal component analysis (PCA) score plot of urine metabolomics analysis. **(A)** ESI+ model. **(B)** ESI- model. PalH: (40 mg/kg).

Glycerophospholipid metabolism, Pentose and glucuronate interconversions, Vitamin B6 metabolism, Pantothenate and CoA biosynthesis, Cysteine and methionine metabolism, Primary bile acid biosynthesis, Arginine and proline metabolism, TCA cycle.

According to the influence value threshold of 0.10, Taurine and hypotaurine metabolism, Glycerophospholipid metabolism, Pentose and glucuronate interconversions are selected as the most relevant pathways. Numerous studies have proved that the disorders of Taurine metabolism play a pivotal pathogenetic role in the initiation and progression of gastrointestinal diseases (Gu et al., 2020). Taurine has been well recognized as an antioxidant both *in vitro* and *in vivo*, and high concentrations of taurine probably contribute to the protection of gastric mucosa from oxidative stress. *H. pylori* infection leads to a decrease in taurine in model rats, indicating that the antioxidant activity decreased in the course of CAG. Glycerophospholipid metabolism was continually disturbed during CAG which has been demonstrated to be closely associated with the immune response. Glycerophospholipid levels are significantly reduced in GCA patients, indicated the disease related dysfunction in glycerophospholipid metabolism (Sun et al., 2020). As one of the subcategories of carbohydrate metabolism, Pentose and glucuronate interconversions is the basis for providing more carbohydrates to the gastrointestinal tract to resist the more complex environment caused by *H. pylori*. In this study, immune dysfunction and energy metabolism disorders together provide a favorable environment for the colonization of *H. pylori*. Pal has a significant callback function on related biomarkers, which may help to improve the CAG induced by *H. pylori*.

Vitamin B6 (VB6) metabolism is necessary to maintain normal physiological functions *in vivo*. Studies have shown that VB6 participates in cellular and humoral immunity during the process of immune response. VB6 deficiency can cause a decline in immunity and affect the expression of certain inflammatory factors (IFN-γ, IL-8), and plays an important role in inflammation caused by gastrointestinal injury (Zhou et al., 2019). As a multifactorial disease, gastrointestinal diseases is ultimately caused by the imbalance between acid secretion and cytoprotective factors. Pantothenate and Pantetheine are important metabolite of Pantothenate and CoA biosynthesis, which are significantly reduced metabolites in gastric ulcers, suggesting Pantothenate and CoA biosynthesis was closely related to the progress of gastrointestinal diseases (Farrokhi et al., 2019). The balance of amino acid metabolism often determines the progression of the disease. In this study, CAG caused an increase in S-adenosylmethionine indicated the imbalance of Cysteine and methionine metabolism and Arginine and proline metabolism. Arginine and proline are considered as potential plasma biomarkers of gastric injury, which can monitor various physiological and pathological conditions of the gastrointestinal tract in real time (Shin et al., 2019). High levels of amino acids is a nutritional requirements for growth of *H. pylori* (Nedenskov, 1994). Turning to another obviously affected amino acid, taurine also affects Primary bile acid biosynthesis. The synthesis and secretion of bile acids are blocked resulting in excessive bacterial growth and impaired epithelial barrier function (AJC and Mcu1), further promoting bacterial transmembrane invasion. It was worth noting that, similar to previous studies, the TCA cycle was down-regulated in this study (Nishiumi et al., 2017). As a critical metabolic checkpoint in the pathological environment, TCA cycle drives a variety of important metabolic pathways and eventually forms a closely related interactive network.

In summary, Pal could reverse the metabolic disorder caused by CAG induced by *H. pylori*, destroy the favorable conditions of *H. pylori* colonization, maintain the gastric mucosal epithelial barrier, restore the immune function of the body, and effectively curb the rapid development of CAG (**Figure 11C**).

CONCLUSION

This study was the first to systematically explore the efficacy and molecular mechanism of Pal in the treatment of CAG induced by *H. pylori* based on serum and urine metabolomics. The results

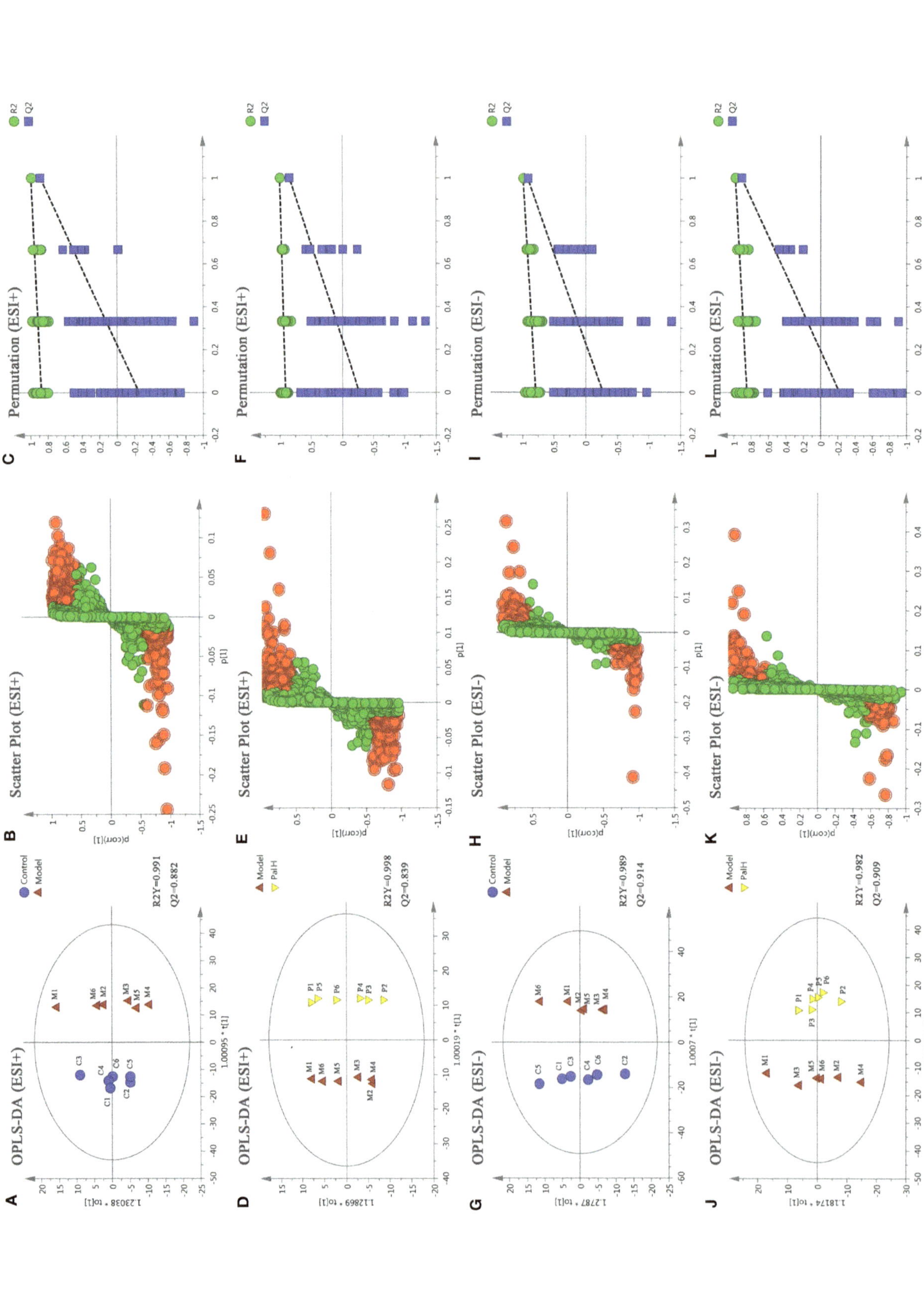

FIGURE 10 | The orthogonal-partial least squares-discriminant analysis (OPLS-DA) score plots, S-plots and 100-permutation test of serum metabolomics analysis. **(A–F)** ESI+ model. **(G–L)** ESI- model. PalH: (40 mg/kg).

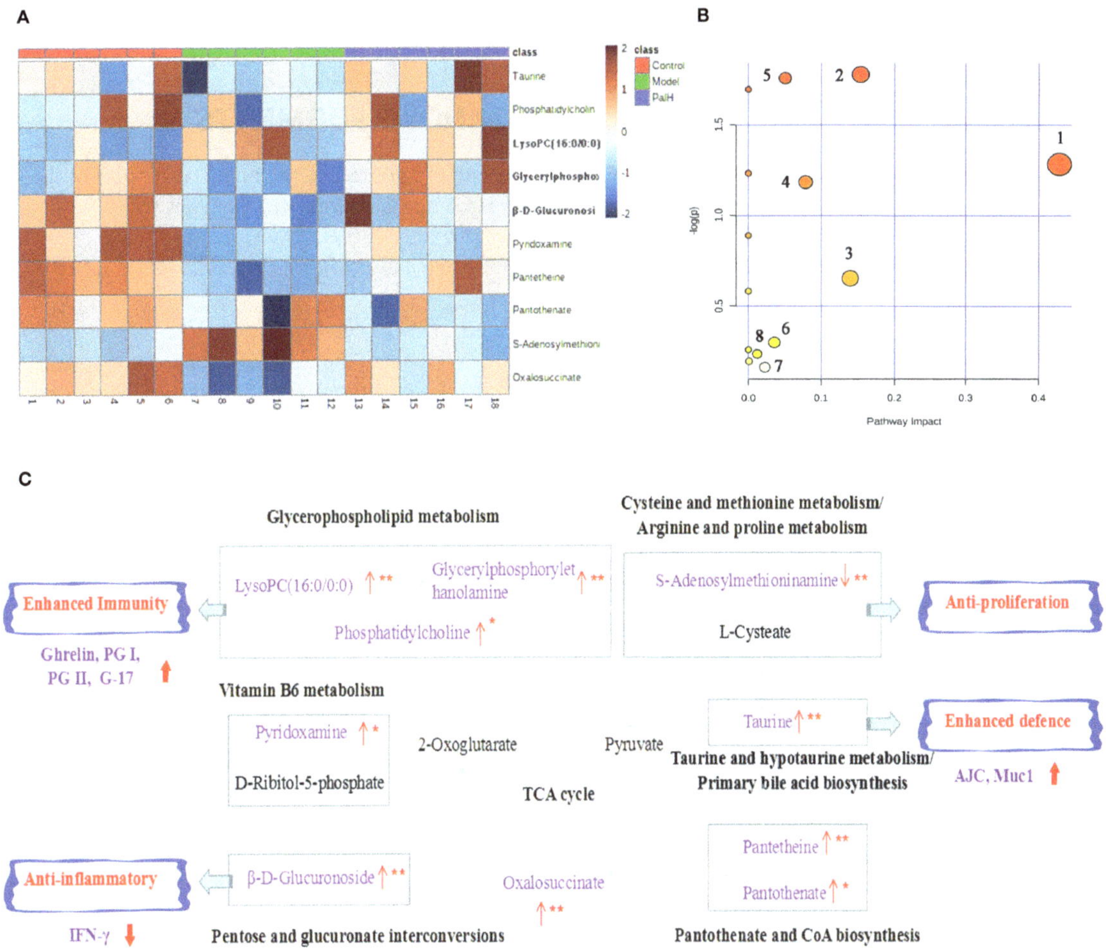

FIGURE 11 | Pathway analysis of Pal treatment. **(A)** The heatmap of 10 potential metabolites. **(B)** Metabolomic pathway construction of the metabolic pathways involved in the effects of Pal on chronic atrophic gastritis (CAG). **(C)** Signaling networks associated with the differentially expressed metabolic pathways. Red represents the detected metabolite.

TABLE 4 | Results of integrating enrichment analysis of biomarkers with MetaboAnalyst 4.0.

No	Pathway	Match status	Raw *p*	− log(p)	Impact
1	Taurine and hypotaurine metabolism	1/8	0.27773	1.2811	0.42857
2	Glycerophospholipid metabolism	3/36	0.16941	1.7754	0.15471
3	Pentose and glucuronate interconversions	1/18	0.52028	0.65339	0.14062
4	Vitamin B6 metabolism	1/9	0.3066	1.1822	0.07843
5	Pantothenate and CoA biosynthesis	2/19	0.1728	1.7556	0.05
6	Cysteine and methionine metabolism	1/33	0.7417	0.29881	0.03514
7	Primary bile acid biosynthesis	1/46	0.84974	0.16283	0.02239
8	Arginine and proline metabolism	1/38	0.79016	0.23552	0.01212
9	Citrate cycle (TCA cycle)	1/20	0.18215	1.7029	0.00

showed that the metabolism of taurine and subtaurine, the metabolism of glycerol phospholipid and the mutual transformation of pentose and glucuronide played a dominant role in the Pal treatment of *H. pylori*–induced CAG. The selected metabolites and metabolic pathways might be served as potential drug targets for CAG diagnosis and treatment, which is of great significance for the development of Pal-related drugs for the treatment of CAG.

ETHICS STATEMENT

The animal study was reviewed and approved by Fifth Medical Center of PLA General Hospital (Approval ID: IACUC-2018-010).

AUTHOR CONTRIBUTIONS

All authors contributed to the article and approved the submitted version. Conceptualization: XC. Methodology: JZ, RW, HL, CB. Investigation: SW, JW, TY, YW, SR, YT. Writing—original draft: XC. Writing—review and editing: XC. Funding acquisition: YZ.

ACKNOWLEDGMENTS

The authors appreciate the financial support of the National key Research and Development Program (No.2018YFC1704500).

REFERENCES

Chen, X., Wang, R. L., Bao, C. M., Zhang, J. Z., Zhang, J. L., Li, R. S., et al. (2020). Palmatine ameliorates Helicobacter pylori-induced chronic atrophic gastritis by inhibiting MMP-10 through ADAM17/EGFR. *Eur. J. Pharmacol.* 882:173267. doi: 10.1016/j.ejphar.2020.173267

Crafa, P., Russo, M., Miraglia, C., Barchi, A., Moccia, F., Nouvenne, A., et al. (2018). From Sidney to OLGA: an overview of atrophic gastritis. *Acta BioMed.* 89, 93–99. doi: 10.23750/abm.v89i8-S.7946

Farrokhi, Y. R., Amiri-Dashatan, N., Koushki, M., Dadpay, M., and Goshadrou, F. (2019). A Metabolomic Study to Identify Potential Tissue Biomarkers for Indomethacin-Induced Gastric Ulcer in Rats. *Avicenna J. Med. Biotechnol.* 11 (4), 299–307.

Gu, J. P., Huang, C. H., Hu, X. M., Xia, J. M., Shao, W., and Lin, D. H. (2020). Nuclear magnetic resonance-based tissue metabolomic analysis clarifies molecular mechanisms of gastric carcinogenesis. *Cancer Sci.* 111 (9), 3195–3209. doi: 10.1111/cas.14443

Jung, J., Choi, J. S., and Jeong, C. S. (2014). Inhibitory Activities of Palmatine from Coptis chinensis Against Helicobactor pylori and Gastric Damage. *Toxicol. Res.* 30, 45–48. doi: 10.5487/TR.2014.30.1.045

Kishikawa, H., Ojiro, K., Nakamura, K., Katayama, T., Arahata, K., Takarabe, S., et al. (2020). Previous Helicobacter pylori infection-induced atrophic gastritis: A distinct disease entity in an understudied population without a history of eradication. *Helicobacter* 25 (1), e12669. doi: 10.1111/hel.12669

Lahner, E., Esposito, G., Pilozzi, E., Purchiaroni, F., Corleto, V. D., Di, G. E., et al. (2015). Occurrence of gastric cancer and carcinoids in atrophic gastritis during prospective long-term follow up. *Scand. J. Gastroenterol.* 50 (7), 856–865. doi: 10.3109/00365521.2015.1010570

Li, C., Huang, P., Wong, K., Xu, Y. F., Tan, L. H., Chen, H. B., et al. (2018). Coptisine-induced inhibition of Helicobacter pylori: elucidation of specific mechanisms by probing urease active site and its maturation process. *J. Enzyme Inhib. Med. Chem.* 33, 1362–1375. doi: 10.1080/14756366.2018.1501044

Ma, H., He, K., Zhu, J. W., Li, X. G., and Ye, X. L. (2019). The anti-hyperglycemia effects of Rhizoma Coptidis alkaloids: A systematic review of modern pharmacological studies of the traditional herbal medicine. *Fitoterapia* 134, 210–220. doi: 10.1016/j.fitote.2019.03.003

Nedenskov, P. (1994). Nutritional requirements for growth of Helicobacter pylori. *Appl. Environ. Microbiol.* 60 (9), 3450–3453. doi: 10.1128/AEM.60.9.3450-3453.1994

Nishiumi, S., Yoshida, M., and Azuma, T. (2017). Alterations in metabolic pathways in stomach of mice infected with Helicobacter pylori. *Microb. Pathog.* 109, 78–85. doi: 10.1016/j.micpath.2017.05.027

Osawa, H., Nakazato, M., Date, Y., Kita, H., Ohnishi, H., Ueno, H., et al. (2005). Impaired production of gastric ghrelin in chronic gastritis associated with Helicobacter pylori. *J. Clin. Endocrinol. Metab.* 90 (1), 10–16. doi: 10.1210/jc.2004-1330

Schulz, C., Schütte, K., Mayerle, J., and Malfertheiner, P. (2019). Helicobacter pyloriThe role of the gastric bacterial microbiome in gastric cancer: and beyond. *Therap. Adv. Gastroenterol.* 12:1756284819894062. doi: 10.1177/1756284819894062

Shin, S. Y., Jeong, H. M., Chung, S. E., Kim, T. H., Thapa, S. K., Lee, D. Y., et al. (2019). Simultaneous analysis of acetylcarnitine, proline, hydroxyproline, citrulline, and arginine as potential plasma biomarkers to evaluate NSAIDs-induced gastric injury by liquid chromatography-tandem mass spectrometry. *J. Pharm. BioMed. Anal.* 165, 101–111. doi: 10.1016/j.jpba.2018.11.051

Strickertsson, J. A., Døssing, K. B., Aabakke, A. J., Nilsson, H. O., Hansen, T. V., Knigge, U., et al. (2011). Interferon-γ inhibits ghrelin expression and secretion via a somatostatin-mediated mechanism. *World J. Gastroenterol.* 17 (26), 3117–3125. doi: 10.3748/wjg.v17.i26.3117

Sun, Y. F., Li, S. S., Li, J., Xiao, X., Hua, Z. L., Wang, X., et al. (2020). A clinical metabolomics-based biomarker signature as an approach for early diagnosis of gastric cardia adenocarcinoma. *Oncol. Lett.* 19 (1), 681–690. doi: 10.3892/ol.2019.11173

Tarabasz, D., and Kukula-Koch, W. (2020). Palmatine: A review of pharmacological properties and pharmacokinetics. *Phytother. Res.* 34 (1), 33–50. doi: 10.1002/ptr.6504

Topi, S., Santacroce, L., Bottalico, L., Ballini, A., Inchingolo, A. D., Dipalma, G., et al. (2020). Gastric Cancer in History: A Perspective Interdisciplinary Study. *Cancers (Basel)* 12 (2), 264. doi: 10.3390/cancers12020264

Wang, X., Sun, H., Zhang, A., Sun, W., Wang, P., and Wang, Z. (2011). Potential role of metabolomics approaches in the area of traditional Chinese medicine: as pillars of the bridge between Chinese and Western medicine. *J. Pharm. BioMed. Anal.* 55, 859–868. doi: 10.1016/j.jpba.2011.01.042

Wang, L., Wang, X., Zhang, S. L., Zhu, X. M., Liu, Y. Q., Song, Z. J., et al. (2017). Gastroprotective effect of palmatine against acetic acid-induced gastric ulcers in rats. *J. Natural Med.* 71 (1), 257–264. doi: 10.1007/s11418-016-1057-2

Wang, K., Chai, L. W., Ding, L. Q., and Qiu, F. (2017). Identification of metabolites of palmatine in rats after oral administration using ultra-high-performance liquid chromatography/quadrupole time-of-flight mass spectrometry. *Rapid Commun. Mass Spectrom.* 31, 523–537. doi: 10.1002/rcm.7819

Werawatganon, D. (2014). Simple animal model of Helicobacter pylori infection. *World J. Gastroenterol.* 20, 6420–6424. doi: 10.3748/wjg.v20.i21.642

Yokozawa, T., Satoh, A., Cho, E. J., Kashiwada, Y., and Ikeshiro, Y. (2005). Protective role of *Coptidis Rhizoma* alkaloids against peroxynitrite-induced damage to renal tubular epithelial cells. *J. Pharm. Pharmacol.* 57, 367–374. doi: 10.1211/0022357055470

Zagari, R. M., Rabitti, S., Greenwood, D. C., Eusebi, L. H., Vestito, A., and Bazzoli, F. (2017). Systematic review with meta-analysis: diagnostic performance of the combination of pepsinogen, gastrin-17 and anti-Helicobacter pylori antibodies serum assays for the diagnosis of atrophic gastritis. *Aliment. Pharmacol. Ther.* 46 (7), 657–667. doi: 10.1111/apt.14248

Zhang, C., Zhang, H. Y., Yu, L., and Cao, Y. (2014). Helicobacter pylori dwelling on the apical surface of gastrointestinal epithelium damages the mucosal barrier through direct contact. *Helicobacter* 19 (5), 330–342. doi: 10.1111/hel.12138

Zhao, W., and Zhang, X. Z. (2011). Inhibitory effect of Palmatine and berberine on the proliferation of HUMAN gastric cancer cell MGC803. *Life Sci. Instrum.* 9 (02), 44–47.

Zhou, J. T., Li, C.-L., Tan, L. H., Xu, Y. F., Liu, Y. H., Mo, Z. Z., et al. (2017). Inhibition of Helicobacter pylori and Its Associated Urease by Palmatine: Investigation on the Potential Mechanism. *PLoS One* 12, e0168944. doi: 10.1371/journal.pone.0168944

Zhou, J., Yao, N., Wang, S. X., An, D. C., Cao, K., Wei, J. L., et al. (2019). Fructus Gardeniae-induced gastrointestinal injury was associated with the inflammatory response mediated by the disturbance of vitamin B6, phenylalanine, arachidonic acid, taurine and hypotaurine metabolism. *J. Ethnopharmacol.* 235, 47–55. doi: 10.1016/j.jep.2019.01.041

6

Novel and Emerging Therapies for Inflammatory Bowel Disease

Badr Al-Bawardy[1]*, *Raina Shivashankar*[2] *and Deborah D. Proctor*[1]

[1]Section of Digestive Diseases, Yale School of Medicine, New Haven, CT, United States, [2]Division of Gastroenterology and Hepatology, Thomas Jefferson University, Philadelphia, PA, United States

Correspondence:
Badr Al-Bawardy
badr.albawardy@yale.edu

Inflammatory bowel diseases (IBD) such as ulcerative colitis and Crohn's disease are chronic, relapsing and remitting disorders of intestinal inflammation with potential systemic manifestations. Despite the availability of current biologics, such as anti-tumor necrosis factor (anti-TNF), anti-integrins, anti-interleukins and small molecules such as tofacitinib, the rates of primary and secondary treatment failure remain high in IBD. This highlights the importance of continued development of new therapeutic targets and modifications of existing ones to improve the treatment response rates and to also improve the safety profile and tolerability of these medications. In this review we will discuss novel treatment target agents including selective janus kinase (JAK) inhibitors, anti-interleukin (IL) (IL-12/IL-23), leukocyte trafficking/migrating inhibitors (such as sphingosine-1-phosphate receptor modulator) and other small molecules currently in development.

Keywords: inflammatory bowel disease, small molecule, biologic, novel therapy, emerging therapy

INTRODUCTION

Inflammatory bowel disease (IBD) is a chronic, progressive disease that can lead to complications including bowel damage, need for hospitalizations and surgery, decreased quality of life, and disability. The incidence rates of IBD have been increasing world-wide. While the highest rates have been noted in North America and Europe, increasing incidence rates have been observed in previously low-incidence regions such as Asia as these countries become more developed (Loftus Jr, 2004; Molodecky et al., 2012; Shivashankar and Lewis, 2017a). The cause for this phenomenon is largely unknown, however it may be related to the complex interplay between genetics and the environment (Shivashankar and Lewis, 2017a). The latter has been implicated in the development of IBD because of the observation that higher incidence rates are seen in industrialized nations; therefore diet, pollution, microbial exposure, and sanitation may be involved (Molodecky and Kaplan, 2010; Shivashankar and Lewis, 2017a).

Since IBD can be a chronic and progressive disease, optimal treatment early in the disease course to prevent complications is paramount. The current treatment paradigm for moderate-severe Crohn's disease (CD) and ulcerative colitis (UC) is to use biologic therapy early to achieve clinical remission and mucosal healing, which will ultimately decrease the risk of corticosteroid use, surgeries, hospitalizations and increase quality of life (Klenske et al., 2019).

The currently available biologic agents include anti-tumor necrosis factor-alpha (TNF-α) agents (infliximab, adalimumab, certolizumab, and golimumab); anti-integrin agents (vedolizumab,

Abbreviations: AE, adverse event; CD, crohn's disease; CRP, C-reactive protein; FDA, food and drug administration; IBD, inflammatory bowel disease; IL, interleukin; IFN, interferon; IV, intravenous; JAK, janus kinase; NF-κB, nuclear transcription factor kappaB; PRO, patient reported outcome; S1P, sphingosine 1-phosphate; SC, subcutaneous; TNF-α, tumor necrosis factor alpha; TYK, tyrosine kinase; UC, ulcerative colitis.

TABLE 1 | Target, mode of delivery and development phase of emerging therapeutic agents in IBD.

Drug class	Agent	Target	Mode of delivery	Crohn's disease	Ulcerative colitis
JAK inhibitors	Tofacitinib	JAK1/JAK3	Oral	N/A	FDA approved
	Filgotinib	JAK1	Oral	Phase III recruiting	Phase IIb/III completed
	Upadacitinib	JAK1	Oral	Phase III recruiting	Phase III recruiting
	TD-1473	Pan-JAK (gut selective)	Oral	Phase II recruiting	Phase IIb/III recruiting
	Brepocitinib (PF-06700841)	TYK2/JAK1	Oral	Phase IIa recruiting	Phase IIb recruiting
	PF-06651600	JAK3	Oral		
	BMS-986165	TYK2	Oral	Phase II recruiting	Phase II recruiting
Anti-trafficking therapies	Vedolizumab SC	α4β7 integrin	SC	N/A	Phase III completed
	Etrolizumab	α4β7 and αEβ7 integrins	SC	Phase III recruiting	Phase III completed
	AJM300	α4 integrin	Oral	N/A	Phase III recruiting
	PF-00547659	MAdCAM	SC	Phase II completed	Phase II completed
IL-23 inhibitors	Risankizumab	IL23/p19 subunit	IV, SC	Phase III active, not recruiting	Phase III enrolling by invitation
	Brazikumab	IL23/p19 subunit	IV, SC	Phase IIb/III recruiting	Phase 2/OLE enrolling by invitation
	Mirikizumab	IL23/p19 subunit	IV, SC	Phase III recruiting	Phase III recruiting
	Guselkumab	IL23/p19 subunit	IV, SC	Phase II/III recruiting	Phase II/III recruiting
S1P receptor modulators	Ozanimod	S1PR1 and S1PR5	Oral	Phase III recruiting	Phase III completed
	Etrasimod	S1PR1, S1PR4 and S1PR5	Oral	Phase II/III recruiting	Phase III recruiting
	Amiselimod (MT-1303)	S1PR1	Oral	Phase II completed	N/A
PDE4 inhibitors	Apremilast	PDE4	Oral	N/A	Phase II completed
TLR9 agonist	Cobitolimod	TLR9	Topical (enema)	N/A	Phase IIb completed, Phase III planned

JAK, janus kinase; TYK 2, tyrosine kinase 2; S1P, sphingosine 1 phosphate; S1PR sphingosine 1 phosphate receptor; PDE4, phosphodiesterase 4; TLR9, toll-like receptor 9; α4β7, alpha4-beta7; αEβ7, alphaE-beta7; α4, alpha4; MAdCAM, mucosal addressin cell adhesion molecule-1; IL-23, interleukin 23; IV, intravenous; SC, subcutaneous; OLE, open label extension.

natalizumab); and an anti-interleukin (IL) 12-23 agent (ustekinumab). Finally, tofacitinib, a non-biologic small molecule is approved for the treatment of moderate-severe UC. The choice between these agents depends on IBD phenotype and behavior, previous biologic exposure and response, potential adverse effects of therapy, patient co-morbidities, and shared-decision making with patients.

Despite the number of available medications, there are appreciable rates of primary non-response, loss of response, or adverse reactions thereby necessitating additional treatment options. Therefore, the purpose of this review article is to describe novel and emerging therapies for IBD. In this review we will discuss novel treatment target agents including selective janus kinase (JAK) inhibitors, anti-interleukin (IL) (IL-12/IL-23), leukocyte trafficking/migrating inhibitors (such as sphingosine-1-phosphate receptor modulator) and other small molecules currently in development (**Table 1**). This review will focus on the pipeline of these new therapeutic agents and will not include other novel and emerging therapeutic modalities such as stem cell therapy or microbiome targeted therapies.

JAK Inhibitors

Cytokine mediators of inflammation in IBD such as IL-9, IL-12, IL-23 and interferon-gamma (IFN-γ) are reliant on the Janus Kinase Signal Transducer and Activator of Transcription (JAK-STAT) pathway signaling (Salas et al., 2020). In addition, genome wide association studies have demonstrated risk loci in the JAK region in IBD (Barrett et al., 2008; Anderson et al., 2011). Therefore, targeting the JAK-STAT is an appealing therapeutic modality in IBD. JAK1, JAK2, JAK3 and tyrosine kinase 2 (TYK2) are all part of the JAK family of tyrosine kinase proteins.

Tofacitinib

Tofacitinib, a non-selective JAK inhibitor, was approved by the US food and drug administration (FDA) in May 2018 for the treatment of UC. The pivotal induction and maintenance clinical trials, OCTAVE 1-3, have demonstrated efficacy of tofacitinib in inducing and maintaining clinical and endoscopic remission in UC (Sandborn et al., 2017b). Notably, tofacitinib was also shown to be effective in the more refractory anti-TNF-α exposed UC patients compared to placebo. On the other hand, a phase IIb randomized clinical trial of tofacitinib in CD failed to meet the primary endpoints (Panés et al., 2017). Multiple factors might have contributed to the negative results of the study including: study design and high placebo response rate. Subsequently, a systematic review and meta-analysis of clinical trials of different JAK inhibitors (tofacitnib, filgotinib, pefecitinib, upadacitinib, TD-1473) in CD demonstrated the effectiveness of JAK inhibitors in inducing clinical remission (Ma et al., 2019).

Tofacitinib provided the advantage being an oral agent compared to current intravenous (IV) or subcutaneous (SC) biologic agent formulations. The rapid onset of action of tofacitinib is a positive feature as improvement in symptoms of rectal bleeding and stool frequency can occur within 3 days of starting treatment in UC patients according to post-hoc analysis of the pivotal trials (Hanauer et al., 2019). Conversely, tofacitinib has been associated with increased risk of herpes zoster infection and hyperlipidemia (Winthrop et al., 2018). In addition, tofacitinib has a black box warning for venous thromboembolism and mortality after risk was noted in a subset of patients with rheumatoid arthritis taking the 10 mg p.o. BID dose (FDA Drug Safety Communication, 2019). Therefore, there has been an increased interest in the development of more selective JAK inhibitors to enhance the effectiveness and the safety profile in IBD.

Filgotinib

Filgotinib is a once daily oral small molecule with higher selectivity for JAK 1 inhibition. JAK 1 (in addition to JAK 3) have been shown to be expressed on both B cells and T cells within the healthy colon mucosa (Salas et al., 2020). The efficacy of filgotinib in CD was evaluated in a phase II, double-blinded, placebo controlled randomized clinical trial, FITZROY. In this trial, patients were randomized to filgotinib 200 mg once a day or placebo and after 10 weeks based on response, patients received either once daily filgotinib 200 mg, filgotinib 100 mg or placebo for another 10 weeks (Vermeire et al., 2017b). A significantly higher proportion of patients in the filgotinib groups achieved the primary endpoint of clinical remission [defined as Crohn's disease activity index (CDAI) < 150] at week 10 compared to placebo (47 vs. 23%; $p = 0.0077$) (Vermeire et al., 2017b). In anti-TNF-α naïve patients, the rate of clinical remission at week 10 was 60% (n = 34) compared to 37% (n = 26) in anti-TNF-α experienced patients. The rate of endoscopic response and mucosal healing in the overall filgotinib group was numerically higher but did not reach statistical significance. However, endoscopic assessment in this trial was limited by short follow up time. In terms of safety, up to 20 weeks follow up, serious infections were noted in 3% in the filgotinib group with none reported in the placebo group.

A phase IIB/III study (SELECTION) evaluating filgotinib for induction and maintenance therapy for moderate to severe UC was recently completed (Feagan et al., 2020b). The induction study included a cohort of biologic exposed and another cohort of biologic naïve patients (Feagan et al., 2020b; Peyrin-Biroulet et al., 2020). In each cohort patients were randomized to either filgotinib 100 mg, filgotinib 200 mg or placebo daily. The composite primary endpoint of endoscopic, rectal bleeding and stool frequency (EBS) remission (defined as Mayo endoscopic subscore ≤1, rectal bleeding subscore of 0, stool frequency subscore decrease of 1 or more points from baseline and ≤1) rates were significantly higher in the 200 mg filgotinib groups (26.1% in the biologic naïve cohort and 11.5% in the biologic experienced cohort) compared to the placebo groups. One case of pulmonary embolism in the filgotinib 200 mg group was noted and four total cases of herpes zoster in filgotinib groups were noted (1 in the 100 mg group and three in the 200 mg group) (Feagan et al., 2020b).

Patients who achieved clinical remission or response after 10 weeks of induction therapy with either filgotinib or placebo were included in the maintenance study (Peyrin-Biroulet et al., 2020). In this study 664 patients with moderate to severe UC who received placebo induction remained in the placebo maintenance arm, while patients randomized to the filgotinib induction were re-randomized to filgotinib induction dose maintenance arm or placebo arm (Peyrin-Biroulet et al., 2020). The composite primary endpoint of EBS remission at week 58 was achieved in 37.2% in the filgotinib 200 mg group vs. 11.2% in the placebo arm ($p < 0.025$) and 23.8% in the filgotinib 100 mg group vs. 13.5% in the placebo arm ($p < 0.05$) (Peyrin-Biroulet et al., 2020). Overall, filgotinib was well tolerated. Two cases of venous thromboembolism were reported in the placebo arm but none in the filgotinib group. Herpes zoster was reported in two patients in the filgotinib arms (one in each of the filgotinib groups) but none in the placebo groups (Peyrin-Biroulet et al., 2020).

A phase III clinical trial of filgotinib in CD is currently in progress (NCT02914561; NCT02914600). In addition, a phase II study evaluating filgotinib in perianal fistulizing CD is ongoing (NCT03077412).

Upadacitinib

Upadacitinib is an oral JAK inhibitor that has high selectivity for JAK 1 inhibition. It is currently approved for the treatment of rheumatoid arthritis with moderate to severe activity who have either failed or are intolerant to methotrexate. In a phase II clinical trial (CELEST), patients with moderate to severe CD (n = 220) who failed immunosuppressants or biologics were assigned to either placebo or upadacitinib at the following doses: 3 mg twice a day (BID), 6 mg BID, 12 mg BID, 24 mg BID for 16-weeks induction (Sandborn et al., 2020c). Post-induction, patients were re-randomized to upadacitinib at the following doses: 3 mg BID, 12 mg BID, 24 mg once daily (QD) for 36 weeks (maintenance). Although clinical remission at week 16 was not significantly different between the treatment groups and placebo, endoscopic remission at week 12/16 was significantly higher in the upadacitinib groups compared to placebo (Sandborn et al., 2020c). Higher doses of upadacitinib were associated with higher rates of endoscopic remission in this trial.

In the phase II UC-ACHIEVE trial, moderate to severe UC patients (n = 250) who failed or were intolerant to immunosuppressive or biologic therapy were assigned to placebo or upadacitinib at the following once daily doses: 7.5, 15, 30, 45 mg (Sandborn et al., 2020e). Clinical remission was significantly higher in the 15 mg (14.3%; $p = 0.013$), 30 mg (13.5%; $p = 0.011$), and the 45 mg groups (19.6%; $p = 0.002$) compared to 0% in the placebo group. Similarly, endoscopic improvement at week 8 (Mayo endoscopic subscore ≤1) was significantly higher in a dose dependent manner in the upadacitinib groups compared to placebo (Sandborn et al., 2020e).

In terms of safety, there were a total of three cases of herpes zoster in the upadacitinib group compared to none in the placebo group in the CELEST trial and 1 case in the upadacitinib group compared to none in the placebo group in the UC-ACHIEVE trial (Sandborn et al., 2020c; Sandborn et al., 2020e). Once case of thromboembolism occurred in a patient on the 45 mg upadacitinib dose in the UC-ACHIEVE trial.

Currently, upadacitinib is in phase III clinical trials for CD (NCT03345836, NCT03345823) and UC (NCT03653026, NCT03006068, NCT02819635).

TD-1473

TD-1473 is an oral pan-JAK inhibitor that is designed to be gut specific to limit systemic toxicity of pan-JAK inhibition. In a phase 1b trial, patients with moderate to severe UC (n = 40) were assigned to placebo or one of the following once daily TD-1473 doses: 20 mg, 80 mg or 270 mg) for 28 days (Sandborn et al., 2020f). Only five of the 40 patients were exposed to anti-TNF therapies in the past. Clinical response rate was 20% in the 20 and 80 mg groups compared to 55% in the 270 mg group while the clinical response rate was 11% in the placebo group (no statistical analyses performed as study not powered for outcomes) (Sandborn et al., 2020f). There were also trends in endoscopic improvement along with reduction in fecal calprotectin and c-reactive protein (CRP) levels with TD-1473. Overall adverse event rates were similar in the placebo group at 44.4 and 38.7% in the TD-1473 groups. Phase IIb/III studies of TD-1473 for moderate to severe UC are currently recruiting (NCT03758443, NCT03920254). In addition, a phase II study of TD-1473 in moderate to severe CD in underway (NCT03635112).

TYK2 Inhibitors

TYK2 is one of the JAK-STAT family proteins. It is involved in intracellular cytokine signaling. Brepocitinib (PF-06700841) is an oral TYK2/JAK1 inhibitor that has been shown to be well tolerated and effective in phase I and phase IIa studies of patients with plaque psoriasis (Banfield et al., 2018; Forman et al., 2020). PF-06651600 is an oral selective JAK3 inhibitor. Phase IIa/IIb trials of combination brepocitinib (PF-06700841) and PF-06651600 are currently recruiting for moderate to severe CD (NCT03395184) and UC (NCT02958865).

BMS-986165 is an oral selective TYK2 inhibitor. Phase II trials of BMS-986165 in CD (NCT03599622) and UC (NCT03934216) are currently recruiting.

IL-12/IL-23 Inhibitors

IL-23 is a regulator of T-helper (Th)-17 cell and type 3 innate lymphoid cell (ILC3) pathways that lead to inflammatory cytokine production and inflammation and polymorphisms of the IL-23 receptor gene may be associated with increased susceptibility to CD (Feagan et al., 2017). IL-23 prevents regulatory T-cell response in the intestine, and therefore increases inflammation in this gut (Feagan et al., 2017; Sands et al., 2017). Ustekinumab, which inhibits both IL-12 and the IL-23 p40 subunit, has been shown to be effective for induction and maintenance of remission in patients with moderate-severe CD and UC (Feagan et al., 2016; Sands et al., 2019a).

However, it is unclear if the effect of ustekinumab is mainly driven by its inhibition of IL-12, IL-23 or both (Deepak and Sandborn, 2017). Selective inhibition of the IL-23 pathway, which leaves the IL-12 pathway intact, carries the potential advantage of less severe infection and decreased malignancy risk (Deepak and Sandborn, 2017; Baker and Isaacs, 2018). A potential benefit of only blocking the p19 subunit of IL-23 is possible increased safety since the IL-12 mediated Th1 response, which is required in the immune response to intracellular pathogens, is left intact (Deepak and Sandborn, 2017).

Risankizumab

Risankizumab is a humanized monoclonal antibody against the p19 subunit of IL-23. The induction dosing is provided intravenously (IV) while the maintenance dosing is a subcutaneous (SC) injection. A phase II trial of induction therapy with risankizumab was conducted in patients with moderate-severe CD; 93% of patients were previously exposed to at least one anti-TNF agent (Deepak and Sandborn, 2017; Feagan et al., 2017). Risankizumab (200 mg or 600 mg IV) was compared to placebo at weeks 0, 4, and 8. The primary outcome was clinical remission (defined as a CDAI <150) at week 12 (Feagan et al., 2017).

At week 12, those treated with risankizumab had significantly higher rates of clinical remission vs. placebo (30.5 vs. 15.4%, p = 0.0489), clinical response (39 vs. 20.5%, 0 = 0.0273), endoscopic remission (17 vs. 3%, p = 0.0015), and deep remission (7 vs. 0, p = 0.0107) (Feagan et al., 2017). There was no difference in the proportion of mucosal healing between those treated with risankizumab (200 mg: 2%, 600 mg 7%) vs. placebo (3%) (200 mg v. placebo, p = 0.97 and 600 mg v. placebo, p = 0.31) (Feagan et al., 2017). Rates of adverse events (AEs) were similar between those treated with placebo and risankizumab. The most common AE was worsening of underlying CD (Feagan et al., 2017). Other AEs included nausea, abdominal pain, arthralgia, and headache (Feagan et al., 2017). There were no dose-related increases in AE in those treated with risankizumab (Feagan et al., 2017).

An open-label extension (OLE) study was completed to study the efficacy and safety of extended IV induction and SC maintenance therapy (Feagan et al., 2018). Those who did not achieve deep remission in the 12-weeks induction phase of the previously described phase II induction study received open-label IV risankizumab 600 mg every 4 weeks for 12 weeks; patients who were in clinical remission at week 26 were included in the maintenance phase and received open-label SC risankizumab 180 mg every 8 weeks for 26 weeks (Feagan et al., 2018). The following definitions were used: clinical remission (CDAI <150), endoscopic response (>50% Crohn's disease Endoscopic Index of Severity [CDEIS] reduction from baseline), endoscopic remission (CDEIS ≤4, or ≤2 for patients with isolated ileitis) (Feagan et al., 2018). One-hundred and one patients received the extended induction dose, and 53% (54/101 patients) were in clinical remission at week 26 (Feagan et al., 2018). Sixty-two patients received risankizumab maintenance therapy, and at week 52 clinical remission was maintained in 71% (44/62 patients), 81% (50/62) had clinical response, 35% (22/62) were in endoscopic remission, 24% (15/62) had mucosal healing, and 29% (18/62) achieved deep remission (Feagan et al., 2018). There were no new safety signals noted and the most frequent AEs included arthralgia, headache, abdominal pain, nasopharyngitis, nausea, and pyrexia (Feagan et al., 2018).

The long-term safety of risankizumab was studied in the phase 2 OLE study and no new safety signals were noted; 92% of patients reported AEs and 35% of patients experienced serious adverse events (Ferrante et al., 2020). The most common AEs included nasopharyngitis (31%), gastroenteritis (23%), and fatigue (20%) (Ferrante et al., 2020). Nine percent of patients had serious infections while 5% of patients reported opportunistic infections. There were no malignancies or deaths (Ferrante et al., 2020).

Overall, risankizumab was well-tolerated and found to be effective compared to placebo in inducing clinical remission, response, and endoscopic remission at week 12. Currently, we are awaiting results from phase III clinical trials (NCT03105128; estimated study completion date February 2021). In addition, a phase II/III clinical trial of risankizumab in ulcerative colitis is currently recruiting (NCT03398148).

Brazikumab (MEDI 2070)

Brazikumab, a human immunoglobulin G2 monoclonal antibody, selectively binds the p19 subunit of IL-23 (Sands et al., 2017). Like risankizumab, the induction dose is an IV infusion while the maintenance dose is a SC injection. A phase IIa trial included 119 patients with moderate-severe CD who either failed or were intolerant to anti-TNF agents; 31% of patients were exposed to at least one anti-TNF. Patients were given either brazikumab 700 mg IV or placebo at weeks 0 and 4, and then received open label brazikumab 210 mg subcutaneously every 4 weeks from weeks 12 to 112 (Sands et al., 2017). The primary outcome was clinical response (CDAI decrease of 100 points from baseline or clinical remission [CDAI <150]) at week 8 (Sands et al., 2017). Compared to placebo, a higher proportion of patients treated with brazikumab achieved clinical response at week 8 (49.2% v. 26.7%, p = 0.01) as well as a composite outcome of clinical response and 50% reduction from baseline in either fecal calprotectin or CRP concentration (42.4% v. 10%, p < 0.001) (Sands et al., 2017). There was no difference in clinical remission at week eight between those treated with brazikumab vs. placebo (27.1 vs. 15%, p = 0.10) (Sands et al., 2017). A similar proportion of patients who received placebo and active treatment during the initial double-blind period achieved clinical response, clinical remission, the composite outcome of clinical response and at least 50% reduction from baseline in either fecal calprotectin or CRP concentration at week 24 (57.7 vs. 53.8%, 40.4 vs. 42.3%, and 48.1 vs. 46.2%, respectively) (Sands et al., 2017). Patients with higher baseline serum concentration of IL-22 were found to be more likely to responds to brazikumab than to placebo (Sands et al., 2017; Sabino et al., 2019).

There was no difference in proportions of patients with treatment-emergent AEs or serious AEs between placebo and brazikumab treated groups (Sands et al., 2017). Equal numbers of clinically significant infections occurred in patients receiving brazikumab in both study periods and in patients receiving placebo in the double-blind period (Sands et al., 2017). The most common AEs included headache, nasopharyngitis, and abdominal pain (Sands et al., 2017).

In summary, two infusions of brazikumab at weeks 0 and 4 achieved a higher rate of clinical response at week 8 compared to placebo and continued SC dosing every 4 weeks led to ongoing clinical response and remission at week 24 (Sands et al., 2017). Brazikumab was generally well-tolerated in this study with follow-up to 24 weeks (Sands et al., 2017). Of note, there was no endoscopic evaluation or imaging as part of this phase 2a study (Sands et al., 2017). Currently, brazikumab is in a phase IIb/III trial in patients with CD (NCT03759288; anticipated completion date Dec 2022) and is in a phase II/open label extension in UC patients (NCT03616821; anticipated completion date april 2023).

Mirikizumab

Mirikizumab is an IV and SC immunoglobulin G4-variant monoclonal antibody, and it binds to the p19 subunit of IL23 (Sandborn et al., 2020d). A phase II study of 249 patients with moderate-severe UC was conducted to assess the efficacy and safety of mirikizumab; 63% of patients were previously exposed to a biologic (Sandborn et al., 2020d). Patients were randomized to either IV placebo, mirikizumab 50 mg, or 200 mg, or mirikizumab 600 mg at weeks 0, 4, and 8 (Sandborn et al., 2020d). Those with clinical response to mirikizumab at week 12 were then randomized to maintenance mirikizumab 200 mg every 4 weeks or every 12 weeks (Sandborn et al., 2020d). The primary endpoint was clinical remission (Mayo rectal bleeding subscore 0, with 1-point decrease from baseline for stool frequency, and 0 or one for endoscopy) (Sandborn et al., 2020d). Clinical remission at week 12 is as follows: 15.9% (95% CI, 6.8–24.9; p = 0.66) in the mirikizumab 50 mg group; 22.6% (12.2–33.0; p = 0.004) in the mirikizumab 200 mg group; and 11.5% (3.5–19.5, p = 0.142) in the 600 mg group vs. 4.8% (0–10) in the placebo groups (Sandborn et al., 2020d). Endoscopic improvement at week 12 was seen in 23.8% (13.3–34.3, p = 0.12) of the mirikizumab 50 mg group; 30.6% (23.3–34.3; p = 0.0007) in the 200 mg group, and 13.1% (4.6–21.6; p = 0.215) in the 600 mg group vs. 6.3% (0.3–12.4) in the placebo treated groups (Sandborn et al., 2020d).

Following the 12 weeks induction period, 93 mirikizumab treated patients achieved clinical response and were randomized to SC mirikizumab at 200 mg every 4 weeks or every 12 weeks (Sandborn et al., 2020d). At week 52, 53.7 and 39.7% of patients treated every 4 weeks and every 12 weeks, achieved clinical remission, respectively (Sandborn et al., 2020d). These rates were similar in those who were both biologic-exposed and biologic-naïve (Sandborn et al., 2020d). Endoscopic remission (Mayo endoscopic subscore = 0) at week 52 were 14.8% (every 4 weeks) and 28.3% (every 12 weeks) (Sandborn et al., 2020d). Durable clinical remission (clinical remission at both weeks 12 and 52) was 61.1% in the every 4 weeks maintenance dose and 38.5% in the every 12 weeks group (Sandborn et al., 2020d).

The most frequent AEs included nasopharyngitis, worsening of UC, headache, anemia, cough, nausea; no dose related increases in AEs were reported (Sandborn et al., 2020d).

An open label extension of this phase II study looked at the outcome of patients treated with mirikizumab who did not respond clinically in the initial induction period (Sandborn et al., 2020a). These patients were randomized to either 600 mg IV mirikizumab or 1,000 mg IV mirikizumab every 4 weeks (Sandborn et al., 2020a). At week 24, those who had a clinical response continued the maintenance period of 200 mg SC mirikizumab (Sandborn et al., 2020a). Endpoints included clinical remission (Mayo rectal bleeding = 0, 0 or 1 with a 1 point decrease from baseline), clinical response, endoscopic remission (Mayo endoscopic subscore = 0), or endoscopic improvement (endoscopic subscore of 0 or 1) at weeks 24 or 52 (Sandborn et al., 2020a). In the 12 weeks extension of the mirikizumab 600 mg dose and 1,000 mg mirikizumab dose, 50 and 43.8%, respectively, achieved clinical response and 15 and 9.4%, respectively, achieved clinical remission (Sandborn et al., 2020a). Endoscopic improvement was seen in 20% of patients in the 600 mg group and 15.6% of patients in the 1,000 mg group (Sandborn et al., 2020a). In those who had clinical response at week 24 and continued to maintenance therapy, 65.8% remained in clinical response, 26.3% had clinical remission, and 34.2% had endoscopic improvement at week 52 (Sandborn et al., 2020a). No new AEs identified.

In summary, the phase II dose ranging study of mirikizumab showed a trend toward inducing clinical remission and response around week 12 in patients with moderate-severe UC (Sandborn et al., 2020d). In those who did not initially respond to induction dosing, extended IV dosing of mirikizumab for 12 additional weeks showed a clinical response in about 50% of patients (Sandborn et al., 2020a).

Given its efficacy in patients with UC, mirikizumab was studied for its safety and efficacy in patients with CD in a phase II study (Sands et al., 2019b). Patients were randomized to mirkizumab 200 mg, 600 mg, 1,000 mg and placebo and this was administered at weeks 0, 4, and 8 (Sands et al., 2019b). The primary endpoint was endoscopic response (50% reduction from baseline in SES-CD) at week 12 (Sands et al., 2019b). Endoscopic response rates were higher in the mirkizumab groups compared to placebo at week 12 [200 mg: 25.8% (95% CI: 10.4–41.2), p = 0.079; 600 mg: 37.5% (20.7–54.3), p = 0.003; 1,000 mg: 43.8 (31.6–55.9), $p < 0.001$; placebo: 10.9 (3.3–18.6)] (Sands et al., 2019b). Additionally, patient reported outcome remission rates and CDAI response rates were greater in the 600 and 1000 mg mirikizumab group compared to placebo (Sands et al., 2019b). The frequencies of serious AEs and treatment-emergent AEs were similar between placebo and treatment groups (Sands et al., 2019b).

Mirikizumab was also evaluated for long-term efficacy and safety over 52 weeks in the phase II maintenance SERENITY study (Sands et al., 2020). Patients who achieved ≥1 point improvement in SES-CD at week 12 on mirikizumab were then re-randomized to maintenance mirikizumab IV or SC every 4 weeks (Sands et al., 2020). The primary endpoints were CDAI remission (<150 points), patient reported outcome (PRO) remission (stool frequency ≤2.5 and abdominal pain ≤1 and not worse than baseline), endoscopic response (50% reduction from baseline in SES-CD), and endoscopic remission (SES-CD score <4 for ileal-colonic disease or <2 for isolated ileal disease, and no subscore >1) (Sands et al., 2020). Endoscopic response rates were 58.5 and 58.7%; PRO remission rates were 46.3 and 45.7% in the IV and SC groups, respectively (Sands et al., 2020). In those who achieved endoscopic response at week 12, 69.6 and 66.7% had an endoscopic response at week 52 in the IV and SC groups, respectively (Sands et al., 2020). Also, in those who had endoscopic remission at week 12, 50 and 64.3% maintained endoscopic remission at week 52, respectively, in the IV and SC groups (Sands et al., 2020). There were similar treatment-emergent AEs and serious AEs in both the IV and SC groups (Sands et al., 2020).

Treatment with mirikizumab did have a dose-dependent improvement in endoscopic response and remission as well as patient-reported response and remission at week 12 in patients with CD (Authors, 2019) (A SPECIAL MEETING REVIEW EDITION: Highlights in Inflammatory Bowel Disease From the 14th Congress of ECCO: A Review of Selected Presentations From the 14th Congress of the European Crohn's and Colitis Organization (ECCO) * March 6–9, 2019 * Copenhagen, DenmarkSpecial Reporting on:* VARSITY: A Double-Blind, Double-Dummy, Randomized Controlled Trial of Vedolizumab vs. Adalimumab in Patients With Active Ulcerative Colitis* Analyses of Data From the VISIBLE 1 and 2 Trials: Vedolizumab in Patients With Ulcerative Colitis or Crohn's Disease* Improved Endoscopic Outcomes and Mucosal Healing of Upadacitinib as an Induction Therapy in Adults With Moderately to Severely Active Ulcerative Colitis: Data From the U-ACHIEVE Study* Long-Term Safety of Vedolizumab in Ulcerative Colitis and Crohn's Disease: Final Results From the GEMINI LTS Study* Pediatric Crohn's Disease Adalimumab Level-Based Optimization Treatment (PAILOT) Randomized Controlled Trial* Maintenance Treatment With Mirikizumab, a P19-Directed IL-23 Antibody: 52-Week Results in Patients With Moderately to Severely Active Ulcerative Colitis* Real-World Effectiveness and Safety of Vedolizumab and Anti-TNF Therapy in Biologic-Naive Patients With Ulcerative Colitis or Crohn's disease: Results From the EVOLVE Study* A Randomized, Multicenter, Double-Blind, Placebo-Controlled Study of a Targeted-Release Oral Cyclosporine Formulation in the Treatment of Mild to Moderate Ulcerative Colitis: Efficacy Results* Real-World Analyses of Patients With IBD Treated With VedolizumabPLUS Meeting Abstract Summaries With Expert Commentary by: Edward V. Loftus Jr, MD Professor of Medicine Division of Gastroenterology and Hepatology Mayo Clinic Rochester, Minnesota, 2019). Mirikizumab also had been shown to have sustained efficacy to week 52 (Sands et al., 2020). Mirkizumab for CD is currently being studied in a phase III trial (NCT03926130). Phase III Induction, maintenance and open label extension studies are currently recruiting for UC (NCT03518086, NCT03524092, NCT03519945).

Guselkumab

Guselkumab is an IV and SC anti-IL23 that is currently approved for the treatment of moderate-severe plaque psoriasis (Sandborn et al., 2020i). GALAXI 1 is a phase II study that evaluated the efficacy and safety of guselkumab in patients with moderate-severe CD who either had intolerance or inadequate response to corticosteroids, immunosuppressive agents and/or biologics (Sandborn et al., 2020i). Patients were randomized to guselkumab 200 mg, 600 mg, or 1,200 mg at weeks 0, 4, and 8; ustekinumab (the reference arm) ~6 mg/kg IV at week 0 and 90 mg SC at week 8; or placebo IV (Sandborn et al., 2020i). Outcomes of interest included change in CDAI scores compared to baseline, clinical remission (CDAI < 150) and response, clinical biomarker response (clinical response and ≥50% reduction from baseline in CRP or fecal calprotectin), endoscopic response, and safety (Sandborn et al., 2020i). Two-hundred and fifty CD patients were included in this study and about 50% had failed biologics (Sandborn et al., 2020i). There were significant decreases of CDAI from baseline in all guselkumab groups compared to placebo at week 12 (Sandborn et al., 2020i). Compared to placebo, there was a higher proportion patients in all guselkumab groups who achieved clinical remission (200 mg: 54%, 600 mg: 56%, 1,200 mg: 50%, placebo: 15.7%), clinical biomarker response (200 mg: 54%, 600 mg: 48%, 1,200 mg: 42%, placebo: 11.8%), and endoscopic response (200 mg: 36%, 600 mg: 40%, 1,200 mg: 36%, placebo: 11.8%) (Sandborn et al., 2020i). In those who failed biologics, 45.5% (35/77) in the guselkumab group and 12.5% (3/24) in the placebo group achieved clinical remission at week 12 (Sandborn et al., 2020i). The rates of AE, infections, and serious AE were similar across all guselkumab treatment arms compared to placebo (Sandborn et al., 2020i).

In summary, in patients with moderate-severe CD, guselkumab was more efficacious in terms of clinical response, remission, endoscopic response, and clinical-biomarker response compared to placebo. There was no clear dose-response in this phase II study (Sandborn et al., 2020i). Guselkumab Is currently in phase II/III trials with an estimated study completion date in October 2024 (NCT03466411).

Additionally, a phase IIb/III study of the safety and efficacy of guselkumab in patients with moderate-severe UC was started in September 2019 (NCT04033445; anticipated completion by July 2025). In addition, a phase IIa study is evaluating combination treatment of guselkumab and golimumab in moderate-severe UC (NCT03662542) (Hanzel and D'Haens, 2020).

IL-6 Inhibitors

PF-04236921

PF-04236921 is a fully human immunoglobulin G2 monoclonal antibody that binds IL-6, which has many pro-inflammatory effects. A phase II study (ANDANTE I) aimed to evaluate the efficacy and safety of PF-04236921 in patients with moderate-to-severe CD who had inadequately responded to anti-TNF therapy (Danese et al., 2019). This study was then followed by an open-label extension study (ANDANTE II) with the primary aim of studying long-term safety, tolerability, and immunogenicity. For the phase II study, patients were randomized 1:1:1:1 to receive placebo or PF-04236921 10, 50, or 200 mg SC on days 1 and 28. The primary endpoint for the induction study was CDAI-70 response at weeks 8 or 12. Secondary endpoints included CDAI-70 and CDAI-100 response rates, CDAI remission (CDAI score <150). The primary aim of the OLE study was safety (Danese et al., 2019).

In the induction study PF-04236921 50 mg was found to have significantly higher CDAI-70 rates compared to placebo at weeks 8 (49.3 vs. 30.6%, $p < 0.05$) and 12 (47.4 vs. 28.6%, $p < 0.05$) (Danese et al., 2019). CDAI remission rates with PF-04236921 50 mg daily were significantly higher at week 12 compared to placebo 27.4 vs. 10.9%, $p < 0.05$) (Danese et al., 2019). The PF-04236921 10 mg dose did not meet the primary end point.

One-hundred and nine one patients entered the OLE study, and 89 (46%) were CDAI responders at OLE baseline. A majority of patients (77.8%) had their PF-04236921 dose escalated to 100 mg between weeks 8 and 48. In those who had been on drug in the induction period (n = 65), the HBI response and remission rates were 40 and 32%, respectively, at week 48 (Danese et al., 2019). It was rare to find antidrug antibodies. One out of 680 serum samples (0.1%) were found to be positive for anti-drug antibody (at week 4 with dose of 50 mg). CRP levels were noted to be suppressed during the OLE treatment period.

The most common serious adverse effects with CD-related, such as worsening of CD and abdominal pain, and nasopharyngitis. In the OLE study, most AEs were mild-moderate in severity. One death occurred in the induction study, and this was in the 50 mg group; the patient died of respiratory failure secondary to pneumonia and was thought to be unrelated to the treatment. Cases of GI perforation and GI abscesses were seen in the induction and OLE studies of patients on PF-04236921; most cases were identified in areas of previous disease involvement or surgery.

In summary, in patients with moderate-severe CD, PF-04236921 50 mg was more efficacious than placebo in inducing response and remission at week 12. In those in the OLE, who were initially on active drug during the induction period, about 40% had an HBI response rate at week 48. There are signals of GI perforation and abscess in the PF-04236921 treatment groups, and therefore this signal will need to be carefully monitored in any future clinical trials. At this time there are no phase three trials of PF-04236921.

Human IL-22Fc Fusion Protein

UTTR1147A

The activation of the IL-22 pathway may help to increase epithelial tight junctions, promote mucus production, and lead to secretion of antimicrobial peptides (Rothenberg et al., 2019). Ultimately this pathway may promote tissue regeneration, and therefore it is a valuable treatment target. UTTR1147A (IL-22Fc) is a fusion protein consisting of a linked human IL-22 and crystallizable fragment (Fc) of the human IgG4 (Rothenberg et al., 2019). A recent phase 1a trial studied single, ascending intravenous (1–120 μg/kg) and subcutaneous (3–120 μg/kg) doses of UTTR1147A on safety and tolerability in healthy volunteers (Rothenberg et al., 2019). The maximum tolerated IV dose was 90 μg/kg and most common AEs were dose-dependent but reversible skin effects. UTTR1147A increased proportionally to the doses given, and this caused elevations of IL-22 signaling biomarkers without causing systemic inflammation. Thus, preliminary data shows that UTTR1147A promotes the IL-22 signaling pathway and may lead to tissue regeneration without immunosuppression. This would be a novel mechanism of action in those with epithelial injury, such as what occurs in patients with IBD.

A phase Ib study analyzed UTTR1147A in healthy volunteers and UC patients. 38 healthy volunteers and 24 UC patients were given UTTR1147A or placebo at doses ranging between 30–90 μg/kg either weekly or monthly (6:2 UTTR1147A: placebo per cohort) (Wagner et al., 2020). The Mayo Clinic score was evaluated at baseline, day 30, and day 85. The study found that UTTR1147A was safe and well tolerated in both groups of patients and most common side effects were dermatologic effects of dry skin, erythema, and pruritis. Interestingly, at the same dose level, UC patients had relatively lower drug exposures than healthy volunteers and this was thought to be due to faster drug clearance (Wagner et al., 2020). Additionally, UC patients had attenuated pharmacodynamics response (production of biomarkers such as CRP) compared to healthy volunteers (Wagner et al., 2020). However, this study showed that there was an adequate safety and PK profile in both cohorts, and UTTR1147A did produce pharmacodynamics biomarkers in both cohorts. Further data would be important to study this novel mechanism of action in the treatment of patients with IBD.

Anti-Adhesion Molecules

Migration of pro-inflammatory T cells into the gut facilitates inflammation which is characteristic of CD and UC (Targan et al., 2007; Lin et al., 2015; Shivashankar and Pardi, 2017b). Interaction between surface-expressed α4β1 and α4β7 integrins on lymphocytes and adhesion molecules [vascular cell adhesion molecule-1 (VCAM-1) or mucosal addressin cell adhesion molecule-1 (MAdCAM-1)], which are present on endothelial cells, allow for activated effector T cells to target the gut (Shivashankar and Pardi, 2017b). This interaction allows for movement of T cells out of the blood stream and into the gastrointestinal tract (Sugiura et al., 2013; Shivashankar and Pardi, 2017b; Sandborn et al., 2020b). Natalizumab (NAT), a humanized IgG4 monoclonal antibody that targets the α4-integrin subunit of α4β1 and α4β7 on the surface of lymphocytes, has been approved for CD and multiple sclerosis since it blocks lymphocyte trafficking to the gut and brain. NAT has been associated with progressive multifocal leukoencephalopathy (PML) (Feagan et al., 2013; Park and Jeen, 2018). On the other hand, vedolizumab (VDZ) is a humanized IgG1 monoclonal antibody that specifically targets the α4β7 integrin, and it has been approved for UC and CD and therefore selectively prevents leukocyte migration to the gut (Feagan et al., 2013; Park and Jeen, 2018). In this section, we will focus on novel anti-adhesion molecules and a novel method of administration of VDZ.

SC Vedolizumab

VDZ, an infusion medication, was approved in 2014 for moderate-severe UC and CD. From clinical trial data, CD patients who responded to induction dosing at week 6 were more likely to achieve clinical remission, clinical response, and corticosteroid-free remission at week 52 compared to placebo (Sandborn et al., 2013). In addition, UC patients treated with VDZ in clinical trials had a significantly higher rate of clinical remission, clinical response, mucosal healing, and corticosteroid-free remission at week 52 compared to placebo (Feagan et al., 2013).

A new SC formulation of VDZ has been studied in those with UC; the benefit of this formulation is its convenient route of administration for patients who would like to avoid maintenance IV infusion therapy. A phase III open-label study (VISIBLE 1) of patients with moderate-severely active UC was conducted to assess the efficacy of SC VDZ as maintenance therapy (Sandborn et al., 2020b). The primary endpoint was clinical remission (total Mayo score ≤2 and no subscore >1) at week 52. VDZ 300 mg IV was administered at weeks 0 and 2 (Sandborn et al., 2020b). Those with clinical response at week 6 were then randomized to maintenance treatment with SC VDZ 108 mg every 2 weeks, IV VDZ 300 mg every 8 weeks, or placebo (Sandborn et al., 2020b). SC VDZ had a higher rate of clinical remission at week 52 compared to placebo in both anti-TNF naïve and anti-TNF exposed patients (53.7 vs. 18.9%, $p < 0.01$ and 33.3 vs. 5.3%, $p = 0.023$, respectively) (Sandborn et al., 2020b). There were also significantly higher rates of endoscopic improvement (56.6 vs. 21.4%, $p < 0.001$) and durable clinical response (64.2 and 28.6%, $p < 0.001$) when SC VDZ was compared to placebo (Sandborn et al., 2020b). There was no significant difference between SC VDZ and placebo in terms of durable clinical remission (15.1 vs. 5.4%, $p = 0.076$) or corticosteroid-free remission (28.9 vs. 8.3%, $p = 0.067$) (Sandborn et al., 2020b). Endpoints were generally similar between SC VDZ and IV VDZ.

There were no new safety signals when SC VDZ was compared to IV VDZ. The most common AE was worsening of UC disease activity, nasopharyngitis, upper respiratory infections, and anemia (Sandborn et al., 2020b). Eleven patients (10.4%) receiving SC VDZ had injection-site reactions characterized by rash, swelling, erythema, and pruritis (Sandborn et al., 2020b). There were no cases of PML or deaths. The VDZ pharmacokinetics achieved with SC VDZ was similar to that of the IV formulation (Sandborn et al., 2020b).

Overall, this study showed that SC vedolizumab was effective and well-tolerated as maintenance therapy for UC following an induction with IV VDZ. Efficacy outcomes were generally similar between maintenance SC VDZ and IV VDZ. Also, the safety profile was encouraging, and no new safety signals were identified. SC VDZ will give patients an option for an alternate mode of administration if they prefer to avoid long-term infusions. SC VDZ for moderate-severe UC will potentially be available in 2022.

Etrolizumab

While VDZ targets only the α4β7 integrin, etrolizumab is a SC humanized monoclonal anti-integrin antibody that selectively binds the β7 subunit of both α4β7 and αEβ7 integrins (Vermeire et al., 2014; Sandborn et al., 2020h). Therefore, etrolizumab controls movement of inflammatory cells into the gastrointestinal tract and also mediates inflammatory effects on the gut mucosa (Vermeire et al., 2014; Sandborn et al., 2020h). The phase II EUCALYPTUS study showed that etrolizumab was beneficial over placebo in patients with moderate-severe UC (Vermeire et al., 2014). In this study, 124 patients were randomized to two doses of SC etrolizumab—either 100 mg at weeks 0, 4, and 8 with placebo at week 2; or 420 mg loading lose (LD) at week 0, followed by 300 mg at weeks 2, 4, and 8—or placebo (Vermeire et al., 2014). The primary endpoint was clinical remission at week 10 (Mayo clinic score ≤2 with no individual subscore >1). Compared to placebo (0 patients in clinical remission), etrolizumab (100 mg: 21%, $p = 0.004$; LD+

300 mg: 10%, $p = 0.048$) treatment was found to lead to a higher proportion of patients in clinical remission at week 10 (Vermeire et al., 2014). Adverse events occurred at a similar frequency across all groups—61% of 100 mg etrolizumab group, 49% in the LD+ 300 mg group, and 72% in the placebo group. No patients developed PML.

Etrolizumab has an extremely active phase III clinical trial program and includes direct comparisons to infliximab and adalimumab. There are currently six randomized controlled trials and two open label extension studies. The aim of HIBISCUS I and II (identical induction trials of etrolizumab 105 mg vs. adalimumab and placebo), GARDENIA (maintenance study studying etrolizumab 105 mg vs. infliximab), and LAUREL (maintenance trial evaluating etrolizumab 105 mg against placebo) is to study UC patients who are anti-TNF naïve. HICKORY is a maintenance trial studying etrolizumab 105 mg vs. placebo in anti-TNF exposed UC patients (Sandborn et al., 2020h). The primary endpoints are based on clinical response (≥3 point decrease and 30% reduction in Mayo clinic score and ≥1 point decrease in rectal bleeding or an absolute rectal bleeding score of 0 or 1), remission (MCS ≤2, with individual subscore ≤1 and rectal bleeding score of 0) at each trial's specified time points (Sandborn et al., 2020h). COTTONWOOD is the open-label extension and safety monitoring study of UC patients treated with etrolizumab who were followed until week 108 (Sandborn et al., 2020h).

Early results from the HICKORY study included 130 UC patients and 45% had previously been exposed to ≥2 anti-TNFs (Peyrin-Biroulet et al., 2017). Stool frequency rates improved from baseline to week 4 in 30% and at week 14 in 50% of patients (Peyrin-Biroulet et al., 2017). Rectal bleeding remission rates were observed from baseline to week 4 in about 30% of patients and at week 14 in about 50% of patients (Peyrin-Biroulet et al., 2017). Biomarkers decreased at week 14 (fecal calprotectin: mean 57% decrease; CRP: 33% decrease) (Peyrin-Biroulet et al., 2017). Therefore, in patients previously exposed to anti-TNFs, etrolizumab led to symptom improvement as early as week 4 (Peyrin-Biroulet et al., 2017).

For patients with CD, the BERGAMOT study is an induction and maintenance trial evaluating anti-TNF naïve and experienced patients (etrolizumab 105 and 210 mg vs. placebo) (Sandborn et al., 2020h). Eligible patients may enter JUNIPER study, which will be the open label extension of etrolizumab 105 mg (Sandborn et al., 2020h). The co-primary endpoint for BERGAMOT is clinical remission (unweighted abdominal pain score ≤1 and stool frequency ≤3) and endoscopic improvement (>50% reduction in SES-CD from baseline) at weeks 14 and 62 (Sandborn et al., 2020h). The primary outcome for JUNIPER is long term efficacy (clinical remission assessed at 12 weeks intervals), endoscopic remission (SES-CD ≤4 [≤2 for pts with ileal disease] with no segment >1) at week 108 and incidence and severity of AEs (Sandborn et al., 2020h).

The BERGAMOT induction cohort included 300 CD patients who were randomized to etrolizumab 105 mg SC every 4 weeks, 210 mg at weeks 0, 2, 4, 8, and 12, or placebo for a 14 weeks induction period (Selinger et al., 2018). Previous anti-TNF exposure was noted in 73% of patients (Selinger et al., 2018). Symptomatic remission was seen in a greater number of patients treated with etrolizumab [105 mg: 20.8% (90% confidence interval 15.4–27.5); 210 mg: 24.8 (18.9–31.8)] compared to placebo (11.9 [6.6–20.5]) at week 14 (Selinger et al., 2018). Similarly, more patients treated with etrolizumab (105 mg: 21 [15.6–27.8] and 210 mg: 17.4 [12.4–23.7] achieved endoscopic improvement compared to placebo (3.4 [1.1–9.7]) at week 14 (Selinger et al., 2018). AEs were comparable between etrolizumab and placebo; there were no cases of PML or death (Selinger et al., 2018).

In addition to providing further data on clinical response, remission, and endoscopic remission data for etrolizumab, these data may help clinicians decide which biologic is an ideal first-line agent for their patient (Sandborn et al., 2020h). The HIBISCUS I and II and GARDENIA studies will be the first phase III trials in UC to study the efficacy of a novel agent directly compared to another agent, i.e., infliximab and adalimumab (Sandborn et al., 2020h).

AJM300

α4 or α4β7 targets have been shown to be possible therapeutic targets in the treatment of IBD since suppression of these integrins have controlled development of colitis in an animal model (Sugiura et al., 2013). A variety of small molecule α4 integrin antagonists have been studied in clinical trials for conditions such as asthma and multiple sclerosis. AJM300 is an oral small molecule that targets α4 integrin, and it is classified as a phenylalanine derivative (Yoshimura et al., 2015). This small molecule's duration of action is very short, within one day of last dose as described in a phase IIa study (Yoshimura et al., 2015). AJM300 has been shown to be effective in experimental colitis model in mice; this study showed that the active metabolite of AJM300 inhibited the binding of α4β1/α4β7 integrin-expressing cells to VCAM-1/MAdCAM-1 *in vitro* (Sugiura et al., 2013). Given the α4 blockade, there may be a potential risk for PML in AJM-300 therapy (Yoshimura et al., 2015).

A phase IIa study including 102 patients with moderate active UC was conducted to assess the primary outcome measure of clinical response (decrease in Mayo score of at least 3 points and decrease of at least 30% from baseline, with decrease in rectal bleeding subscore of at least 1 point or an absolute rectal bleeding score of 0 or 1) at week 8 (Yoshimura et al., 2015). Patients who had inadequate response or intolerance to mesalamine or corticosteroids were given AJM300 960 mg orally or placebo three times daily for 8 weeks (Yoshimura et al., 2015). Compared to placebo, those treated with AJM300 had higher rates of clinical response (62.7 vs. 25.5%, $p = 0.0002$), clinical remission (23.5 vs. 3.9%, $p = 0.0099$), and mucosal healing (58.8 vs. 29.4%, $p = 0.0014$) (Yoshimura et al., 2015).

There was a significant increase in peripheral leukocyte count as would be expected from an anti-α4 integrin; this increase was seen as early as week 2 (Yoshimura et al., 2015). However, this finding normalized the day after the last dose given at week 8 thereby suggesting a short duration of action (Yoshimura et al., 2015). The most common adverse events were nasopharyngitis and UC, with higher AEs seen with UC in the placebo group (Yoshimura et al., 2015). Overall, however, there were similar rates of AEs observed between the treatment and placebo arms (Sabino et al., 2019). There were no serious AEs observed, and infection, and PML were not seen in this study (Yoshimura et al., 2015).

In summary, AJM-300 was more effective than placebo in inducing clinical response, clinical remission, and mucosal healing in moderately active UC patients who had only been exposed to mesalamine or steroids in the past. However, the study was limited by a small sample size and a short study duration (8 weeks) (Yoshimura et al., 2015). Unfortunately, there were extremely low number of patients who were intolerant or inadequately responding to steroids in this study, and there was no information on exposure to immunomodulators and anti-TNFs (Yoshimura et al., 2015). AJM300 is currently in phase III trials for UC patients, and the estimated study completion date is February 2021 (NCT03531892).

Abrilumab (AMG 181or MEDI 7183)

Abrilumab is an injectable fully human monoclonal immunoglobulin G2 antibody that targets the α4β7 integrin and prevents interaction with MADCAM-1 (Sandborn et al., 2017a). Abrilumab has a high bioavailability after SC dosing and a long half-life (about 31 days) (Sandborn et al., 2019).

A phase IIb study in patients with CD who had inadequate or loss of response or intolerance to immunosuppressives, anti-TNFs, or corticosteroids were randomized to receive placebo or abrilumab (21 mg or 70 mg) SC on day 1, weeks 2 and 4, and then every 4 for 24 weeks, or one dose of abrilumab 210 mg SC on day 1 (Sandborn et al., 2017a). The primary endpoint was clinical remission (CDAI < 150) at week 8 (Sandborn et al., 2017a). There was no significant difference in clinical remission at week 8 between abrilumab at any dose when compared to placebo (Sandborn et al., 2017a). Of note, there were higher rates of clinical remission at week 12 in those treated with a single dose of abrilumab 210 mg when compared to placebo in those who previously failed anti-TNF therapy (Sandborn et al., 2017a). AE rates were similar among all groups through week 24, and there were no cases of PML or death (Sandborn et al., 2017a).

A phase II induction and sustained remission study of abrilumab was conducted in patients with active moderate-severe UC who did not respond or lost response to usual medical therapy (Sandborn et al., 2019). Patients were randomized to SC placebo or abrilumab (7, 21, 70 mg) on day 1, week 2, week 4, and then every 4 weeks thereafter until week 24 or a single dose of 210 mg abrilumab on day 1 followed by placebo at the same dosing scheduled noted previously until week 24 (Sandborn et al., 2019). An open-label phase of the study involved administration of abrilumab 210 mg once every 3 months (Sandborn et al., 2019). The primary endpoint was remission (total Mayo score ≤2 points with no individual sub-score >1 point) at week 8 (Sandborn et al., 2019). There were significantly higher odds of achieving clinical remission, clinical response, and mucosal healing at week 8 in those treated with abrilumab 70 and 210 mg compared to placebo (Sandborn et al., 2019). In those with prior anti-TNF failure, there were greater clinical remission rates at week 8 in the abrilumab 70 and 210 mg dose (Sandborn et al., 2019).

However, there were no clear benefits of abrilumab treatment at week 24—in this study, patients continued their initial treatment regardless of whether they responded after the induction period (Sandborn et al., 2019). The odds of sustained remission did increase in patients who continued to take multiple doses of abrilumab 70 mg every 4 weeks compared to placebo (Sandborn et al., 2019).

There were no differences in AEs across treatment groups through week 24. The most common AE were non-serious infections, gastrointestinal effects, headache, and arthralgia (Sandborn et al., 2019). The only serious AE noted in more than one patient in the abrilumab treated group was worsening of UC (Sandborn et al., 2019). There were no cases of PML or death. Ten patients (8.6%) in the placebo group and 9 (3.8%) in the abrilumab group reported neoplasms (Sandborn et al., 2019). A limitation of this phase II study of abrilumab in UC include its short duration; phase III studies are needed to assess the long-term response of the 70 mg dose after 24 weeks (Sandborn et al., 2019).

In conclusion, while the phase II study of abrilumab in CD failed to meet its primary endpoint, the study in UC patients showed efficacy at week 8 with higher rates of clinical remission, clinical response, and mucosal healing. Since there was no clear benefit of abrilumab at week 24 in UC patients, longer term phase III studies are required to better assess this finding. Phase 3 studies have not yet started.

PF-00547659 (SHP647)

PF-00547659 is a SC fully human monoclonal antibody that binds to MAdCAM, thereby decreasing lymphocyte trafficking to the gut and leading to decreased gastrointestinal inflammation (Sandborn et al., 2018). A phase II dose ranging study of PF-00547659 was conducted in patients with moderate-severe CD who have a history of failure or intolerance to immunosuppressives and/or anti-TNF therapy (Sandborn et al., 2018). This study included 265 patients who were randomized to PF-00547659 22.5, 75 mg, or 225 mg or placebo (Sandborn et al., 2018). The primary endpoint was a CDAI 70-point decrease from baseline at week eight or 12 (Sandborn et al., 2018). There was no significant difference in CDAI response between the treatment group and placebo at week 8 (22.5 mg: 52.7%, 75 mg: 60.1%, 225 mg: 62.7%) or 12 (22.5 mg: 62%, 75 mg: 64.7%, 225 mg: 57.5%); this was likely due to a high clinical response in the placebo group (47.7% at week 8 and 58.6% at week 12) (Sandborn et al., 2018).

In a post-hoc analysis, the proportions of patients who achieved clinical remission were higher in all PF-00547659 dose groups than in placebo at weeks 8 and 12 in those with higher inflammatory burden as evidenced by higher median high sensitivity CRP values (>5 mg/L or >18.8 mg/L) or higher baseline SES-CD scores (>17) at baseline (Sandborn et al., 2018). The incidence of AEs, serious AEs, and discontinuation was similar across all treatment groups.

The long-term safety and efficacy portion of the study followed patients for a further 6 months (D'Haens et al., 2018a). The most common AEs with treatment included nasopharyngitis (5.6%), arthralgia (6.0%), and headache (5.2%) (D'Haens et al., 2018a).

There were two deaths (multiorgan failure after postoperative aspiration following resection of the terminal ileum and metastatic adenocarcinoma of unknown primary) however neither were thought to be drug related (D'Haens et al., 2018a). Harvey Bradshaw Index response rates were sustained over 6 months of treatment (D'Haens et al., 2018a).

A post-hoc analysis also looked at endoscopic outcomes following induction therapy with PF-00547659 (D′Haens et al., 2018b). Mean total SES-CD scores across four colon and one ileal segments were found to trend toward a decrease across all treatment arms (except for the 75 mg dose) (D′Haens et al., 2018b). The 22.5 mg dose showed the largest trend toward improvement in endoscopic disease severity (mean change from baseline to week 10 at 22.5 mg dose: 4.0; 75 mg: 0; 225 mg: −1; placebo: 1.5) (D′Haens et al., 2018b). However, no consistent association between clinical and endoscopic improvement was observed (D′Haens et al., 2018b).

In patients with moderate-severe UC, a phase II study that evaluated the efficacy and safety of PF-00547659 in 357 patients who had failed or were intolerant to at least one usual therapy found the drug to be superior to placebo (Vermeire et al., 2017a; Sabino et al., 2019). The primary endpoint was clinical remission (Mayo score ≤2 with no individual subscore >1 and rectal bleeding subscore ≤1) at week 12 (Vermeire et al., 2017a). The remission rates in those treated with PF-00547659 (7.5 mg: 11.3%; 22.5 mg: 16.7%; 75 mg: 15.5%; 225 mg: 5.7%) were higher than placebo (2.7%) at week 12; the 225 mg dosing did not achieve statistical significance compared to placebo (Vermeire et al., 2017a). Similar to the findings from the CD trial, PF-00547659 was overall well-tolerated (Vermeire et al., 2017a).

In conclusion, in patients with CD, PF00547659 was not significantly different compared to placebo in achieving clinical response at weeks 8 or 12 likely due to high placebo response rates (Sabino et al., 2019). On the other hand, three out of four doses of PF00547659 did achieve significantly higher rates of clinical remission than placebo in patents with UC. Phase III studies in patients with IBD have not yet been announced.

Oral Anti-tumor Necrosis Factor Agents

Anti-TNF agents were the first class of biologics approved for the treatment of moderate to severe UC and CD. They have revolutionized the treatment paradigm of IBD and have proven to be effective (Sands et al., 2004; Rutgeerts et al., 2005; Hanauer et al., 2006; Sandborn et al., 2007; Schreiber et al., 2007). One of the limitations of current anti-TNF agents is that they are currently administered by IV or as SC injectables only. This is associated with risk of infusion/injection reactions, systemic side effects and increased cost of repeated infusions/injections. An oral and intestinally restricted anti-TNF agent would help overcome some of these challenges of current anti-TNF agents.

AVX-470

AVX-470 is an oral polyclonal immunoglobulin that is derived from the colostrum of cows that have been immunized with human recombinant anti-TNF. In the first human study, 36 patients with UC received either AVX-470 (pH dependent delayed release capsules) at doses of 0.2, 1.6, and 3.5 g/day or placebo (Harris et al., 2016). In terms of safety, AVX-470 was well tolerated and the total rate of AEs was 52% compared to 78% in the placebo group. At 4 weeks, the overall clinical response and remission rates were 25.9 and 3.7% in the AVX-470 group compared to 11.1 and 0% in the placebo group, respectively. Endoscopic remission was achieved in 7.4% in the AVX-470 group compared to none in the placebo group. In term of immunogenicity, no human anti-bovine antibodies were detected.

OPRX-106

OPRX-106 is an oral anti-TNF agent. It is a combination of plant cell-expressed human anti-TNF receptor II fused to IgG1 Fc domain. The plant cells function as a delivery mechanism. A phase II randomized, 2-arm, open label clinical trial of 25 patients with UC treated with OPRX-106 at 2 or 8 mg daily for 8 weeks was performed (Almon et al., 2020). A total of 18 patients completed the study. Clinical response defined as a decrease in the Mayo score by at least 3 points was achieved in 67% and clinical remission (Mayo score ≤2 without sub-score being greater than 1) was achieved in 28%. Mucosal healing (Mayo endoscopic score ≤1) was achieved in 33% (Almon et al., 2020). In terms of immunogenicity, no anti-drug antibodies were detected.

Oral anti-TNF agents have the potential of enhanced safety, decreased immunogenicity and higher patient acceptance. Although promising, the current available data on efficacy and safety of oral anti-TNF agents is limited and future larger trials are needed to evaluate efficacy, safety, feasibility and cost effectiveness.

Sphingosine-1-Phosphate Receptor Modulators

Sphigosine-1-phosphate is a sphingolipid ligand of G protein coupled receptors (S1P1-S1P5) which are responsible for controlling the egress of lymphocytes from lymphoid organs. The S1P/S1PR interaction can also result in internalization of the S1PR which leads to decrease lymphocyte release from the lymphoid tissue into the circulation. Fingolimod was the first S1P receptor modulator approved for the treatment of multiple sclerosis in 2010 (Cohen et al., 2010; Kappos et al., 2010). Fingolimod is a non-selective S1P receptor modulator and has high affinity for S1PR 1 and S1PR3-5. Although overall well tolerated, fingolimod has been associated with adverse events such as bradycardia, hypertension, infection and elevated liver tests (Danese et al., 2018).

Ozanimod

Ozanimod is a S1P receptor modulator with selective affinity for S1PR1 and S1PR5. It was approved by the US FDA in 2020 for the treatment of relapsing MS (Cohen et al., 2016; Cohen et al., 2019; Comi et al., 2019).

TOUCHSTONE is a phase II double blind, randomized clinical trial of ozanimod 0.5 or 1 mg vs. placebo daily in moderate to severe UC (n = 197). The primary outcome was clinical remission at 8 weeks (Mayo clinic score ≤2; No sub-score > 1). The primary outcome was achieved in 16% in the ozanimod 1 mg group vs. 14% in the ozanimod 0.5 mg group vs. 6% in the placebo group ($p = 0.048$ and $p = 0.14$, respectively) (Sandborn et al., 2016). Mucosal healing at week 8 (defined as Mayo endoscopy sub-score ≤1) was achieved in 34% in the 1 mg group vs. 28% in the 0.5 mg group compared to 12% in the placebo group ($p = 0.002$ and $p = 0.03$, respectively). At week 32, clinical remission was 21% in the 1 mg group and 26% in the 0.5 mg group compared to 6% in the placebo group ($p = 0.01$ and $p = 0.002$, respectively). Mucosal and histologic healing rates were similarly significantly higher in the ozanimod groups compared to placebo at 32 weeks (Sandborn et al., 2016). In the ozanimod groups, one patient developed bradycardia (patient had previous history of bradycardia) and four patients developed elevated liver enzymes.

TRUE-NORTH is a phase III randomized, double-blind, placebo-controlled trial of induction and maintenance ozanimod in UC completed in 2020 (Danese et al., 2020a; Sandborn W. et al., 2020). In the induction phase of 10 weeks, moderately to severely active UC patients received either ozanimod 1 mg or placebo daily. The primary endpoint of clinical remission (based on 3-component Mayo score) was met in 18.4% in the ozanimod group vs. 6% in the placebo group ($p < 0.0001$) (Sandborn W. et al., 2020). Clinical remission was numerically higher then placebo but did not achieve statistical significance in the anti-TNF exposed patients who received ozanimod (10 vs. 4.6%; $p = 0.195$). Secondary outcomes of clinical response, endoscopic improvement and mucosal healing (both endoscopy and histology) rates were significantly in the total ozanimod group compared to placebo. The reported rate of bradycardia was 0.5% in the ozanimod group.

In the maintenance trial, 457 moderate to severe UC patients who achieved clinical response after 10 weeks of ozanimod induction therapy were then re-randomized at 1:1 to either ozanimod 1 mg or placebo and outcomes assessed at week 52 (Sandborn W. et al., 2020). Clinical remission (based on 3-component Mayo score) rates were significantly higher in the ozanimod group at 37% compared to 18.5% in the placebo group ($p < 0.0001$) (Danese et al., 2020a). Anti-TNF exposed patients who received ozanimod also had a significantly higher rate of clinical remission compared to placebo (28.9% vs. 10.1; $p = 0.0053$). All secondary endpoints of the trial were also met in the ozanimod group including: clinical response, endoscopic improvement, corticosteroid-free remission, maintenance of clinical remission, durable clinical remission and mucosal healing (both endoscopic and histologic) (Danese et al., 2020a). In this trial, ozanimod was also well tolerated with the most common reported AEs being abnormal liver tests and headaches. Elevation of alanine aminotransferase (ALT) was noted in 4.8% in the ozanimod group compared to 0.4% in the placebo group (Danese et al., 2020a).

For CD, ozanimod was evaluated in a phase II multicenter, uncontrolled, prospective observer-blinded endpoint trial, STEPSTONE (Feagan et al., 2020a). The trial had a 12-weeks induction period followed by a 100-weeks extension study. Patients with moderately to severely active CD (n = 69) received a 7-days dose escalation of ozanimod followed by 11 weeks of ozanimod 1 mg oral capsule daily. The primary endpoint was reduction in the Simple Endoscopic Score for Crohn's disease (SES-CD) at 12 weeks from baseline. The mean change of SES-CD at week 12 was − 2.2 ± 6 and 23.2% of patients achieved endoscopic response (defined as SES-CD decrease by ≥ 50%) (Feagan et al., 2020a). Clinical remission (defined as CDAI <150) was noted in 39.1% of patients. The most common AE was CD flare and there were no cases of bradycardia or arrhythmias reported (Feagan et al., 2020a).

Phase III, placebo-controlled induction and maintenance studies of ozanimod in moderate to severe CD are currently recruiting (NCT03440372, NCT03440385, NCT03464097, NCT03467958).

Etrasimod

Etrasimod is an oral S1P receptor modulator with selectivity for S1PR1, S1PR4 and S1PR5. A phase II (OASIS; proof of concept), double-blinded trial randomized moderate to severe UC patients (n = 156) to either etrasimod 1 mg, etrasimod 2 mg or placebo in a 1:1:1 fashion for 12 weeks (Sandborn et al., 2020g). The primary endpoint was improvement in the modified Mayo Clinic score at 12 weeks from baseline and secondary endpoints included: the improvement in the total Mayo Clinic score, improvement in the two component Mayo Clinic score (rectal bleeding and endoscopy) and endoscopic improvement (endoscopy sub-score ≤ 1). The primary endpoint was achieved in the etrasimod 2 mg group compared to placebo (least square mean difference, 0.99; 90% CI, 0.30–1.68; $p = 0.009$) but not in the etrasimod 1 mg group. Compared to placebo, the etrasimod 2 mg group had higher rates of: endoscopic improvement (41.8 vs. 17.8%; $p = 0.003$), improvement in the total Mayo score ($p = 0.010$) and improvement in the 2 component Mayo score ($p = 0.002$) (Sandborn et al., 2020g). Histologic remission (defined as Geboes score <2) was an exploratory endpoint of the trial and was significantly higher in the etrasimod 2 mg group compared to placebo (19.5 vs. 6.1%; $p = 0.03$) (Sandborn et al., 2020g).

In this trial there was significantly higher rates of discontinuation of drug due to AEs in the etrasimod groups (n = 7) compared to placebo (n = 0) (Sandborn et al., 2020g). The most common AEs other than disease worsening are upper respiratory tract infections, nasopharyngitis and anemia. In etrasimod 2 mg group, transient first-degree heart block occurred in two patients and type 1 s degree heart block was noted in one patient. The authors report that all three patients had evidence of atrioventricular block noted on electrocardiography prior to receiving the study drug (Sandborn et al., 2020g).

Phase III induction and maintenance trials of etrasimod for moderate to severe UC are currently recruiting (NCT03996369, NCT03945188, NCT03950232, NCT04176588). A phase II/III study of etrasimod induction and maintenance in CD has recently opened and is currently recruiting (NCT04173273).

Amiselimod (MT-1303)

Amiselimod is an oral S1P receptor modulator with higher selectivity for S1PR1 than other S1P receptors. Phase II study of amiselimod demonstrated that is well tolerated and potentially effective for multiple sclerosis (Kappos et al., 2016). A phase II randomized, placebo-controlled trial of amiselimod in CD (NCT02378688) was completed and at this time results are not published. A proof of concept study randomized 78 patients to either amiselimod 0.4 mg (n = 40) or placebo (n = 38) (D'Haens et al., 2019). The primary outcomes of clinical response (decrease in CDAI by 100 points) at week 12 was achieved in 48.7 vs. 54.1% in the placebo group. No significant differences were noted in the fecal calprotectin and CRP in the two groups (D'Haens et al., 2019).

Phosphodiesterase 4 Inhibitors

Phosphodiesterases (PDE1-PDE11) are a group of intracellular enzymes that catalyze the breakdown of cyclic adenosine monophosphate (cAMP) and cyclic guanosine monophosphate (cGMP). PDE4 catalyzes the breakdown of 3, 5′ cAMP in multiple cell types including T-cells, macrophages and monocytes. This leads to activation of nuclear transcription factor kappaB (NF-κB) which eventually promotes downstream proinflammatory effects. Therefore, inhibition of PDE4 can lead to suppression of NF-κB and subsequently reduce TNF-α mRNA expression and production of nitric oxide and also increase synthesis of anti-inflammatory cytokines such as IL-10 and IL-6 (Ollivier et al., 1996; Gobejishvili et al., 2008; Kwak et al., 2005; Platzer et al., 1999). Therefore, there has been interest in developing PDE4 inhibitors as therapeutic agents in IBD.

Apremilast

Apremilast is an oral PDE4 inhibitor that is currently approved by the US FDA for the treatment of psoriasis and psoriatic arthritis. A double-blind, phase II trial randomized UC patients to apremilast 30 mg (n = 57), apremilast 40 mg (n = 55) or placebo (n = 58) twice daily (Danese et al., 2020b). The primary endpoint of clinical remission (defined as total Mayo UC score ≤2; no individual score >1) was achieved in 31.6% in the 30 mg group ($p = 0.01$ compared to placebo), 21.8% in the 40 mg group compared to 12.1% in the placebo group ($p = 0.27$) (Danese et al., 2020b). Endoscopic response (defined as a decrease in the Mayo endoscopic subscore by ≥ 1) was achieved in 41.4% of patients in the placebo group compared to 73.7% in the 30 mg group ($p < 0.0001$) and 47.3% in the 40 mg group ($p = 0.69$). Both the 30 and 40 mg apremilast groups showed greater reduction in CPR and fecal calprotectin compared to placebo. Although the primary endpoint was not reached in this trial, post hoc analysis demonstrated that a significantly higher proportion of patient in both apremilast groups had a Mayo endoscopic subscore of ≤1 compared to placebo (Danese et al., 2020b).

In terms of safety, the most common side effect reported in the apremilast groups were headaches at 25.5% in the 40 mg group and 21.1% in the 30 mg group compared to 6.9% in the placebo group. Serious AE rate was 2.4% in the placebo group and 1.8% in the 40 mg apremilast group (1 patient who experienced pancreatitis but thought not to be related to study drug) (Danese et al., 2020b). Currently, a phase III UC trial of apremilast has not been registered.

Cobitolimod

Cobitolimod is an oligodeoxynucleotide that is DNA-based and binds to Toll-like receptor 9 (TLR9) on lymphocytes and antigen presenting cells. It activates TLR 9 which lead to induction of regulatory T-cells that produce anti-inflammatory IL-10 in addition to suppressing proinflammatory TH-17 cells. Cobitolimod is a topical agent and is supposed to have low systemic absorption.

A double-blind study (COLLECT) randomized 131 patients with moderate to severe UC to two topically administered doses (during colonoscopy) of cobitolimod 30 mg (n = 87) or placebo (n = 44) (Atreya et al., 2016). The primary endpoint of induction of clinical remission at week 12 (defined as Clinical Activity Index (CAI) ≤4) was 44.4% in the cobitolimod group vs. 46.5% in the placebo group ($p = 0.91$) (Atreya et al., 2016). However, the study did meet multiple secondary endpoints including symptomatic remission, clinical remission with mucosal healing and histologic improvement.

A dose ranging, double-blinded phase IIb study (CONDUCT) randomized 213 patients with moderate to severe left-sided UC into five different treatment arms that received drug or placebo via rectal enemas: cobitolimod 31 mg, 125 mg, or 250 mg at weeks 0 and 3; cobitolimod 125 mg at weeks 0, 1,2 and 3 or placebo (Atreya et al., 2020). The primary endpoint of clinical remission at 6 weeks (defined as Mayo subscore of 0 for rectal bleeding, 0 or 1 for stool frequency + ≥ 1-point decrease from baseline, endoscopy subscore of 0 or 1-excluding friability) was achieved in the cobitolimod 250 mg group at 21% (n = 9) vs. 7% (n = 3) in the placebo group ($p = 0.025$) (Atreya et al., 2020). The rest of the dosing groups did not achieve the primary endpoint compared to placebo. Cobitolimod was well tolerated with an adverse event rate across the dosing groups from 25 to 43% compared to 48% in the placebo group (Atreya et al., 2020). Phase 3 studies are planned for UC (not yet registered at this time).

CONCLUSION

In conclusion, the armamentarium of IBD therapeutic agents is ever expanding. This review highlights some of these novel and emerging therapies. For example, there has been significant development in the small molecules class of agents such as JAK inhibitors and S1P receptor modulators. These agents offer the advantages of ease of administration as they are oral agents and do not have the downside of immunogenicity and antibody formation seen with some of the IV/SC biologics. Some of these agents such might also have the possibility of more rapid onset of action as seen with tofacitinib. In addition, some of these agents will likely have the potential of having a more favorable safety profile compared to anti-TNF agents. This includes for example the development of the intestinally restricted pan-JAK inhibitor (TD-1473), anti-integrins/ anti-MAdCAM therapies and IL-23 therapies. In the era of increasing therapeutic agents to treat IBD, the challenge will the ability to select the best agent for the individual patient. This calls for the development of precision/personalized medicine approach to the treatment of IBD.

DISCLOSURES

BA-B is on the Speaker Bureau of Takeda and AbbVie. RS is on the Speaker Bureau of and received clinical research grant support from AbbVie, and is on the advisory board of Pfizer. DP has no conflicts to disclose.

AUTHOR CONTRIBUTIONS

BA-B, Literature search, manuscript draft, final review and editing. RS, Literature search, manuscript draft, manuscript review. DP, Manuscript draft, critical review and final editing.

REFERENCES

Almon, E., Shaaltiel, Y., Sbeit, W., Fich, A., Schwartz, D., Waterman, M., et al. (2020). Novel orally administered recombinant anti-TNF alpha fusion protein for the treatment of ulcerative colitis: results from a phase 2a clinical trial. *J. Clin. Gastroenterol.* 55(2). 134–140. doi:10.1097/MCG.0000000000001314

Anderson, C. A., Boucher, G., Lees, C. W., Franke, A., D'Amato, M., Taylor, K. D., et al. (2011). Meta-analysis identifies 29 additional ulcerative colitis risk loci, increasing the number of confirmed associations to 47. *Nat. Genet.* 43, 246–252. doi:10.1038/ng.764

Atreya, R., Bloom, S., Scaldaferri, F., Gerardi, V., Admyre, C., Karlsson, Å., et al. (2016). Clinical effects of a topically applied toll-like receptor 9 agonist in active moderate-to-severe ulcerative colitis. *Eccojc* 10, 1294–1302. doi:10.1093/ecco-jcc/jjw103

Atreya, R., Peyrin-Biroulet, L., Klymenko, A., Augustyn, M., Bakulin, I., Slankamenac, D., et al. (2020). Cobitolimod for moderate-to-severe, left-sided ulcerative colitis (CONDUCT): a phase 2b randomised, double-blind, placebo-controlled, dose-ranging induction trial. *Lancet Gastroenterol. Hepatol.* 5, 1063–1075. doi:10.1016/s2468-1253(20)30301-0

Authors (2019). A SPECIAL MEETING review EDITION: highlights in inflammatory bowel disease from the 14th congress of ECCO: a review of selected Presentations from the 14th congress of the European Crohn's and colitis organisation (ECCO) * March 6-9, 2019 * copenhagen, DenmarkSpecial reporting on:* VARSITY: a double-blind, double-dummy, randomized controlled trial of vedolizumab versus adalimumab in patients with active ulcerative colitis* analyses of data from the VISIBLE 1 and 2 trials: vedolizumab in patients with ulcerative colitis or Crohn's disease* improved endoscopic outcomes and mucosal healing of upadacitinib as an induction therapy in Adults with moderately to severely active ulcerative colitis: data from the U-achieve study* long-term safety of vedolizumab in ulcerative colitis and Crohn's disease: final results from the GEMINI LTS study* pediatric Crohn's disease adalimumab level-based optimization treatment (PAILOT) randomized controlled trial* maintenance treatment with mirikizumab, a P19-directed IL-23 antibody: 52-week results in patients with moderately to severely active ulcerative colitis* real-world effectiveness and safety of vedolizumab and anti-TNF therapy in biologic-naive patients with ulcerative colitis or Crohn's disease: results from the EVOLVE study* A randomized, multicenter, double-blind, placebo-controlled study of a targeted-release oral cyclosporine formulation in the treatment of mild to moderate ulcerative colitis: efficacy results* real-world analyses of patients with IBD treated with VedolizumabPLUS meeting Abstract Summaries with Expert commentary by: edward V. Loftus Jr, MDProfessor of MedicineDivision of Gastroenterology and HepatologyMayo ClinicRochester, Minnesota. *Gastroenterol. Hepatol. (N Y)* 15, 1–24.

Baker, K. F., and Isaacs, J. D. (2018). Novel therapies for immune-mediated inflammatory diseases: what can we learn from their use in rheumatoid arthritis, spondyloarthritis, systemic lupus erythematosus, psoriasis, Crohn's disease and ulcerative colitis? *Ann. Rheum. Dis.* 77, 175–187. doi:10.1136/annrheumdis-2017-211555

Banfield, C., Scaramozza, M., Zhang, W., Kieras, E., Page, K. M., Fensome, A., et al. (2018). The safety, tolerability, pharmacokinetics, and pharmacodynamics of a TYK2/JAK1 inhibitor (PF-06700841) in healthy subjects and patients with plaque psoriasis. *J. Clin. Pharmacol.* 58, 434–447. doi:10.1002/jcph.1046

Barrett, J. C., Hansoul, S., Nicolae, D. L., Cho, J. H., Duerr, R. H., Rioux, J. D., et al. (2008). Genome-wide association defines more than 30 distinct susceptibility loci for Crohn's disease. *Nat. Genet.* 40, 955–962. doi:10.1038/ng.175

Cohen, J. A., Arnold, D. L., Comi, G., Bar-Or, A., Gujrathi, S., Hartung, J. P., et al. (2016). Safety and efficacy of the selective sphingosine 1-phosphate receptor modulator ozanimod in relapsing multiple sclerosis (RADIANCE): a randomised, placebo-controlled, phase 2 trial. *Lancet Neurol.* 15, 373–381. doi:10.1016/s1474-4422(16)00018-1

Cohen, J. A., Barkhof, F., Comi, G., Hartung, H.-P., Khatri, B. O., Montalban, X., et al. (2010). Oral fingolimod or intramuscular interferon for relapsing multiple sclerosis. *N. Engl. J. Med.* 362, 402–415. doi:10.1056/nejmoa0907839

Cohen, J. A., Comi, G., Selmaj, K. W., Bar-Or, A., Arnold, D. L., Steinman, L., et al. (2019). Safety and efficacy of ozanimod versus interferon beta-1a in relapsing multiple sclerosis (RADIANCE): a multicentre, randomised, 24-month, phase 3 trial. *Lancet Neurol.* 18, 1021–1033. doi:10.1016/s1474-4422(19)30238-8

Comi, G., Kappos, L., Selmaj, K. W., Bar-Or, A., Arnold, D. L., Steinman, L., et al. (2019). Safety and efficacy of ozanimod versus interferon beta-1a in relapsing multiple sclerosis (SUNBEAM): a multicentre, randomised, minimum 12-month, phase 3 trial. *Lancet Neurol.* 18, 1009–1020. doi:10.1016/s1474-4422(19)30239-x

Danese, S., Feagan, B. G., Wolf, D. C., et al. (2020a), Ozanimod as maintenance therapy in patients with moderate-to-severe ulcerative colitis: results from the phase 3, randomized, double-blind, placebo-controlled true north study. UEG week, virtual conference

Danese, S., Furfaro, F., and Vetrano, S. (2018). Targeting S1P in inflammatory bowel disease: new avenues for modulating intestinal leukocyte migration. *J. Crohns Colitis* 12, S678–S686. doi:10.1093/ecco-jcc/jjx107

Danese, S., Neurath, M. F., Kopoń, A., Zakko, S. F., Simmons, T. C., Fogel, R., et al. (2020b). Effects of apremilast, an oral inhibitor of phosphodiesterase 4, in a randomized trial of patients with active ulcerative colitis. *Clin. Gastroenterol. Hepatol.* 18, 2526–2534. doi:10.1016/j.cgh.2019.12.032

Danese, S., Vermeire, S., Hellstern, P., Panaccione, R., Rogler, G., Fraser, G., et al. (2019). Randomised trial and open-label extension study of an anti-interleukin-6 antibody in Crohn's disease (ANDANTE I and II). *Gut* 68, 40–48. doi:10.1136/gutjnl-2017-314562

Deepak, P., and Sandborn, W. J. (2017). Ustekinumab and anti-interleukin-23 agents in Crohn's disease. *Gastroenterol. Clin. North America* 46, 603–626. doi:10.1016/j.gtc.2017.05.013

D'Haens, G., Danese, S., Davies, M., and Hibi, T (2019). DOP48 Amiselimod, a selective S1P receptor modulator in Crohn's disease patients: a proof-of-concept study. *J. Crohn's Colitis* 13, S055–S056. doi:10.1093/ecco-jcc/jjy222.082

D'Haens, G. R., Reinisch, W., Lee, S. D., Tarabar, D, Louis, E, Kłopocka, M., et al. (2018a). OP024 Long-term safety and efficacy of the anti-MAdCAM monoclonal antibody SHP647 for the treatment of Crohn's disease: the OPERA II study. *J. Crohn's Colitis* 12, S017–S018. doi:10.1093/ecco-jcc/jjx180.023

D'Haens, G. R., Gorelick, K., Wang, Y., Cataldi, F., and Sandborn, W J. (2018b). DOP062 the anti-MAdCAM antibody SHP647 in Crohn's disease: endoscopic effects of induction therapy. *J. Crohn's Colitis* 12, S073. doi:10.1093/ecco-jcc/jjx180.099

FDA Drug Safety Communication (2019). *FDA approves boxed warning about increased risk of blood clots and death with higher dose of arthritis and ulcerative colitis medicine tofacitinib.* XeljanzXeljanz XR).

Feagan, B. G., Panés, J., Ferrante, M., Kaser, A., D'Haens, G. R., Sandborn, W. J., et al. (2018). Risankizumab in patients with moderate to severe Crohn's disease:

an open-label extension study. *Lancet Gastroenterol. Hepatol.* 3, 671–680. doi:10.1016/s2468-1253(18)30233-4

Feagan, B. G., Rutgeerts, P., Sands, B. E., Hanauer, S., Colombel, J.-F., Sandborn, W. J., et al. (2013). Vedolizumab as induction and maintenance therapy for ulcerative colitis. *N. Engl. J. Med.* 369, 699–710. doi:10.1056/nejmoa1215734

Feagan, B. G., Sandborn, W. J., D'Haens, G., Panés, J., Kaser, A., Ferrante, M., et al. (2017). Induction therapy with the selective interleukin-23 inhibitor risankizumab in patients with moderate-to-severe Crohn's disease: a randomised, double-blind, placebo-controlled phase 2 study. *Lancet* 389, 1699–1709. doi:10.1016/s0140-6736(17)30570-6

Feagan, B. G., Sandborn, W. J., Danese, S., Wolf, D. C., Liu, W. J., Hua, S. Y., et al. (2020a). Ozanimod induction therapy for patients with moderate to severe Crohn's disease: a single-arm, phase 2, prospective observer-blinded endpoint study. *Lancet Gastroenterol. Hepatol.* 5, 819–828. doi:10.1016/s2468-1253(20)30188-6

Feagan, B. G., Sandborn, W. J., Gasink, C., Jacobstein, D., Lang, Y., Friedman, J. R., et al. (2016). Ustekinumab as induction and maintenance therapy for Crohn's disease. *N. Engl. J. Med.* 375, 1946–1960. doi:10.1056/nejmoa1602773

Feagan, B. G., Loftus, E. V., Jr, Danese, S., Vermeire, S., Sandborn, W J., Ritter, T., Mehta, R., et al. (2020b), Efficacy and safety OF filgotinib as induction therapy for patients with moderately to severely active ulcerative colitis: results from the phase 2B/3 SELECTION study. UEG, virtual conference *Journal of the Canadian Association of Gastroenterology.* 4(Supplement_1):18-20. doi:10.1093/jcag/gwab002.014

Ferrante, M., Feagan, B. G., Panés, J., Baert, F., Louis, E., Dewit, O., et al. (2020). OP27 Long-term safety and efficacy of risankizumab treatment in patients with Crohn's disease: final results from the Phase 2 open-label extension study. *J. Crohn's Colitis* 14, S024–S025. doi:10.1093/ecco-jcc/jjz203.026

Forman, S. B., Pariser, D. M., Poulin, Y., Vincent, M. S., Gilbert, S. A., Kieras, E. M., et al. (2020). TYK2/JAK1 inhibitor PF-06700841 in patients with plaque psoriasis: phase IIa, randomized, double-blind, placebo-controlled trial. *J. Invest. Dermatol.* 140(12):2359–2370.e5 .doi:10.1016/j.jid.2020.03.962

Gobejishvili, L., Barve, S., Joshi-Barve, S., and McClain, C. (2008). Enhanced PDE4B expression augments LPS-inducible TNF expression in ethanol-primed monocytes: relevance to alcoholic liver disease. *Am. J. Physiology-Gastrointestinal Liver Physiol.* 295, G718–G724. doi:10.1152/ajpgi.90232.2008

Hanauer, S. B., Sandborn, W. J., Rutgeerts, P., Fedorak, R. N., Lukas, M., MacIntosh, D., et al. (2006). Human anti-tumor necrosis factor monoclonal antibody (adalimumab) in Crohn's disease: the CLASSIC-I trial. *Gastroenterology* 130, 323–333. quiz 591. doi:10.1053/j.gastro.2005.11.030

Hanauer, S., Panaccione, R., Danese, S., Cheifetz, A., Reinisch, W., Higgins, P. D. R., et al. (2019). Tofacitinib induction therapy reduces symptoms within 3 Days for patients with ulcerative colitis. *Clin. Gastroenterol. Hepatol.* 17, 139–147. doi:10.1016/j.cgh.2018.07.009

Hanzel, J., and D'Haens, G. R. (2020). Anti-interleukin-23 agents for the treatment of ulcerative colitis. *Expert Opin. Biol. Ther.* 20, 399–406.

Harris, M. S., Hartman, D., Lemos, B. R., Erlich, E. C., Spence, S., Kennedy, S., et al. (2016). AVX-470, an orally delivered anti-tumour necrosis factor Antibody for treatment of active ulcerative colitis: results of a first-in-human trial. *Eccojc* 10, 631–640. doi:10.1093/ecco-jcc/jjw036

Kappos, L., Arnold, D. L., Bar-Or, A., Camm, J., Derfuss, T., Kieseier, B. C., et al. (2016). Safety and efficacy of amiselimod in relapsing multiple sclerosis (MOMENTUM): a randomised, double-blind, placebo-controlled phase 2 trial. *Lancet Neurol.* 15, 1148–1159. doi:10.1016/s1474-4422(16)30192-2

Kappos, L., Radue, E.-W., O'Connor, P., Polman, C., Hohlfeld, R., Calabresi, P., et al. (2010). A placebo-controlled trial of oral fingolimod in relapsing multiple sclerosis. *N. Engl. J. Med.* 362, 387–401. doi:10.1056/nejmoa0909494

Klenske, E., Bojarski, C., Waldner, M., Rath, T., Neurath, M. F., Atreya, R., et al. (2019). Targeting mucosal healing in Crohn's disease: what the clinician needs to know. *Therap Adv. Gastroenterol.* 12, 1756284819856865. doi:10.1177/1756284819856865

Kwak, H. J., Song, J. S., No, Z. S., Song, J. H., Yang, S. D., and Cheon, H. G. (2005). The inhibitory effects of roflumilast on lipopolysaccharide-induced nitric oxide production in RAW264.7 cells are mediated by heme oxygenase-1 and its product carbon monoxide. *Inflamm. Res.* 54, 508–513. doi:10.1007/s00011-005-1386-1

Lin, L., Liu, X., Wang, D., and Zheng, C. (2015). Efficacy and safety of antiintegrin antibody for inflammatory bowel disease. *Medicine (Baltimore)* 94, e556. doi:10.1097/md.0000000000000556

Loftus, E. V., Jr. (2004). Clinical epidemiology of inflammatory bowel disease: incidence, prevalence, and environmental influences. *Gastroenterology* 126, 1504–1517. doi:10.1053/j.gastro.2004.01.063

Ma, C., Lee, J. K., Mitra, A. R., Teriaky, A., Choudhary, D., Nguyen, T. M., et al. (2019). Systematic review with meta-analysis: efficacy and safety of oral Janus kinase inhibitors for inflammatory bowel disease. *Aliment. Pharmacol. Ther.* 50, 5–23. doi:10.1111/apt.15297

Molodecky, N. A., and Kaplan, G. G. (2010). Environmental risk factors for inflammatory bowel disease. *Gastroenterol. Hepatol. (N Y)* 6, 339–346.

Molodecky, N. A., Soon, I. S., Rabi, D. M., Ghali, W. A., Ferris, M., Chernoff, G., et al. (2012). Increasing incidence and prevalence of the inflammatory bowel diseases with time, based on systematic review. *Gastroenterology* 142, 46–54. e42; quiz e30. doi:10.1053/j.gastro.2011.10.001

Ollivier, V., Parry, G. C. N., Cobb, R. R., de Prost, D., and Mackman, N. (1996). Elevated cyclic AMP inhibits NF-κB-mediated transcription in human monocytic cells and endothelial cells. *J. Biol. Chem.* 271, 20828–20835. doi:10.1074/jbc.271.34.20828

Panés, J., Sandborn, W. J., Schreiber, S., Sands, B. E., Vermeire, S., D'Haens, G., et al. (2017). Tofacitinib for induction and maintenance therapy of Crohn's disease: results of two phase IIb randomised placebo-controlled trials. *Gut* 66, 1049–1059. doi:10.1136/gutjnl-2016-312735

Park, S. C., and Jeen, Y. T. (2018). Anti-integrin therapy for inflammatory bowel disease. *Wjg* 24, 1868–1880. doi:10.3748/wjg.v24.i17.1868

Peyrin-Biroulet, L., Feagan, B. G., Mansfield, J., Rubin, D. T., Arulmani, U., Maciuca, R., et al. (2017). OP011 Etrolizumab treatment leads to early improvement in symptoms and inflammatory biomarkers in anti-TNF-refractory patients in the open-label induction cohort of the phase 3 HICKORY study. *J. Crohn's Colitis* 11, S6–S7. doi:10.1093/ecco-jcc/jjx002.010

Peyrin-Biroulet, L., Loftus, E. V., Jr, Danese, S., Vermeire, S., Sandborn, W. J., Fogel, R., Nijhawan, S., et al. (2020), Efficacy and safety OF filgotinib as maintenance therapy for patients with moderately to severely active ulcerative colitis: results from the phase 2B/3 SELECTION study. UEG, virtual conference *Journal of the Canadian Association of Gastroenterology.* 4(Supplement_1):21-23. doi:10.1093/jcag/gwab002.016

Platzer, C., Fritsch, E., Elsner, T., Lehmann, M. H., Volk, H.-D., and Prösch, S. (1999). Cyclic adenosine monophosphate-responsive elements are involved in the transcriptional activation of the human IL-10 gene in monocytic cells. *Eur. J. Immunol.* 29, 3098–3104. doi:10.1002/(sici)1521-4141(199910)29:10<3098::aid-immu3098>3.0.co;2-h

Rothenberg, M. E., Wang, Y., Lekkerkerker, A., Danilenko, D. M., Maciuca, R., Erickson, R., et al. (2019). Randomized phase I healthy volunteer study of UTTR 1147A (IL -22Fc): a potential therapy for epithelial injury. *Clin. Pharmacol. Ther.* 105, 177–189. doi:10.1002/cpt.1164

Rutgeerts, P., Sandborn, W. J., Feagan, B. G., Reinisch, W., Olson, A., Johanns, J., et al. (2005). Infliximab for induction and maintenance therapy for ulcerative colitis. *N. Engl. J. Med.* 353, 2462–2476. doi:10.1056/nejmoa050516

Sabino, J., Verstockt, B., and Vermeire, S., (2019). New biologics and small molecules in inflammatory bowel disease: an update. *Therap Adv. Gastroenterol.* 12, 1756284819853208. doi:10.1177/1756284819853208

Salas, A., Hernandez-Rocha, C., Duijvestein, M., Faubion, W., McGovern, D., Vermeire, S., et al. (2020). JAK-STAT pathway targeting for the treatment of inflammatory bowel disease. *Nat. Rev. Gastroenterol. Hepatol.* 17, 323–337. doi:10.1038/s41575-020-0273-0

Sandborn, W. J., Ferrante, M., Bhandari, B. R., Berliba, E., Hibi, T., D'Haens, G. R., et al. (2020a). Efficacy and safety of continued treatment with mirikizumab in a phase 2 trial of patients with ulcerative colitis. *Clin. Gastroenterol. Hepatol.* doi:10.1016/j.cgh.2020.09.028

Sandborn, W. J., Baert, F., Danese, S., Krznarić, Ž., Kobayashi, T., Yao, X., et al. (2020b). Efficacy and safety of vedolizumab subcutaneous formulation in a randomized trial of patients with ulcerative colitis. *Gastroenterology* 158, 562–572. doi:10.1053/j.gastro.2019.08.027

Sandborn, W. J., Cyrille, M., Berner Hansen, M., Feagan, B. G., Loftus, E. V., Vermeire, S., et al. (2017a). OP035 Efficacy and safety of abrilumab (AMG 181/MEDI 7183) therapy for moderate to severe Crohn's disease. *J. Crohn's Colitis* 11, S22–S23. doi:10.1093/ecco-jcc/jjx002.034

Sandborn, W. J., Cyrille, M., Hansen, M. B., Feagan, B. G., Loftus, E. V., Rogler, G., et al. (2019). Efficacy and safety of abrilumab in a randomized, placebo-controlled trial for moderate-to-severe ulcerative colitis. *Gastroenterology* 156, 946–957. doi:10.1053/j.gastro.2018.11.035

Sandborn, W. J., Feagan, B. G., Loftus, E. V., Jr., Peyrin-Biroulet, L., Van Assche, G., D'Haens, G., et al. (2020c). Efficacy and safety of upadacitinib in a randomized trial of patients with Crohn's disease. *Gastroenterology* 158, 2123–2138. doi:10.1053/j.gastro.2020.01.047

Sandborn, W. J., Feagan, B. G., Rutgeerts, P., Hanauer, S., Colombel, J.-F., Sands, B. E., et al. (2013). Vedolizumab as induction and maintenance therapy for Crohn's disease. *N. Engl. J. Med.* 369, 711–721. doi:10.1056/nejmoa1215739

Sandborn, W. J., Feagan, B. G., Wolf, D. C., D'Haens, G., Vermeire, S., Hanauer, S. B., et al. (2016). Ozanimod induction and maintenance treatment for ulcerative colitis. *N. Engl. J. Med.* 374, 1754–1762. doi:10.1056/nejmoa1513248

Sandborn, W. J., Ferrante, M., Bhandari, B. R., Berliba, E., Feagan, B. G., Hibi, T., et al. (2020d). Efficacy and safety of mirikizumab in a randomized phase 2 study of patients with ulcerative colitis. *Gastroenterology* 158, 537–549. doi:10.1053/j.gastro.2019.08.043

Sandborn, W. J., Ghosh, S., Panes, J., Schreiber, S., D'Haens, G., Tanida, S., et al. (2020e). Efficacy of upadacitinib in a randomized trial of patients with active ulcerative colitis. *Gastroenterology* 158, 2139–2149. doi:10.1053/j.gastro.2020.02.030

Sandborn, W. J., Hanauer, S. B., Rutgeerts, P., Fedorak, R. N., Lukas, M., MacIntosh, D. G., et al. (2007). Adalimumab for maintenance treatment of Crohn's disease: results of the CLASSIC II trial. *Gut* 56, 1232–1239. doi:10.1136/gut.2006.106781

Sandborn, W. J., Lee, S. D., Tarabar, D., Louis, E., Klopocka, M., Klaus, J., et al. (2018). Phase II evaluation of anti-MAdCAM antibody PF-00547659 in the treatment of Crohn's disease: report of the OPERA study. *Gut* 67, 1824–1835. doi:10.1136/gutjnl-2016-313457

Sandborn, W. J., Nguyen, D. D., Beattie, D. T., Brassil, P., Krey, W., Woo, J., et al. (2020f). Development of gut-selective pan-janus kinase inhibitor TD-1473 for ulcerative colitis: a translational medicine programme. *J. Crohns Colitis* 14, 1202–1213. doi:10.1093/ecco-jcc/jjaa049

Sandborn, W. J., Peyrin-Biroulet, L., Zhang, J., Chiorean, M., Vermeire, S., Lee, S. D., et al. (2020g). Efficacy and safety of etrasimod in a phase 2 randomized trial of patients with ulcerative colitis. *Gastroenterology* 158, 550–561. doi:10.1053/j.gastro.2019.10.035

Sandborn, W. J., Su, C., Sands, B. E., D'Haens, G. R., Vermeire, S., Schreiber, S., et al. (2017b). Tofacitinib as induction and maintenance therapy for ulcerative colitis. *N. Engl. J. Med.* 376, 1723–1736. doi:10.1056/nejmoa1606910

Sandborn, W. J., Vermeire, S., Vermeire, S., Tyrrell, H., Hassanali, A., Lacey, S., et al. (2020h). Etrolizumab for the treatment of ulcerative colitis and Crohn's disease: an overview of the phase 3 clinical program. *Adv. Ther.* 37, 3417–3431. doi:10.1007/s12325-020-01366-2

Sandborn, W. J., Chan, D., and Johanns, J., (2020i). The efficacy and safety OF guselkumab induction therapy IN patients with moderately to severely active CROHN'S disease: week 12 interim analyses from the phase 2 GALAXI 1 study. UEG, virtual conference

Sandborn, W., D'Haens, G. R., and Wolf, D. C., (2020), Ozanimod as induction therapy IN moderate-to-severe ulcerative colitis: results from the phase 3, randomized, double-blind, placebo-controlled true north study. UEG, virtual conference

Sands, B. E., Anderson, F. H., Bernstein, C. N., Chey, W. Y., Feagan, B. G., Fedorak, R. N., et al. (2004). Infliximab maintenance therapy for fistulizing Crohn's disease. *N. Engl. J. Med.* 350, 876–885. doi:10.1056/nejmoa030815

Sands, B. E., Chen, J., Feagan, B. G., Penney, M., Rees, W. A., Danese, S., et al. (2017). Efficacy and safety of MEDI2070, an antibody against interleukin 23, in patients with moderate to severe Crohn's disease: a phase 2a study. *Gastroenterology* 153, 77–86. doi:10.1053/j.gastro.2017.03.049

Sands, B. E., Sandborn, W. J., Panaccione, R., O'Brien, C. D., Zhang, H., Johanns, J., et al. (2019a). Ustekinumab as induction and maintenance therapy for ulcerative colitis. *N. Engl. J. Med.* 381, 1201–1214. doi:10.1056/nejmoa1900750

Sands, B. E., Sandborn, W. J., Peyrin-Biroulet, L., Higgins, P. D., Hirai, F., Belin, R., et al. (2019b). 1003 - efficacy and safety of mirikizumab (LY3074828) in a phase 2 study of patients with Crohn's disease. *Gastroenterology* 156, S. doi:10.1016/s0016-5085(19)37335-4

Sands, B. E., Sandborn, W. J., and Peyrin-Biroulet, L., (2020), Efficacy and safety OF mirikizumab after 52-WEEKS maintenance treatment IN patients with moderate-to-severe CROHN'S disease. UEG virtual conference 2020.

Schreiber, S., Khaliq-Kareemi, M., Lawrance, I. C., Thomsen, O. Ø., Hanauer, S. B., McColm, J., et al. (2007). Maintenance therapy with certolizumab pegol for Crohn's disease. *N. Engl. J. Med.* 357, 239–250. doi:10.1056/nejmoa062897

Selinger, C., Sandborn, W., Panes, J., Jones, J., Hassanali, A., Jacob, R., et al. (2018). OTU-003 Etrolizumab as induction therapy in moderate to severe crohn's disease: results from bergamot cohort 1. *Gut* 67, A53. doi:10.1136/gutjnl-2018-bsgabstracts.106

Shivashankar, R., and Lewis, J. D. (2017a). The role of diet in inflammatory bowel disease. *Curr. Gastroenterol. Rep.* 19, 22. doi:10.1007/s11894-017-0563-z

Shivashankar, R., and Pardi, D. S. (2017b). Use of anti-tumor necrosis factors and anti-integrins in the treatment of Crohn's disease. *Gastroenterol. Clin. North America* 46, 589–601. doi:10.1016/j.gtc.2017.05.012

Sugiura, T., Kageyama, S., Andou, A., Miyazawa, T., Ejima, C., Nakayama, A., et al. (2013). Oral treatment with a novel small molecule alpha 4 integrin antagonist, AJM300, prevents the development of experimental colitis in mice. *J. Crohn's Colitis* 7, e533–e542. doi:10.1016/j.crohns.2013.03.014

Targan, S. R., Feagan, B. G., Fedorak, R. N., Lashner, B. A., Panaccione, R., Present, D. H., et al. (2007). Natalizumab for the treatment of active Crohn's disease: results of the ENCORE Trial. *Gastroenterology* 132, 1672–1683. doi:10.1053/j.gastro.2007.03.024

Vermeire, S., O'Byrne, S., Keir, M., Williams, M., Lu, T. T., Mansfield, J. C., et al. (2014). Etrolizumab as induction therapy for ulcerative colitis: a randomised, controlled, phase 2 trial. *Lancet* 384, 309–318. doi:10.1016/s0140-6736(14)60661-9

Vermeire, S., Sandborn, W. J., Danese, S., Hébuterne, X., Salzberg, B. A., Klopocka, M., et al. (2017a). Anti-MAdCAM antibody (PF-00547659) for ulcerative colitis (TURANDOT): a phase 2, randomised, double-blind, placebo-controlled trial. *The Lancet* 390, 135–144. doi:10.1016/s0140-6736(17)30930-3

Vermeire, S., Schreiber, S., Petryka, R., Kuehbacher, T., Hebuterne, X., Roblin, X., et al. (2017b). Clinical remission in patients with moderate-to-severe Crohn's disease treated with filgotinib (the FITZROY study): results from a phase 2, double-blind, randomised, placebo-controlled trial. *Lancet* 389, 266–275. doi:10.1016/s0140-6736(16)32537-5

Wagner, F., Mansfield, J., Geier, C., Dash, A., Wang, Y., Li, C., et al. (2020). P420 A randomised, observer-blinded phase Ib multiple, ascending dose study of UTTR1147A, an IL-22Fc fusion protein, in healthy volunteers and ulcerative colitis patients. *J. Crohn's Colitis* 14, S382–S383. doi:10.1093/ecco-jcc/jjz203.549

Winthrop, K. L., Melmed, G. Y., Vermeire, S., Long, M. D., Chan, G., Pedersen, R. D., et al. (2018). Herpes zoster infection in patients with ulcerative colitis receiving tofacitinib. *Inflamm. Bowel Dis.* 24, 2258–2265. doi:10.1093/ibd/izy131

Yoshimura, N., Watanabe, M., Motoya, S., Tominaga, K., Matsuoka, K., Iwakiri, R., et al. (2015). Safety and efficacy of AJM300, an oral antagonist of α4 integrin, in induction therapy for patients with active ulcerative colitis. *Gastroenterology* 149, 1775–1783. doi:10.1053/j.gastro.2015.08.044

7

AICAR, an AMP-Activated Protein Kinase Activator, Ameliorates Acute Pancreatitis-Associated Liver Injury Partially Through Nrf2-Mediated Antioxidant Effects and Inhibition of NLRP3 Inflammasome Activation

Lijun Kong[1], Hewei Zhang[1], Chaosheng Lu[2], Keqing Shi[3], Hongjian Huang[1], Yushu Zheng[1], Yongqiang Wang[1], Dan Wang[2], Hongwei Wang[1] and Wei Huang[4]**

[1]Key Laboratory of Diagnosis and Treatment of Severe Hepato-Pancreatic Diseases of Zhejiang Province, The First Affiliated Hospital of Wenzhou Medical University, Wenzhou, China, [2]Department of Pediatrics, The First Affiliated Hospital of Wenzhou Medical University, Wenzhou, China, [3]Translational Medicine Laboratory, The First Affiliated Hospital of Wenzhou Medical University, Wenzhou, China, [4]Department of Nutrition, The First Affiliated Hospital of Wenzhou Medical University, Wenzhou, China

***Correspondence:**
Hongwei Wang
15258085168@163.com
Wei Huang
hw120418@163.com

Acute pancreatitis (AP) is a highly fatal acute inflammation and is often accompanied by multiple organ dysfunction syndrome (MODS). The liver, one of the most vulnerable extrapancreatic organs in AP, is the major organ involved in the evolution of the disease and correlates strongly with the occurrence of MODS. However, the etiology of pancreatitis-associated liver injury (PALI) has not been clarified and currently lacks an effective treatment. 5-Aminoimidazole-4-carboxamide ribonucleotide (AICAR) is a cell permeable nucleoside with pleiotropic effects on anti-inflammatory and antioxidant stress that binds with adenosine monophosphate protein kinase (AMPK) and induces AMPK activation. However, the role of AICAR in PALI remains elusive. Here, we show that activation of AMPK by AICAR, a direct AMPK agonist, significantly ameliorates sodium taurocholate-induced PALI in rats, whereas treatment of PALI rats with the AMPK antagonist Compound C profoundly exacerbates the degree of liver injury, suggesting that hepatic AMPK activation exerts an essential protective role in PALI. Mechanistically, AICAR induces AMPK activation, which in turn activates nuclear factor erythroid 2-related factor 2(Nrf2) -regulated hepatic antioxidant capacity and inhibits NLRP3 inflammasome-mediated pyrolysis, protecting rats from sodium taurocholate-induced PALI. In addition, Nrf2 deficiency strikingly weakens the beneficial effects of AICAR on alleviation of liver injury, oxidative stress and NLRP3 inflammasome activation in L-arginine-induced PALI mice. Thus, AICAR protects against PALI in rodents by triggering AMPK, which is mediated at least in part by Nrf2-modulated antioxidant effects and NLRP3 inflammasome activation.

Keywords: pancreatitis, liver injury, AMPK, Nrf2, NLRP3 inflammasome

INTRODUCTION

Acute pancreatitis (AP) is a highly fatal acute inflammation with rapid progression. (Argaiz and de Moraes, 2021). There is an increasing prevalence of AP, with an estimated 33.74 cases per 100,000 people worldwide each year (Garg and Singh, 2019). The high mortality of AP is largely attributed to multiple organ dysfunction syndrome (MODS), such as liver or lung injury (Shi et al., 2020). The liver, a major organ involved in the evolution of AP, is strikingly vulnerable to inflammatory cytokines and correlates strongly with the occurrence of MODS (Li S. et al., 2019; Mei et al., 2019). Pancreatitis-associated liver injury (PALI) is a serious and even fatal complication in the development of AP (Wang et al., 2018). Mechanistically, a series of endogenous vasoactive substances released during AP lead to hepatic microcirculation disturbance, which is the essential cause of liver injury (Wenhong et al., 2012). Liver injury in turn triggers a systemic inflammatory response by affecting toxin metabolism and releasing massive inflammatory mediators (Rios et al., 2010; Ou et al., 2017). The PALI phenomenon has been observed in both clinical and experimental settings (Wang et al., 2006; Wenhong et al., 2012; Lv et al., 2015; Bakır et al., 2016; Ou et al., 2017). Notably, Curbey et al. reported that 80% of AP patients had liver damage and the liver injury aggravates the degree of pancreatitis if it is not intervened in time, which significantly prolongs the course of pancreatitis (Ou et al., 2017; Li X. et al., 2019). To date, the etiology of PALI has not been clarified, and no effective treatment has been developed. Thus, finding a promising therapeutic way to prevent or treat this devastating and fatal disease is urgently needed.

Adenosine monophosphate protein kinase (AMPK) is the main energy receptor regulating cell metabolism (Yang et al., 2021; Zhao et al., 2021). The activation of AMPK depends on the phosphorylation of Thr172 of the α subunit (Garcia and Shaw, 2017). In general, AMPK is activated under energy stress by sensing an increase in the ratios of AMP/ATP and ADP/ATP, thereby stimulating the catabolic process and maintaining energy homeostasis (Lin and Hardie, 2018). In addition to its role in energy dynamic balance, activated AMPK is also associated with reducing redox stress, inhibiting inflammation or limiting cell proliferation (Zimmermann et al., 2015; Liu et al., 2020; Chin et al., 2021). Recent studies indicate that AMPK activation plays an inhibitory role in mediating ethanol-induced oxidative stress in human pancreatic acinar cells, whereas AMPK inhibition can aggravate liver inflammation in mice with hepatic ischemia-reperfusion (Zhou et al., 2018; Srinivasan et al., 2020). Although the anti-inflammatory and antioxidant stress functions of AMPK activation have been well characterized, little is known about the pathophysiological roles in PALI, and the potential mechanism whereby AMPK activation protects against PALI remains poorly defined.

Under physiological conditions, serine 374, 408 and 433 of nuclear factor erythroid related factor 2 (Nrf2) are hyperphosphorylated with the activation of AMPK (Matzinger et al., 2020). Early studies have reported that AMPK activation enhances cellular antioxidant potential by activating the transcriptional activity of Nrf2 (Garcia and Shaw, 2017; Xu et al., 2020). Nrf2 is a member of the Cap'n'Collar (CNC) family of basic leucine zipper (bZIP) transcription factors, which activates the endogenous antioxidant defense system through translocation into the nucleus, thus combating inflammation and oxidative stress (Tonelli et al., 2018; Lyu et al., 2020; Gong et al., 2021; Tan et al., 2021). Inflammation causes oxidative stress; in turn, oxidative stress also boosts the production of inflammatory cytokines through activation of proinflammatory pathways, including the known Nod-like Receptor Protein 3 (NLRP3) inflammasome pathway (Zeng et al., 2017). It consists of NLRP3 scaffold, adaptor protein apoptosis-associated speck-like protein (ASC) and proinflammatory caspase-1 (Zou et al., 2021). When NLRP3 is activated, the p20 subunit and p10 subunit are heterodimerized to form bioactive caspase-1, which processes the release of IL-1β and induces a unique inflammatory type of cell death called pyroptosis (Chen et al., 2017; Unamuno et al., 2021). Growing evidence has established that NLRP3 inflammasome activation leads to hepatocyte pyroptosis and severe liver inflammation (Han et al., 2018; Wree et al., 2018). Recently, the inverse correlation between the activated Nrf2 and NLRP3 inflammasome pathway that inhibits inflammation through augmenting antioxidant capacity in mice have been proved in acute lung injury (Liu et al., 2017). Nonetheless, whether the activation of AMPK plays an antioxidative and anti-inflammatory role through Nrf2-mediated antioxidant effects and inhibition of the NLRP3 inflammasome pathway in PALI remain to be determined.

5-Aminoimidazole-4-formamide ribonucleotide (AICAR) is a kind of cellular permeable nucleoside that activates AMPK to play anti-inflammatory and antioxidant stress effects (Swinnen et al., 2005; Bone et al., 2017; Kaphalia et al., 2019). AICAR is converted into ZMP (an AMP mimic) in cells to bind to the γ subunit of AMPK, causing conformational changes in the enzyme and promoting the phosphorylation of Thr172 of the AMPKα subunit by liver kinase B1 (LKB1) or other upstream AMPK kinases (AMPKK) (Sun et al., 2007; Hill et al., 2016; Lane et al., 2020; Višnjić et al., 2021). Emerging evidence indicates that the activation of AMPK by AICAR attenuates high glucose-induced oxidative stress in rat cardiomyocytes (Shen et al., 2019). Moreover, the direct AMPK agonist AICAR negatively regulates the IL-6-stimulated inflammatory response in human liver cells by suppressing the phosphorylation of STAT3 (Nerstedt et al., 2010). However, it is not clear whether pharmacological activation of AMPK by the direct AMPK small molecule agonist AICAR is a therapeutic strategy for PALI.

In the present study, we investigated whether activation of AMPK by AICAR limits the inflammatory response and oxidative stress in the progression of PALI in two rodent models of severe acute pancreatitis (SAP) *via* Nrf2-mediated antioxidant effects and NLRP3 inflammasome activation. Our results provide the first direct evidence of the beneficial effects of pharmacological activation of AMPK by AICAR against the progression of PALI, including reduced redox stress and decreased NLRP3 inflammasome activation. Moreover, Nrf2 deficiency dramatically weakened these beneficial effects of AICAR in L-arginine-induced PALI mice. Thus, AICAR protects against PALI at least in part through Nrf2-mediated antioxidant effects and inhibition of NLRP3 inflammasome activation.

MATERIALS AND METHODS

Animal Experiments

Male SD rats (220–250 g, age 7–8 weeks) were obtained from the Experimental Animal Center of Wenzhou Medical University. Nrf2-knockout (Nrf2$^{-/-}$) mice on C57BL/6 background were procured from Jackson Laboratory (Bar Harbor, Maine, United States). These homozygous Nrf2$^{-/-}$ mice were backcrossed with C57BL/6 wild type mice. Heterozygous offspring were then further bred to gain wild type and Nrf2$^{-/-}$ littermates. Genotypes of Nrf2$^{-/-}$ mice were identified by PCR. All rats and mice were fed randomly at 24 ± 2°C and 40–60% humidity with a 12 h dark cycle before the experiment. All animal procedures were reviewed and approved by the Animal Ethics Committee of Wenzhou Medical University.

Wild-type rats were randomly divided into four groups: the control group (n = 10), severe acute pancreatitis (SAP) group (n = 10), AMPK agonist (AICAR) group (n = 8) and AMPK inhibitor (Compound C, CC) group (n = 8). Sham operation was performed in the control group. Pancreatitis was induced in the SAP, AICAR and CC groups by retrograde injection of 3% sodium taurocholate (STC, 0.1 ml/100 g of body weight, YZ-110815, Solarbio, Beijing, China) *via* the pancreatic duct using a syringe pump as previously described (Fang et al., 2020). The AICAR group received intraperitoneal injection of AICAR (400 mg/kg) 1 h before the operation. In the CC group, CC (13.8 mg/kg) was also injected intraperitoneally 1 h before the operation. AMPK agonist (AICAR) and AMPK inhibitor (CC) were purchased from MedChemExpress (HY-13417, HY-13418A, MedChemExpress, New Jersey, United States). The specific dosages of AICAR and CC used in this study based in the description in previous studies with minor modifications (Saito et al., 2012; Guo et al., 2014; Martin et al., 2019). 24 h after injection of sodium taurocholate, the rats were anesthetized with isoflurane (in 4% for induction and 3% for maintenance; R510, RWD Life Science, Shenzhen, China) on the anesthetic machine. Rats were sacrificed, and pancreatic tissues, liver tissues and blood samples were collected for further study.

Male C57BL/6 mice or Nrf2$^{-/-}$ mice were randomly divided into three groups: the control group (n = 6), SAP group (n = 6) and AMPK agonist (AICAR) group (n = 6). The control group mice were intraperitoneally injected with 0.9% normal saline. In the SAP and AICAR groups, the pancreatitis model was established by intraperitoneal injection of 8% L-arginine (pH = 7.0, 4.0 g/kg, A5006, Sigma, Missouri, United States) twice at an interval of 1 h as previously described (Liu et al., 2016). In the AICAR group, mice were intraperitoneally injected with AICAR (400 mg/kg) twice: 1 h before and 24 h after model establishment. 48 h after the injection of L-arginine, the mice were anesthetized with isoflurane (in 3.5% for induction and 2.5% for maintenance) on the anesthesia machine. Finally, the mice were sacrificed, and pancreatic tissues, liver tissues and blood samples were collected for subsequent experiments.

Histopathological Analysis

Pancreatic and liver tissues were collected, fixed immediately in 4% paraformaldehyde for 24 h, dehydrated in a graded ethanol series, and then embedded in paraffin. The tissue blocks were cut into 4.5 μm-thick sections, dewaxed, and hydrated. Then, pancreatic and liver sections were stained with hematoxylin and eosin (H&E) staining (G1120, Solarbio, Beijing, China) according to the manufacturer's instructions. After observation under an Olympus BX-51 microscope (Olympus Corporation, Tokyo, Japan), histological scores were obtained to evaluate the degree of pancreatic and liver injury with Image-Pro Plus 6.0 software (Media Cybernetics, Bethesda, United States) as described elsewhere (Rongione et al., 1997; Elshal et al., 2019).

Immunohistochemistry Analysis

Immunohistochemistry was used to qualitatively analyze the expression of phenotypic markers. The liver sections (4.5 μm) were boiled in antigen retrieval buffer containing citrate-hydrochloric acid (C8532, Sigma, Missouri, United States) for 15 min. Then, hydrogen peroxide (3%) was used for 10 min to block the activity of endogenous peroxidase and subsequently blocked with 5% bovine serum albumin (A1933, Sigma, Missouri, United States) for 30 min at 37°C. Primary antibodies for IL-6 (1:200; MB9296, Bioworld Technology, Minnesota, United States), IL-1β (1:200; BS6067, Bioworld Technology, Minnesota, United States), TNF-α (1:200; BS6000, Bioworld Technology, Minnesota, United States), MCP-1 (1:200; DF7577, Affinity, Ohio, United States), HO-1 (1:200; ab13243, Abcam, Massachusetts, United States) and NQO-1 (1:200; ab28947, Abcam, Massachusetts, United States) were added and incubated at 4°C overnight. After washing, the sections were incubated with secondary antibodies (1:200; A0277, Beyotime Institute of Biotechology; Goat anti-rabbit IgG-HRP) for 1 h at 37 °C. Finally, the slides were stained using diaminobenzidine (DAB, P0202, Beyotime, Shanghai, China) for color visualization. Images of representative tissue spots were captured with an Olympus BX-51 microscope (Olympus Corporation, Tokyo, Japan) and analyzed with Image-Pro Plus 6.0 software (Media Cybernetics, Bethesda, United States).

Biochemical Indexes Assay

Fresh pancreatic and liver tissues and blood samples were collected for biochemical analysis. The levels of serum amylase and lipase were measured by assay kit (C016-1-1, A054-1-1, Nanjing Jiancheng Bioengineering Institute, Nanjing, China) to evaluate the degree of pancreatitis. The serum levels of alanine aminotransferase (ALT) and aspartate aminotransferase (AST) were measured with commercial kit (C009-2-1, C010-2-1, Nanjing Jiancheng Bioengineering Institute, Nanjing, China) to evaluate the degree of liver injury and function. The contents of malondialdehyde (MDA) and superoxide dismutase (SOD) in pancreas and liver homogenate were determined with commercial kit (A003-1-2, A001-3-2, Nanjing Jiancheng Bioengineering Institute, Nanjing, China). The contents of myeloperoxidase (MPO) were measured with commercial kit (A044-1-1, Nanjing Jiancheng Bioengineering Institute, Nanjing, China). All measurements were conducted according to the manufacturer's instructions of the assay kit.

Western Blot Analysis

The liver tissues were homogenized in RIPA lysis buffer (P0013C, Beyotime, Shanghai, China), and then the extract was transferred to a centrifuge tube and centrifuged at 12,000 rpm for 20 min. After testing the total protein concentration with a BCA protein analysis kit (P0012S, Beyotime, Shanghai, China), 40 μg of protein sample was separated on a 10% sodium dodecyl sulfate-polyacrylamide gel and transferred to a PVDF membrane. The membrane was blocked with 5% skim milk for 1 h and then incubated with specific primary antibodies against *p*-AMPK (Thr172; 1:1,000; 8208S, Cell Singling Technology, Boston, United States), AMPK (1:1,000; 5832S, Cell Singling Technology, Boston, United States), CD68 (1:1,000; ab125212, Abcam, Massachusetts, United States), NLRP3 (1: 1,000; ab263899, Abcam, Massachusetts, United States), Caspase-1 (1:1,000; 22915-1-AP, Proteintech, Wuhan, China), cleaved IL-1β (1:1,000; AF4006, Proteintech, Wuhan, China), Nrf2 (1:1,000; 20733S, Cell Singling Technology, Boston, United States), HO-1 (1:1,000; ab13243, Abcam, Massachusetts, United States), NQO-1 (1:1,000; ab28947, Abcam, Massachusetts, United States), Lamin B (1:1,000; 12987-1-AP, Proteintech, Wuhan, China) and GAPDH (1:5,000; A00227-1, Boster, Wuhan, China) at 4°C overnight. All membranes were washed with TBST 3 times and incubated with horseradish peroxidase-conjugated secondary antibody (1: 5,000; A25012, Abbkine Scientific Co., Ltd, Wuhan, China) for 1 h. Finally, the bands were visualized using enhanced chemiluminescence (WP20005, Thermo Fisher Scientific, California, United States), and densitometry analysis was performed using VisionWorks imaging software (Eastman Kodak Company, New York, United States).

Nuclear Protein Extraction

Nuclear components were extracted from fresh liver tissues using a nuclear protein extraction kit (P0027, Beyotime, Shanghai, China) according to the manufacturer's instructions.

RNA Extraction and qRT-PCR

Total RNA was extracted from liver tissues with TRIzol Reagent (15596026, Thermo Fisher Scientific, California, United States) according to the manufacturer's specifications. Reverse transcription was completed by a Prime-Script RT Master Mix transcription kit (RR036A, TaKaRa, Tokyo, Japan). mRNA-specific primers (Sangon Biotech, China) were used to detect the RNA expression of IL-6, IL-1β and TNF-α. A 7500 Fast system (Applied Biosystems, United States) was used for qRT-PCR analysis. The results were analyzed using the $2^{-\Delta\Delta Ct}$ method, and GAPDH was amplified as an internal standard. The primer sequences are listed in **Supplementary Table S1**.

Statistical Analysis

All experiments were independently repeated three times. Values are presented as the mean ± SD (standard deviation). Statistical analysis was performed using GraphPad Prism 7.0 software (GraphPad Software, Inc., La Jolla, CA United States). Statistical significance was assessed by Student's t-test and one-way analysis of variance. Multiple comparisons between groups were analyzed using Tukey's post hoc test. $p < 0.05$ was considered statistically significant.

RESULTS

Direct AMPK Agonist AICAR Attenuates Pancreatitis-Associated Liver Injury and Restores Liver Function in Sodium Taurocholate-Induced SAP Rats

We investigated whether the direct AMPK activator AICAR (400 mg/kg) alleviates pancreatitis-associated liver injury by AMPK activation in a rat model of sodium taurocholate-induced SAP. We first validated the AMPK activator activity of AICAR in liver tissues of sodium taurocholate-induced SAP rats. Interestingly, the ratio of *p*-AMPK/AMPK in liver tissues significantly decreased after sodium taurocholate treatment. However, administration of AICAR by intraperitoneal injection into sodium taurocholate-treated rats resulted in a dramatic elevation of this ratio, suggesting that the reduced AMPK phosphorylation levels in the liver tissues of SAP rats were effectively activated by AICAR (**Figure 1A**). Hematoxylin and eosin staining demonstrated that the pancreas in SAP rats presented with notable interstitial edema, inflammatory cell infiltration and hemorrhagic necrosis, with the pancreatitis score analysis indicating a >5-fold increase over the control (**Figures 1B,D**). Likewise, the liver tissues of SAP rats were accompanied by obvious hepatocyte edema, necrosis, liver sinusoid congestion and dramatically damaged hepatic lobular structure, with the liver score analysis indicating a >4-fold increase compared with the control groups (**Figures 1C,D**). However, these negative changes were markedly reduced in the AICAR treatment groups (**Figures 1B–D**). Consistent with our histologic findings, the plasma levels of amylase and lipase, two common clinical indicators for assessing pancreatic injury (Steinberg et al., 2017), were elevated in SAP rats compared with control rats, whereas AICAR treatment prevented these increases (**Figure 1E**). Meanwhile, the increased levels of MDA and decreased concentrations of SOD in the pancreas of SAP rats indicated oxidative stress injury and downregulated antioxidant ability of the pancreas; however, administration of AICAR in rats significantly decreased the levels of MDA and increased the concentrations of SOD in pancreatic tissues of SAP rats, suggesting that AICAR supplementation restores the antioxidant ability of the pancreas in sodium taurocholate-induced SAP rats (**Figure 1F**). Correspondingly, evaluation of liver function in the SAP rats indicated that both the serum values of ALT and AST were significantly increased. In the presence of the AMPK activator AICAR, liver function was improved (**Figure 1G**). Taken together, the above results suggest that sodium taurocholate infusion established a successful rat model of PALI and that supplementation with AICAR not only reduces the severity of pancreatitis but also attenuates PALI and restores liver function in sodium taurocholate-induced SAP rats.

AICAR Prevents SAP-Induced Hepatic Inflammation in a Sodium Taurocholate-Induced SAP Rat Model

We explored the hypothesis that the molecular basis of AICAR in improving PALI is attributed to its anti-inflammatory

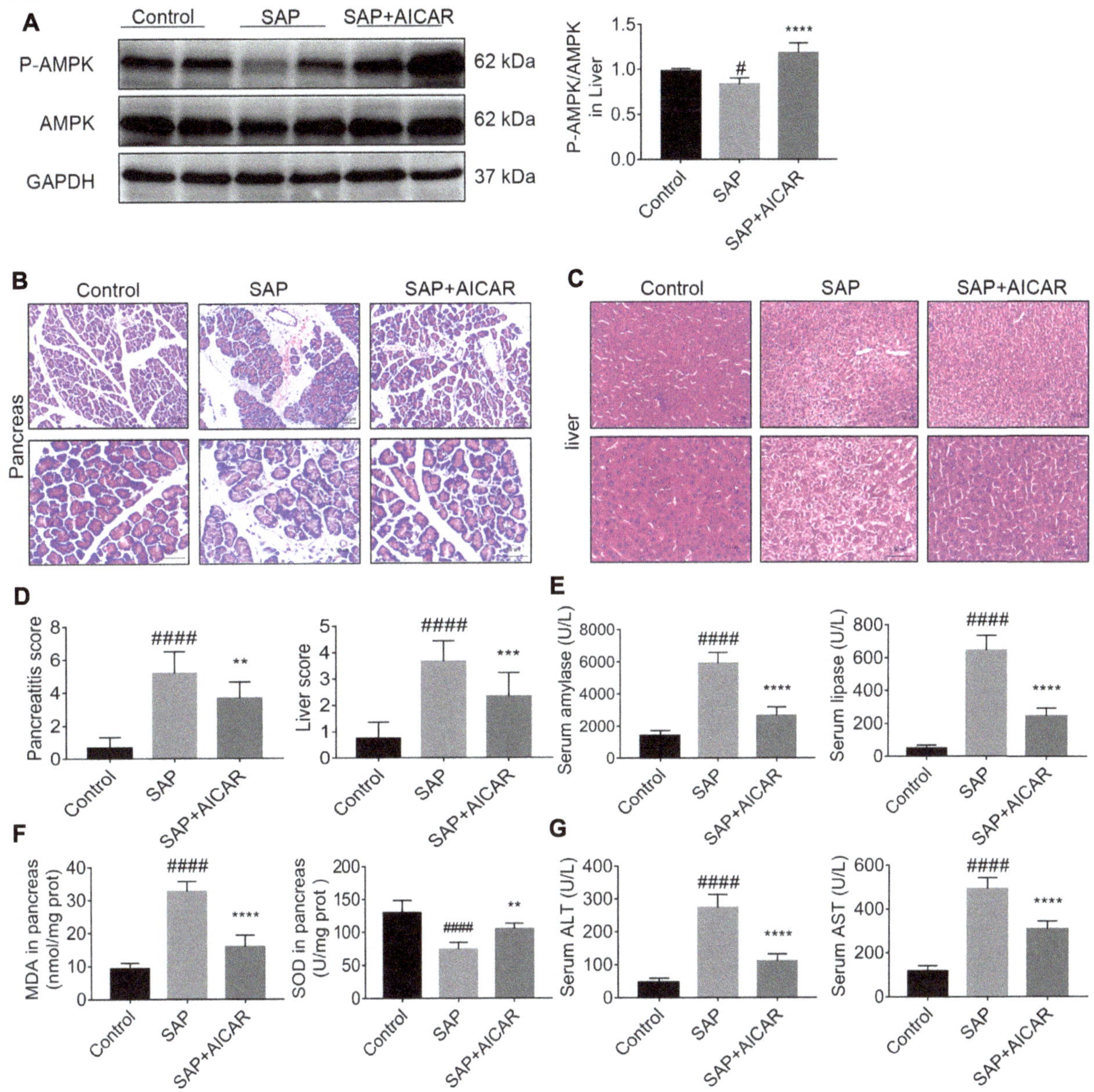

FIGURE 1 | The therapeutic effects of AICAR on pancreatitis-associated liver injury (PALI) in sodium taurocholate-induced SAP rats. 7–8 week-old wild-type male SD rats were randomly divided into three groups: the control group (control, n = 10) was treated with sham operation and injected with 0.9% normal saline; the severe acute pancreatitis (SAP) group (n = 10) was infused with 3% sodium taurocholate (0.1 ml/100 g); and the AMPK agonist (AICAR) group (n = 8) received intraperitoneal injection of AICAR (400 mg/kg) 1 h before the operation. **(A)** The protein expression levels of phosphorylated AMPK (*p*-AMPK) and AMPK were detected by Western blot, and the relative ratios of *p*-AMPK/AMPK were quantified by VisionWorks imaging software. The normalized values are indicated in the histogram. GAPDH expression was used as loading control. **(B,C)** Representative pathological images of the pancreas and liver (200x and 400x) under a light microscope (H&E staining, Bar = 50 μm). **(D)** Histological scores were obtained to evaluate the degree of pancreas and liver injury from H&E staining. **(E)** Serum amylase and lipase levels in rats. **(F)** The MDA and SOD contents in pancreatic tissues of rats in each group. **(G)** Detection of serum ALT and AST activity. Data are presented as the mean ± SD of three independent experiments. $^{\#}p < 0.05$, $^{\#\#}p < 0.01$, $^{\#\#\#}p < 0.001$, $^{\#\#\#\#}p < 0.0001$ vs. control group; $^{*}p < 0.05$, $^{**}p < 0.01$, $^{***}p < 0.001$, $^{****}p < 0.0001$ vs. SAP group.

capability. Our results indicated that the SAP rats exhibited higher hepatic expression of monocyte chemotactic protein 1 (MCP-1, a protein that specifically affects chemotaxis and activates macrophages) and CD68 (a rat macrophage marker) as well as increased concentrations of MPO (a functional and activation marker of neutrophils) in liver tissues compared with the control groups, whereas AICAR treatment profoundly downregulated the expression levels of these inflammatory mediators (**Figures 2A,B,D,E**). In addition, immunohistochemical staining and qRT-PCR indicated that

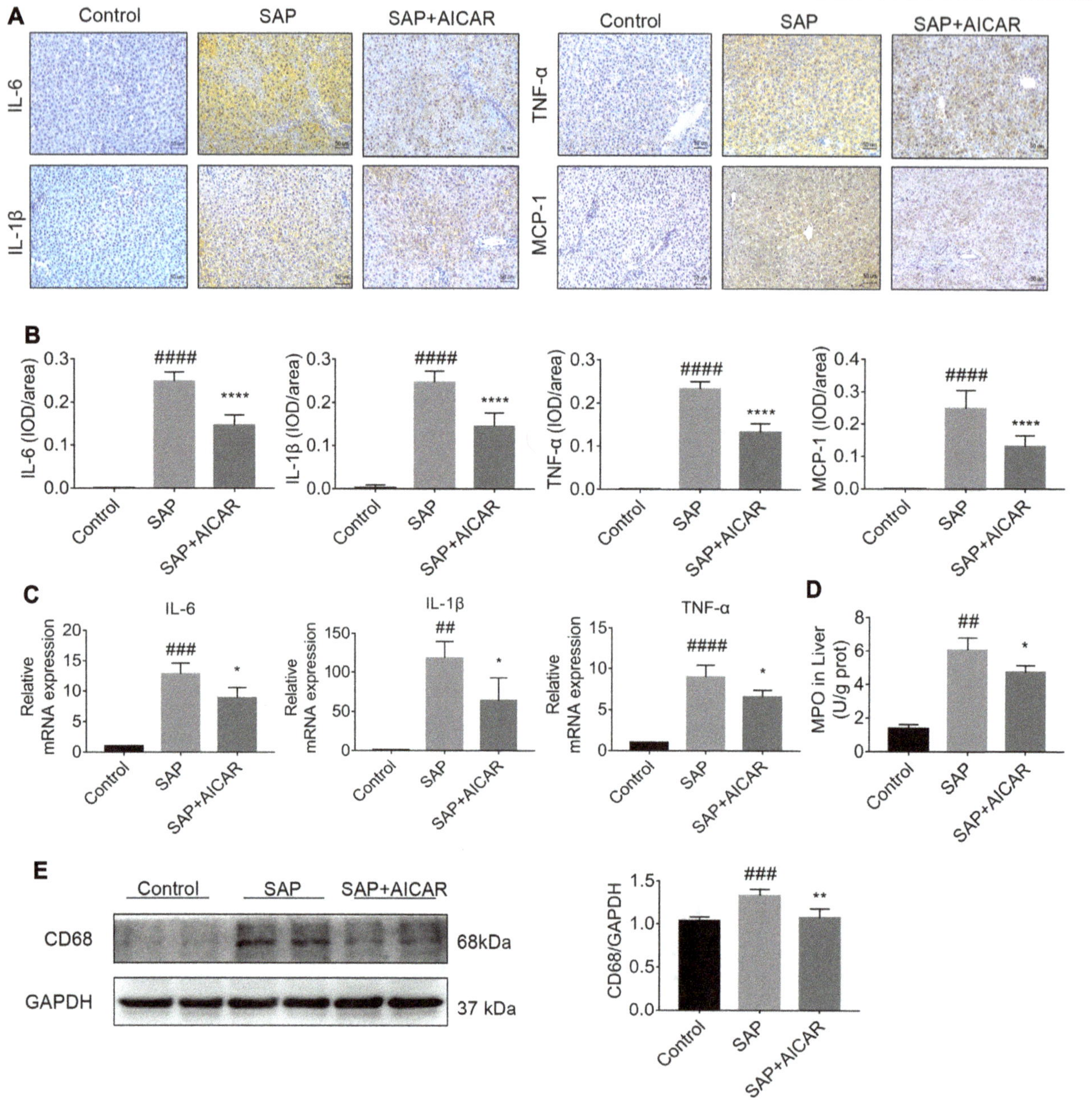

FIGURE 2 | AICAR protects against SAP-induced hepatic inflammation in a sodium taurocholate-induced PALI rat model. 7–8 week-old wild-type male SD rats were randomly divided into three groups: the control group (control, n = 10) was treated with sham operation and injected with 0.9% normal saline; the severe acute pancreatitis (SAP) group (n = 10) was infused with 3% sodium taurocholate (0.1 ml/100 g); and the AMPK agonist (AICAR) group (n = 8) received intraperitoneal injection of AICAR (400 mg/kg) 1 h before the operation. **(A,B)** The protein expression of IL-6, IL-1β, TNF-α and MCP-1 in liver sections was detected by immunohistochemistry (original magnification ×200, Bar = 50 μm). Image-Pro Plus 6.0 software was used for statistical analysis. **(C)** The mRNA levels of IL-6, IL-1β, and TNF-α in liver tissues were measured by RT-qPCR. **(D)** MPO contents in liver tissues. **(E)** The protein expression of CD68 was assessed by Western blot and quantified by densitometry using VisionWorks imaging software. GAPDH expression was used as a loading control. Each value represents the mean ± SD. $^{\#}p < 0.05$, $^{\#\#}p < 0.01$, $^{\#\#\#}p < 0.001$, $^{\#\#\#\#}p < 0.0001$ vs control group; $^{*}p < 0.05$, $^{**}p < 0.01$, $^{***}p < 0.001$, $^{****}p < 0.0001$ vs. SAP group.

the protein and messenger RNA (mRNA) expression levels of IL-6, IL-1β and TNF-α were significantly elevated in the liver tissues of SAP rats compared with the control group; however, replenishment of AICAR inhibited the increased expression of these inflammatory cytokines (**Figures 2A–C**). These observations confirm that AICAR treatment protects against PALI in sodium taurocholate-induced SAP rats, likely by inhibiting the inflammatory response in the liver.

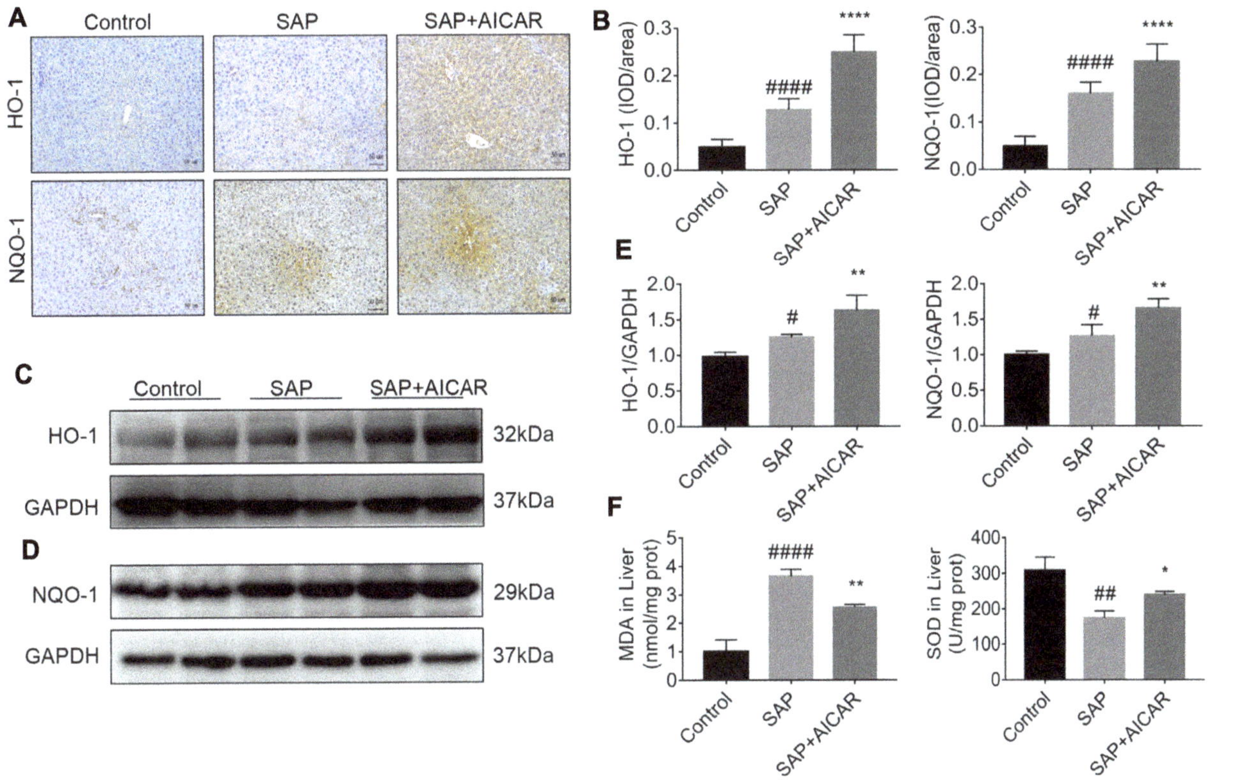

FIGURE 3 | AICAR prevents hepatic oxidative stress in a sodium taurocholate-induced PALI rat model. 7–8 week-old wild-type male SD rats were randomly divided into three groups: the control group (control, n = 10) was treated with sham operation and injected with 0.9% normal saline; the severe acute pancreatitis (SAP) group (n = 10) was infused with 3% sodium taurocholate (0.1 ml/100 g); and the AMPK agonist (AICAR) group (n = 8) received intraperitoneal injection of AICAR (400 mg/kg) 1 h before the operation. **(A,B)** Liver sections were collected and stained with antibodies against HO-1 and NQO-1, and the average integrated optical density (IOD)/area of HO-1 and NQO-1 was quantified using Image-Pro Plus 6.0 software (original magnification ×200, Bar = 50 μm). **(C–E)** The protein expression levels of HO-1 and NQO-1 in liver tissues were assessed by Western blot and quantified by densitometry using VisionWorks imaging software. The level of GAPDH was used as a loading control. **(F)** MDA and SOD contents were measured in liver tissues. Data are presented as the mean ± SD obtained from three independent experiments. $^{\#}p < 0.05$, $^{\#\#}p < 0.01$, $^{\#\#\#}p < 0.001$, $^{\#\#\#\#}p < 0.0001$ vs control group; $^{*}p < 0.05$, $^{**}p < 0.01$, $^{***}p < 0.001$, $^{****}p < 0.0001$ vs. SAP group.

AICAR Treatment Markedly Increases the Antioxidant Abilities of the Liver in Sodium Taurocholate-Induced SAP Rats

To further determine the roles of AICAR in PALI, we next investigated whether replenishment of AICAR can rescue the damaged antioxidant system in sodium taurocholate-induced SAP rats. Not surprisingly, immunohistochemical staining and Western blot results indicated that the hepatic expression levels of antioxidant proteins heme oxygenase-1 (HO-1) and NADPH quinone oxidoreductase 1 (NQO-1) were slightly upregulated in sodium taurocholate-induced SAP rats, which may represent a stress protection for the liver to defend against pancreatitis-induced liver injury. Notably, AICAR supplementation further augmented the hepatic expression levels of HO-1 and NQO-1 after sodium taurocholate treatment in rats (**Figures 3A–E**). Furthermore, the detection results of hepatic tissues in sodium taurocholate-induced SAP rats showed that the levels of MDA were significantly elevated, whereas the concentrations of SOD were strikingly decreased, suggesting that the antioxidant capacity of the liver in sodium taurocholate-induced SAP rats was disrupted. However, treatment with AICAR significantly restored the antioxidant abilities of the liver, as evidenced by an obvious elevation in hepatic concentrations of SOD and a marked decline in the hepatic levels of MDA (**Figure 3F**). These data suggest that AICAR supplementation prevents sodium taurocholate-induced PALI in rats by increasing antioxidant activities in the liver.

AICAR Treatment Activates the AMPK/Nrf2 Signaling Pathway and Inhibits NLRP3 Inflammasome Activation in the Liver Tissues of Sodium Taurocholate-Induced SAP Rats

Next, we focused on dissecting the deeper molecular mechanism by which AICAR inhibits oxidative stress and inflammation in the liver tissues of sodium taurocholate-induced SAP rats by activating AMPK phosphorylation. We performed Western blot to test the nuclear translocation of Nrf2 and the protein expression of NLRP3 as well as its downstream proteins caspase-1 and cleaved IL-1β in hepatic tissues of sodium

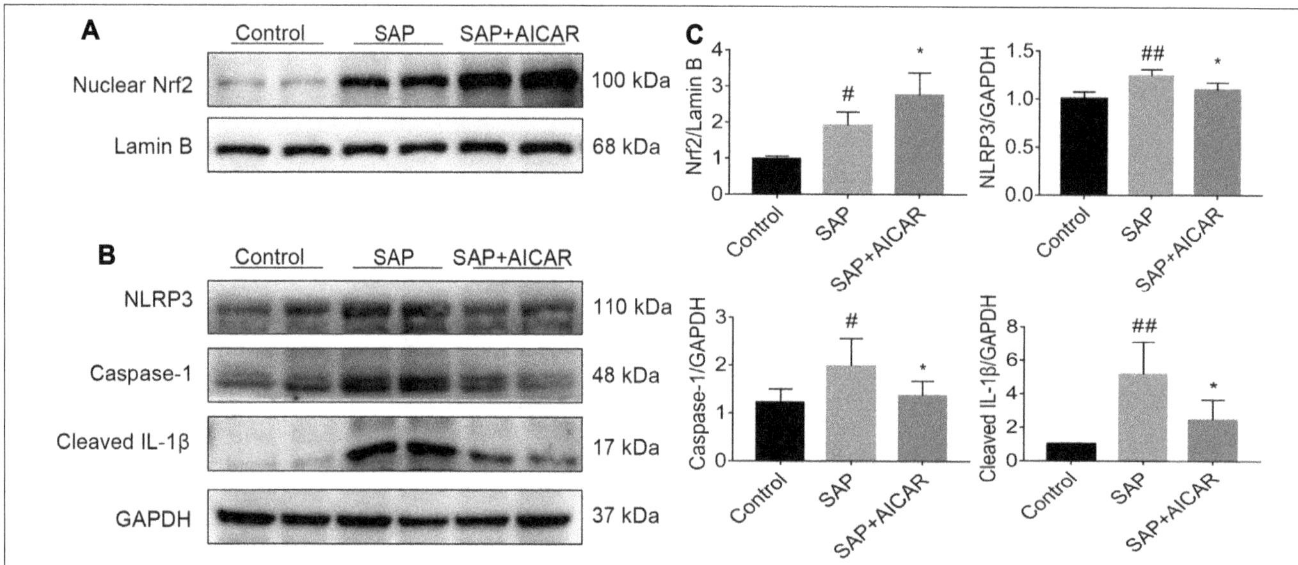

FIGURE 4 | The effects of AICAR on the activation of the AMPK/Nrf2 signaling pathway and inhibition of NLRP3 inflammasome activation in the liver tissues of sodium taurocholate-induced SAP rats. 7–8 week-old wild-type male SD rats were randomly divided into three groups: the control group (control, n = 10) was treated with sham operation and injected with 0.9% normal saline; the severe acute pancreatitis (SAP) group (n = 10) was infused with 3% sodium taurocholate (0.1 ml/100 g); and the AMPK agonist (AICAR) group (n = 8) received intraperitoneal injection of AICAR (400 mg/kg) 1 h before the operation. **(A)** The levels of nuclear accumulation of Nrf2 in liver tissues of each group were detected by Western blot analysis. For the internal control, Lamin B was used. **(B)** The protein expression levels of NLRP3, caspase-1, and cleaved IL-1β in liver tissues were measured by Western blot using anti-NLRP3, anti-caspase-1 and anti-cleaved IL-1β antibodies. GAPDH was used as an internal control. **(C)** Relative band densities were quantified using VisionWorks imaging software, and the results are expressed in the histogram. Data are presented as the mean ± SD obtained from three independent experiments. $^{\#}p < 0.05$, $^{\#\#}p < 0.01$, $^{\#\#\#}p < 0.001$, $^{\#\#\#\#}p < 0.0001$ vs control group; $^{*}p < 0.05$, $^{**}p < 0.01$, $^{***}p < 0.001$, $^{****}p < 0.0001$ vs. SAP group.

taurocholate-induced SAP rats after treatment with AICAR. The nuclear translocation of Nrf2 was increased following sodium taurocholate treatment, whereas AICAR supplementation further promoted the nuclear accumulation of Nrf2 (**Figures 4A,C**). Moreover, sodium taurocholate treatment significantly increased the hepatic expression of NLRP3, caspase-1 and cleaved-IL-1β, while AICAR supplementation reversed this phenomenon (**Figures 4B,C**). These findings suggest that AICAR markedly alters the nuclear accumulation of Nrf2 and inhibits NLRP3 inflammasome activation in sodium taurocholate-induced PALI rats by activating AMPK phosphorylation. Thus, we speculate that Nrf2 and NLRP3 inflammasome pathway may mediate essential parts in the protective roles of AICAR against oxidative stress and inflammation in sodium taurocholate-induced PALI rats.

Inhibition of AMPK Activation by Compound C Markedly Aggravates PALI in Sodium Taurocholate-Induced SAP Rats

To further elucidate the role of AMPK in PALI, we treated rats with the AMPK inhibitor Compound C (CC, 13.8 mg/kg) by intraperitoneal injection to block the phosphorylation of AMPK in liver tissues, followed by sodium taurocholate infusion. Unsurprisingly, Western blot results showed that sodium taurocholate infusion significantly reduced the ratio of *p*-AMPK/AMPK in liver tissues. As expected, this ratio was further reduced by CC treatment, suggesting that CC treatment successfully inhibited AMPK phosphorylation levels in the liver tissues of SAP rats (**Figure 5A**). Interestingly, treatment with CC significantly exacerbated sodium taurocholate-induced pancreatic injury in rats, as evidenced by further increased acinar necrosis and inflammatory cell infiltration (**Figure 5B**). Evaluation of the pancreatitis score in pancreatic sections also revealed that CC treatment was accompanied by more severe pancreatic injury than SAP (**Figure 5D**). We also observed that administration of CC in rats augmented SAP-induced edema, necrosis and structural disorder in hepatic lobules with further increased liver injury scores compared with SAP rats (**Figures 5C,D**). In addition, the amplitude of SAP-induced elevation of serum levels of both ALT and AST, two markers of liver injury, in CC-treated rats was higher than that in the SAP groups (**Figure 5E**). The above results indicate that inhibition of AMPK phosphorylation by CC enhances sodium taurocholate-induced PALI in rats.

AMPK Inhibition by Compound C Enhances Hepatic Oxidative Stress and NLRP3 Inflammasome Activation in Sodium Taurocholate-Induced PALI Rats

We next explored whether inhibition of AMPK activation by CC could promote hepatic oxidative stress and inflammation levels in sodium taurocholate-induced SAP rats. We found that the increase in the nuclear translocation of Nrf2 in the hepatic tissues of SAP rats was markedly reduced after CC treatment

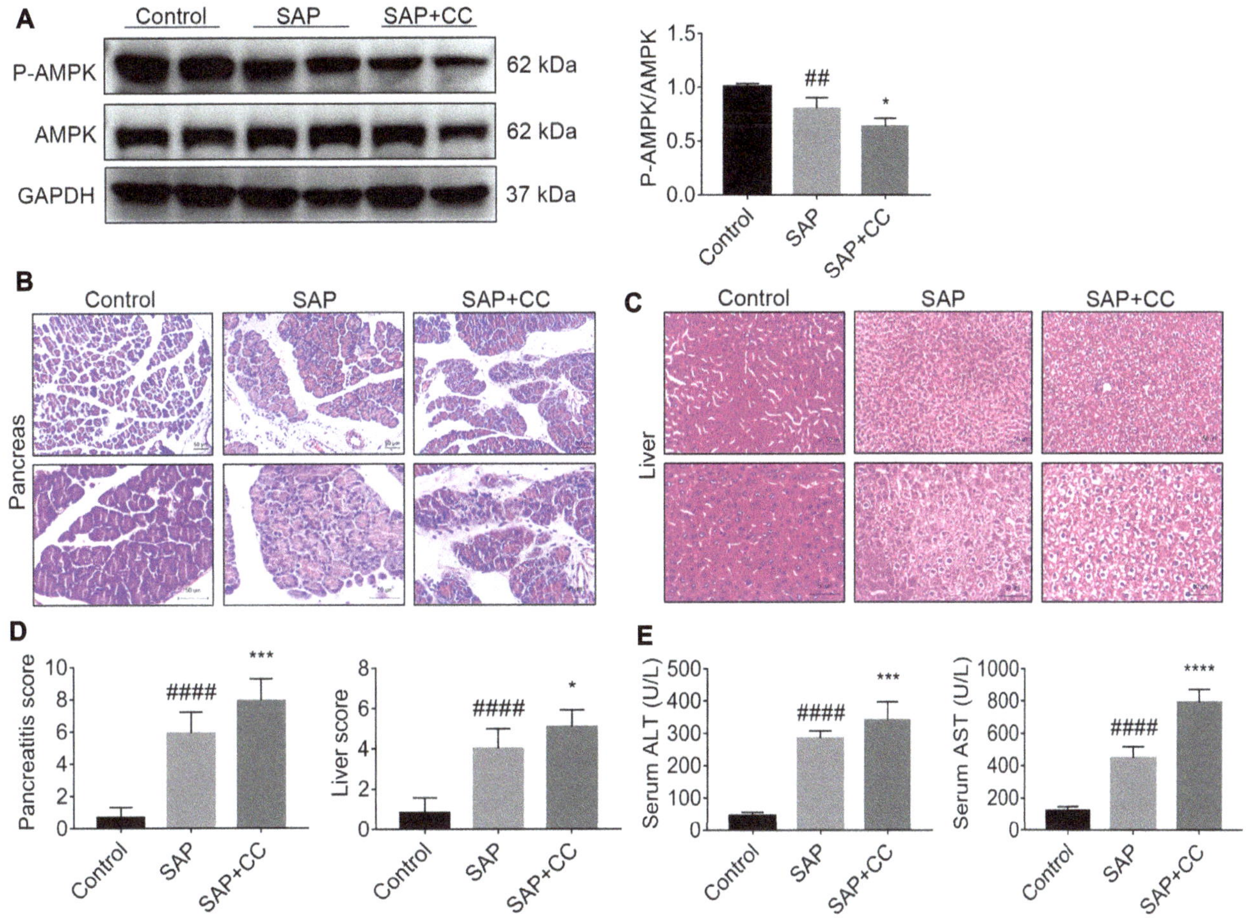

FIGURE 5 | Inhibition of AMPK phosphorylation by Compound C markedly aggravates PALI in sodium taurocholate-induced SAP rats. Seven-to eight-week-old wild-type male SD rats were randomly divided into three groups: the control group (control, n = 10) was treated with a sham operation and injected with 0.9% normal saline; the severe acute pancreatitis (SAP) group (n = 10) was infused with 3% sodium taurocholate (0.1 ml/100 g); and the AMPK inhibitor (CC) group (n = 8) received intraperitoneal injection of CC (Compound C, 13.8 mg/kg) 1 h before the operation. **(A)** The protein expression levels of AMPK and phosphorylated AMPK (*p*-AMPK) in liver tissues were detected by Western blot using anti-AMPK and anti-*p*-AMPK antibodies. GAPDH was used as the internal reference control. Data are presented as mean ± SD of three independent experiments. **(B,C)** Histological images of H&E staining in pancreas and liver tissues (200x and 400x) under a light microscope (Bar = 50 μm). **(D)** Histological scores were obtained to evaluate the degree of pancreas and liver injury from H&E staining. **(E)** Serum ALT and AST concentrations were detected. Data are presented as the mean ± SD of three independent experiments. $^{\#}p < 0.05$, $^{\#\#}p < 0.01$, $^{\#\#\#}p < 0.001$, $^{\#\#\#\#}p < 0.0001$ vs control group; $^{*}p < 0.05$, $^{**}p < 0.01$, $^{***}p < 0.001$, $^{****}p < 0.0001$ vs. SAP group.

(**Figures 6A,B**). We further measured MDA and SOD levels, which are indicators of oxidative damage, in the liver tissues of each group. The levels of hepatic MDA in rats treated with CC were significantly augmented compared to those in the SAP groups (**Figure 6C**). Alternatively, treatment with CC had a reduced effect on the magnitude of sodium taurocholate-induced decline in hepatic SOD levels (**Figure 6D**). Moreover, these changes in CC-treated SAP rats were accompanied by significantly increased hepatic expression of NLRP3, caspase-1 and cleaved IL-1β compared with SAP rats (**Figures 6E,F**), which results in a certain type of inflammatory response-related cell death called pyroptosis (Guo et al., 2021). Thus, we next compared the levels of IL-6, IL-1β and TNF-α in the liver tissues of SAP rats by q-PCR analysis with or without CC treatment. Consistent with our previous findings, the expression of these inflammatory cytokines was upregulated in the SAP groups, whereas CC treatment led to a further increase in the mRNA abundance of the aforementioned inflammatory genes (**Figure 6G**). Ultimately, our data suggest that inhibition of AMPK phosphorylation by CC aggravates PALI in sodium taurocholate-induced SAP rats, likely by repressing Nrf2-mediated antioxidant stress and anti-inflammatory roles.

Nrf2 Knockout Weakens the Protective Effects of AICAR on PALI in L-Arginine-Induced SAP Mice

Since the aforementioned data indicate that the anti-inflammatory and antioxidant stress effects of AICAR may be related to the induction of Nrf2 nuclear translocation, we further investigated whether Nrf2 deficiency would affect the protective effects of AICAR against PALI in L-arginine-

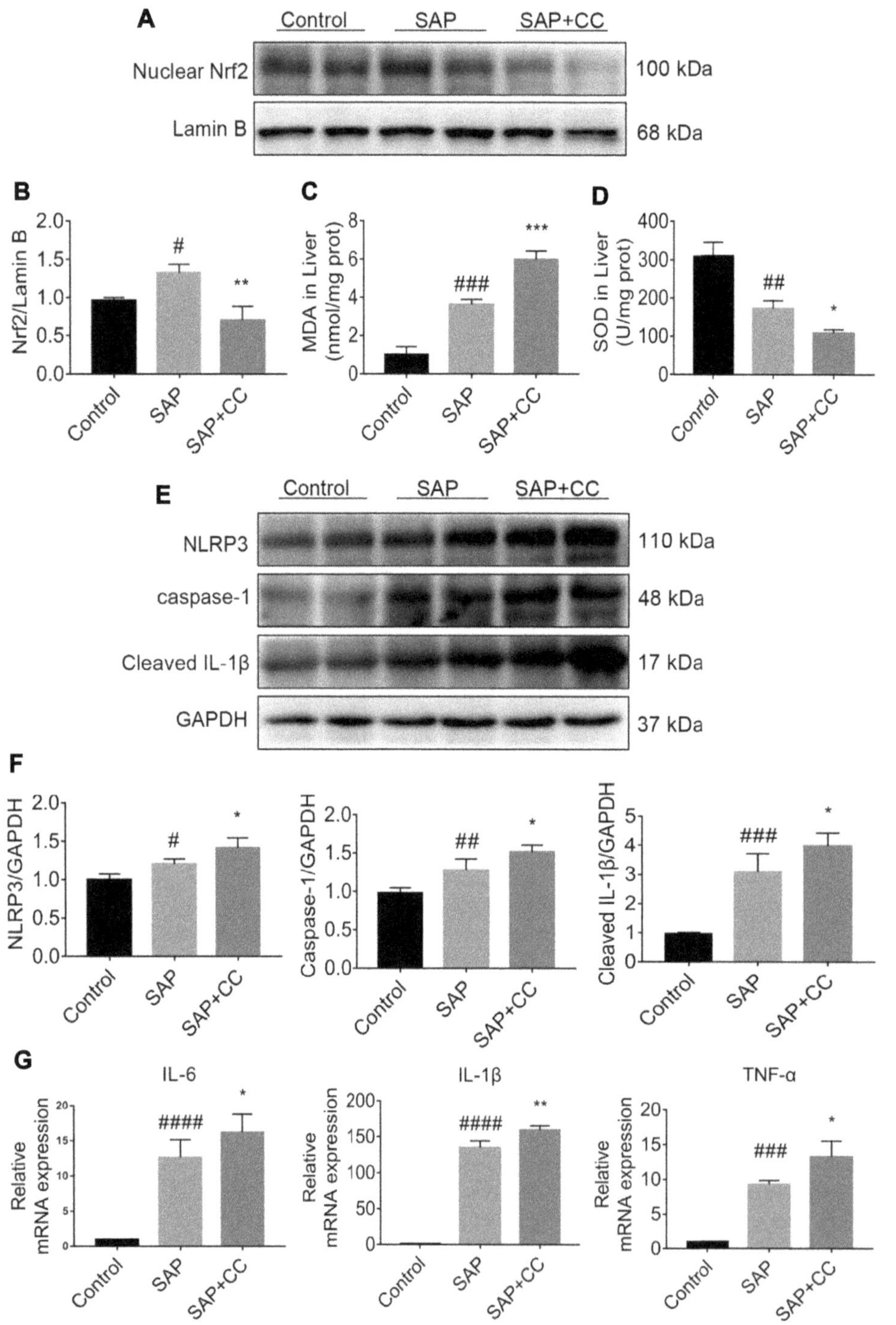

FIGURE 6 | Inhibition of AMPK phosphorylation by Compound C enhances hepatic oxidative stress and inflammation levels in sodium taurocholate-induced SAP rats. Seven-to eight-week-old wild type male SD rats were randomly divided into three groups: the control group (control, n = 10) was treated with a sham operation and injected with 0.9% normal saline; the severe acute pancreatitis (SAP) group (n = 10) was infused with 3% sodium taurocholate (0.1 ml/100 g); and the AMPK inhibitor (CC) group (n = 8) received intraperitoneal injection of CC (Compound C, 13.8 mg/kg) 1 h before the operation. **(A)** The nuclear translocation levels of Nrf2 in liver tissues were determined by Western blot. For the internal control, Lamin B was used. **(C,D)** The contents of MDA and SOD in liver tissues were determined. **(E)** The protein expression of NLRP3, caspase-1, and cleaved IL-1β was detected by Western blot. GAPDH was used as the internal reference control. **(B,F)** The relative ratios of Nrf2, NLRP3, caspase-1, and cleaved IL-1β were quantified using VisionWorks imaging software. **(G)** The mRNA levels of IL-6, IL-1β, and TNF-α in liver tissues were measured by RT-qPCR. Data are presented as the mean ± SD of three independent experiments. $^{\#}p < 0.05$, $^{\#\#}p < 0.01$, $^{\#\#\#}p < 0.001$, $^{\#\#\#\#}p < 0.0001$ vs control group; $^{*}p < 0.05$, $^{**}p < 0.01$, $^{***}p < 0.001$, $^{****}p < 0.0001$ vs. SAP group.

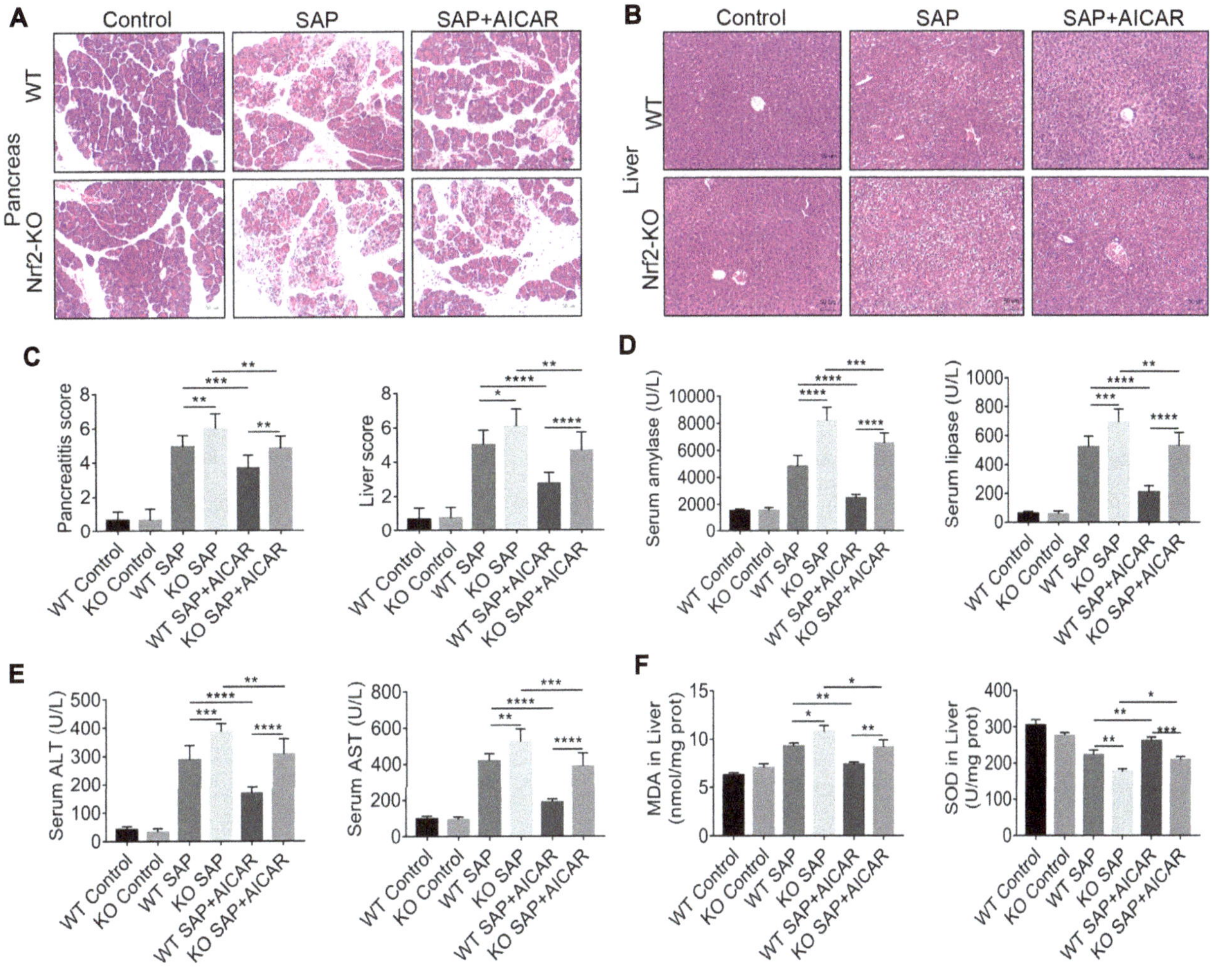

FIGURE 7 | Nrf2 knockout attenuates the protective effects of AICAR on PALI and the inhibitory effects of hepatic oxidative stress in L-arginine-induced SAP mice. Male wild-type mice or Nrf2$^{-/-}$ mice were divided into three groups: the control group (control, n = 6) was intraperitoneally injected with 0.9% normal saline; the SAP group (n = 6) was intraperitoneally injected with 8% L-arginine hydrochloride (pH = 7.0, 4 g/kg) twice at an interval of 1 h; and the AMPK agonist (AICAR, n = 6) group was intraperitoneally injected with AICAR (400 mg/kg) twice: 1 h before and 24 h after L-arginine hydrochloride administration. **(A,B)** Representative pathological images of the pancreas and liver (200x) under a light microscope (H&E staining, Bar = 50 μm). **(C)** Histological scores were obtained to evaluate the degree of pancreas and liver injury from H&E staining. **(D)** The concentrations of serum amylase and lipase were detected. **(E)** The levels of serum ALT and AST were measured to evaluate liver function. **(F)** Concentrations of MDA and SOD in liver tissues from different groups. Data are presented as the mean ± SD of three independent experiments. Data are presented as mean ± SD of three independent experiments. $^*p < 0.05$, $^{**}p < 0.01$, $^{***}p < 0.001$, $^{****}p < 0.0001$.

induced SAP mice. L-arginine-induced elevations in serum levels of pancreas injury enzymes (amylase and lipase) and the pathological changes as well as pancreatitis scores analyzed in H&E-stained pancreas sections in Nrf2 knockout (KO) mice were higher than those in WT SAP mice (**Figures 7A–D**). Meanwhile, the beneficial effects of AICAR against L-arginine-induced pancreatic injury reflected by the above indicators were significantly attenuated in Nrf2 KO mice compared with WT littermates (**Figures 7A,C**). Likewise, the pathological changes in liver sections of the Nrf2 KO SAP mice were more severe than those in the WT SAP groups by H&E staining (**Figure 7B**). Additionally, treatment of WT SAP mice with AICAR markedly reduced these negative pathological changes (**Figure 7B**); however, these protective effects mediated by AICAR were weakened in Nrf2 KO mice (**Figure 7B**). The liver injury scores, consistent with the pathological appearance in each group, further confirmed our findings (**Figure 7C**). Moreover, the serum levels of ALT and AST in both WT and Nrf2 KO mice were augmented after L-arginine administration. Notably, the levels of these two markers indicated that liver injury in Nrf2 KO mice was higher than that in WT mice (**Figure 7E**). Alternatively, AICAR treatment markedly attenuated the L-arginine-induced elevation in the serum levels of ALT and AST in WT SAP mice, while these phenomena were significantly inhibited in Nrf2 KO mice (**Figure 7E**). Therefore, these results indicate that Nrf2 plays an important role in the protective effects of AICAR against L-arginine-induced PALI in mice.

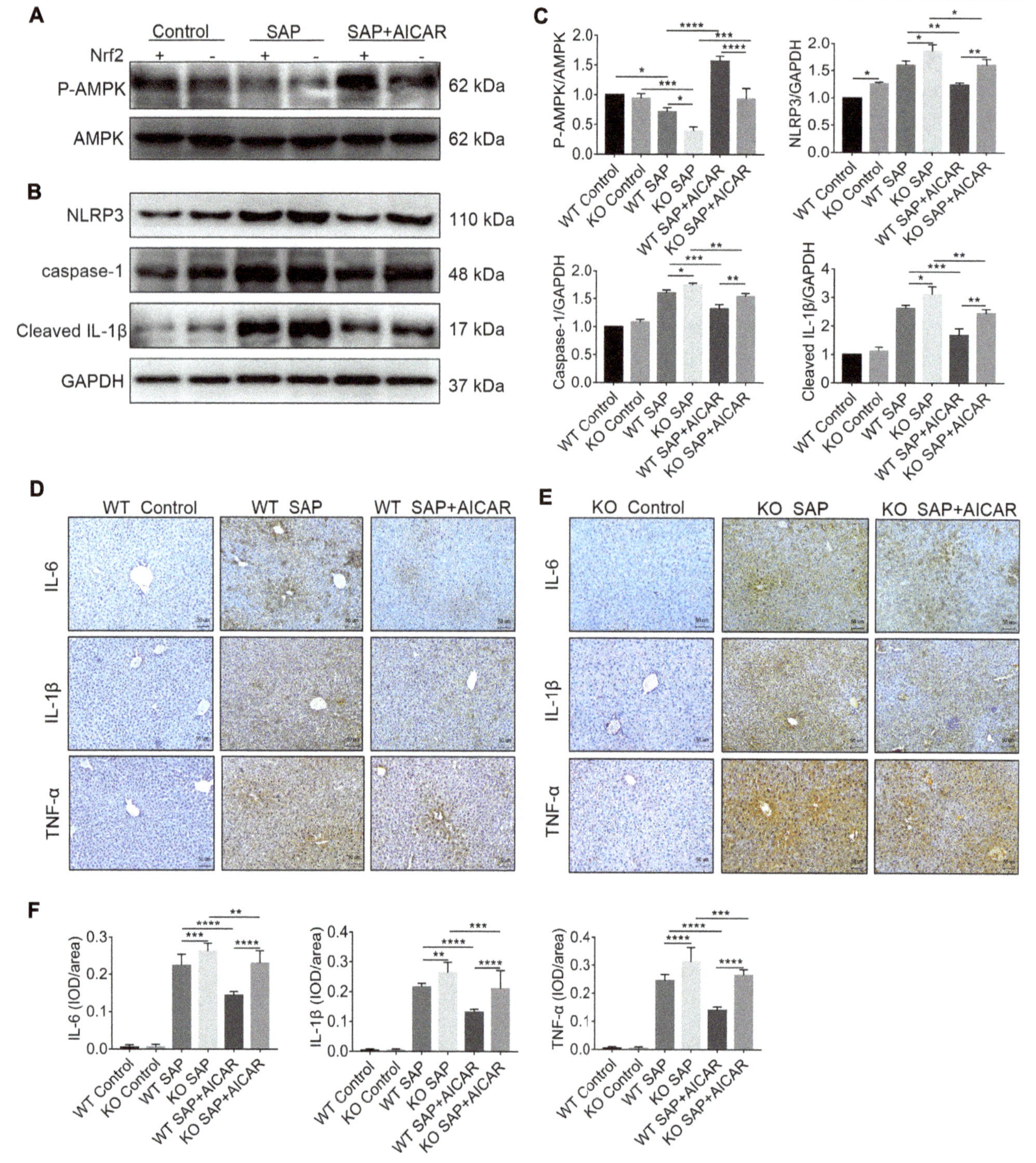

FIGURE 8 | Nrf2 deficiency impairs the inhibitory effects of AICAR against hepatic NLRP3 inflammasome activation in L-arginine-induced SAP mice. Male wild type mice or Nrf2$^{-/-}$ mice were divided into three groups: the control group (control, n = 6) was intraperitoneally injected with 0.9% normal saline; the SAP group (n = 6) was intraperitoneally injected with 8% L-arginine hydrochloride (pH = 7.0, 4 g/kg) twice at an interval of 1 h; and the AMPK agonist (AICAR, n = 6) group wasintraperitoneally injected with AICAR (400 mg/kg) twice: 1 h before and 24 h after L-arginine hydrochloride administration. **(A–C)** The protein expression levels of phosphorylated AMPK, total AMPK, NLRP3, caspase-1, and cleaved IL-1β were measured by Western blot, and the relative ratios of *p*-AMPK/AMPK and band densities of Nrf2, NLRP3, caspase-1, and cleaved IL-1β were quantified using VisionWorks imaging software. GAPDH was used as an internal reference. **(D–F)** The protein expression of IL-6, IL-1β and TNF-α in liver sections was detected by immunohistochemistry (original magnification ×200, Bar = 50 μm). Image-Pro Plus 6.0 software was used for statistical analysis. Data are presented as the mean ± SD of three independent experiments. $^{*}p < 0.05$, $^{**}p < 0.01$, $^{***}p < 0.001$, $^{****}p < 0.0001$.

Nrf2 Deficiency Impairs the Inhibitory Effects of AICAR Against PALI-Related Hepatic Oxidative Stress and NLRP3 Inflammasome Activation in L-Arginine-Induced SAP Mice

To further clarify whether the beneficial effect of AICAR on antioxidant stress was Nrf2 dependent, we measured MDA and SOD levels in the liver tissues of L-arginine-treated Nrf2 KO mice and WT littermates with or without AICAR supplementation. After L-arginine treatment, the production of MDA in liver tissues was conspicuously increased, and the levels of SOD were significantly decreased in Nrf2 KO mice compared to WT mice. Additionally, administration of AICAR was associated with markedly reduced MDA levels, and the concentrations of SOD were significantly augmented compared to those in the WT SAP group. However, these beneficial antioxidant effects of AICAR were largely blocked in Nrf2 KO mice compared to WT littermates (**Figure 7F**). These observations indicate that the antioxidant ability of AICAR in the liver tissues of L-arginine-induced PALI mice was partially dependent on Nrf2.

We next determined whether induction of Nrf2 is required for the inhibition of the NLRP3 inflammasome-associated inflammatory response in the liver tissues of L-arginine-induced PALI mice. Thus, we performed Western blot to compare the hepatic expression levels of NLRP3, caspase-1 and cleaved-IL-1β between L-arginine-treated Nrf2 KO mice and WT littermates with or without AICAR administration. The results showed that the hepatic expression of NLRP3, caspase-1 and cleaved-IL-1β in Nrf2 KO mice was higher than that in WT littermates after L-arginine treatment (**Figures 8A–C**). Furthermore, replenishment of AICAR profoundly decreased the expression of these indicators in the liver tissues of WT littermates compared with the WT SAP group; however, these observed trends were significantly reversed in Nrf2 KO mice (**Figures 8B,C**). Thus, our findings suggest that Nrf2 deficiency impairs the inhibitory effect of AICAR against NLRP3 inflammasome activation in L-arginine-induced PALI mice. To further elucidate the role of Nrf2 in the anti-inflammatory effects of AICAR, we detected the expression levels of several inflammatory factors, including IL-6, IL-1β and TNF-α, in each group of Nrf2 KO mice and WT littermates. Immunohistochemistry analysis showed that L-arginine induced the expression of these inflammatory factors in the liver tissues of both Nrf2 KO mice and WT littermates, resulting in a further increase in their expression (**Figures 8D–F**). Moreover, replenishment of AICAR decreased L-arginine-induced hepatic inflammatory factor accumulation in WT littermates, while these anti-inflammatory effects of AICAR were markedly reversed in Nrf2 KO mice compared with WT controls (**Figures 8D–F**). Taken together, our results suggest that Nrf2 deficiency largely eliminates the negative regulation of AICAR on the NLRP3 inflammasome activation associated inflammatory response in the liver tissues of L-arginine-induced PALI mice.

DISCUSSION

The central goal of this study was to investigate the pharmacological activation of AMPK by AICAR as a therapeutic strategy for the treatment of PALI. Our findings demonstrated that AICAR activates AMPK, which leads to Nrf2-mediated antioxidant stress and inhibition of NLRP3-related inflammation, and thus improving PALI. This study indicated that AMPK exerted an essential role in the pathological processes of PALI and presented the first evidence that pharmacological activation of AMPK by AICAR ameliorates PALI, suggesting that AICAR may be a promising therapeutic agent for the treatment of PALI.

In the current study, we demonstrated that both 1 day after sodium taurocholate infusion in rats and 2 days after intraperitoneal injection of L-arginine in mice successfully induced rodent models of PALI, as evidenced by marked elevation in the plasma levels of amylase, lipase, ALT and AST as well as severe pathological injury of the pancreas and liver in the two experimental SAP models (**Figures 1B–G, Figures 7A–F**). This study provided novel evidence that SAP caused a drastic reduction in hepatic expression levels of phosphorylated AMPK in sodium taurocholate- and L-arginine-induced rodent SAP models, suggesting that AMPK may be involved in the pathogenesis of PALI (**Figure 1A, Figures 8A,C**). Herein, we obtained two lines of evidence to demonstrate our hypothesis. On the one hand, administration of the direct AMPK activator AICAR led to a dramatic elevation in hepatic expression levels of phosphorylated AMPK and prevented PALI in sodium taurocholate- and L-arginine-induced rodent SAP models (**Figures 1A–G, Figures 7A–E, Figures 8A,C**). On the other hand, inhibiting the activity of AMPK in liver tissues by using the AMPK inhibitor Compound C profoundly exacerbated PALI in sodium taurocholate-induced SAP rats (**Figures 5A–E**). Although previous studies have shown that compound C may play roles independent of AMPK inhibition, such as anti-glioma and inhibition of Bone morphogenetic protein (BMP) pathway, it is still the only available cell permeability AMPK antagonist (Yu et al., 2008; Liu et al., 2014). Similar to our findings, AMPK activation by AICAR has been shown to protect the kidney from overt damage in a rat model of kidney ischemia-reperfusion injury (Lempiäinen et al., 2012). In addition, a Compound C-induced reduction in myocardial AMPK activity impaired cardiac function and aggravated oxidative stress in cardiomyocytes in DOX-induced acute cardiotoxicity mice (Liu et al., 2018).

In the pathogenesis of PALI, the uncontrollable hepatic inflammatory response and elevated oxidative stress triggered by SAP will continue to damage hepatocytes, which are central mediators for accelerating the development of PALI (Yang et al., 2003; Moniaux et al., 2011). According to previous reports, AMPK activation is involved in the inhibition of the

IL-6-stimulated inflammatory response in human liver cells and mediates the antioxidant stress ability of fibroblast growth factor (FGF) one in a mouse model of nonalcoholic fatty liver disease (Nerstedt et al., 2013; Liu et al., 2020). Therefore, we explored the hypothesis that the molecular basis of AICAR in improving PALI is attributed to its anti-inflammatory capability and reduction of hepatic oxidative stress by AMPK activation. Our findings demonstrated that AMPK was required for the regulation of hepatic inflammation and oxidative stress in sodium taurocholate-induced PALI rats and that AICAR ameliorated PALI by AMPK activation in this rat model, which was associated with its anti-inflammatory and antioxidative actions.

Next, we focused on dissecting the molecular mechanism to explain how AMPK activation by AICAR reduced hepatic inflammation and oxidative stress in PALI. In response to inflammatory reaction, Nrf2 is released from Keap1 and translocates to the nucleus, thus activating the endogenous antioxidant defense system by enhancing the transcription of a variety of antioxidant enzymes, such as HO-1 and NQO-1, presenting a superior effect in oxygen reduction balance. In particular, oxidative stress and inflammation are closely connected, and increased levels of proinflammatory cytokines induce oxidative stress. In turn, oxidative stress overactivation further exacerbates the inflammatory response (Dandekar et al., 2015; Antonucci et al., 2017). Furthermore, studies have also shown that the activation of Nrf2 can inhibit inflammation-mediated injury *via* its antioxidant cascade (Joo Choi et al., 2014; Saha et al., 2020). Notably, several recent studies have demonstrated that Nrf2 negatively regulates the activity of the NLRP3 inflammasome, which is a central regulator of inflammation required for PALI (Hou et al., 2018; Chen et al., 2019). Upon stimulation, NLRP3 collects ASC protein and converts procaspase-1 into active caspase-1, which cleaves pro-IL-β or pro-IL-18 into mature forms, ensuing and promoting hepatic inflammatory injury (Mridha et al., 2017). However, the crosstalk between Nrf2 and the NLRP3 inflammasome pathway in PALI remains to be determined. In addition, previous reports found that AMPK also inhibits NLRP3 inflammasome activation in a mouse model of diabetic cardiomyopathy and acute pancreatitis (Chen et al., 2020; Yang et al., 2020). In fact, AMPK phosphorylates Nrf2 at serine 374, 408, and 433, moves Nrf2 from the cytoplasm to the nucleus, and binds to the antioxidant response element (ARE) gene to exert its antioxidant effect (Matzinger et al., 2020). In the current study, rats treated with AMPK agonists (AICAR) and inhibitors (CC) demonstrated that AMPK plays an important role in activating Nrf2 signaling and inhibiting NLRP3 inflammasome pathways in PALI and that hepatic Nrf2 may act as a key mediator of AICAR protection against PALI-associated oxidative stress and NLRP3 inflammasome activation. Therefore, we speculate that the direct activation of AMPK by AICAR exerts its antioxidant and anti-inflammatory roles to prevent PALI through Nrf2-mediated antioxidant effects and inhibition of the NLRP3 inflammasome pathway.

To verify our hypothesis, we used Nrf2 KO mice and WT mice to conduct a comparative study in an L-arginine-induced PALI model with or without AICAR treatment. We found that knockout of Nrf2 limited the ability of AICAR to reduce the severity of PALI in mice (**Figures 7A–E**). Most importantly, Nrf2 gene deletion markedly weakened the protective effects of AICAR to prevent SAP-induced oxidative stress and NLRP3 inflammasome activation in the liver tissues of L-arginine-induced PALI mice (**Figure 7F**, **Figures 8B,C**). However, AICAR still had a slight protective effect on PALI in Nrf2 KO mice. AMPK can regulate a variety of physiological and pathological effects through multiple pathways to affect cell metabolism and survival (Carling, 2017; Ramirez Reyes et al., 2021). This result may be attributed to the activation of AMPK by AICAR leading to other pathway modulations independent of Nrf2 signaling in PALI and resulting in other biological effects, such as AMPK-related mitochondrial homeostasis, ferroptosis and necroptosis, which are worthy of further exploration in our future research (Herzig et al., 2018; Song et al., 2018; Lee et al., 2020). Nonetheless, our findings indicate that activation of Nrf2 by AICAR mediates important roles in ameliorating hepatic oxidative stress and inhibiting NLRP3 inflammasome pathway activation in PALI mice regardless of whether Nrf2 is the master pathway.

Despite our novel findings, the current study has some limitations. First, our observations are only based on two rodent PALI models. AICAR has been used clinically for myocardial protection in coronary artery bypass grafting and myocardial ischemic injury (Rao et al., 2016). We should further determine the role of AICAR in PALI in humanoid large animals and in clinical studies. Second, our results demonstrated that AICAR protects against PALI partially through Nrf2-mediated antioxidant effects and inhibition of NLRP3 inflammasome activation, whether AICAR plays these positive roles mainly depends on reducing the activation of inflammatory cells, such as macrophages and neutrophils, exerting a protective effect on hepatocytes or inducing other hepatoprotective factors requires further investigation. Third, although AICAR is a widely used AMPK agonist, it also plays important AMPK-independent effects including regulating gluconeogenesis and oxidative phosphorylation (OXPHOS). Therefore, in addition to its inhibitory effects on inflammation and oxidative stress by activating ampk, AICAR may play protective roles of PALI through these AMPK-independent pathways which need to be further explored (Višnjić et al., 2021). Fourth, this study predominantly focuses on the AMPK/Nrf2 signaling pathway. However, there are also many other important regulatory pathways involved in the course of PALI such as Toll like receptor 4 (TLR4) signaling pathway, transforming growth factor β1 (TGF-β1) and p38 mitogen-activated protein kinase (MAPK) signaling pathway (TGF-β1-p38 MAPK), which need to be investigated in our future study (Wang et al., 2018). Fifth, given the powerful therapeutic effect of AICAR in PALI, the potential effect of AICAR in other organ dysfunctions including respiratory, renal, and cardiovascular of SAP needs to be further explored.

In summary, our data indicate that AICAR, a direct AMPK activator, exhibits significant therapeutic effects against PALI in sodium taurocholate- and L-arginine-induced rodent models by promoting AMPK phosphorylation by effectively inhibiting hepatic oxidative stress and inflammation. Thus, as a cell permeable nucleoside, AICAR has high therapeutic value for

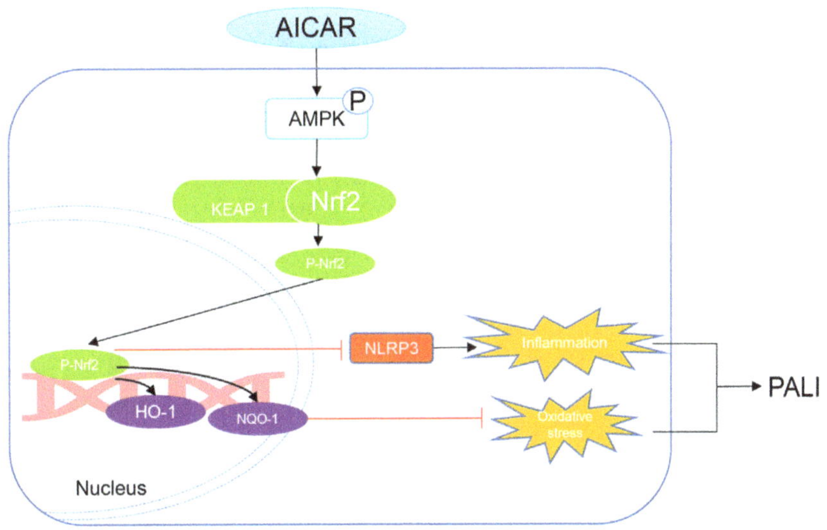

FIGURE 9 | Mechanistic illustration of the basis of AICAR protection against pancreatitis-associated liver injury (PALI). AICAR inhibits hepatic oxidative stress and inflammation by promoting AMPK phosphorylation partially *via* Nrf2-mediated antioxidant effects and inhibition of NLRP3 inflammasome activation, resulting in protection against PALI in sodium taurocholate- and L-arginine-induced SAP models.

the treatment of PALI. Importantly, this study provides new insight into the mechanisms underlying the improvement of hepatic oxidative stress and inflammation in PALI by AICAR. AMPK activation promotes the nuclear accumulation of Nrf2, which partially mediates antioxidant effects and inhibits NLRP3 inflammasome activation and thus is important for AICAR protection against PALI (**Figure 9**). We conclude that because AICAR is already used in the clinic, the development of novel therapies using AICAR to promote AMPK phosphorylation is promising for future medical interventions of PALI.

ETHICS STATEMENT

The animal study was reviewed and approved by the Animal Ethics Committee of Wenzhou Medical University.

AUTHOR CONTRIBUTIONS

WH and HW designed the experiments. LK, HZ, and CL conducted the experiments and co-wrote the manuscript. KS, HH, YZ, YW, and DW analyzed the data. All authors contributed to the article and approved the submitted version.

FUNDING

This work was supported by grants from Wenzhou Science and Technology Bureau (No. Y20180506), the Research incubation Project of the first affiliated Hospital of Wenzhou Medical University (No. FHY2019032 and No. FHY2019058) and National Natural Science Foundation of China (No. 82070834; 81800567).

REFERENCES

Antonucci, L., Porcu, C., Iannucci, G., Balsano, C., and Barbaro, B. (2017). Non-Alcoholic Fatty Liver Disease and Nutritional Implications: Special Focus on Copper. *Nutrients* 9, 1137. doi:10.3390/nu9101137

Argaiz, E. R., and de Moraes, A. G. (2021). Acute Pancreatitis. *Lancet* 397, 279. doi:10.1016/s0140-6736(21)00092-1

Bakır, M., Geyikoglu, F., Colak, S., Turkez, H., Bakır, T. O., and Hosseinigouzdagani, M. (2016). The Carvacrol Ameliorates Acute Pancreatitis-Induced Liver Injury via Antioxidant Response. *Cytotechnology* 68, 1131–1146. doi:10.1007/s10616-015-9871-z

Bone, N. B., Liu, Z., Pittet, J. F., and Zmijewski, J. W. (2017). Frontline Science: D1 Dopaminergic Receptor Signaling Activates the AMPK-Bioenergetic Pathway in Macrophages and Alveolar Epithelial Cells and Reduces Endotoxin-Induced ALI. *J. Leukoc. Biol.* 101, 357–365. doi:10.1189/jlb.3HI0216-068RR

Carling, D. (2017). AMPK Signalling in Health and Disease. *Curr. Opin. Cel Biol* 45, 31–37. doi:10.1016/j.ceb.2017.01.005

Chen, H., Ning, X., and Jiang, Z. (2017). Caspases Control Antiviral Innate Immunity. *Cell Mol Immunol* 14, 736–747. doi:10.1038/cmi.2017.44

Chen, H., Tran, D., Yang, H. C., Nylander, S., Birnbaum, Y., and Ye, Y. (2020). Dapagliflozin and Ticagrelor Have Additive Effects on the Attenuation of the Activation of the NLRP3 Inflammasome and the Progression of Diabetic Cardiomyopathy: an AMPK-mTOR Interplay. *Cardiovasc. Drugs Ther.* 34, 443–461. doi:10.1007/s10557-020-06978-y

Chen, Z., Zhong, H., Wei, J., Lin, S., Zong, Z., Gong, F., et al. (2019). Inhibition of Nrf2/HO-1 Signaling Leads to Increased Activation of the NLRP3 Inflammasome in Osteoarthritis. *Arthritis Res. Ther.* 21, 300. doi:10.1186/s13075-019-2085-6

Chin, W. Y., He, C. Y., Chow, T. W., Yu, Q. Y., Lai, L. C., and Miaw, S. C. (2021). Adenylate Kinase 4 Promotes Inflammatory Gene Expression via Hif1α and AMPK in Macrophages. *Front. Immunol.* 12, 630318. doi:10.3389/fimmu.2021.630318

Dandekar, A., Mendez, R., and Zhang, K. (2015). Cross Talk between ER Stress, Oxidative Stress, and Inflammation in Health and Disease. *Methods Mol. Biol.* 1292, 205–214. doi:10.1007/978-1-4939-2522-3_15

Elshal, M., Abu-Elsaad, N., El-Karef, A., and Ibrahim, T. (2019). Retinoic Acid Modulates IL-4, IL-10 and MCP-1 Pathways in Immune Mediated Hepatitis and Interrupts CD4+ T Cells Infiltration. *Int. Immunopharmacol* 75, 105808. doi:10.1016/j.intimp.2019.105808

Fang, D., Lin, Q., Wang, C., Zheng, C., Li, Y., Huang, T., et al. (2020). Effects of Sildenafil on Inflammatory Injury of the Lung in Sodium Taurocholate-Induced Severe Acute Pancreatitis Rats. *Int. Immunopharmacol* 80, 106151. doi:10.1016/j.intimp.2019.106151

Garcia, D., and Shaw, R. J. (2017). AMPK: Mechanisms of Cellular Energy Sensing and Restoration of Metabolic Balance. *Mol. Cel* 66, 789–800. doi:10.1016/j.molcel.2017.05.032

Garg, P. K., and Singh, V. P. (2019). Organ Failure Due to Systemic Injury in Acute Pancreatitis. *Gastroenterology* 156, 2008–2023. doi:10.1053/j.gastro.2018.12.041

Gong, C., Yang, H., Wang, S., Liu, J., Li, Z., Hu, Y., et al. (2021). hTERT Promotes CRC Proliferation and Migration by Recruiting YBX1 to Increase NRF2 Expression. *Front Cel Dev Biol* 9, 658101. doi:10.3389/fcell.2021.658101

Guo, X., Hu, S., Liu, J. J., Huang, L., Zhong, P., Fan, Z. X., et al. (2021). Piperine Protects against Pyroptosis in Myocardial Ischaemia/reperfusion Injury by Regulating the miR-383/RP105/AKT Signalling Pathway. *J. Cel Mol Med* 25, 244–258. doi:10.1111/jcmm.15953

Guo, Y., Zhang, Y., Hong, K., Luo, F., Gu, Q., Lu, N., et al. (2014). AMPK Inhibition Blocks ROS-Nfκb Signaling and Attenuates Endotoxemia-Induced Liver Injury. *PLoS One* 9, e86881. doi:10.1371/journal.pone.0086881

Han, C. Y., Rho, H. S., Kim, A., Kim, T. H., Jang, K., Jun, D. W., et al. (2018). FXR Inhibits Endoplasmic Reticulum Stress-Induced NLRP3 Inflammasome in Hepatocytes and Ameliorates Liver Injury. *Cell Rep* 24, 2985–2999. doi:10.1016/j.celrep.2018.07.068

Hennig, P., Garstkiewicz, M., Grossi, S., Di Filippo, M., French, L. E., and Beer, H. D. (2018). The Crosstalk between Nrf2 and Inflammasomes. *Int. J. Mol. Sci.* 19, 562. doi:10.3390/ijms19020562

Herzig, S., and Shaw, R. J. (2018). AMPK: Guardian of Metabolism and Mitochondrial Homeostasis. *Nat. Rev. Mol. Cel Biol* 19, 121–135. doi:10.1038/nrm.2017.95

Hill, J. L., Kobori, N., Zhao, J., Rozas, N. S., Hylin, M. J., Moore, A. N., et al. (2016). Traumatic Brain Injury Decreases AMP-Activated Protein Kinase Activity and Pharmacological Enhancement of its Activity Improves Cognitive Outcome. *J. Neurochem.* 139, 106–119. doi:10.1111/jnc.13726

Hou, Y., Wang, Y., He, Q., Li, L., Xie, H., Zhao, Y., et al. (2018). Nrf2 Inhibits NLRP3 Inflammasome Activation through Regulating Trx1/TXNIP Complex in Cerebral Ischemia Reperfusion Injury. *Behav. Brain Res.* 336, 32–39. doi:10.1016/j.bbr.2017.06.027

Joo Choi, R., Cheng, M. S., and Shik Kim, Y. (2014). Desoxyrhapontigenin Up-Regulates Nrf2-Mediated Heme Oxygenase-1 Expression in Macrophages and Inflammatory Lung Injury. *Redox Biol.* 2, 504–512. doi:10.1016/j.redox.2014.02.001

Kaphalia, L., Srinivasan, M. P., Kakumanu, R. D., Kaphalia, B. S., and Calhoun, W. J. (2019). Ethanol Exposure Impairs AMPK Signaling and Phagocytosis in Human Alveolar Macrophages: Role of Ethanol Metabolism. *Alcohol. Clin. Exp. Res.* 43, 1682–1694. doi:10.1111/acer.14131

Lane, S. L., Houck, J. A., Doyle, A. S., Bales, E. S., Lorca, R. A., Julian, C. G., et al. (2020). AMP-activated Protein Kinase Activator AICAR Attenuates Hypoxia-Induced Murine Fetal Growth Restriction in Part by Improving Uterine Artery Blood Flow. *J. Physiol.* 598, 4093–4105. doi:10.1113/jp279341

Lee, H., Zandkarimi, F., Zhang, Y., Meena, J. K., Kim, J., Zhuang, L., et al. (2020). Energy-stress-mediated AMPK Activation Inhibits Ferroptosis. *Nat. Cel Biol* 22, 225–234. doi:10.1038/s41556-020-0461-8

Lempiäinen, J., Finckenberg, P., Levijoki, J., and Mervaala, E. (2012). AMPK Activator AICAR Ameliorates Ischaemia Reperfusion Injury in the Rat Kidney. *Br. J. Pharmacol.* 166, 1905–1915. doi:10.1111/j.1476-5381.2012.01895.x

Li, S., Zhou, J., Xu, S., Li, J., Liu, J., Lu, Y., et al. (2019). Induction of Nrf2 Pathway by Dendrobium Nobile Lindl. Alkaloids Protects against Carbon Tetrachloride Induced Acute Liver Injury. *Biomed. Pharmacother.* 117, 109073. doi:10.1016/j.biopha.2019.109073

Li, X., Cao, Y., Liu, Z., Chen, H., and Mao, H. (2019). The Relationship between Liver Injury and Serum Levels of C-Reactive Protein and Procalcitonin in Patients with Acute Pancreatitis. *J. Coll. Physicians Surg. Pak* 29, 287–289. doi:10.29271/jcpsp.2019.03.287

Lin, S. C., and Hardie, D. G. (2018). AMPK: Sensing Glucose as Well as Cellular Energy Status. *Cell Metab* 27, 299–313. doi:10.1016/j.cmet.2017.10.009

Liu, B., Huang, J., and Zhang, B. (2016). Nobiletin Protects against Murine L-Arginine-Induced Acute Pancreatitis in Association with Downregulating p38MAPK and AKT. *Biomed. Pharmacother.* 81, 104–110. doi:10.1016/j.biopha.2016.03.051

Liu, C. Y., Zhou, Y., Chen, T., Lei, J. C., and Jiang, X. J. (2020). AMPK/SIRT1 Pathway Is Involved in Arctigenin-Mediated Protective Effects against Myocardial Ischemia-Reperfusion Injury. *Front. Pharmacol.* 11, 616813. doi:10.3389/fphar.2020.616813

Liu, D., Ma, Z., Di, S., Yang, Y., Yang, J., Xu, L., et al. (2018). AMPK/PGC1α Activation by Melatonin Attenuates Acute Doxorubicin Cardiotoxicity via Alleviating Mitochondrial Oxidative Damage and Apoptosis. *Free Radic. Biol. Med.* 129, 59–72. doi:10.1016/j.freeradbiomed.2018.08.032

Liu, Q., Lv, H., Wen, Z., Ci, X., and Peng, L. (2017). Isoliquiritigenin Activates Nuclear Factor Erythroid-2 Related Factor 2 to Suppress the NOD-like Receptor Protein 3 Inflammasome and Inhibits the NF-Kb Pathway in Macrophages and in Acute Lung Injury. *Front. Immunol.* 8, 1518. doi:10.3389/fimmu.2017.01518

Liu, X., Chhipa, R. R., Nakano, I., and Dasgupta, B. (2014). The AMPK Inhibitor Compound C Is a Potent AMPK-independent Antiglioma Agent. *Mol. Cancer Ther.* 13, 596–605. doi:10.1158/1535-7163.Mct-13-0579

Lv, P., Fan, L. J., Li, H. Y., Meng, Q. S., and Liu, J. (2015). Protective Effect of Thalidomide on Liver Injury in Rats with Acute Pancreatitis via Inhibition of Oxidative Stress. *Ann. Clin. Lab. Sci.* 45, 508–514.

Lyu, H., Wang, H., Li, L., Zhu, J., Chen, F., Chen, Y., et al. (2020). Hepatocyte-specific Deficiency of Nrf2 Exacerbates Carbon Tetrachloride-Induced Liver Fibrosis via Aggravated Hepatocyte Injury and Subsequent Inflammatory and Fibrogenic Responses. *Free Radic. Biol. Med.* 150, 136–147. doi:10.1016/j.freeradbiomed.2020.02.015

Martin, L. M., Möller, M., Weiss, U., Russe, O. Q., Scholich, K., Pierre, S., et al. (2019). 5-Amino-1-β-D-Ribofuranosyl-Imidazole-4-Carboxamide (AICAR) Reduces Peripheral Inflammation by Macrophage Phenotype Shift. *Int. J. Mol. Sci.* 20, 3255. doi:10.3390/ijms20133255

Matzinger, M., Fischhuber, K., Pölöske, D., Mechtler, K., and Heiss, E. H. (2020). AMPK Leads to Phosphorylation of the Transcription Factor Nrf2, Tuning Transactivation of Selected Target Genes. *Redox Biol.* 29, 101393. doi:10.1016/j.redox.2019.101393

Mei, F., Yu, J., Li, M., Xiang, M., Hong, Y., Zhou, Y., et al. (2019). Magnesium Isoglycyrrhizinate Alleviates Liver Injury in Obese Rats with Acute Necrotizing Pancreatitis. *Pathol. Res. Pract.* 215, 106–114. doi:10.1016/j.prp.2018.10.030

Moniaux, N., Song, H., Darnaud, M., Garbin, K., Gigou, M., Mitchell, C., et al. (2011). Human Hepatocarcinoma-Intestine-Pancreas/pancreatitis-Associated Protein Cures Fas-Induced Acute Liver Failure in Mice by Attenuating Free-Radical Damage in Injured Livers. *Hepatology* 53, 618–627. doi:10.1002/hep.24087

Mridha, A. R., Wree, A., Robertson, A. A. B., Yeh, M. M., Johnson, C. D., Van Rooyen, D. M., et al. (2017). NLRP3 Inflammasome Blockade Reduces Liver Inflammation and Fibrosis in Experimental NASH in Mice. *J. Hepatol.* 66, 1037–1046. doi:10.1016/j.jhep.2017.01.022

Nerstedt, A., Cansby, E., Amrutkar, M., Smith, U., and Mahlapuu, M. (2013). Pharmacological Activation of AMPK Suppresses Inflammatory Response

Evoked by IL-6 Signalling in Mouse Liver and in Human Hepatocytes. *Mol. Cel Endocrinol* 375, 68–78. doi:10.1016/j.mce.2013.05.013

Nerstedt, A., Johansson, A., Andersson, C. X., Cansby, E., Smith, U., and Mahlapuu, M. (2010). AMP-activated Protein Kinase Inhibits IL-6-stimulated Inflammatory Response in Human Liver Cells by Suppressing Phosphorylation of Signal Transducer and Activator of Transcription 3 (STAT3). *Diabetologia* 53, 2406–2416. doi:10.1007/s00125-010-1856-z

Ou, Z. B., Miao, C. M., Ye, M. X., Xing, D. P., He, K., Li, P. Z., et al. (2017). Investigation for Role of Tissue Factor and Blood Coagulation System in Severe Acute Pancreatitis and Associated Liver Injury. *Biomed. Pharmacother.* 85, 380–388. doi:10.1016/j.biopha.2016.11.039

Ramirez Reyes, J. M. J., Cuesta, R., and Pause, A. (2021). Folliculin: A Regulator of Transcription through AMPK and mTOR Signaling Pathways. *Front. Cel Dev Biol* 9, 667311. doi:10.3389/fcell.2021.667311

Rao, E., Zhang, Y., Li, Q., Hao, J., Egilmez, N. K., Suttles, J., et al. (2016). AMPK-dependent and Independent Effects of AICAR and Compound C on T-Cell Responses. *Oncotarget* 7, 33783–33795. doi:10.18632/oncotarget.9277

Rios, E. C., Moretti, A. I., de Souza, H. P., Velasco, I. T., and Soriano, F. G. (2010). Hypertonic saline Reduces Metalloproteinase Expression in Liver during Pancreatitis. *Clin. Exp. Pharmacol. Physiol.* 37, 35–39. doi:10.1111/j.1440-1681.2009.05220.x

Rongione, A. J., Kusske, A. M., Kwan, K., Ashley, S. W., Reber, H. A., and McFadden, D. W. (1997). Interleukin 10 Reduces the Severity of Acute Pancreatitis in Rats. *Gastroenterology* 112, 960–967. doi:10.1053/gast.1997.v112.pm9041259

Saha, S., Buttari, B., Panieri, E., Profumo, E., and Saso, L. (2020). An Overview of Nrf2 Signaling Pathway and its Role in Inflammation. *Molecules* 25, 5474. doi:10.3390/molecules25225474

Saito, S., Furuno, A., Sakurai, J., Park, H. R., Shin-ya, K., and Tomida, A. (2012). Compound C Prevents the Unfolded Protein Response during Glucose Deprivation through a Mechanism Independent of AMPK and BMP Signaling. *PLoS One* 7, e45845. doi:10.1371/journal.pone.0045845

Shen, Z., Chen, Q., Jin, T., Wang, M., Ying, H., Lu, J., et al. (2019). Theaflavin 3,3'-digallate Reverses the Downregulation of Connexin 43 and Autophagy Induced by High Glucose via AMPK Activation in Cardiomyocytes. *J. Cel Physiol* 234, 17999–18016. doi:10.1002/jcp.28432

Shi, N., Liu, T., de la Iglesia-Garcia, D., Deng, L., Jin, T., Lan, L., et al. (2020). Duration of Organ Failure Impacts Mortality in Acute Pancreatitis. *Gut* 69, 604–605. doi:10.1136/gutjnl-2019-318241

Song, X., Zhu, S., Chen, P., Hou, W., Wen, Q., Liu, J., et al. (2018). AMPK-mediated BECN1 Phosphorylation Promotes Ferroptosis by Directly Blocking System Xc- Activity. *Curr. Biol.* 28, 2388. doi:10.1016/j.cub.2018.05.094

Srinivasan, M. P., Bhopale, K. K., Caracheo, A. A., Amer, S. M., Khan, S., Kaphalia, L., et al. (2020). Activation of AMP-Activated Protein Kinase Attenuates Ethanol-Induced ER/oxidative Stress and Lipid Phenotype in Human Pancreatic Acinar Cells. *Biochem. Pharmacol.* 180, 114174. doi:10.1016/j.bcp.2020.114174

Steinberg, W. M., Buse, J. B., Ghorbani, M. L. M., Ørsted, D. D., and Nauck, M. A. (2017). Amylase, Lipase, and Acute Pancreatitis in People with Type 2 Diabetes Treated with Liraglutide: Results from the LEADER Randomized Trial. *Diabetes Care* 40, 966–972. doi:10.2337/dc16-2747

Sun, Y., Connors, K. E., and Yang, D. Q. (2007). AICAR Induces Phosphorylation of AMPK in an ATM-dependent, LKB1-independent Manner. *Mol. Cel Biochem* 306, 239–245. doi:10.1007/s11010-007-9575-6

Swinnen, J. V., Beckers, A., Brusselmans, K., Organe, S., Segers, J., Timmermans, L., et al. (2005). Mimicry of a Cellular Low Energy Status Blocks Tumor Cell Anabolism and Suppresses the Malignant Phenotype. *Cancer Res.* 65, 2441–2448. doi:10.1158/0008-5472.Can-04-3025

Tan, X., Jiao, P. L., Sun, J. C., Wang, W., Ye, P., Wang, Y. K., et al. (2021). β-Arrestin1 Reduces Oxidative Stress via Nrf2 Activation in the Rostral Ventrolateral Medulla in Hypertension. *Front. Neurosci.* 15, 657825. doi:10.3389/fnins.2021.657825

Tonelli, C., Chio, I. I. C., and Tuveson, D. A. (2018). Transcriptional Regulation by Nrf2. *Antioxid. Redox Signal.* 29, 1727–1745. doi:10.1089/ars.2017.7342

Unamuno, X., Gómez-Ambrosi, J., Ramírez, B., Rodríguez, A., Becerril, S., Valentí, V., et al. (2021). NLRP3 Inflammasome Blockade Reduces Adipose Tissue Inflammation and Extracellular Matrix Remodeling. *Cel Mol Immunol* 18, 1045–1057. doi:10.1038/s41423-019-0296-z

Višnjić, D., Lalić, H., Dembitz, V., Tomić, B., and Smoljo, T. (2021). AICAr, a Widely Used AMPK Activator with Important AMPK-independent Effects: A Systematic Review. *Cells* 10, 1095. doi:10.3390/cells10051095

Wang, Q., Zhang, X., Lei, S., Wang, Y., Zhuang, Y., Chen, Y., et al. (2018). RNA Sequence Analysis Reveals Pathways and Candidate Genes Associated with Liver Injury in a Rat Pancreatitis Model. *Pancreatology* 18, 753–763. doi:10.1016/j.pan.2018.08.006

Wang, X., Zhao, X., Shi, C., Börjesson, A., Chen, Z., Axelsson, J., et al. (2006). Potential Mechanisms and Significance of Acute Pancreatitis-Associated Liver Injury. *Scand. J. Gastroenterol.* 41, 604–613. doi:10.1080/00365520500347105

Wenhong, D., Jia, Y., Weixing, W., Xiaoyan, C., Chen, C., Sheng, X., et al. (2012). Zerumbone Attenuates the Severity of Acute Necrotizing Pancreatitis and Pancreatitis-Induced Hepatic Injury. *Mediators Inflamm.* 2012, 156507. doi:10.1155/2012/156507

Wree, A., McGeough, M. D., Inzaugarat, M. E., Eguchi, A., Schuster, S., Johnson, C. D., et al. (2018). NLRP3 Inflammasome Driven Liver Injury and Fibrosis: Roles of IL-17 and TNF in Mice. *Hepatology* 67, 736–749. doi:10.1002/hep.29523

Xu, W., Zhao, T., and Xiao, H. (2020). The Implication of Oxidative Stress and AMPK-Nrf2 Antioxidative Signaling in Pneumonia Pathogenesis. *Front. Endocrinol. (Lausanne)* 11, 400. doi:10.3389/fendo.2020.00400

Yang, J., Fier, A., Carter, Y., Liu, G., Epling-Burnette, P. K., Bai, F., et al. (2003). Liver Injury during Acute Pancreatitis: the Role of Pancreatitis-Associated Ascitic Fluid (PAAF), P38-MAPK, and Caspase-3 in Inducing Hepatocyte Apoptosis. *J. Gastrointest. Surg.* 7, 200–208. doi:10.1016/s1091-255x(02)00134-8

Yang, J., Zhou, Y., and Shi, J. (2020). Cordycepin Protects against Acute Pancreatitis by Modulating NF-Kb and NLRP3 Inflammasome Activation via AMPK. *Life Sci.* 251, 117645. doi:10.1016/j.lfs.2020.117645

Yang, M., Luo, S., Jiang, N., Wang, X., Han, Y., Zhao, H., et al. (2021). DsbA-L Ameliorates Renal Injury through the AMPK/NLRP3 Inflammasome Signaling Pathway in Diabetic Nephropathy. *Front. Physiol.* 12, 659751. doi:10.3389/fphys.2021.659751

Yu, P. B., Hong, C. C., Sachidanandan, C., Babitt, J. L., Deng, D. Y., Hoyng, S. A., et al. (2008). Dorsomorphin Inhibits BMP Signals Required for Embryogenesis and Iron Metabolism. *Nat. Chem. Biol.* 4, 33–41. doi:10.1038/nchembio.2007.54

Zeng, J., Chen, Y., Ding, R., Feng, L., Fu, Z., Yang, S., et al. (2017). Isoliquiritigenin Alleviates Early Brain Injury after Experimental Intracerebral Hemorrhage via Suppressing ROS- And/or NF-Kb-Mediated NLRP3 Inflammasome Activation by Promoting Nrf2 Antioxidant Pathway. *J. Neuroinflammation* 14, 119. doi:10.1186/s12974-017-0895-5

Zhao, Y., Ye, S., Lin, J., Liang, F., Chen, J., Hu, J., et al. (2021). NmFGF1-Regulated Glucolipid Metabolism and Angiogenesis Improves Functional Recovery in a Mouse Model of Diabetic Stroke and Acts via the AMPK Signaling Pathway. *Front. Pharmacol.* 12, 680351. doi:10.3389/fphar.2021.680351

Zhou, H., Wang, H., Ni, M., Yue, S., Xia, Y., Busuttil, R. W., et al. (2018). Glycogen Synthase Kinase 3β Promotes Liver Innate Immune Activation by Restraining AMP-Activated Protein Kinase Activation. *J. Hepatol.* 69, 99–109. doi:10.1016/j.jhep.2018.01.036

Zimmermann, K., Baldinger, J., Mayerhofer, B., Atanasov, A. G., Dirsch, V. M., and Heiss, E. H. (2015). Activated AMPK Boosts the Nrf2/HO-1 Signaling axis--A Role for the Unfolded Protein Response. *Free Radic. Biol. Med.* 88, 417–426. doi:10.1016/j.freeradbiomed.2015.03.030

Zou, J., Wang, S. P., Wang, Y. T., and Wan, J. B. (2021). Regulation of the NLRP3 Inflammasome with Natural Products against Chemical-Induced Liver Injury. *Pharmacol. Res.* 164, 105388. doi:10.1016/j.phrs.2020.105388

8

Cichorium pumilum Jacq Extract Inhibits LPS-Induced Inflammation via MAPK Signaling Pathway and Protects Rats From Hepatic Fibrosis Caused by Abnormalities in the Gut-Liver Axis

*Chang Han[1†], Xi Wu[2†], Nan Zou[3], Yunsheng Zhang[4], Jinqi Yuan[3], Yuefeng Gao[5], Wen Chen[1], Jia Yao[1], Cong Li[1], Jinqiu Hou[1] and Dongmei Qin[1]**

[1]Key Laboratory of Xinjiang Phytomedicine Resource and Utilization, Ministry of Education, School of Pharmacy, Shihezi University, Shihezi, China, [2]Dongfang Hospital, Beijing University of Chinese Medicine, Beijing, China, [3]First Affiliated Hospital, School of Medicine, Shihezi University, Shihezi, China, [4]Husbandry Research Institute, Xinjiang Academy of Animal Science, Urumqi, China, [5]State Key Laboratory of Animal Nutrition, College of Animal Science and Technology, China Agricultural University, Beijing, China

***Correspondence:**
Dongmei Qin
qdm_pha@shzu.edu.cn

[†]These authors share first authorship

The development of liver fibrosis is closely related to the gut microbiota, and the "gut-liver axis" is the most important connection between the two. ethyl acetate extract of *Cichorium pumilum* Jacq (CGEA) is an herbal extract consisting mainly of sesquiterpenoids. The anti-inflammatory and hepatoprotective effects of CGEA have been reported, but the anti-fibrotic effects of CGEA via intestinal microbes and the "gut-liver axis" cycle have rarely been reported. In this study, we observed that CGEA not only directly attenuated inflammatory factor levels in inflamed mice, but also attenuated liver inflammation as well as liver fibrosis degeneration in rats with liver fibrosis caused by colitis. We observed *in vitro* that CGEA significantly promoted the growth of Bifidobacterium adolescentis. Similarly, fecal 16S rDNA sequencing of liver fibrosis rats showed that CGEA intervention significantly altered the composition of the intestinal microbiota of liver fibrosis rats. CGEA increased the abundance of intestinal microbiota, specifically, CGEA increased the ratio of Firmicutes to Bacteroidetes, CGEA could significantly increase the levels of Ruminococcus. In addition, CGEA intervention significantly protected intestinal mucosal tissues and improved intestinal barrier function in rats. Lactucin is the main sesquiterpenoid in CGEA, and HPLC results showed its content in CGEA was up to 6%. Lactucin has been reported to have significant anti-inflammatory activity, and in this study, we found that Lactucin decreased p38 kinases (p38), phosphorylation of the extracellular signal-regulated kinase (ERK) and protein kinase B (AKT) protein phosphorylation in lipopolysaccharide (LPS)-activated RAW264.7 cells, thereby reducing mRNA expression and protein expression of pro-inflammatory factors inducible nitric oxide synthase (iNOS) and cyclooxygenase-2 (COX-2), and inhibiting the release of inflammatory factors interleukin (IL)-6 and nitric oxide (NO), exerting anti-inflammatory effects. In summary, the prevention of liver fibrosis caused by intestinal inflammation by CGEA may be achieved by regulating the intestinal microbiota and restoring the intestinal barrier thereby improving the "gut-liver axis" circulation, reducing liver inflammation, and ultimately alleviating liver fibrosis. Notably, the direct anti-inflammatory effect of CGEA may be due to its content of Lactucin, which can exert anti-inflammatory effects by inhibiting the phosphorylation of Mitogen-activated protein kinase (MAPK) and Akt signaling pathways.

Keywords: liver fibrosis, *Cichorium pumilum* Jacq, gut microbiota, inflammation, lactucin

INTRODUCTION

Hepatic fibrosis is a chronic liver disease that can lead to end-stage liver disease or cirrhosis and eventually to liver cancer. This causes a serious threat to human health. Extensive researches have been devoted to analyze the mechanisms underlying the pathogenesis of liver fibrosis in recent years, but there are fewer studies on the resistance to liver fibrosis from the perspective of intestinal microbiota and the "gut-liver axis" circulation.

In recent years, the relationship between gut microbes and the liver is receiving increasing attention (Bajaj et al., 2012; Ling et al., 2015). Marshall's (Marshall, 1998) concept of the "gut-liver axis" points out that when the intestinal mucosa is damaged, the permeability of the intestine increases and harmful bacteria and their metabolites [lipopolysaccharide (LPS) and endotoxins] enter the portal vein and move to the liver with blood circulation ("leaky gut") (Marshall, 1998; Kamada et al., 2013; Nakamoto et al., 2017), activate the liver's immune response, and release inflammatory cytokines such as IL-6, IL-1β, TNF-α, etc., thereby accelerate the progression of liver fibrosis (Lau et al., 2015).

In addition, LPS is a key factor in triggering intestinal inflammation (Hu et al., 2016a), which can further affect liver function through the "gut-liver axis" (Li et al., 2018). Also, LPS can directly activate intrahepatic and extrahepatic mononuclear-macrophages, releasing large amounts of inflammatory factors such as nitric oxide (NO), tumor necrosis factor (TNF)-α, interleukin (IL)-1β, interleukin (IL)-6 (Ribeiro et al., 2015; Liu et al., 2017), etc., occurrence of these inflammatory events is regulated by non-receptor-type tyrosine kinases, such as Janus kinase (JAK) 2, phosphoinositide 3-kinase (PI3K), protein kinase B (Akt), and mitogen-activated protein kinases (MAPKs) (Van Dort et al., 2015; Hu et al., 2016b). Especially up-regulating activated MAPK protein expression, including extracellular signal-regulated kinases (ERK), c-Jun N-terminal kinase (JNK), and p38 are closely related to intestinal inflammation (Xie et al., 2019). As reported earlier (Zanello et al., 2011), the inflammatory response of swine intestine caused by E.*coli* infection is closely related to the MAPK signaling pathway, and the Astilbin improves inflammatory bowel disease through PI3K, STAT3, and MAPK signaling pathways (Han et al., 2020). Published work suggests that regulation of gut microbial composition, reduces the phosphorylation of MAPK and AKT proteins (Serreli et al., 2020; Zhang et al., 2020). In summary, by modulating the gut microbial composition and reducing intestinal inflammation, pathogenic bacteria and their metabolites in the liver can be inhibited, thereby reducing liver fibrosis.

Cichorium pumilum Jacq (CG) is a traditional herb in Uighur medicine and is often used in folklore as a remedy for liver disease (Tong et al., 2017). Substantial studies on CG were carried out by our group and it was found that *Cichorium pumilum* Jacq ethyl acetate extract (CGEA) reduces CCl_4 and thioacetamide-induced liver fibrosis in rats via the TGF β/Smad signaling pathway (Qin et al., 2013; Qin et al., 2014). CGEA was also found to have significant growth inhibitory effects on both *Staphylococcus aureus* and *Enterococcus faecalis* (Han et al., 2019). According to Lee CG can significantly promote the growth of probiotic bacteria and reduce the growth of harmful bacteria in the intestine, indicating that CG has a significant "probiotic-like effect" (Lee et al., 2015). Therefore, we predict that CGEA may reduce inflammation by modulating intestinal microbes to combat liver fibrosis.

Studies have shown that the main components of CGEA are sesquiterpene lactones, and the main components are Lactucin and Lactucopicrin (Pyrek, 1985). Our group isolated a total of 25 compounds from CGEA, 14 of which were sesquiterpene lactones (**Supplementary Table S3**), and preliminary experimental results showed that Lactucin has extremely strong anti-inflammatory activity (Dang et al., 2019). Lactucin is the most abundant terpenoid in CGEA with significant antibacterial, adipogenesis-inhibiting effects (Wang et al., 2020). Although Lactucin exhibits excellent anti-inflammatory activity, however, its anti-inflammatory mechanism of action has not been much reported, so we investigated the anti-inflammatory effects of Lactucin in MAPK and AKT signaling pathways at the cellular and molecular biological levels to elucidate the mechanism of Lactucin's anti-inflammatory effects.

On these indications, we predicted that CGEA could improve liver fibrosis through the "gut-liver axis" by reducing intestinal inflammation and promoting probiotic growth, with Lactucin playing a major anti-inflammatory role. Altogether, in the present study, we demonstrated that CGEA can promote probiotic growth and prevent liver fibrosis caused by 2,4,6-trinitrobenzen sulfonic acid (TNBS)-induced intestinal inflammation. We then validated the anti-inflammatory effect of Lactucin *in vitro* using RAW264.7 cells.

MATERIALS AND METHODS

Preparation of CGEA and Lactucin

CGEA and Lactucin were prepared by our research team as follows: 1 kg of dried roots of CG (Xinjiang Medicines Co., Ltd., Xinjiang, China. identified by Prof. Mehmet Nur Ayhoi at Xinjiang Uygur Medical College) was soaked in 95% ethanol for 5 times at room temperature (2 L each time for 3 days), the extract was suspended in water, extracted 1:1 with ethyl acetate and water, and the solvent was volatilized at room temperature to obtain CGEA (7.644 g). The CGEA fraction was fractionated by a silica gel column chromatograph (CC) eluting with a gradient of CH_2Cl_2-MeOH (from 30:1 to 3:1) to give subfractions B. Fraction B was subjected to a MCI CC to remove pigment eluted excessively with 70, 80, 90 and 100% methyl alcohol to give subfractions B1. Fraction B1 was separated by an RP C18 silica gel CC to give compound 10 (38 mg), and the compound 10 was identified by ^{1}H NMR and ^{13}C NMR spectroscopy as Lactucin (Dang et al., 2019) (**Supplementary Figure S1**).

High Performance Liquid Chromatography Analysis

The composition of CGEA was analyzed using Agilent 1,290 Infinity II HPLC (Agilent, Germany), and the retention time of the detected peaks was compared to that of the Lactucin standard (The standard was prepared by the research group with a purity of ≥95%) for comparison and determination of the Lactucin composition and content in CGEA. HPLC was equipped with a (4.6 × 150 mm, 5 μm) Agilent TC-C18 liquid chromatography column (Agilent, Germany). Mobile phase: Methanol (A)-0.1% formic acid (B), Elution gradient: 0–10 min, 25% A-30% A; 10–20 min, 30% A-70% A; 20–30 min, 70% A-70% A, flow rate 1.0 ml/min, column temperature 30°C, detection wavelength 275 nm, injection volume 5 μL.

Protocol of Animal Experiments *in vivo*

Thirty adult male Sprague Dawley (SD) rats, weighing 180 ± 10 g, were provided by the Xinjiang medical university Experimental Animal center (Xinjiang China) [No. SCXK (Xin) 2016-0004]. The rats reared in alternate light and dark environments at approximately 22°C. All experimental procedures were approved by the Ethics Committee of First Affiliated Hospital, Shihezi University School of Medicine (Approval No. 2020-035-01).

After 7 days of adaptive feeding, the rats were randomly divided into five baskets. The rats fasting the night before modeling, drinking water normally, the rats were given intraperitoneal injection of 10% chloral hydrate (ShangHai Macklin Biochemical Co., Ltd., ShangHai, China) the next day, and the rats except blank control group were inverted after anesthesia to insert a 2 mm-diameter silicone hose with solution (The blank control group was fed with normal saline and the remaining 5% 2,4,6-trinitrobenzensulphonic acid (TNBS, BeiJing OuHe Technology Co., Ltd., BeiJing, China) were mixed with 50% ethanol, 60 mg kg^{-1} TNBS) into the intestinal depth of about 8 cm from the anus. Twice a week for 12 weeks, starting at week 13, except for the blank control group, the rats were randomly divided into model group, positive group (Sulfasalazine, Shanghai Xinyi Tianping Pharmaceutical Co., Ltd., ShangHai, China), high dose group of CGEA-I (CGEA-I, 150 mg kg^{-1}), low dose group of CGEA-II (CGEA-II, 100 mg kg^{-1}), the dosage is set based on the previous research basis of our research team (Qin et al., 2019a). Dose groups were fed with the respective medicine. The blank control group and the model group were given normal saline of equal volume once a day for 14 days.

At the end of the experimental period, after fasting for 12 h, all rats were weighed, collected blood by abdominal aorta after anesthetization by injection with 10% chloral hydrate solution and sacrificed. Subsequently, serum was separately prepared by centrifuge at the temperature of 4°C for 15 min for biochemical detection. Rat livers and colon were collected and then a small portion of liver and intestinal tissue samples immediately dissected and fixed in 4% paraformaldehyde (Biosharp Life Sciences Technology Co., Ltd., BeiJing, China). The remaining tissues and the freshly collected feces were rapidly frozen in liquid nitrogen and preserved at −80°C for Tissue homogenate kit analysis and 16S rDNA Gene Sequencing Analysis.

Determination of Serum Biomarkers

According to the manufacturer's commercially available kit instructions (Nanjing Jiancheng Bioengineering Institute, Nanjing, China), the activities of alanine aminotransferase (ALT), aspartate aminotransferase (AST), lactate dehydrogenase (LDH), Albumin (Alb) and gamma-glutamyl transferase (γ-GT) in serum were determined by an enzymatic colorimetric method (Wu et al., 2019).

Assay of IL-6 and TNF-α in Liver

Weigh about 1 g of liver tissue, and add 9 times ice of normal saline, cut the tissue as much as possible with small ophthalmic scissors, use tissue homogenizer to grind into 10% tissue homogenate. The prepared homogenate was prepared with centrifuge at 4°C, 3,000 r/min, 15min centrifugation for supernatant. The levels of IL-6 and TNF-α in liver tissues were determined according to the enzyme-linked immunosorbent assay (ELISA) kit instructions (Shanghai Yaji Biological Co., Ltd., Shanghai, China).

Pathological Assessment of Liver and Colon Tissue

The liver tissues and colon tissues were fixed in 4% paraformaldehyde. The tissues were subsequently dehydrated in a graded ethanol series (75–100%) and embedded in paraffin wax. The tissues were sectioned at 4 μm thickness, liver tissue was stained with hematoxylin and eosin (HE) and Masson, and colon tissue was stained with HE, digitally photographed by light microscopic at total magnifications of ×100.

Determination of Fecal Microbial Composition by16S rDNA Gene Sequencing Analysis

Total Bacterial DNA was isolated from rat fecal samples by TIANamp Stool DNA Kit (TianGen Biotech Co., Ltd., BeiJing, China) and the quality of DNA extraction was detected by 1.2% agarose gel electrophoresis. Design primers based on conserved regions in sequences and add sample specific Barcode sequence. Then the 16S V3-V4 regions were PCR amplified. PCR amplified recovery products were quantified by fluorescence, and each sample was mixed according to the corresponding proportion according to the requirement of sequencing quantity of each sample according to the fluorescence quantitative results. The sequencing library was prepared using the TruSeq Nano DNA LT Library Prep Kit of Illumina company. Finally, high-throughput sequencing. All procedures, analysis of sequencing and the extracted DNA was subjected to Illumina Miseq PE250 platform. The content of the sequencing was commissioned to Shaanxi Irun Biotechnology Co., China.

In vivo Anti-Inflammatory Effect Study of CGEA

Twenty-four healthy Kunming mice, weighing 25 ± 2 g, were provided by the Xinjiang medical university Experimental Animal center (Xinjiang China) [No. SCXK (Xin) 2016-0004], and all experimental procedures were approved by the Ethics Committee of First Affiliated Hospital, Shihezi University School of Medicine (Approval No. 2020-035-01).

After one week of adaptive feeding, the mice were randomly divided into four groups, namely Normal group, Model group, Treatment group, and Positive group, with six mice in each group. The mice were numbered and weighed, and the Treatment group was given 100 mg kg^{-1} CGEA by oral gavage, the Normal group and the Model group were given saline by oral gavage in equal amounts, and the Positive group was treated with 10 mg kg^{-1} dexamethasone sodium phosphate injection (Hubei Qianjiang Pharmaceutical Co., Ltd., Qianjiang, China) by intraperitoneal injection. All mice were treated twice daily for 7 days, and all mice were fasted but not water after the last dose on the seventh day. Except for the normal group, a single intraperitoneal injection of LPS at a dose of 15 mg kg^{-1} was administered to all groups on day 8 for the establishment of an acute inflammatory model in mice, and blood was obtained immediately after 3 h by removing the eyeballs.

Biochemical Indexes Detection

After the blood was removed from the eyeball, it was left for 30 min, then centrifuged at 4°C, 3,000 r·min^{-1} for 20 min, and the serum was removed, and the content of IL-1β and IL-6 in the serum was measured in strict accordance with the instructions of ELISA kit (Shanghai Yaji Biological Co., Ltd., Shanghai, China).

Determination of Liver and Spleen Index

After blood collection, cervical dislocation and execution of each group of mice, the spleen and thymus were removed intact, washed with saline, swabbed dry, weighed the mass, and calculated the spleen and thymus index.

Organ index (mg·g^{-1}) = Organ mass (mg)/Body mass (g).

Evaluation of CGEA in Promoting Probiotic Growth *in vitro*

Bifidobacterium (BBL) adolescentis [ATCC15703] and *Lactobacillus* acidophilus [ATCC4356] suspensions (10^7 CFU mL^{-1}) were transferred to BBL and DeMan-Rogosa-Sharpe (MRS) liquid medium containing 50, 25, 12.5, 6.25, 3.125, 1.56, 0.78, 0.39, 0.195, and 0.0975 mg mL^{-1} CGEA extracts, respectively, and the initial bacterial volume was adjusted to 10^6 CFU mL^{-1}. The same volume of bacterial suspension without CGEA was used as a normal control, and the wells containing only liquid medium were used as a reference control, and incubated for 12 h at 37°C under anaerobic conditions, and then the optical density value (OD value) of bacterial suspensions at 600 nm were measured with a microplate reader (Thermo Scientific, United States) to determine the optimal growth-promoting concentrations.

The Growth Curve Method was Utilized to Observe the Bacterial Growth Status

The bacteria were treated with the same operation as above, and the optimal concentration of CGEA was added respectively. Under anaerobic conditions, the bacteria were incubated at 37°C for 24 h, and the OD value of the bacteria suspended at 600 nm wavelength was measured every 2 h with a microplate reader, and the bacterial growth curve was plotted with the measurement time and its corresponding OD value to evaluate the effect of CGEA on the growth process of the strain.

Cell Culture and Processing

RAW 264.7 cells were donated by Xinjiang Uygur Autonomous Region Institute of Medicine, Maintain the cells in DMEM/High Glucose medium (HyClone, Logan, Utah, United States) supplemented with 10% v/v fetal bovine serum (FBS, Gibco, United States) and 1% penicillin-streptomycin solution (HyClone, Logan, Utah, United States), and put them into 25 cm^2 culture flasks, and then place them in a constant temperature incubator (Thermo Fisher Scientific, United States) at 37°C and 5% CO_2, Subculture every 2–3 days to maintain logarithmic growth. DMSO (Beijing Solarbio Technology Co., BeiJing, China) was used to prepare Lactucin solutions of different concentrations and added to the cell culture fluid. The proportion of DMSO in the cell culture fluid was 0.1% (v/v).

Cell Viability

MTT (Beijing Solarbio Technology Co., BeiJing, China) was used to determine the effect of Lactucin on cell viability. Cells were propagated in a 96-well flat-bottom plate at a cell density of 1 × 10^5 and combined for 16 h, the cells were counted using a hemocytometer. Then, the medium in the wells was discarded, and medium containing different concentrations of Lactucin was used to treat the cells for 24 h. At the end of incubation, each well was added with 10% MTT solution and the cells were cultured for another 4 h. Then carefully aspirate the culture solution, add 110 μL of formazan solution to each well, shake on a shaker at low speed for 10 min, and measure each wavelength at 490 nm by a microplate reader the absorbance (OD) value of the well.

Determination of NO, IL-6 and TNF-α Production

Cells were implanted in 96-well flat-bottom plates at a cell density of 1 × 10^5 for 16 h, and then the culture solution was discarded. The cells in the normal group and the model group were added with DMEM/High Glucose medium, and the drug intervention group was added with low (12.5 μmol L^{-1}), medium

(25 μmol L^{-1}) and high (50 μmol L^{-1}) doses of Lactucin medium to pre-protect the cells for 30 min. Except for the normal group, LPS (Solarbio Technology Co., BeiJing, China) (1 μg mL^{-1}) was added to each well, and the culture was continued for 24 h. To measure NO, mix 100 μL of cell supernatant with an equal volume of Griess reagent (Hu et al., 2016a), measure the absorbance of each well at a wavelength of 550 nm using a microplate reader within 5 min, and calculate the content of NO in the cell culture solution. The levels of IL-6 and TNF-α (Shanghai Yaji Biological Co., Ltd., Shanghai, China) in the culture medium were measured using Elisa kit.

RNA Extraction and Quantitative Real Time-PCR Analysis

Cells were implanted in 6-well plate at a density of 1×10^6 and incubated for 16 h. Then, the drug intervention group was added with low (12.5 μmol L^{-1}), medium (25 μmol L^{-1}) and high doses (50 μmol L^{-1}) of Lactucin medium to pre-protect the cells for 30 min. Except for the normal group, LPS (1 μg mL^{-1}) was added to each well, and the culture was continued for 6 h, and then, according to the manufacturer's instructions, total cell RNA was extracted using Trizol reagent (Invitrogen, Carlsbad, CA, United States). First-strand cDNA was synthesized from the total RNA (1 μg) was used the PrimeScript™ RT reagent Kit with gDNA Eraser (TaKaRa Corporation, Japan). Then use the LightCycler 480 PCR fluorescence quantifier (Roche, Germany) to amplify the target gene according to the method reported previously. The conditions for qPCR were 95°C for 10 min followed by 45 cycles at 95°C for 15 s, 57°C for 15 s, and 72°C for 15 s, with a final extension at 72°C for 10 min. GAPDH was used as the house-keeping genes, and the relative expression change factor of each target gene was calculated by $2^{-\triangle\triangle CT}$ method (Hu et al., 2016b). **Table 1** lists the oligonucleotide primers of the target gene.

Western Blot Analysis

A total of 1×10^6 cells plated in a 6-well plate for 16 h and then exposed to Lactucin for 30 min before stimulation with LPS for indicated time. After washing the cells twice with cold PBS, the cells were scraped to collect the cells, 100 μL of radio immunoprecipitation assay (RIPA) lysis buffer (CoWin Biosciences Co., BeiJing, China) was added, shaken thoroughly and placed in a refrigerator at 4°C, lyzed for 30 min, and then centrifuged at 4°C and 12,000 r/min for 10 min, extracted the total protein of the cell, and used the bicinchoninic acid (BCA) protein concentration determination kit (Solarbio Life Sciences, BeiJing, China) for concentration determination. Sodium dodecyl sulfate-polyacrylamide gel electrophoresis (SDS-PAGE) was used to separate the proteins (50 μg) in each sample and transferred onto polyvinylidene fluoride (PVDF, Millipore, Billerica, MA, United States) membranes. The PVDF membranes were then incubated overnight at 4 °C with primary antibodies including iNOS antibody (1:1,000, Cell Signaling Technology, United States), COX-2 antibody (1:1,000, Bioworld, NanJing China), P-Akt antibody (1:1,000), Akt antibody (1:2000) all from (Boster Biological technology, WuHan, China), p38 antibody (1:2000), P-p38 antibody (1:2000), ERK1/2 antibody (1: 2000), P-ERK1/2 antibody (1:2000), JNK antibody (1:2000), P-JNK antibody (1: 2000), GAPDH antibody (1:2000), Actin antibody (1:2000), all from (Beyotime Biotechnology, ShangHai, China). The membranes were then incubated for 1 h with horseradish peroxidase (HRP)-conjugated goat anti-rabbit/mouse IgG antibody (1:5,000, Zhongshan Jinqiao Biotechnology Co., Beijing, China), and the immunoreactive proteins were visualized using the enhanced chemiluminescence reagent (ECL, Solarbio Technology Co., Beijing, China). The images were obtained using ChemiDoc™ Omnimaging System (Bio-Rad, Hercules, CA, United States) and developed using ImageJ (NIH, United States) Software for quantification.

Statistical Analysis

Each group of experiments was independently repeated 3 times, and the data were expressed as mean ± standard deviation (SD). All date were analyzed with Graph Pad Prism 6.0 software (California, United States). One-way analysis of variance (ANOVA) was used to compare differences among multiple groups, and unpaired Student's t-test was used to analyze the significance between two groups. Values of $p < 0.05$ was considered statistically significant.

RESULTS

HPLC Analysis

By comparing the retention times of CGEA and Lactucin in the chromatograms, we found that the major component and the observed peak at 275 nm were identified as Lactucin (**Figure 1**) at a concentration of 6%.

CGEA Attenuates Liver Fibrosis in Rats

In the process of establishing the animal model, the rats showed thin feces, blood feces, which showed obvious characteristics of colitis. From the fourth week, we used orbital blood collection to determine AST and ALT indicators in some of the rats, and at 6 weeks, AST and ALT in the rats' serum began to appear abnormal compared with the normal group, indicating that the rats began to show liver damage. Our previous experimental results have shown that liver damage lasting more than 6 weeks can cause liver fibrosis (Qin et al., 2019a; Qin et al., 2019b). Therefore, we continued to give rats enemas with TNBS for up to 12 weeks to promote the formation of liver fibrosis in rats. The results showed that no distinct edema lesions or abnormal color was observed in liver tissue of the control group. In contrast, the model group significantly resulted in ischemia and abnormal color of rat liver tissue, however, both CGEA and Sulfasalazine significantly improved the liver congestion function and normalized the color of the liver (**Figure 2A**). The AST, ALB and γ-GT in serum were significantly increased in the model group compared with those of normal group ($p < 0.05$) and ALT, LDH was significantly increased ($p < 0.01$) (**Figures 2B–F**). CGEA-I can significantly reduce the levels of AST (**Figure 2B**) and γ-GT (**Figure 2F**) ($p < 0.05$), CGEA-II also significantly reduced the level of γ-GT ($p < 0.01$) (**Figure 2F**). In conclusion, we successfully created a new liver injury-hepatic fibrosis model

TABLE 1 | Primer sequences.

Gene	Forward primer 5′-3′	Reverse primer 5′-3′	Amplified fragment
GAPDH	AGGAGAGTGTTTCCTCGTCC	TGAGGTCAATGAAGGGGTCG	145 bp
IL-6	CCGGAGAGGAGACTTCACAG	TCCACGATTTCCCAGAGAAC	121 bp
IL-1β	TGCAGAGTTCCCCAACTGGTACA	GTGCTGCCTAATGTCCCCTTG	102 bp
TNF-α	TCAGCCTCTTCTCATTCCTG	TGAAGAGAACCTGGGAGTAG	136 bp
iNOS	CCCTTCCGAAGTTTCTGGCAGCAG	GGCTGTCAGAGCCTCGTGGCTTTGG	108 bp
COX-2	CACTACATCCTGACCCACTT	ATGCTCCTGCTTGAGTATGT	258 bp

using TNBS-ethanol enemas, and CGEA mitigated liver fibrosis in this model.

CGEA Significantly Improves Histopathological Changes in Liver Fibrosis in Rats

The results of HE staining showed that, compared with those of the normal group, the liver lobules of the model group were blurred in outline, the structure was obviously damaged, the central veins were dilated, the arrangement of the hepatic cord was disordered, and there was a large number of inflammatory cells infiltrating the hepatic lobules and confluent area (**Figure 2A**). Masson's staining results showed that collagen fibrous tissue proliferation and collagen deposition increased around the central vein and in the confluent area of the liver of the model group rats, forming obvious fibrous intervals with typical histological features of liver fibrosis. Compared with those of the normal group, collagen fibers were mainly distributed in the liver interstitium in the CGEA group and were significantly reduced, especially in the CGEA-I group (**Figure 2A**). In conclusion, the rats in this experiment have typical liver fibrosis characteristics, and CGEA can significantly reduce the collagen fibrillar content in the liver, with significant anti-fibrotic activity.

CGEA Reduces Inflammatory Factor Levels in Rat Liver

In order to verify that the effect of CGEA on liver fibrosis in experimental rats is achieved by reducing liver inflammation, we determined the levels of IL-6 and TNF-α in rat liver tissue using the ELISA method. TNF-α and IL-6, are important inflammatory response factors in the organism that promotes fibrosis formation by inducing inflammatory responses in the liver. The results of this study showed that CGEA-II group could significantly reduce the level of IL-6 ($p < 0.001$) (**Figure 2G**), the effect of CGEA on the level of TNF-α was not significant ($p > 0.05$) (**Figure 2H**).

CGEA Improves Colonic Tissue Changes in Rats With Colitis

The results showed that the colon in the control group had no obvious edema and no ulceration, while the colonic tissue in the model group showed obvious ulceration and tissue necrosis, and the CGEA intervention could significantly improve the lesions in the colonic tissue (**Figure 3**). Similarly, the results of HE staining showed that there was no damage to the colon tissue of the normal group of rats, and the glandular structure in the colon was intact. In the model group, the mucosal layer of the colonic tissue was severely damaged, with loss of microvilli and glandular fragmentation. The colon of the treated group had a large amount of granulation tissue proliferation and epithelial regeneration, especially the CGEA-I group had the best repair effect (**Figure 3**). It means that CGEA treatment can significantly improve the damage of colon tissue and reduce the inflammation of colon.

CGEA Alters the Composition of the Microbiota in the Gut of Rats With Hepatic Fibrosis

The Chao1 index and Simpson index represent the richness and diversity of microbes in the gut. Compared with those of the normal group, the enrichment of gut microorganisms in the TNBS group increased slightly and the diversity decreased, while the CGEA and positive drug groups corrected this change, but there was no significant difference among all groups ($p > 0.05$) (**Figures 4A,B**). In order to observe specific changes in microorganisms in the gut, we genetically sequenced microorganisms in intestinal feces by 16S rDNA, and it is noteworthy that the TNBS group and the administration intervention group caused changes in bacterial communities at the level of phylum and genus, and at the taxonomic level of phylum, Proteobacteria, Firmicutes and Bacteroidetes represent the majority of the total sequence of bacteria. Compared with those of the normal group, the abundance of Firmicutes in the intestines of rats in the TNBS group was significantly reduced and the abundance of Bacteroidetes was significantly increased, while the CGEA group and the positive drug group improved this situation by increasing the abundance of Firmicutes, Proteobacteria and Acidobacteria and reducing the abundance of Abundance of Bacteroidetes. (**Figure 4D**); at the level of genus, compared with those of the normal group, after TNBS modeling, the abundance of Prevotella in the intestines of rats was reduced, and the abundance of *Pseudomonas* and Ochrobactrum was increased, and the CGEA intervention could reduce the abundance of Ochrobactrum and increase the abundance of Ruminococcus and *Acinetobacter*, making the intestinal flora more to the normal level (**Figure 4C**).

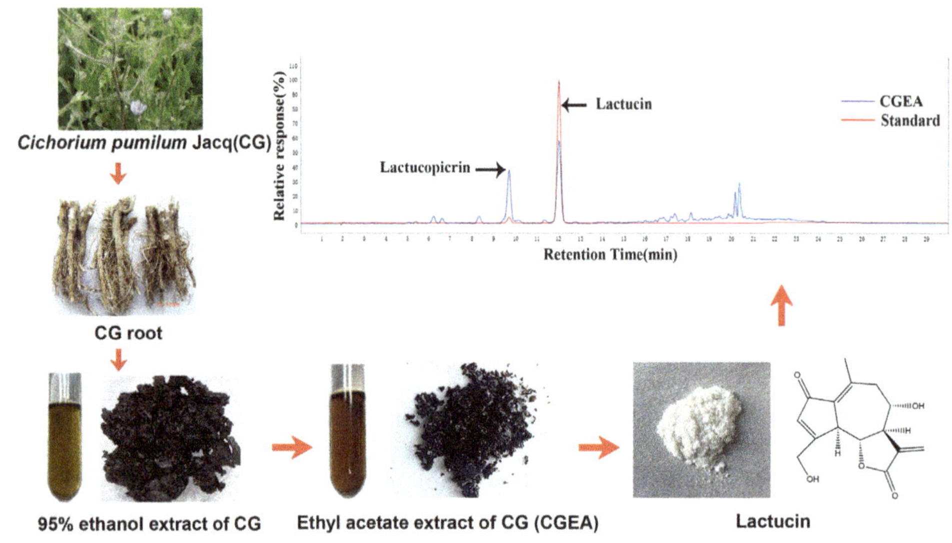

FIGURE 1 | Preparation of CGEA and Lactucin and their analysis by HPLC, HPLC chromatogram of CGEA at 275 nm, peaks is Lactucin.

CGEA Reduces the Level of Inflammation and Improves the Organ Index in Mice

Compared with the normal group, IL-1β and IL-6 in the serum of mice in the model group were highly significantly elevated ($p < 0.001$). Compared with the model group, CGEA significantly reduced the level of IL-6 in the serum of mice ($p < 0.01$). Although CGEA could not significantly reduce the level of IL-1β, the results could indicate that CGEA had a decreasing effect on IL-1β (**Figure 5**). Similarly, CGEA also reduced the spleen index and thymus index in mice (**Table 2**).

CGEA Promotes the Growth of Bifidobacterium Adolescentis

Compared with the Normal group, high concentrations of CGEA significantly inhibited the growth of Bifidobacterium adolescentis and *Lactobacillus acidophilus*, and as the concentration decreased, CGEA showed some microbial growth promoting effects, especially at a concentration of 0.78 mg mL^{-1}, the growth promoting effect of CGEA on Bifidobacterium adolescentis was the most obvious (**Figure 6A**). Further, the growth curve results showed that with the decrease of CGEA concentration, CGEA at 0.78 mg mL^{-1} concentration could significantly promote the growth of Bifidobacterium adolescentis after 16 h of co-interaction ($p < 0.01$), and when the concentration continued to decrease, this promotion effect started to weaken again (**Figure 6C**); the effect of CGEA on the growth promoting effect of CGEA on *Lactobacillus acidophilus* was not significant, but the toxic effect of low concentration of CGEA on *Lactobacillus acidophilus* was also very weak and basically did not affect the normal growth of *Lactobacillus acidophilus* (**Figure 6D**).

Lactucin Significantly Reduces LPS-Induced Levels of Inflammatory Mediator Production in RAW264.7 Cells

To further clarify the potent anti-inflammatory activity of CGEA, we investigated the mechanism of anti-inflammatory action of its main compound, Lactucin, *in vitro*. First, the toxic effect of Lactucin on RAW264.7 cells was determined by MTT, and the results showed that when Lactucin was 50 μmol L^{-1}, the cell viability was recovered 88.08%, which can be considered as no significant cytotoxicity. Similarly, DMSO at a final concentration of 0.1% was not cytotoxic, whereas 100, 200, and 400 μmol L^{-1} all showed significant cytotoxicity with cell survival rates of 55.64, 23.40, and 7.66%, respectively (**Figure 7A**); therefore, subsequent experiments were performed using Lactucin at non-cytotoxic concentrations of 12.5, 25, and 50 μmol L^{-1}, providing a basis for the variation in the experimental data not due to cytotoxicity. The results showed that 50 μmol L^{-1}, 25 μmol L^{-1} Lactucin could significantly inhibit the level of NO production in RAW264.7 cells ($p < 0.01$), and 12.5 μmol L^{-1} Lactucin could also significantly inhibit NO production ($p < 0.05$) (**Figure 7B**); 50 μmol L^{-1}, 25 μmol L^{-1} Lactucin could significantly inhibit IL-6 production ($p < 0.001$), 12.5 μmol L^{-1} Lactucin could also significantly inhibit IL-6 production ($p < 0.01$) (**Figure 7C**); and the inhibitory effect of Lactucin on TNF-α was not significant ($p > 0.05$) (**Figure 7D**).

Lactucin Significantly Inhibits LPS-Induced Inflammatory mRNA Expression Levels in RAW264.7 Cells

It is well known that iNOS is a key enzyme for cellular production of large amounts of NO (Cassini-Vieira et al., 2015), and in addition, COX-2 is an inflammatory gene that catalyzes the production of PGE_2 and is involved in promoting the

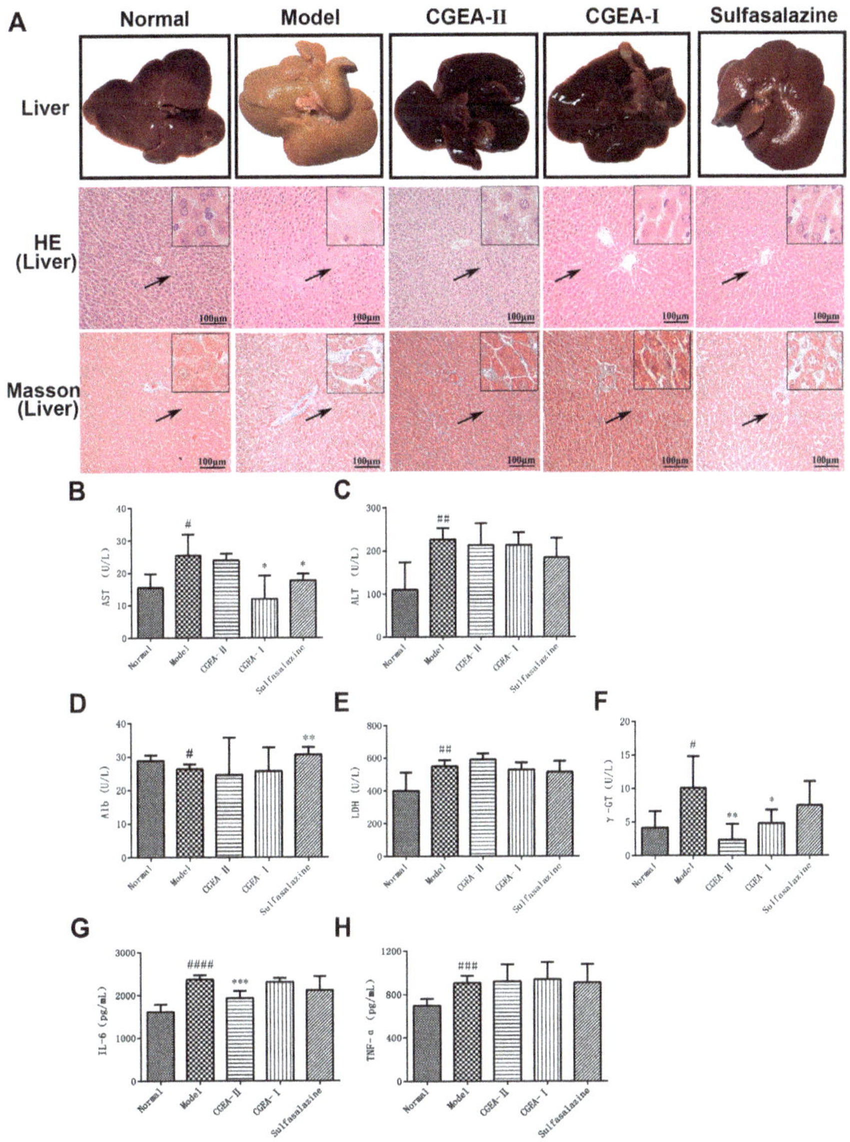

FIGURE 2 | CGEA reduces liver index and inflammation index of liver fibrosis rats. **(A)** Typical images of representative liver pathology for HE staining and Masson staining. **(B–F)** Effects of CGEA on serum AST, ALT, Alb, LDH, and γ-GT activities. **(G–H)** Statistic analysis of liver inflammation scoring (IL-6, TNF-α). Data are shown as mean ± SD in each group (*$p < 0.05$, **$p < 0.01$, ***$p < 0.001$ with the Model Group; #$p < 0.05$, ##$p < 0.01$, ###$p < 0.001$, ####$p < 0.0001$ with the Normal Group; $n = 6$). Abbreviations: Normal, Healthy rats; Model, Rats with enteritis and liver fibrosis; CGEA-II, CGEA low-dose treatment group; CGEA-I, CGEA high-dose treatment group; AST, aspartate transaminase; ALT, alanine transaminase; Alb, albumin; LDH, lactate dehydrogenase; γ-GT, γ-glutamyl transpeptidase.

inflammatory response process (He et al., 2020). To further investigate whether the inhibitory effects of lactucin on NO, PGE_2, IL-6, TNF-α, and IL-1β are related to the genes responsible for regulation, we determined the effects of lactucin on the expression of mRNA with relevant targets. The results showed that the mRNA levels of the target genes were undetectable in the unstimulated RAW264.7 cells. After LPS stimulation, the mRNA expression of iNOS, COX-2, IL-6, IL-1β and TNF-α was significantly increased. Lactucin significantly inhibited the mRNA expression of these genes in a concentration-dependent manner, in which 50 $\mu mol\,L^{-1}$ of Lactucin significantly inhibited the mRNA expression of IL-6, IL-1β and COX-2 ($p < 0.05$) (**Figure 8A,B,E**) and extremely significantly inhibited the mRNA expression of iNOS ($p < 0.01$), and 25 $\mu mol\,L^{-1}$ of Lactucin had a significant inhibitory effect on the mRNA expression of iNOS ($p < 0.05$) (**Figure 8D**), Lactucin had an inhibitory effect on TNF-α mRNA expression, but there was no significant difference ($p > 0.05$) (**Figure 8C**). These results suggest that the inhibition of inflammatory mediators in LPS-stimulated macrophages by Lactucin can be explained by the inhibition of the mRNA expression achieved in the production of inflammatory mediators.

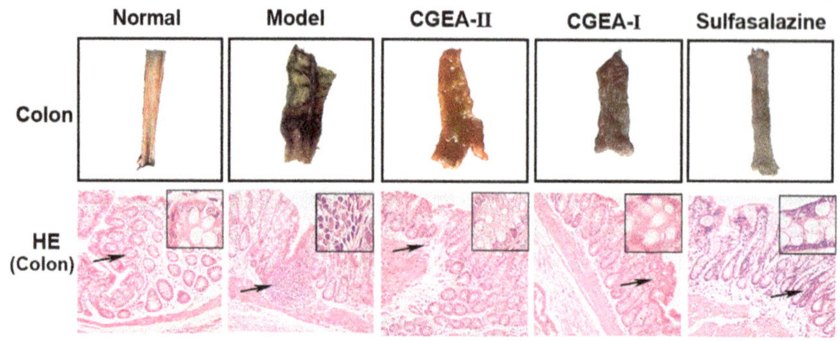

FIGURE 3 | CGEA restores the colonic barrier function of rats with liver fibrosis. Representative colon tissue images and HE-stained images(Normal: Healthy rats, Model: Rats with enteritis and liver fibrosis, CGEA-II: CGEA low-dose treatment group, CGEA-I: CGEA high-dose treatment group.)

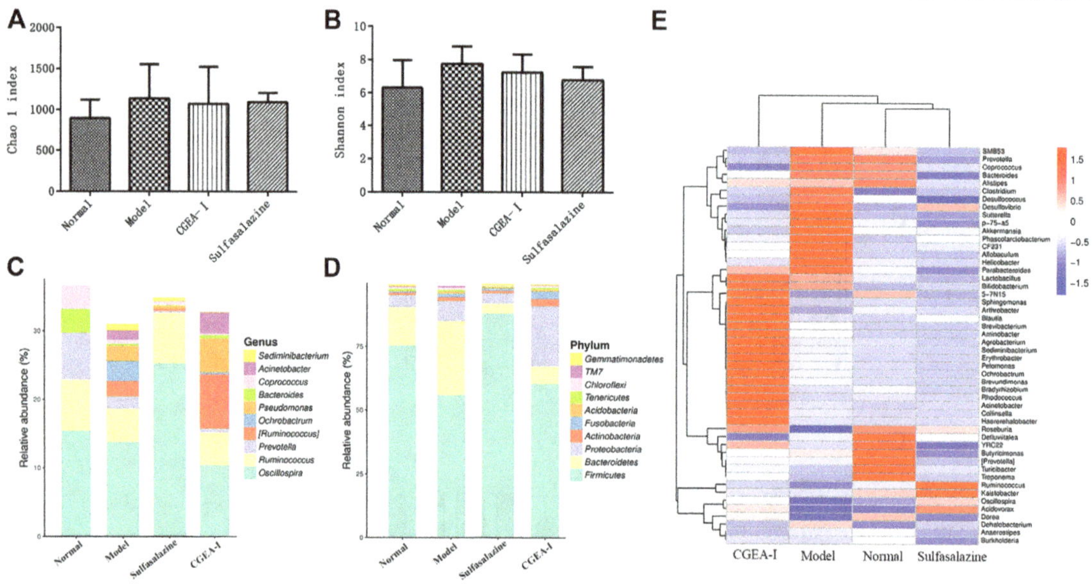

FIGURE 4 | CGEA reverses the changes of intestinal microbes. **(A–B)** Effects of CGEA on the observed species Chao one index and Shannon index in fecal microbiota after long-term TNBS exposure, respectively. **(C)** CGEA significantly ameliorated the relative abundance changes of fecal microbial composition at the genus level due to TNBS intake. **(D)** CGEA dramatically modified TNBS-induced relative abundance alterations of fecal microbial composition at the phylum level. **(F)** Heat map analysis of the gut microbiota. Data are shown as mean ± SD from three independent experiments (Normal: Healthy rats, Model: Rats with enteritis and liver fibrosis, CGEA-I: CGEA high-dose treatment group).

Lactucin Significantly Inhibits iNOS, COX-2 Protein Expression

To further investigate whether the inhibitory effect of Lactucin on inflammatory mediators is related to its associated proteins, Western Blot was used to determine protein expression of iNOS and COX-2. The results showed that after 12 h of LPS stimulation, iNOS and COX-2 proteins were highly expressed in the cells, whereas iNOS and COX-2 proteins were hardly expressed in normal cells, 50 $\mu mol\,L^{-1}$ of lactucin could extremely significantly inhibit iNOS and COX-2 protein expression ($p < 0.01$), and 25 $\mu mol\,L^{-1}$ of lactucin could also extremely significantly inhibit iNOS protein expression ($p < 0.01$), in addition, it is evident that 0.1% of DMSO had no effect on protein expression (**Figure 9A**).

Lactucin Significantly Inhibits AKT, MAPKs Protein Phosphorylation

Dysregulation of MAPK signaling pathway is one of the key factors that induce inflammation. Inhibition of MAPK signaling pathway can ameliorate many inflammatory diseases (Gong et al., 2014). At the same time, inhibition of Akt protein phosphorylation also prevents NF-κB p50 subunit movement toward the cell nucleus, which in turn inhibits inflammatory factor production (Lai et al., 2015). The results showed that the phosphorylation of MAPKs and AKT proteins could be induced by LPS stimulation for 30 min 50 $\mu mol\,L^{-1}$ of Lactucin significantly reduced the phosphorylation of p38, ERK1/2 (**Figure 9B**) and AKT proteins ($p < 0.05$) (**Figure 9C**), had no significant effect on the phosphorylation of JNK proteins, and

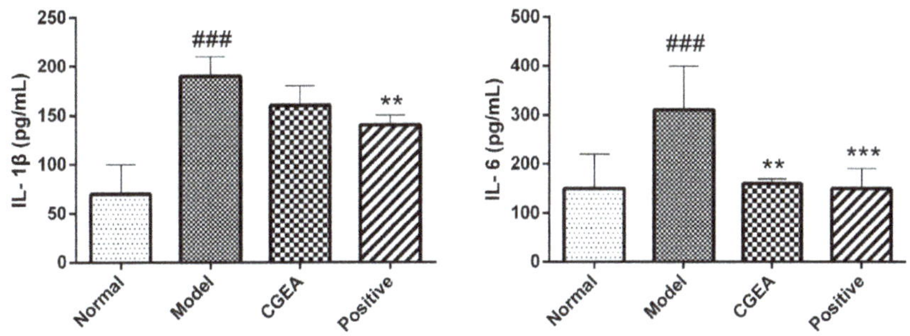

FIGURE 5 | CGEA reduces the serum levels of IL-1β and IL-6 in inflamed mice. Data are shown as mean ± SD in each group (**$p < 0.01$, ***$p < 0.001$ with the Model Group; ###$p < 0.001$ with the Normal Group; $n = 6$). Abbreviations: Normal, Healthy mice; Model, LPS-induced inflammation model mice; CGEA, 100 mg ml^{-1} dose treatment group; Positive, dexamethasone sodium phosphate injection treatment group.

TABLE 2 | Effect of CGEA on spleen index and thymus index in mice with LPS-induced acute inflammation ($x \pm s$, $n = 6$).

Group	Dosage ($mg \cdot kg^{-1}$)	Spleen index ($mg \cdot g^{-1}$)	Thymus index ($mg \cdot g^{-1}$)
Normal	–	3.08 ± 0.49	1.37 ± 0.39
Model	–	4.00 ± 0.85	1.66 ± 0.96
CGEA	100	3.00 ± 0.46	1.57 ± 0.51
Positive	10	2.62 ± 0.87*	1.39 ± 0.16

** P < 0.05 with the Model Group.*

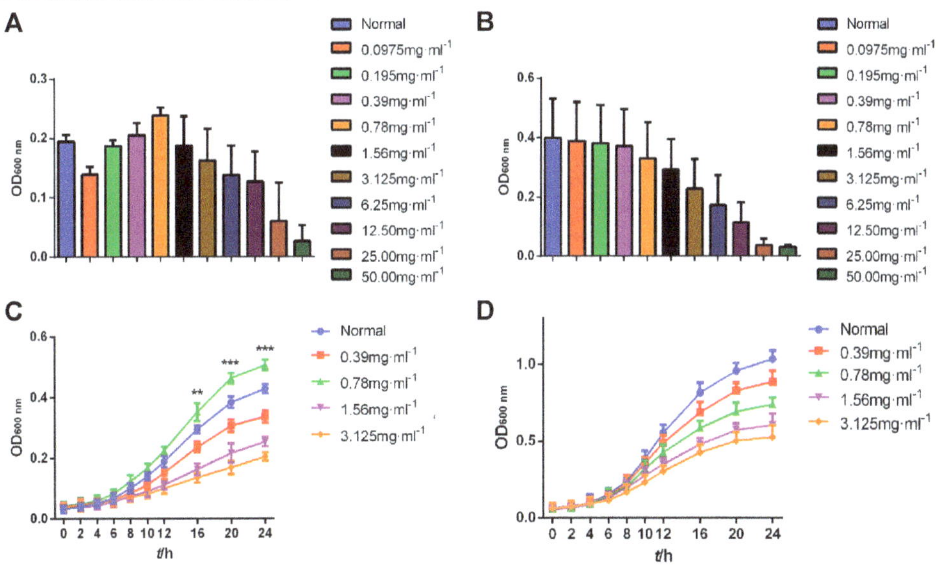

FIGURE 6 | Growth curve of Bifidobacterium adolescentis and *Lactobacillus* acidophilus. Data are shown as mean ± SD in each group (**$p < 0.01$, ***$p < 0.001$ with the Normal Group; $n = 3$). **(A, C)** Bifidobacterium adolescentis. **(B, D)** *Lactobacillus* acidophilus. Abbreviations: Normal, The bacterial suspension without CGEA.

almost no effect on the non-phosphorylated AKT, p38, ERK1/2, and JNK protein content.

DISCUSSION

In this study, we demonstrated that CGEA significantly ameliorated liver fibrosis induced by chronic colitis in rats. Promoting the growth of bifidobacteria. Interestingly, we found that CGEA could alter the composition of microorganisms in the rat intestine, and the gut-liver axis has been reported to be closely associated with liver fibrosis, however, intestinal microbes and intestinal barrier are two key factors associated with liver fibrosis (Tripathi et al., 2018). Our results found that persistent colitis disturbed microbial populations in the rat gut, as evidenced by up-regulating of

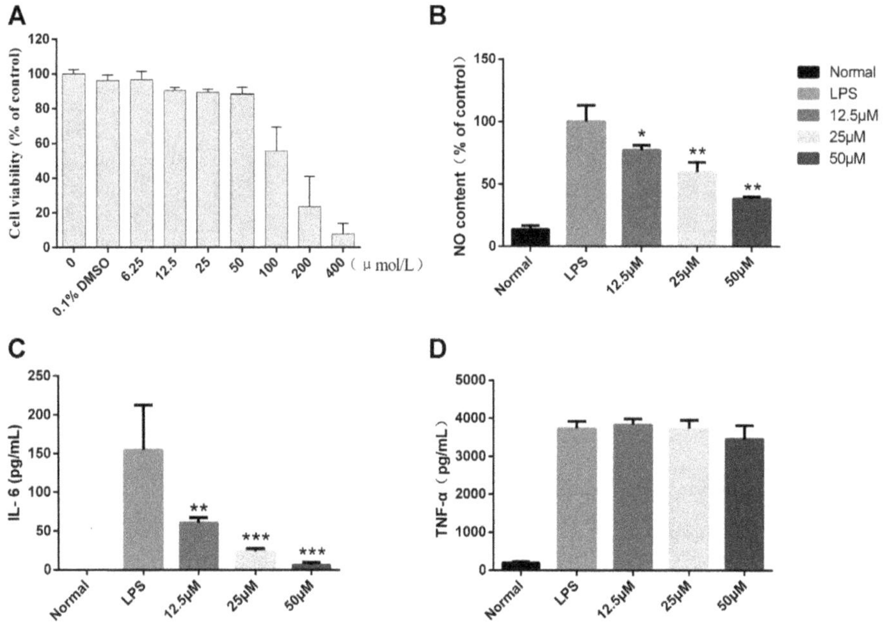

FIGURE 7 | *In vitro* anti-inflammatory effect of Lactucin in LPS-activated RAW 264.7 cells. **(A)** The cell viability of RAW264.7 cells were assessed by MTS assay. **(B)** The concentrations of NO were measured using the Griess reaction, and Lactucin significantly inhibited NO production. **(C, D)** The levels of IL-6 and TNF-α in the culture supernatants were determined by ELISAs, and Lactucin significantly inhibited IL-6 production. Data are shown as mean ± SD in each group (*$p < 0.05$, **$p < 0.01$, ***$p < 0.001$ with the LPS Group, $n = 3$. Normal Group: RAW264.7 cells without LPS activation).

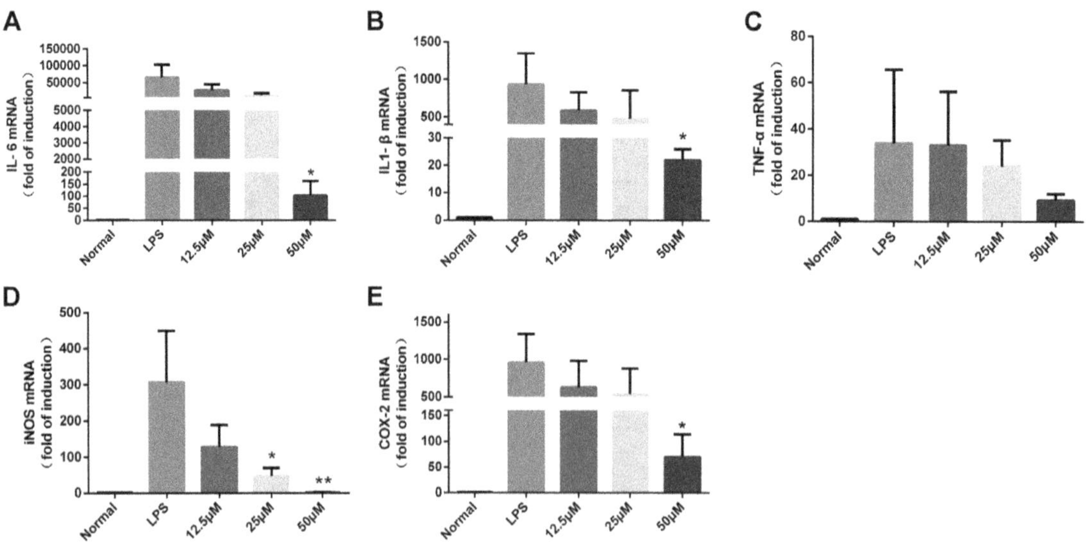

FIGURE 8 | The effect of Lactucin on mRNA expression of a set of inflammatory genes. and Lactucin significantly inhibited IL-6, IL1-β, iNOS, and COX-2 mRNA expression. Data are shown as mean ± SD for each group (*$p < 0.05$, **$p < 0.01$ with the LPS Group, $n = 3$. Normal Group: RAW264.7 cells without LPS activation).

the abundance of Bacteroidetes and down-regulating the abundance of Firmicutes in the intestine, which is consistent with a report by Frank (Frank et al., 2011), and the Bacteroidetes and Firmicutes, as the two main dominant groups in the intestine, participated in the metabolism and absorption of nutrients in the body. Firmicutes can help the body absorb more energy from food (Ley et al., 2006), thus increasing the body's resistance, while patients with liver fibrosis have abnormal liver function and generally weak immunity. CGEA may improve the body's immunity against liver fibrosis by reconfiguring microbial populations in the intestine.

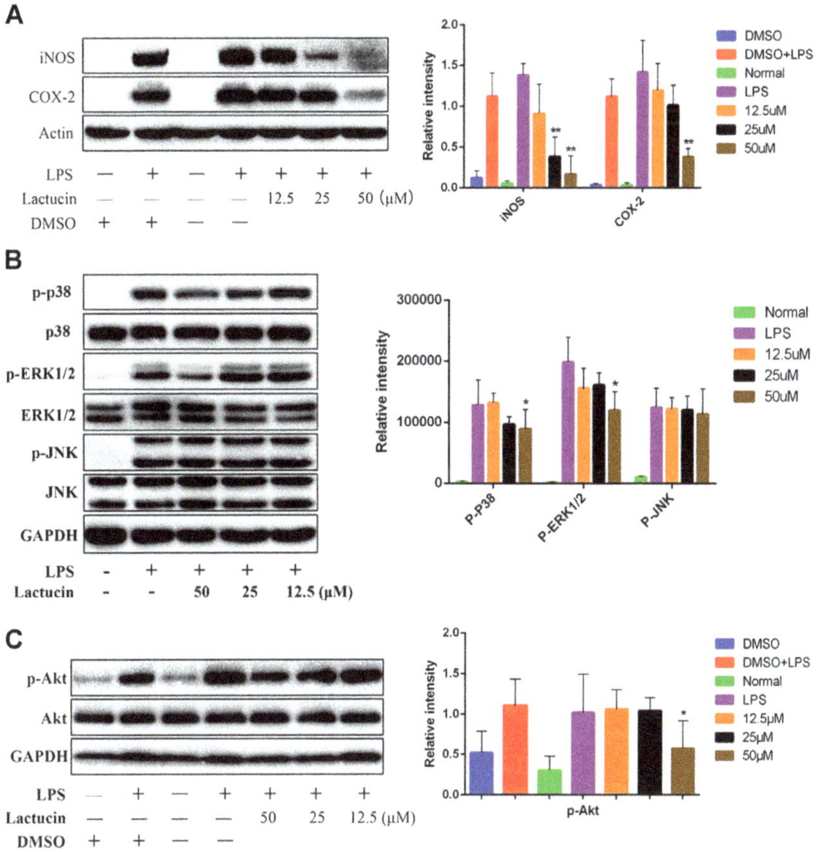

FIGURE 9 | Effect of Lactucin on the activation of signaling pathways. **(A)** The whole-cell lysates were extracted for immunoblotting to determine the level of iNOS, COX-2. **(B, C)** The whole-cell lysates were extracted for immunoblotting to determine the levels of phospho- or total MAPKs (ERK, p38, and JNK) and AKT identified based on their antibodies. Data are shown as mean ± SD for each group (*$p < 0.05$ with the LPS Group, $n = 3$. Normal Group: RAW264.7 cells without LPS activation).

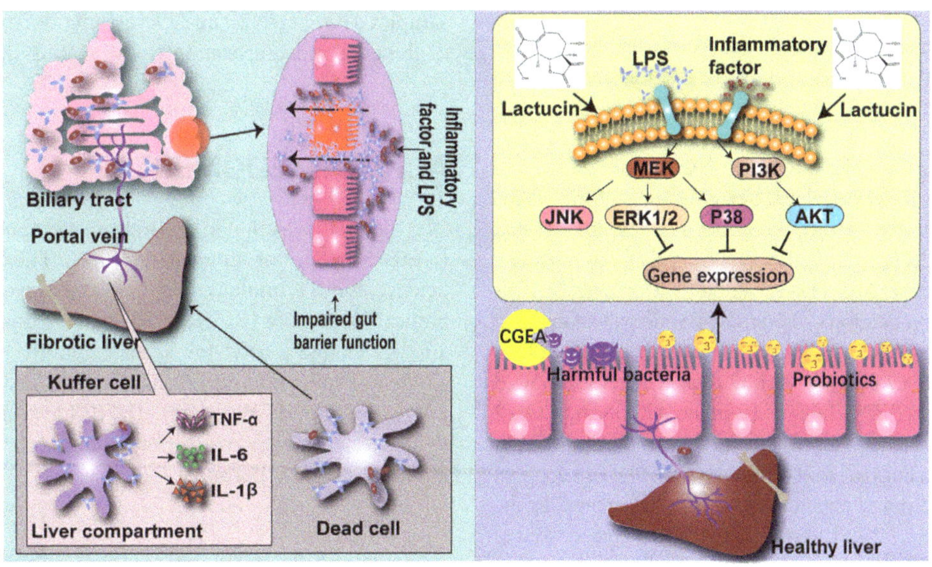

FIGURE 10 | CG confers anti-inflammatory effects by inhibiting the phosphorylation pathway of MAPK signaling pathway, thereby improving the intestinal microenvironment and reducing the production of liver fibrosis through the "gut-liver axis".

On the other hand, when intestinal inflammation persists, the intestinal villi become sparse and damaged, the intestinal barrier function is disrupted, and the metabolites of microorganisms in the gut with harmful flora enter the liver with the enterohepatic axis, stimulating inflammation in the liver. Our results show that increased expression of inflammatory factors in the liver of rats with colitis reveals that functionally impaired intestinal microbes can stimulate intrahepatic inflammation and enter the enterohepatic circulation through the damaged intestinal barrier, exacerbating the development of liver fibrosis. The metabolism of short-chain fatty acids (SCFAs) produced by the Ruminococcus is one of the richest families of Fusobacteria under the Firmicutes (Sagheddu et al., 2016), which enhances the protective effect of the intestinal barrier (Kang et al., 2017; Porras et al., 2017). Therefore, we speculate that the protective effect of CGEA on the rat intestinal barrier may be related to its promotion of the growth of Ruminococcus, however, its specific mechanism of action needs to be further investigated.

Almost all liver diseases are accompanied by inflammation (Bai et al., 2017), and sustained inflammatory stimuli lead to substantial loss of hepatocytes and loss of liver function (Wu et al., 2019), thus reducing the production of inflammatory factors is important to reduce liver injury and fibrosis (O'Reilly et al., 2014; Seki and Schwable, 2015). IL-6 is a proinflammatory cytokine produced after immune activation that can exacerbate chronic inflammation (Cha et al., 2015). And our results table that CGEA significantly reduced serum levels of IL-6 both in acutely inflamed mice and in rats with liver fibrosis. In conclusion, our results suggest that CGEA can reduce the expression of inflammatory factors not only directly, but also indirectly by regulating microorganisms and improving the circulation of the enterohepatic axis.

Earlier experiments demonstrated the most significant anti-inflammatory activity of Lactucin in CGEA (Dang et al., 2019). In the present experiments we further determined the content of Lactucin and the HPLC results showed that the content of Lactucin in CGEA was 6%.Lactucin being the major compound in CGEA, we predict that the anti-inflammatory activity exhibited by CGEA is mainly due to the anti-inflammatory effect exerted by Lactucin. It is well known that dysregulation of MAPK signaling pathway is a key factor in triggering inflammation (Jeong et al., 2014; Duan et al., 2017). Moreover, MAPKs and PI3K/Akt signaling pathways can directly promote DNA binding activity, leading to the up-regulation of iNOS and TNF-α mRNA expression in RAW 264.7 cells (Hu et al., 2016a). The results showed that Lactucin could significantly inhibit LPS-induced iNOS and COX-2 mRNA expression and protein expression in RAW264.7 cells, which is consistent with the findings of Lee et al. (Lee et al., 2010). This suggests to us that Lactucin exert anti-inflammatory effects by suppressing the phosphorylation of ERK1/2 and p38 signaling pathways, which lead to the inhibition of NO production in RAW 264.7 cells.

PI3K/Akt is a serine/threonine-specific protein kinase that plays a key role in many cell growth processes and is closely related to the MAPK signaling pathway, which can both activate and inhibit each other (Meng et al., 2009; Aksamitiene et al., 2012). Our results indicate that Lactucin can significantly inhibit the mRNA expression of IL-6 and IL-1β in RAW264.7 cells and significantly inhibit the phosphorylation of AKT protein. In conclusion, the results here indicate that Lactucin is anti-inflammatory by inhibiting the activation of the MAPK-AKT signaling pathway in RAW264.7 cells, thereby inhibiting the production of inflammatory factors such as NO and IL-6.

CONCLUSION

Taken together, our results indicated that CGEA can ameliorate liver fibrosis induced by 5% TNBS-50% ethanol solution. The mechanism of action may combine the modulation of ERK1/2, p38 and AKT signaling pathways with improvement of the "gut-liver axis" circulation to inhibit inflammation and thus exert an anti-fibrotic effect (**Figure 10**).

ETHICS STATEMENT

The animal study was reviewed and approved by the Animal Experimental Ethical Inspection of First Affiliated Hospital, Shihezi University School of Medicine.

AUTHOR CONTRIBUTIONS

All the authors devoted much effort to the paper. DQ, CH was responsible for experimental design. DQ, CH, XW and NZ were in charge of completing the experiments and writing the paper. DQ, JY, YZ, CL and JH assisted with the acquisition of the samples. DQ, CH, NZ and YG were involved in critical evaluation of the data and preparation of the manuscript.

ACKNOWLEDGMENTS

We thank the National Natural Science Foundation of China (NO.81560680) for financial support. The authors thank the Science and Technology Research and Development Project of Shihezi University (RCZK 2018C12) for financial support. The authors thank the Major science and technology project of Xinjiang Production and Construction Corps (2020AA005) for financial support. We thank Dr B Thyagarajan of School of Pharmacy, University of Wyoming for his analysis and guidance of the experiment.

REFERENCES

Aksamitiene, E., Kiyatkin, A., and Kholodenko, B. N. (2012). Cross-talk between Mitogenic Ras/MAPK and Survival PI3K/Akt Pathways: a Fine Balance. *Biochem. Soc. Trans.* 40 (1), 139–146. doi:10.1042/BST20110609

Bai, X., Yang, P., Zhou, Q., Cai, B., Buist-Homan, M., Cheng, H., et al. (2017). The Protective Effect of the Natural Compound Hesperetin against Fulminant Hepatitisin Vivoandin Vitro. *Br. J. Pharmacol.* 174 (1), 41–56. doi:10.1111/bph.13645

Bajaj, J. S., Hylemon, P. B., Ridlon, J. M., Heuman, D. M., Daita, K., White, M. B., et al. (2012). Colonic Mucosal Microbiome Differs from Stool Microbiome in Cirrhosis and Hepatic Encephalopathy and Is Linked to Cognition and Inflammation. *Am. J. Physiology-Gastrointestinal Liver Physiol.* 303 (6), G675–G685. doi:10.1152/ajpgi.00152.2012

Cassini-Vieira, P., Araújo, F. A., da Costa Dias, F. L., Russo, R. C., Andrade, S. P., Teixeira, M. M., et al. (2015). iNOS Activity Modulates Inflammation, Angiogenesis, and Tissue Fibrosis in Polyether-Polyurethane Synthetic Implants. *Mediators Inflamm.* 2015, 1–9. doi:10.1155/2015/138461

Cha, B.-J., Park, J.-H., Shrestha, S., Baek, N.-I., Lee, S. M., Lee, T. H., et al. (2015). Glycosyl Glycerides from Hydroponic Panax Ginseng Inhibited No Production in Lipopolysaccharide-Stimulated raw264.7 Cells. *J. Ginseng Res.* 39 (2), 162–168. doi:10.1016/j.jgr.2014.10.005

Dang, T., Zheng, G., Zhang, Q., Jin, P., Zhang, H., Su, L., et al. (2019). Sesquiterpenoids with Diverse Carbon Skeletons from the Roots of Cichorium Glandulosum and Their Anti-inflammatory Activities. *Fitoterapia* 136, 104170. doi:10.1016/j.fitote.2019.104170

Duan, X., Gao, S., Li, J., Wu, L., Zhang, Y., Li, W., et al. (2017). Acute Arsenic Exposure Induces Inflammatory Responses and CD4+ T Cell Subpopulations Differentiation in Spleen and Thymus with the Involvement of MAPK, NF-kB, and Nrf2. *Mol. Immunol.* 81, 160–172. doi:10.1016/j.molimm.2016.12.005

Frank, D. N., Robertson, C. E., Hamm, C. M., Kpadeh, Z., Zhang, T., Chen, H., et al. (2011). Disease Phenotype and Genotype Are Associated with Shifts in Intestinal-Associated Microbiota in Inflammatory Bowel Diseases. *Inflamm. Bowel Dis.* 17 (1), 179–184. doi:10.1002/ibd.21339

Gong, X. W., Yang, Q. H., Yan, H. Z., Zhang, Y. P., Liang, Y. J., Liu, Y. Z., et al. (2014). [Effects of Soothing Liver and Invigorating Spleen Recipes on LPS-Induced Hepatocytes Injury of Rats and TLR4/p38MAPK Signal Pathway]. *Zhongguo Zhong Yao Za Zhi* 39 (20), 4027–4033. doi:10.4268/cjcmm20142024

Han, C., Dang, T., Wang, R., Yao, J., Qin, D. M., and Zhang, Y. S. (2019). Study on Differences in Antibacterial Activity of Ethanol Extracts from Chicory Roots and Stems against *staphylococcus Aureus* and *enterococcus Faecalis*. *Chin. Pharmacol. Bull.* 35 (04), 540–545. doi:10.3969/j.issn.1001-1978.2019.04.019

Han, S., Lin, Z., Wen, J., Wu, K., Xu, Y., Zhang, Y., et al. (2020). Astilbin Promotes the Induction of Regulatory NK1.1− CD4+ NKG2D+ T Cells through the PI3K, STAT3, and MAPK Signaling Pathways. *Int. Immunopharmacol.* 81, 106143. doi:10.1016/j.intimp.2019.106143

He, R., Hua, K., Zhang, S., Wan, Y., Gong, H., Ma, B., et al. (2020). COX-2 Mediated Crosstalk between Wnt/β-Catenin and the NF-Kb Signaling Pathway during Inflammatory Responses Induced by *Haemophilus* Parasuis in PK-15 and NPTr Cells. *Developmental Comp. Immunol.* 105, 103588. doi:10.1016/j.dci.2019.103588

Hu, W., Wang, X., Wu, L., Shen, T., Ji, L., Zhao, X., et al. (2016b). Apigenin-7-O-β-d-glucuronide Inhibits LPS-Induced Inflammation through the Inactivation of AP-1 and MAPK Signaling Pathways in RAW 264.7 Macrophages and Protects Mice against Endotoxin Shock. *Food Funct.* 7 (2), 1002–1013. doi:10.1039/c5fo01212k

Hu, W., Wu, L., Qiang, Q., Ji, L., Wang, X., Luo, H., et al. (2016a). The Dichloromethane Fraction from Mahonia Bealei (fort.) Carr. Leaves Exerts an Anti-inflammatory Effect Both In Vitro and In Vivo. *J. Ethnopharmacol.* 188, 134–143. doi:10.1016/j.jep.2016.05.013

Jeong, J.-J., Jang, S.-E., Hyam, S. R., Han, M. J., and Kim, D.-H. (2014). Mangiferin Ameliorates Colitis by Inhibiting IRAK1 Phosphorylation in NF-Kb and MAPK Pathways. *Eur. J. Pharmacol.* 740, 652–661. doi:10.1016/j.ejphar.2014.06.013

Kamada, N., Seo, S.-U., Chen, G. Y., and Núñez, G. (2013). Role of the Gut Microbiota in Immunity and Inflammatory Disease. *Nat. Rev. Immunol.* 13 (5), 321 335. doi:10.1038/nri3430

Kang, C., Wang, B., Kaliannan, K., Wang, X., Lang, H., Hui, S., et al. (2017). Gut Microbiota Mediates the Protective Effects of Dietary Capsaicin against Chronic Low-Grade Inflammation and Associated Obesity Induced by High-Fat Diet. *MBio* 8 (3). doi:10.1128/mBio.00470-17

Lai, W., Tian, X., Xiang, Q., Chu, K., Wei, Y., Deng, J., et al. (2015). 11β-HSD1 Modulates LPS-Induced Innate Immune Responses in Adipocytes by Altering Expression of PTEN. *Mol. Endocrinol.* 29 (4), 558–570. doi:10.1210/me.2014-1287

Lau, E., Carvalho, D., and Freitas, P. (2015). Gut Microbiota: Association with Nafld and Metabolic Disturbances. *Biomed. Res. Int.* 2015, 1–9. doi:10.1155/2015/979515

Lee, H. J., Lim, H. J., Lee, D. Y., Jung, H., Kim, M.-R., Moon, D.-C., et al. (2010). Carabrol Suppresses LPS-Induced Nitric Oxide Synthase Expression by Inactivation of P38 and JNK via Inhibition of I-Kbα Degradation in RAW 264.7 Cells. *Biochem. Biophysical Res. Commun.* 391 (3), 1400–1404. doi:10.1016/j.bbrc.2009.12.073

Lee, S.-M., Han, H. W., and Yim, S. Y. (2015). Beneficial Effects of Soy Milk and Fiber on High Cholesterol Diet-Induced Alteration of Gut Microbiota and Inflammatory Gene Expression in Rats. *Food Funct.* 6 (2), 492–500. doi:10.1039/c4fo00731j

Ley, R. E., Turnbaugh, P. J., Klein, S., and Gordon, J. I. (2006). Human Gut Microbes Associated with Obesity. *Nature* 444 (7122), 1022–1023. doi:10.1038/4441022a

Li, Y., Liu, T., Yan, C., Xie, R., Guo, Z., Wang, S., et al. (2018). Diammonium Glycyrrhizinate Protects against Nonalcoholic Fatty Liver Disease in Mice through Modulation of Gut Microbiota and Restoration of Intestinal Barrier. *Mol. Pharmaceutics* 15 (9), 3860–3870. doi:10.1021/acs.molpharmaceut.8b00347

Ling, Z., Liu, X., Cheng, Y., Jiang, X., Jiang, H., Wang, Y., et al. (2015). Decreased Diversity of the Oral Microbiota of Patients with Hepatitis B Virus-Induced Chronic Liver Disease: A Pilot Project. *Sci. Rep.* 5, 17098. doi:10.1038/srep17098

Liu, X., Xie, J., Jia, S., Huang, L., Wang, Z., Li, C., et al. (2017). Immunomodulatory Effects of an Acetylated Cyclocarya Paliurus Polysaccharide on Murine Macrophages raw264.7. *Int. J. Biol. Macromolecules* 98, 576–581. doi:10.1016/j.ijbiomac.2017.02.028

Marshall, J. C. (1998). The Gut as a Potential Trigger of Exercise-Induced Inflammatory Responses. *Can. J. Physiol. Pharmacol.* 76 (5), 479–484. doi:10.1139/cjpp-76-5-47910.1139/y98-049

Meng, J., Peng, H., Dai, B., Guo, W., Wang, L., Ji, L., et al. (2009). High Level of Akt Activity Is Associated with Resistance to Mek Inhibitor Azd6244 (Arry-142886). *cbt* 8 (21), 2073–2080. doi:10.4161/cbt.8.21.9844

Nakamoto, N., Amiya, T., Aoki, R., Taniki, N., Koda, Y., Miyamoto, K., et al. (2017). Commensal Lactobacillus Controls Immune Tolerance during Acute Liver Injury in Mice. *Cel Rep.* 21 (5), 1215–1226. doi:10.1016/j.celrep.2017.10.022

O'Reilly, S., Ciechomska, M., Cant, R., and van Laar, J. M. (2014). Interleukin-6 (IL-6) Trans Signaling Drives a STAT3-dependent Pathway that Leads to Hyperactive Transforming Growth Factor-β (TGF-β) Signaling Promoting SMAD3 Activation and Fibrosis via Gremlin Protein. *J. Biol. Chem.* 289 (14), 9952–9960. doi:10.1074/jbc.M113.545822

Porras, D., Nistal, E., Martínez-Flórez, S., Pisonero-Vaquero, S., Olcoz, J. L., Jover, R., et al. (2017). Protective Effect of Quercetin on High-Fat Diet-Induced Non-alcoholic Fatty Liver Disease in Mice Is Mediated by Modulating Intestinal Microbiota Imbalance and Related Gut-Liver axis Activation. *Free Radic. Biol. Med.* 102, 188–202. doi:10.1016/j.freeradbiomed.2016.11.037

Pyrek, J. S. (1985). Sesquiterpene Lactones of Cichorium Intybus and Leontodon Autumnalis. *Phytochemistry* 24 (1), 186–188. doi:10.1016/S0031-9422(00)80838-9

Qin, D.-M., Hu, L.-P., Zhang, Y., Kang, Y., Han, C., Dang, T., et al. (2019a). Studies on the Protective Effect of Total Flavonoids from Cichorium Glandulosum Roots against Carbon Tetrachloride-Induced Liver Fibrosis in Rats. *Trop. J. Pharm. Res.* 18 (2), 311–319. Available at: https://www.ajol.info/index.php/tjpr/article/view/184523. doi:10.4314/tjpr.v18i2.13

Qin, D.-M., Wang, X.-B., Zou, N., Han, C., and Xu, J. (2019b). Gas chromatography-mass spectrometry (gc-ms) analysis of the volatile oil of cichorium glandulosum boiss et huet and its effects on carbon tetrachloride-induced liver fibrosis in rats. *Med. Sci. Monit.* 25, 3591–3604. doi:10.12659/MSM.913445

Qin, D. M., Nie, Y. R., and Wen, Z. P. (2014). Protection of Rats from Thioacetamide-Induced Hepatic Fibrosis by the Extracts of a Traditional

Uighur Medicine Cichorium Glandulosum. *Iran J. Basic Med. Sci.* 17 (11), 879–885. doi:10.3739/ijbms.18739

Qin, D., Wen, Z., Nie, Y., and Yao, G. (2013). Effect of Cichorium Glandulosum Extracts on Ccl4-Induced Hepatic Fibrosis. *Iran Red Crescent Med. J.* 15 (12), e10908. doi:10.5812/ircmj.10908

Ribeiro, D., Freitas, M., Lima, J. L. F. C., and Fernandes, E. (2015). Proinflammatory Pathways: The Modulation by Flavonoids. *Med. Res. Rev.* 35 (5), 877–936. doi:10.1002/med.21347

Sagheddu, V., Patrone, V., Miragoli, F., Puglisi, E., and Morelli, L. (2016). Infant Early Gut Colonization by Lachnospiraceae: High Frequency of Ruminococcus Gnavus. *Front. Pediatr.* 4, 57. doi:10.3389/fped.2016.00057

Seki, E., and Schwabe, R. F. (2015). Hepatic Inflammation and Fibrosis: Functional Links and Key Pathways. *Hepatology* 61 (3), 1066–1079. doi:10.1002/hep.27332

Serreli, G., Melis, M. P., Zodio, S., Naitza, M. R., Casula, E., Peñalver, P., et al. (2020). Altered Paracellular Permeability in Intestinal Cell Monolayer Challenged with Lipopolysaccharide: Modulatory Effects of Pterostilbene Metabolites. *Food Chem. Toxicol.* 145, 111729. doi:10.1016/j.fct.2020.111729

Tong, J., Mo, Q.-G., Ma, B.-X., Ge, L.-L., Zhou, G., and Wang, Y.-W. (2017). The Protective Effects of Cichorium Glandulosum Seed and Cynarin against Cyclophosphamide and its Metabolite Acrolein-Induced Hepatotoxicity In Vivo and In Vitro. *Food Funct.* 8 (1), 209–219. doi:10.1039/c6fo01531j

Tripathi, A., Debelius, J., Brenner, D. A., Karin, M., Loomba, R., Schnabl, B., et al. (2018). Publisher Correction: The Gut-Liver axis and the Intersection with the Microbiome. *Nat. Rev. Gastroenterol. Hepatol.* 15 (12), 785. doi:10.1038/s41575-018-0031-8

Van Dort, M. E., Galbán, S., Wang, H., Sebolt-Leopold, J., Whitehead, C., Hong, H., et al. (2015). Dual Inhibition of Allosteric Mitogen-Activated Protein Kinase (MEK) and Phosphatidylinositol 3-kinase (PI3K) Oncogenic Targets with a Bifunctional Inhibitor. *Bioorg. Med. Chem.* 23 (7), 1386–1394. doi:10.1016/j.bmc.2015.02.053

Wang, X., Liu, M., Cai, G. H., Chen, Y., Shi, X. C., Zhang, C. C., et al. (2020). A Potential Nutraceutical Candidate Lactucin Inhibits Adipogenesis through Downregulation of Jak2/stat3 Signaling Pathway-Mediated Mitotic Clonal Expansion. *Cells* 9 (2), 331. doi:10.3390/cells9020331

Wu, M., Wang, C., Mai, C., Chen, J., Lai, X., He, L., et al. (2019). Flavonoids from livistona Chinensis Fruit Ameliorates Lps/d-Galn-Induced Acute Liver Injury by Inhibiting Oxidative Stress and Inflammation. *J. Funct. Foods* 61, 103460. doi:10.1016/j.jff.2019.103460

Xie, C., Li, X., Zhu, J., Wu, J., Geng, S., and Zhong, C. (2019). Magnesium Isoglycyrrhizinate Suppresses LPS-Induced Inflammation and Oxidative Stress through Inhibiting NF-Kb and MAPK Pathways in RAW264.7 Cells. *Bioorg. Med. Chem.* 27 (3), 516–524. doi:10.1016/j.bmc.2018.12.033

Zanello, G., Berri, M., Dupont, J., Sizaret, P.-Y., d'Inca, R., Salmon, H., et al. (2011). *Saccharomyces cerevisiae* Modulates Immune Gene Expressions and Inhibits Etec-Mediated Erk1/2 and P38 Signaling Pathways in Intestinal Epithelial Cells. *PloS One* 6 (4), e18573, doi:10.1371/journal.pone.0018573

Zhang, J., Hoedt, E. C., Liu, Q., Berendsen, E., Teh, J. J., Hamilton, A., et al. (2021). Elucidation of proteus Mirabilis as a Key Bacterium in Crohns Disease Inflammation. *Gastroenterology* 160 (1), 317–330. doi:10.1053/j.gastro.2020.09.036

GLOSSARY

AKT (protein kinase B)

ALT (Alanine aminotransferase)

Alb (Albumin)

AST (Aspartate aminotransferase)

CG (Cichorium pumilum Jacq)

CGEA (Ethyl Acetate Extract of Cichorium pumilum Jacq)

COX-2 (Cyclooxygenase-2)

DMSO (dimethyl sulfoxide)

Elisa (enzyme-linked immunosorbent assay)

ERK1/2 (Extracellular signal-regulated kinase)

IL (Interleukin)

iNOS (Inducible nitric oxide synthase)

JNK (Jun-N-terminal kinase)

LDH (Lactate dehydrogenase)

LPS (Lipopolysaccharide)

MAPKs (Mitogen activated protine kinase)

MTT [3-(4,5-dimethylthiazol-2-yl)-2,5-diphenyltetrazolium bromide]

NO (Nitic oxide)

p38 (p38 kinases)

qPCR (Real-time Quantitative polymerase chain reaction)

γ-GT (gamma-glutamyl transferase)

TNBS (2,4,6-trinitrobenzene sulfonic acid)

TNF-α (Tumor necrosis factor-α)

(BBL) Bifidobacterium

(MRS) DeMan-Rogosa-Sharpe

(RIPA) Radio Immunoprecipitation Assay

(BCA) Bicinchoninic Acid

9

The Genus *Alistipes*: Gut Bacteria with Emerging Implications to Inflammation, Cancer and Mental Health

Bianca J. Parker[1], Pamela A. Wearsch[1], Alida C. M. Veloo[2] and Alex Rodriguez-Palacios[3,4]*

[1] Department of Pathology, Case Western Reserve University School of Medicine, Cleveland, OH, United States, [2] Department of Medical Microbiology, University Medical Centre Groningen, University of Groningen, Groningen, Netherlands, [3] Division of Gastroenterology and Liver Disease, Case Western Reserve University School of Medicine, Cleveland, OH, United States, [4] Germ-Free and Gut Microbiome, Digestive Health Research Institute, Case Western Reserve University, Cleveland, OH, United States

***Correspondence:**
Alex Rodriguez-Palacios
axr503@case.edu

Alistipes is a relatively new genus of bacteria isolated primarily from medical clinical samples, although at a low rate compared to other genus members of the *Bacteroidetes* phylum, which are highly relevant in dysbiosis and disease. According to the taxonomy database at The National Center for Biotechnology Information, the genus consists of 13 species: *Alistipes finegoldii*, *Alistipes putredinis*, *Alistipes onderdonkii*, *Alistipes shahii*, *Alistipes indistinctus*, *Alistipes senegalensis*, *Alistipes timonensis*, *Alistipes obesi*, *Alistipes ihumii*, *Alistipes inops, Alistipes megaguti, Alistipes provencensis,* and *Alistipes massiliensis. Alistipes communis* and *A. dispar*, and the subspecies *A. Onderdonkii* subspecies vulgaris (vs. *onderdonkii* subsp.) are the newest strains featured outside that list. Although typically isolated from the human gut microbiome various species of this genus have been isolated from patients suffering from appendicitis, and abdominal and rectal abscess. It is possible that as *Alistipes* spp. emerge, their identification in clinical samples may be underrepresented as novel MS-TOF methods may not be fully capable to discriminate distinct species as separate since it will require the upgrading of MS-TOF identification databases. In terms of pathogenicity, there is contrasting evidence indicating that *Alistipes* may have protective effects against some diseases, including liver fibrosis, colitis, cancer immunotherapy, and cardiovascular disease. In contrast, other studies indicate *Alistipes* is pathogenic in colorectal cancer and is associated with mental signs of depression. Gut dysbiosis seems to play a role in determining the compositional abundance of *Alistipes* in the feces (*e.g.*, in non-alcoholic steatohepatitis, hepatic encephalopathy, and liver fibrosis). Since *Alistipes* is a relatively recent sub-branch genus of the *Bacteroidetes* phylum, and since *Bacteroidetes* are commonly associated with chronic intestinal inflammation, this narrative review illustrates emerging immunological and mechanistic implications by which *Alistipes* spp. correlate with human health.

Keywords: *Alistipes finegoldii*, inflammatory bowel diseases, *A. putredinis*, *A. onderdonkii*, *A. shahii*, *A. indistinctus*, *A. senegalensis*, *A. timonensis*

INTRODUCTION

The human gut microbiome is acquired at birth and as individual go through life, their gut becomes a home to trillions of microorganisms, namely bacteria. With the use of 16S rRNA gene sequencing a diverse profile of bacterial phyla has been identified, with the two most common being *Bacteroidetes* and *Firmicutes*. Collectively, the composition of the gut microbiota amounts to a massive number of cells and functions that equate (even surpass) to that of an additional organ (1). The human microbiota plays a critical role in regulation of the immune response, protection against pathogens, aiding in digestion, as well as in neurologic signaling and vascularization (2). Notably, the microbiota has been found to be involved in health and disease. The imbalance, or dysbiosis, of the intestinal microbiota has been attributed to numerous diseases such as cancer (3), cardiovascular disease (4), inflammatory bowel disease (5), and nervous system disorders (6). Investigators have examined various genera and species that make up the microbiome trying to decipher their role as a collective trying to identify individual microbial species with the ability to modulate diseases.

Taxonomically, *Alistipes* (a. li. sti'pes) is a genus described in 2003 after being discovered in tissue samples of children with appendicitis (7). *Alistipes* are anaerobic bacteria found mostly in the healthy human gastrointestinal (GI) tract microbiota (8). According to the taxonomy database at The National Center for Biotechnology Information (NCBI, txid239759), as of April 2020, *Alistipes* consists of 13 species: *Alistipes finegoldii, Alistipes putredinis, Alistipes onderdonkii, Alistipes shahii, Alistipes indistinctus, Alistipes senegalensis, Alistipes timonensis, Alistipes obesi, Alistipes ihumii, Alistipes inops, Alistipes megaguti, Alistipes provencensis,* and *Alistipes massiliensis* (the latter strain reported as "unpublished by Lacroix et al., as of March 4, 2004, NCBI:txid265312" remains unpublished under that name). However, a case study in 2017 from the same group of scientists reported a novel species called *Tidjanibacter massiliensis* Marseille-P3084, isolated from the colon of a person with irritable bowel syndrome, with 92.1% sequence homology to *A. putredinis* (9), but the strain has not been officially recognized or deposited in public strain biorepositories. To date it is unclear if the *Tidjanibacter* is the same *Alistipes* isolate, or what occurred with the publication of the *Alistipes massiliensis* for which there is no genome or 16S RNA gene sequences available in NCBI. Three newer species were added to the the "List of Prokaryotic names with Standing in Nomenclature" database in January 2020: *A. communis* (strain 5CBH24; DSM 108979; JCM 32850), *A. dispar* (5CPEGH6; DSM 108978; JCM 32848), and the sub-speciation scheme for *A. Onderdonkii* as subsp. *vulgaris* subsp. nov. and the subsp. *onderdonkii* subsp. nov. (https://lpsn.dsmz.de/genus/alistipes, which listed only 11 species on May 12, 2020) (10).

Anecdotally, the first species of *Alistipes* to be discovered was *A. finegoldii* (fi.ne.gol'di.i) which was then named after Sydney M. Finegold (born in 1921; died on September 27, 2018, age 97), a contemporary American researcher in anaerobic bacteriology and infectious diseases clinician who held several Emeritus academic positions at the UCLA and the Wardsworth VA Hospital in Los Angeles since the year 2000 (7, 11). Several recent articles commemorate Dr. Finegold's career in anaerobic microbiology, who greatly contributed to our understanding of anaerobes, which led to the species of *Alistipes* being named after him (12). With a remarkable productivity, Dr. Finegold left a legacy with 819 publications on various aspects of medicine and anaerobic microbiology (13). Alongside *A. finegoldii*, in 2003, *Bacteroides putredinis* was reclassified as *A. putredinis* based on 16S rRNA gene sequencing and biochemical features that showed this species did not belong to the genus *Bacteroides*, but to the genus *Alistipes* (7). Dr. Finegold's charisma is illustrated with the species *A. onderdoinklii*, which was named to honour Andrew B. Onderdonk, a contemporary American microbiologist, Professor of Pathology at Harvard Medical School, for his contribution to intestinal and anaerobic microbiology.

In recent years, several studies have investigated the alterations in bacterial abundance for *Alistipes* in human patients and mouse models during disease. Studies have shown that *Alistipes* dysbiosis can be either beneficial, or harmful. *Alistipes* has been implicated in liver fibrosis (14), colorectal cancer (15), cardiovascular disease (16), and mood disorders (17), among other potential diseases. Additionally, the unique way of fermenting amino acids, putrefaction, has implicated *Alistipes* to play a critical role in inflammation and disease (18). The objective of this review is to expound upon the relationship between *Alistipes* and several non-communicable diseases and to highlight the implications of *Alistipes* dysbiosis.

PHENOTYPING, CULTURE, AND SPECIATION

Alistipes is classified as gram-negative, rod-shaped, anaerobic, and non-spore forming. The species within this genus are non-motile except for *A. obesi*. The genus consists of 12-published species (*A. massiliensis* is not yet published, see above). *Alistipes finegoldii* (type strain AHN 2437^T; CCUG 46020) has circular colonies (0.3–1.0 mm; raised, gray to opaque on sheep blood agar). Despite supplementation, its growth is difficult in liquid media. *Alistipes finegoldii* is bile-resistant and esculin-negative. This bacterium is catalase-negative and nitrogen-reductase negative; and it cannot liquefy gelatin in liquefaction test. This bacterium can hydrolyze tryptophan to indole. In peptone yeast glucose (PYG) broth the major acid produced is succinic acid with a minor amount of acetic and propionic acid produced. The main fatty acid is 13-metyltetradecanoic acid (iso-C15:0). These strains of *A. finegoldii* are resistant to vancomycin, kanamycin, and colistin, as it is expected for *Bacteroides,* according to the Wadsworth manual (19) (named after the hospital where Dr. Finegold worked as a physician and scientist). For the primary identification of anaerobic bacteria, the further use of a bile susceptibility test combined with the antimicrobial resistance helps in differentiating *Alistipes* species as illustrated for some species below (for comparison, *Bacteroides* are resistant to bile) (20), although the precise definition of a species is a subject of constant debate (21). The phenotypic characteristics

TABLE 1 | Summary of first 10 *Alistipes* species and their characteristics.

	A. finegoldii: human appendiceal tissue	***A. putredinis:*** feces, appendicitis, abdom/rectal abscess foot rot sheep, farm soil	***A. onderdonkii:*** abdominal abscess	***A. shahii:*** appendix tissue, urine	***A. indistinctus:*** human feces	***A. timonensis:*** feces, healthy patients Senegal	***A. senegalensis:*** feces, healthy patients Senegal	***A. obesi:*** fecal flora of a French patient suffering from obesity	***A. ihumii:*** fecal flora of female French patient; severe anorexia nervosa	***A. inops:*** human feces
Gram stain	–	–	–	–	–	–	–	–	–	–
Motile	–	–	–	–	–	–	–	+	–	–
Bile resistant	+	–	+	+	–	/	/	/	/	/
Pigment	+	–	+	+	–	+	+	/	/	/
Esculin	–	/	/	/	/	/	/	/	/	/
Gelatin	+	/	/	/	/	/	/	/	/	/
Catalase	–	+	–	–	+	+	+	+	–	–
Nitrogen red.	–	–	–	–	–	/	/	–	–	–
Indole	+	+	+	+	–	+	+	–	–	+
Fermentative	F	NF	F	F	/	NF	F	NF	/	NF
Urease	/	–	–	–	–	/	/	–	–	–

Antibiotic Resistance. A. finegoldii, vancomycin, kanamycin, and colistin. A. putredinis, his strain is sensitive to clindamycin, cefoxitin, chloramphenicol, erythromycin, and metronidazole and moderately resistant to tetracycline and doxycycline. A. timonensis, susceptible to penicillin G, amoxicillin + clavulanic acid, imipenem and clindamycin; A. timonensis is susceptible to metronidazole. A. senegalensis, susceptible to penicillin G, amoxicillin + clavulanic acid, imipenem and clindamycin; A. senegalensis is resistant to metronidazole. A. obesi, susceptible to imipenem, ciprofloxacin, metronidazole, nitrofurantoin, and rifampicin, but resistant to penicillin G, amoxicillin, amoxicillin-clavulanic acid, erythromycin, vancomycin, gentamicin, doxycycline, ceftriaxone, and trimethoprim/sulfamethoxazole. A. ihummi, susceptible to amoxicillin, imipenem, and clindamycin, but resistant to vancomycin. /, not reported; F, fermentative; NF, non-fermentative.

of 10 *Alistipes* spp. in culture media are summarized in **Table 1**.

From a clinical perspective, it is reasonable to expect that bile-resistant strains are more likely to be present or abundant than bile-susceptible strains in the terminal ileum where most bile reabsorption takes place in several mammalian species including humans (22) and where chronic inflammatory bowel conditions are more likely to occur due to alterations in bile-mediated T-cell immunoreactivity (23). However, with the recent discovery of this genus, and the emerging complexity of the genus speciation, it will be necessary to determine if the resistance to bile acids indeed determines the *Alistipes* abundance regionally within the GI, or clinically in diseases characterized by alterations in bile production, which originates in the liver, or their recirculation pathways through the small intestine. Also, clinically relevant, some strains produce beta-lactamases (7), which enhance their antimicrobial resistance to beta-lactam antibiotics including penicillin and cephalosporins.

The species *A. putredinis* (type strain ATCC 29800^T) has been isolated from various specimens such as feces, appendiceal tissue of a patient with acute appendicitis, abdominal and rectal abscesses, foot rot in sheep, and even farm soil (7). This species has circular to slightly irregular convex colonies (pinpoint to 0.5 mm; smooth, translucent to gray). This is a non-pigment producing species and is not 20% bile-resistant. It is catalase-positive and nitrate reductase- and urease-negative. This bacterium can hydrolyze tryptophan to indole. This species is non-fermentative. In 6-day old PYG broth only trace amount of acid was produced, however, in 24-h chopped meat carbohydrate broth succinic acid was produced as a major acid product with minor amounts of acetic, isobutyric, isovaleric, and propionic acid. This strain is sensitive to clindamycin, cefoxitin, chloramphenicol, erythromycin, and metronidazole and moderately resistant to tetracycline and doxycycline (7).

Alistipes onderdonkii (type strain WAL 8169^T; CCUG 48946^T; ATCC BAA-1178^T) and *A. shahii* (type strain WAL 8301^T; CCUG 48947^T; ATCC BAA-1179^T) were isolated from abdominal abscess and appendix tissue respectively, as well as urine (24). They have circular colonies (0.5–0.8 mm and 0.5–1 mm, respectively; gray to opaque on blood agar) and are pigment producing, non-fluorescing when grown on rabbit blood agar. Both species are resistant to 20% bile and hydrolyze tryptophan to indole. They are catalase-, nitrogen reductase-, and urease-negative. Mannose and raffinose are fermented when using the API rapid ID 32A system. Succinic acid is the major metabolic end-product with minor production of acetic and propionic acid. The primary long-chain fatty acid is iso-C15:0 (24). Details for *A. onderdonkii* subspeciation as *vulgaris* subsp. nov. (3BBH6T = JCM 32839T = DSM 108977T, isolated from human feces) for can be found at https://lpsn.dsmz.de/genus/alistipes.

Alistipes indistinctus (type strain YIT 12060^T; DSM 22520^T; JCM 16068^T) was the next species to be discovered. It was isolated from human feces. This species is slightly different, since its shape is more coccoid than rod-shaped, as well as its inability to hydrolyze tryptophan to indole. Its colonies are circular (0.1–0.5 mm slight opaque and gray on modified GAM agar). This bacterium is susceptible to 20% bile, catalase-positive, and urease- and nitrogen reductase-negative. The major products in PYG broth are succinic and acetic acid. The major cellular fatty acid is iso-C15:0 (25).

Two other species, *A. senegalensis* (type strain JC50^T; CSUR P156; DSM 25460) and *A. timonensis* (type strain *JC136^T; CSUR P148; DSM 25383),* were initially isolated from the fecal flora of healthy patients in Senegal. They have circular colonies (0.2–0.3 mm) and are pigment producing. They are catalase and can hydrolyze tryptophan to indole. *A. senegalensis* does ferment mannose, and *A. timonensis* does not. These strains of bacteria are susceptible to penicillin G, amoxicillin plus clavulanic acid, imipenem, and clindamycin. Furthermore, *A. senegalensis* strains are resistant to metronidazole and *A. timonensis* strains are susceptible to metronidazole (21, 26).

Alistipes obesi (type strain ph8^T; CSUR; P186;DSM 25724) was isolated from the fecal microbiota of a French patient suffering from obesity (27). It is a pigment producing species with colonies that are 0.5 mm in diameter; translucent and light gray on blood enriched Columbia agar. It is catalase-positive, nitrogen reductase-, and urease-negative as well as non-fermentative. This bacterium cannot hydrolyze tryptophan to indole. These strains are susceptible to imipenem, ciprofloxacin, metronidazole, nitrofurantoin, and rifampicin, but resistant to penicillin G, amoxicillin, amoxicillin-clavulanic acid, erythromycin, vancomycin, gentamicin, doxycycline, ceftriaxone, and trimethoprim/sulfamethoxazole (27).

Alistipes ihumii (type strain AP11^T; CSUR P204; DSM 26107) was isolated from the fecal microbiota of a female French patient suffering from severe anorexia nervosa. This species forms colonies that are 0.2 mm and translucent on blood-enriched Columbia agar. This bacterium is non-fermentative. It is negative for urease, nitrate reduction, and catalase activity. This bacterium cannot hydrolyze tryptophan to indole. *A. ihumii* strains are susceptible to amoxicillin, imipenem, and clindamycin, but resistant to vancomycin (28).

The species *Alistipes inops* (type strain 627^T; 5DSM 28863^T; VKM B-2859^T) was isolated from human feces. The colonies are circular (0.18–0.30 mm; light gray, with a pale brown center). It has scanty growth on liquid media. It is positive for indole production and negative for catalase, nitrate reductase, and urease. This bacterium is non-fermentative. The major metabolic end products in PYG broth are succinic and acetic acid. The major fatty acid is iso C15:0 (8).

Recently, between November 2019–January 2020, four, new species of *Alistipes* were discovered, *A. megaguti*, *A. provencensis*, *A. communis* (type strain 5CBH24; DSM 108979; JCM 32850, commonly in human feces) and *A. dispar* (5CPEGH6; DSM 108978; JCM 32848, from human feces). *A. megaguti* (type strain Marseille-P5997^T) was isolated from a fresh fecal sample of a young healthy female. This species forms colonies that are 0.2–0.9 mm in diameter on blood-enriched Columbia agar. *A. megaguti* are catalase, urease, and oxidase negative. *A. provencensis* (type strain Marseille-P2431^T) was isolated from a male patient with hypertension and diabetes. This species forms colonies that are 0.4–0.64 mm in diameter on blood-enriched Columbia agar. This species is oxidase and urease negative, and catalase positive (29).

The phenotypic identification of *Alistipes* species is feasible (**Table 1**), yet challenging. A more suitable way to identify *Alistipes* spp. is via NGS (next generation sequencing-based microbiome studies) (30). However, most studies for the classification of new species, which cannot be fully sequenced have been based on Sanger sequencing of the full gene or parts of the 16S rRNA gene. For reference, the specificity of various primers employed for the identification of *Alistipes* species are listed and referenced in **Table 2**, while the details in nucleotide sequence homology and genetic distances within the genus are depicted in **Figure 1**. Compared to culture techniques, the NGS method is more powerful for bacterial identification. However, it does not provide information on the metabolic functions of the organism. Another form of bacterial identification is through metagenomic studies. In this approach, bacterial DNA is processed and sequenced along with host DNA. A new clinical approach that is faster and more effective than Sanger sequencing for bacterial classification is based on mass-spectrometry. Specifically, new rapid high-through put strategies based on matrix assisted laser desorption/ionization time-of-flight mass spectrometry (MALDI-TOF MS) have become widely adapted and common in clinical microbiological settings, which require the constant update of databases to incorporate the spectral of new bacterial strains, primarily of clinical relevance.

MASS SPECTROSCOPY FOR IDENTIFICATION OF BACTERIAL SPECIES

Since the innovative use of MALDI-TOF MS to expedite the identification of microbes in clinical microbiology, there has been a major increase in our understanding of the presence and prevalence of *Alistipes* spp. in clinical medicine. MALDI-TOF MS is a method based on protein spectra, enabling identification of an unknown bacterium within minutes. Due to the introduction of this method in diagnostic microbiology laboratories, fastidious organisms which could previously only be identified using molecular methods, are now identified with ease. With the advancement of MALDI-TOF MS, there has been collaborative initiatives to improve microbial identification, including the European Network of Rapid Identification of Anaerobes (ENRIA), which is multi-national consortium of laboratories in Europe with the goal of unifying the MALDI-TOF MS database for the rapid identification of clinical anaerobes. According to the ENRIA validation study, conducted in 2018 (38), at present 5 *Alistipes* species are represented in the MALDI-TOF MS database: *A. finegoldii*, *A. onderdonkii*, *A. shahii*, *A. indistinctus*, and *A. putredinis*.

TABLE 2 | Referent partial Sanger 16S rRNA gene sequences and primers for *Alistipes* spp.

Species (strain)	Accession	F-primer 5′-3′
A. finegoldii (30) CIP 107999	AY643083 AY643084 1,446 bp	fD1 ccgaattcgtcgacaacAGAGTTTGATCCTGGCTCAG* rP2-cccgggatccaagcttACGGCTACCTTGTTACGACTT*
A. putredinis (31) ATCC 29800	NR_025909 1,468 bp	
A. onderdonkii (24) WAL 8169	NR_043318 1,440 bp	
A. shahii (24) WAL 8301	AY974072 1,433 bp	
A. indistinctus (25) YIT 12060	NR_112896 1,482 bp	
A. timonensis (32) JC136	NR_125589 1,423 bp	
A. senegalensis (32) JC50	NR_118219 1,423 bp	
A. obesi (32) ph8	NR_133025 1,388 bp	
A. ihumii (28) AP11	NR_144706 1,494 bp	
A. inops (8) *627*	NR_145882 1,237 bp	
A. megaguti (29) Marseille-P5997	fig|2364787.3.rna.19 Complete 1,534 bp** LS999984 1,525 bp	
A. provencensis (29) Marseille-P2431	LT223566 1,491 bp	
Tidjanibacter massiliensis	LT598563 1,492 bp	
A. Onderdonkii subsp vulgaris	LC468789 1456bp	LC468802*** 558bp
A. dispar	LC468801 1464bp	LC46889*** 558bp
A. communis	LC468799 1484bp	LC468808*** 558bp

Position Sequence for most *Bacteroides* subgroup
104–121 GTTACTCACCCGTGCGCC[(a)]
288–307 ACCTTCCTCTCAGAACCCCT [(b)]
344–358 ACTGCTGCCTCCCGT
519–536 GWATTACCGCGGCKGCTG
553–572 TAAACCCAATAAATCCGGAT[(c)]
786–803 CTACCAGGGTATCTAATC
907–926 CCGTCAATTCMTTTRAGTTT[(c)]
1092–1114 GGGTTGCGCTCGTTATGGCACTT [(c)]
1225–1242 CCATTGTAACACGTGTGT GGCGGTGTGTRC [(c)]
1487–1505 CCTTGTTACGACTTAGCCC
Standard IUB codes for bases and ambiguity

Inset table, See details in Paster et al. (31). Primer sequence specificity slightly varying across gene positions [(a)] *Bacteroides* + *Prevotella* except *Prevotella nigrescens, P. intermedia*. No porphyromonas. [(b)] *Bacteroides* + *Prevotella*, but also for *Parabacteroides distasonis*, butyric acid-producing *Odoribacter splanchnicus* comb. nov. (33, 34), and periodontitis-associated *Tannerella forsythia* (formerly, *Bacteroides forsythus*), and biofilm-associated *Rikenella microfusus* (35). [(c)] Most bacteria with some exceptions for *P. saccharolytica* (35) and periodontitis associated *Porphyromona endodontalis* (36), *A. putredinis*, *O. splanchnicus*, and *R. microfusus*

**Primers (upper case) used by Weisburg et al. (37) and designed for most eubacteria. f, forward; r, reverse; D, distal; P, proximal. Linker sequences containing restriction sites for cloning are designated in lower case. The "f" series of linkers contain EcoRI and SalI sites, and the "r" series contain HindIJI, BamHI, and XmaI recognition sequences. Reverse primers produce sequences complimentary to the rRNA. Primers rPI, rP2, and rP3 are identical except for the 17th base from the 3′ end. The P2 primer was determined as the sequence providing the greatest diversity of bacteria. FASTA files available for download at https://www.ncbi.nlm.nih.gov/search/all/?term=NR__125589 **complete sequence extracted from complete genome available in PATRIC https://docs.patricbrc.org.*

****Phylogenetic analysis for speciation can also be conducted for Alistipes using the heat shock protein 60 gene (hsp60) as reported by Sakamoto in 2020. Accession numbers for the whole genome sequences of strains 3BBH6T, 5CBH24T, 5CPEGH6T, 5CPYCFAH4, 5NYCFAH2 and 6CPBBH3 are AP019734-AP019739, respectively.*

To contextualize the current relevance of the genus in clinical diagnostics, we conducted a screening of the number of *Alistipes* isolates recovered from human clinical samples at the University Medical Center Groningen, Groningen, the Netherlands, within the 7 years prior to submission of this manuscript. Keeping in mind that only species represented in MALDI-TOF MS databases have been identified using this method, it is noteworthy to mention that only 11 ($n = 11$) clinical isolates belonged to the *Alistipes* genus. Of relevance, these isolates were identified only as either *A. onderdonkii* ($n = 7$) or *A. finegoldii* ($n = 4$). The *Alistipes* isolates were recovered from pus, blood, ascites fluid or from an unspecified specimen. Considering that there have been at least 13 different species identified as distinct according to the NCBI lineage database (as of November 2019), it is interesting that only few species ($n = 5$) have been identified in clinical settings screened by ENRIA. The lack of identification of the other species (e.g., *A. senegalensis, A. timonensis, A. obesi, A. ihumii*, and *A. inops*) in this population indicated that either: (i) *Alistipes* may have specific patterns of geographically-restricted distribution, (ii) that their prevalence in the environment and patients is rather low, (iii) that they are comparatively more difficult to be cultured from clinical specimens using media that apparently facilitates the recovery of the other *Alistipes* spp. (namely, *A onderdonkii* and *A. finegoldii*), (iv) that the MS profile used

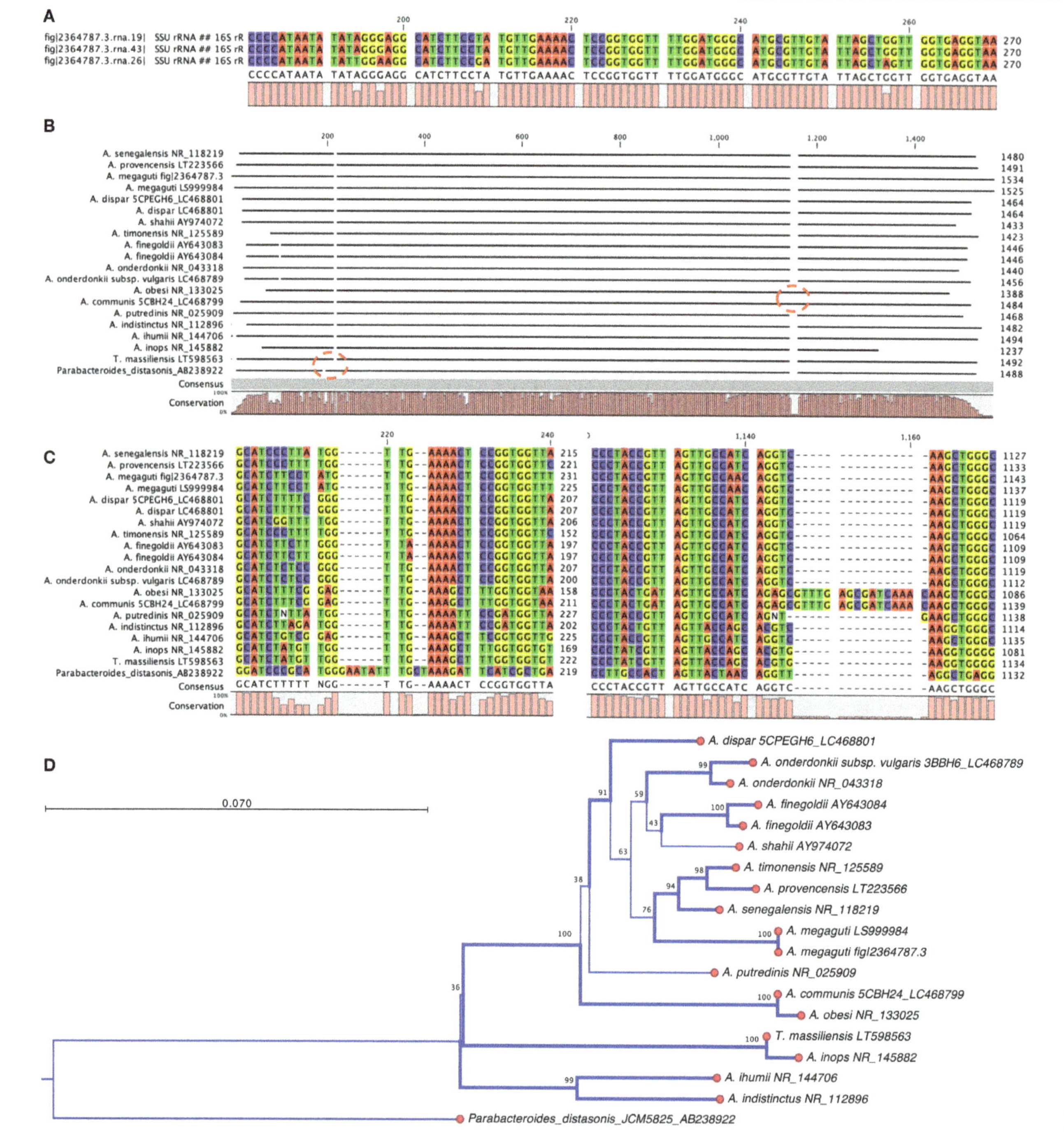

FIGURE 1 | Nucleotide and phylogram of 16S rRNA gene DNA sequences from thirteen strains described in the genus *Alistipes*. **(A)** *Alsitipes megaguti* complete 16S rRNA gene sequences derived from PATRIC complete genome illustrates slight differences between three gene copies contained within three operons in a single genome. Only the most divergent parts of the genes are shown. **(B)** Overview of complete alignment for the 13 strains. Notice the *A. obesi* insertion at around 1,100 bp position. **(C)** Detail of sequence insertion in the *A. obesi* starting at position 1,137 bp position. **(D)** Overview of the distance tree with 10,000 bootstrap branch values depicted if value >90%. Branching set at 60% threshold. Notice that differences may occur in part due to uneven partial gene sequences. Analysis conducted with CLC genomics viewer. Notice position of *T. massiliensis* vs. *A. inops* and *A. putredinis*.

to differentiate species is still suboptimal to discriminate such species as separate, or (v) that the original species descriptions may not be reproducible descriptions in the context of culture and mass spectrometry profiles.

ECOLOGY IN DISEASES

According to the NCBI, the full lineage of *Alistipes* is Bacteria; *Bacteroidetes*; *Bacteroidia*; *Bacteroidales*; *Rikenellaceae* (NCBI:

txid239759). Therefore, *Alistipes* is a genus member of the *Rikenellaceae* family (NCBI:t xid171550), which is a small family within the *Bacteroidales* order that is composed of eight genera: *Acetobacteroides, Alistipes, Anaerocella, Millionella, Mucinivorans, Rikenella, Ruminofilibacter*, and *Tidjanibacter*. These genera are commonly found in the intestinal tract of various animals and humans, where they are believed to have symbiotic relationships with the host. One of the most commonly detected species from the genus *Alistipes*, that can be isolated from human feces, is *A. onderdonkii* (39).

From an ecological perspective, *Alistipes* is found primarily in the gut of healthy humans (8). However, *Alistipes* has also been isolated from the blood stream, as well as appendicular, abdominal, perirectal and brain abscesses highlighting their potential opportunistic pathogenic role in human diseases. *Alistipes* has been found in other body fluids, namely, urine and peritoneal fluid (8). Of contrasting interest within this genus, *A. ihumii* has been isolated from the feces of a patient suffering from anorexia nervosa, while *A. obesi* was isolated from a patient suffering from morbid obesity. Combining the later observations with the fact that *Alistipes finegoldii* has been considered a growth promoter in broiler chickens (40), and *A. putredinis* has been observed to increase with cruciferous vegetable intake in humans (41), it is reasonable to assume that different *Alistipes* species may have different roles in nutrition and health, depending on the host, and the bodily system influenced. Although the NCBI taxonomy database has a disclaimer stating that it is not an authoritative source for nomenclature or classification, the NCBI recommend the database users to consult the relevant scientific literature for the most reliable information, which is summarized below and in **Table 3**.

ALISTIPES IN LIVER DISEASE AND SHORT-CHAIN FATTY ACIDS

Hepatocellular carcinoma (HCC) is the second deadliest form of cancer worldwide (55).

HCC is often developed from advanced liver fibrosis that is caused by cirrhosis, non-alcoholic fatty liver disease (NAFLD), or non-alcoholic steatohepatitis (NASH). These liver diseases have been associated with the "microbiota-liver axis," indicating that dysbiosis as one of the potential causes (56). In studies done on the microbiota composition and liver fibrosis. It is seen that throughout the advancement of the fibrosis that *Alistipes* is decreased.

For example, in patients with compensated and decompensated liver cirrhosis (LC), a paired-end metagenomic sequence of the gut microbiome from fresh stool samples of healthy volunteers and patients with various types of LC. This study showed a decrease of *A. shahii* and *A. putredinis* when compared to healthy controls. This finding of an increase in the abundance of *Alistipes* in healthy control patients in comparison to patients with LC has also been seen in studies focusing on feces and biopsies of LC patients (57). Moreover, a decrease of *A. indistinctus* was observed as the disease progressed from compensated to decompensated (43). Once an individual has decompensated liver cirrhosis, the patient begins to generate a multitude of severe complications, such as hepatic encephalopathy. Another study showed that when comparing stool microbiome between patients suffering from decompensated liver cirrhosis with acute hepatic encephalopathy, *Alistipes* has a protective role and the decrease in its abundance correlates to an increase of hepatic encephalopathy recurrence (44). Thus, a decrease in *Alistipes* spp. correlates with the progression of liver cirrhosis into the decompensated state.

Additionally, the reduction in *Alistipes* abundance in patients with liver fibrosis can be seen in other fibrotic diseases such NASH and NAFLD. Rau et al. (14) showed that patients with NAFLD with substantial fibrosis had a reduction in fecal concentration of acetate and propionate, with no significant difference in butyrate concentration. When comparing healthy controls with patients suffering from NASH, there is a significant reduction in *A. finegoldii* with the normalized count mean reduced from 542 to 19 (fold-change of −1.829). Moreover, in NAFLD patients with significant fibrosis, a major reduction in *A. onderdonkii* was observed from 285 to 31 (fold change of −2.566). It is noteworthy that *Alistipes* spp. decreases in these advanced fibrotic patients as well as fecal acetate and propionate levels. This correlates with a study done by Polansky et al. (58) where they showed that in the cecal microbiota of chickens that *Alistipes* is a propionate producer expressing methylmalonyl-CoA epimerase, in which the gene for this enzyme is located on an operon with the acetyl-CoA carboxylase gene. It has also been shown that *Alistipes* is an acetate producer (59). Due to previous studies suggesting that short chain fatty acids (SCFAs) have anti-inflammatory mechanisms, it can be suggested that this decrease in *Alistipes* contributes to the decrease in SCFA and therefore contributes to the advanced fibrosis seen in these NAFLD patients.

Moreover, a study performed on mice with HCC showed the potential anti-inflammatory effects of a health-beneficial bacteria probiotic. It was believed that T-regs would be induced in patients with HCC thus suppressing the Th17 expression. A probiotic entitled Prohep was used, and after 38 days a reduction in tumor growth and Th17 cells was observed. Moreover, there was an increase in Treg/Tr1 cells, an anti-inflammatory cell subset. *Alistipes* was shown to increase in abundance in the mice cohort receiving the probiotic (45, 60). At the species level it is shown that *A. shahii* was one of the species that was significantly increased in the probiotic group. They hypothesize that *A. shahii* was playing a role in tumor suppression similar to what was is seen in cancer immunotherapy (61). Additionally, the investigators noted a significant increase in acetate and propionate metabolic potential in the probiotic group correlating with an increase in SCFAs-producing bacteria, such as *Alistipes* contributing to the suppression of Th17 cells in the gut, ultimately reducing the recruitment of Th17 cells to the liver (45). Also, in past studies it has been shown that SCFAs derived from fermented dietary fibers increase the levels of propionate found within the portal vein ultimately preventing cancer cell proliferation in liver tissue (62). Ultimately, *Alistipes*

TABLE 3 | Summary of studies reporting the experimental or observational associations between *Alistipes* spp. and various non-communicable diseases (2003–2019).

Disease	Study model	Study design	*Alistipes* effects
Inflammation Colitis (42) (Protective)*	Mice: BALB/c	Oral DSS-colitis. 16S microbiome and oral infection.	Pglyrp1-4 (antibacterial immunomodulator gene) KO mice have less *Alistipes* spp. Oral *A. finegoldii* attenuates antibiotic > DSS-colitis in WT mice
Inflammation Liver cirrhosis (43) (Protective)	Humans: China	Meta-omics-based study analyzing urine and stool samples from health controls, compensated and decompensated LC patients	In both compensated and decompensated LC patients *A. shahii* and *A. putredinis* decrease and during progression from compensated to decompensated *A. indistinctus* further decreased
Inflammation Acute hepatic encephalopathy (44) (Protective)	Humans: Taiwan	Longitudinal cohort before treatment, 2–3 d after, and 2–3 mo after	*Alistipes* decreases during AHE compared to healthy controls, compensated, and decompensated cirrhosis. Also associated with recurrence at 1 year
Inflammation NASH/NAFLD (14) (Protective)	Humans: Germany	16S rRNA sequencing of stool	*A. finegoldii* decreased in NASH when compared to healthy controls. *A. onderdonkii* was reduced in patients with NAFLD
Inflammation Hepatocellular carcinoma, HCC (45) (Protective)	Mice: Male C57BL6/N	Metagenomic study using the stool of control mice vs. mice with tumor. The mice were fed probiotic [mixture (1:1:1) of *Lactobacillus rhamnosus* GG, *Escherichia coli* Nissle 1917 and heat inactive VSL#3]	*Alistipes* spp. and *A. shahii* increased in mice receiving the probiotic, in which there was modulation in pro-inflammatory cytokines in tumor microenvironment
Cancer Colorectal cancer (46) (Pathogenic)	Mice: C57BL/6J	qPCR/16S rRNA seq. to identify *Alistipes* in $Lcn2^{-/-}$, $Il10^{-/-}$ mice. $Il10^{-/-}$ mice gavaged with *A. finegoldii* to determine tumor localization.	*Alistipes* promotes colorectal cancer via IL-6/STAT3 pathway causing right sided tumorigenesis
Cardiovascular Atrial fibrillation (16) (Protective)	Humans: China	Metagenomic and metabolomic analyses of fecal samples extracted from patients with non-vascular atrial fibrillation or HC	*Alistipes* decreases in abundance in atrial fibrillation group when compared to HC
Cardiovascular Hypertension (47, 48) (Pathogenic)	Humans: America	Metagenomics of DNA extracted from fecal samples. High blood pressure (HBP) vs. controls.	*A. finegoldii* and *A. indistinctus* increase in HBP; LPS increase, Th17 cells, and inflammation; in HBP decrease in butyrate-producing cells; increase plasma intestinal fatty acid binding protein (I-FABP); and gut epithelial tight junction Zonulin
Cardiovascular Congestive heart failure (49) (Protective)	Humans: China	Metagenomics of DNA extracted from fecal samples	*Alistipes* decreased together with *Faecalibacterium* and *Oscillibacter*, while *Ruminococcus*, *Acinetobacter*, and *Veillonella* increased
Cardiovascular atherosclerosis cardiovascular disease (50) (Protective)	Humans: China	Metagenomics of DNA extracted from fecal samples	*Alistipes shahii* decreases together with *Bacteroides* spp., *Prevotella copri*, in ACVD
Mental health Anxiety (17) (Pathogenic)	Mice: BALB/c	Stress induced by grid floor housing. DGGE,16S Microbiome, Triple test, tail suspension test, and burrowing	*Alistipes* spp. increased after 2 weeks on grid floor housing. There was also significant change in the mice behavior
Mental health Myalgic encephal. Chronic fatigue (51) (Pathogenic)	Humans: Belgium Norway	16S rRNA sequencing of stool.	3.8-fold increase of *Alistipes* spp. in Norwegian patients vs. Norwegian controls
Mental health depression (52) (Pathogenic)	Humans: China	Pyrosequencing of DNA from feces of either healthy controls of patients with active- and responded-major depressive disorder (MMD).	*Alistipes* increases in both A-MDD and R-MDD groups when compared to HC; due to being indole positive decrease in serotonin availability. *Faecalibacterium* decreases in MMD
Mental health Autism spectrum disorder (53) (Protective)	Humans: Italy	Pyrosequencing using 16S rRNA from stool samples of 40 autistic and 40 neurotypical pediatric patients	*Alistipes* decreased with *Bilophila*, *Dialister, Parabacteroides, Veillonella. Collinsella, Dorea Corynebacterium,* and *Lactobacillus* increased
Mental health PDD-NOS (autism) (54) (Pathogenic)	Humans: Italian children	bTEFAP analysis on DNA and cDNA samples from each patient and pyrosequencing of 16S rDNA and rRNA	*Alistipes* was found at the highest abundance in AD and PDD-NO; possibly due to high production of propionic acid which has been shown to have neurobiological effects in rats

**Protective; overall interpretation of results with respect to outcome for each disease.*

can be seen as a potential SCFA producer and their decrease contributes to these hepatic fibrotic conditions due to a decrease in anti-inflammatory cytokines and inability to suppress Th17 cells. Further studies will be important in the near future to better define the role of this genus in liver pathologies and health.

ALISTIPES IN CARDIOVASCULAR DISEASE, HYPERTENSION, AND THE EPITHELIUM

Cardiovascular disease (CVD) is the leading cause of mortality and morbidity in both developing and developed countries (5). With CVDs projected to rise in the future as the global population ages, the evaluation of the relationship with the gut microbiota has been investigated more extensively. *Alistipes* has been linked with CVD risk factors such as hypertension, as well as several CVDs such as atrial fibrillation (AF), congestive heart failure (CHF), and atherosclerosis cardiovascular disease (ACVD) (50).

In hypertension, it is believed that *Alistipes* contributes to inflammation and epithelium alterations. Kim et al. (48) demonstrated the relationship between the gut barrier dysfunction in patients with hypertension and the gut microbiota in humans. They used shotgun metagenomic analysis studying fecal samples from 22 patients with high blood pressure and 18 control patients. The data revealed an increase in *A. finegoldii* and *A. indistinctus* that was positively correlated with systolic blood pressure. Additionally, it was shown that *A. finegoldii*, known to trigger intestinal inflammation, had an increased number and functional genes in the high blood pressure cohort. Overall, the increase in *A. finegoldii* was observed to be positively correlated with systolic blood pressure (SBP), suggesting that this species is a potential driver for gut barrier dysfunction and inflammation in patients with high blood pressure. Also, it is believed that the hypotensive phenotype of inflammation is caused by the lipopolysaccharide (LPS) in *Alistipes*, which is known to be pro-inflammatory, leading to an increase in Th17 cells expressing CD161 and CCR6/integrin Beta7, as well as the decrease in butyrate-producing bacteria, which are known to be anti-inflammatory (47). Despite such argument, it is important to highlight that several other types of anaerobic bacteria, including species within the *Bacteroides* genus, may also contribute to the complexity of disease attributes conferred to date to the *Alistipes* genus. Further studies will be critical to elucidate more precise mechanisms.

Various studies have indicated that *Alistipes* plays a protective role in CVDs. Additionally, *Alistipes* has been associated directly with CVDs such as atrial fibrillation (AF). Atrial fibrillation is the most common arrhythmia and is prevalent in patients with hypertension, heart failure, and obesity (63). Atrial fibrillation is characterized on an EKG by the absence of P waves with irregular R-R intervals due to irregular beating of the atria leading to irregular conduction of impulses to the ventricles (64). In a study by Zuo et al. (16), conducted to quantify the relationship between the gut microbiome and AF, a whole-metagenomic shotgun sequence performed on 100 stool samples from Chinese participants, showed a drastic decrease in *Alistipes* spp. in the intestinal tract of patients with AF. However, bacteria that drastically increased during AF, such as *Streptococcus*, were proposed in the study to be the cause of the decline in *Alistipes*, suggesting a potential antagonistic effect between *Alistipes* and *Streptococcus*. This trend was commonly seen in other heart conditions, such as ACVD (50) and CHF (49). Evidence for the involvement of *Alistipes* in CVD is contradictory; that is, it is unclear if associations are protective or beneficial or pathogenic. Because most CVDs share common pathophysiological characteristics, such as endothelial dysfunction (16), it is possible that the role of *Alistipes* may depend on disease mechanisms shared across several CDVs. Therefore, more studies on the gut-heart axis could lead to the future understanding of microbiome-related diseases and potential therapies.

ALISTIPES IN GUT INFLAMMATION AND OTHER *BACTEROIDETES*

Due to the diverse microbial community in the gastrointestinal tract, there is a strong correlation between dysbiosis and inflammatory bowel disease (IBD). The most common IBDs within the human population are Crohn's disease (CD) and ulcerative colitis (UC). UC is a chronic inflammatory disease that primarily targets the colon. It has been suggested that *A. finegoldii* is a protective species against colitis since *A. finegoldii* is decreased in mice with colitis. Due to this fact, a study was performed in which microbiota-depleted mice were treated with oral DSS to induce colitis. When gavaged with *A. finegoldii*, the severity of colitis was similar to that of the WT mice (42). Mice developed colitis when *A. finegoldii* was added with *Bacteroides eggerthii*, a colitis- inducing bacteria, but the severity of the colitis was significantly decreased compared to that of mice with *B. eggerthii* alone or added with other bacteria such as *Parabacteroides distasonis*, or *Prevotella falsenii*. This further indicates that *A. finegoldii* is a colitis-attenuating bacteria (42). Of contrasting clinical interest, A. finegoldii has been isolated in association with other Bacteroides from gut-wall cavernous fistulous tract (CavFT) microlesions in severe Crohn's disease. The causal-effect and their prevalence in such lesions are currently under investigation in our laboratory (65–67).

A study by Butera et al. (68) showed 8 weeks old NOD2 knockout mice had an enrichment of *Alistipes*, anti-inflammatory cytokines (TGF-beta and IL-10), and $CD4^+LAP^+FoxP3^-$ regulatory T cells. A possible connection for these observations comes from studies with curcumin, a spice that has been shown to modulate bowel inflammation by increasing $CD4^+LAP^+FoxP3^-$ cells via IL-10 (69). To test to see the severity of the NOD2 knock-out in mice with colitis, they induced colitis via intra-rectal administration of 2,4,6-Trinitrobenzene sulfonic acid (TNBS) and used the expression of anti-inflammatory cytokine mRNA to determine the severity. It was found that the NOD2 knock-out mice had less severe colitis than the wild-type. Also, it was noted that the severity of the colitis was related to the different proportion of $CD4^+LAP^+FoxP3^-$ cells observed prior to the TNBS treatment. Moreover, previous studies have shown a common trend of *Alistipes* abundance in NOD2 knock-out murine microbiota profiles (70). Of interest, *Alistipes* has been observed increasing among patients taking probiotics in an anti-inflammatory effect background (45). To date, it remains unclear what mechanisms of interaction exist between this genus and the other microorganisms in the gut, including food and probiotic strains, and the intramural fistulizing lessions we reported in surgical patients with CD. Metagenomic studies of fecal samples from the mouse model of spontaneous CD ileitis (SAMP1/YitFc, characterized by a fully penetrant 3D- stereomicroscopic pattern of segmental cobblestone ileitis resembling human CD) revealed an enrichment of Alistipes compared to the parental AKR/J mouse colony (cohabiting for >10 years in the same room), suggesting that Alistipes spp. could be associated with the promotion of segmental ileitis (65, 71, 72).

ALISTIPES AND CANCER VIA BENEFICIAL IMMUNOMODULATION

Cancer, like cardiovascular disease, causes high rates of mortality and morbidity worldwide. Colorectal cancer (CRC) is one of the most common types of cancer typically targeting older individuals, as well as African Americans. CRC is also a form of cancer that has been linked to dysbiosis of the gut microbiota. *Alistipes* has been found to contribute to the pathogenesis, acting as a potential pathogen. Moschen et al. (15) showed that *A. finegoldii* promotes right sided colorectal cancer via the IL-6/STAT 3 pathway. Lipocalin 2 (LCN 2), an anti-microbial protein that binds to siderophores ultimately reduces iron availability (73). In patients with IBD LCN 2 is found in high concentrations in mucosal and fecal samples. Essentially, this can reduce the prevalence of *Alistipes*, as iron is a regulatory factor for the growth of *A. finegoldii*. However, Moschen et al. (15) went on to show that *A. finegoldii* caused intestinal inflammation after 1 week of being orally administered in WT, LCN 2 KO, and IL-10 KO C57BL/6J mice. Therefore, the paper concluded that *Alistipes* thrives in an inflamed environment that lacks LCN 2 and promotes inflammation and tumor formation. Moreover, they showed that *Alistipes finegoldii* was found in higher abundance in the ceca than other locations within the large intestine.

Despite the pathogenic effects observed for *Alistipes* in CRC, this genus has been shown to have a beneficial role in cancer immunotherapy by modulating the tumor microenvironment. One of the main hallmarks of cancers is to evade the immune system. Therefore, one form of anti-cancer treatment has been to manipulate the tumor microenvironment. An example of immunotherapy is to manipulate the microenvironment by inducing tumor necrosis factor (TNF) production by tumor-associated myeloid cells which ultimately leads to tumor eradication. One way to do this is to use a combination of intra-tumoral CpG-oligodeoxynucleotides (ODN) to activate TLR9, and inhibitory IL-10R antibodies. This immunotherapy typically halts tumor growth and induces TNF-dependent hemorrhagic necrosis by tumor-associated myeloid cells leading to tumor suppression.

In a study performed by Iida et al. (61) C57Bl/6 mice were injected subcutaneously with MC38 colon carcinoma cells and pre-treated with antibiotics (vancomycin, imipenem, and neomycin). The study initially determined whether antibiotics affected cancer immunotherapy. The authors found that antibiotics led to a decrease in efficiency of the tumor eradication due to a reduction in TNF production. The investigators then determined if those results depended on the bacterial load in the intestinal tract. Therefore, germ free (GF) mice with the MC38 tumors received anti-IL-10R/CpG-ODN treatment. Treated GF mice produced a significantly lower amount of TNF than specific pathogen free (SPF) mice. This suggests that the tumor-associated innate myeloid cells are primed by microbiota for inflammatory cytokine production in response to anti-IL-10R/CpG-ODN and that the reduced bacterial load from either the antibiotic treatment or germ-free status reduces this response and the TNF-dependent early-tumor necrosis. To better understand the role of antibiotics and the role of the gut microbiota, MC38 tumor bearing mice were gavaged with LPS and the TNF expression was reestablished. When they examined the microbiota involved via fecal microbiota composition, there was a positive correlation between *Alistipes* genus and a role for TLR4-priming/TNF production. Iida et al. (61) believed the TNF restoration was due to the role of pro-inflammatory gram-negative bacteria, *A. shahii*, binding to TLR4, priming the expression of TNF production. To further prove their hypothesis, authors then showed a delay in the recovery of *A. shahii* following antibiotic treatment, which also paralleled an ~4-week phase of TNF restoration after the antibiotic administration. Furthermore, they showed that when mice that were pre-treated with antibiotic and gavaged with *A. shahii*, the tumor-associated myeloid cells function to produce TNF was restored. Clinically relevant, the study indicated that when there is a reduction in *Alistipes*, there is a parallel reduction in optimal responses to cancer immunotherapy (61).

Others have also identified a role for *Alistipes* in cancer immunotherapy. For instance, non-small cell lung carcinoma (NSCLC) has a poor prognosis and no current therapy. Recently checkpoint inhibitors for PD-1 have been proposed as a potential immunotherapy for NSCLC. However, a major number of patients still persist with poor prognosis. Nivolumab is a fully human Immunoglobulin G4 monoclonal antibody against PD-1, therefore it blocks T cells from binding to the ligand PD-1L, typically expressed by the tumor, preventing T cell exhaustion. A study to find a potential correlation between gut microbiota and patients with NSCLC responding favorably to Nivolumab was conducted that presented evidence that *A. putredinis* was increased in patients who responded well to Nivolumab correlating with the study mentioned above (74).

MENTAL HEALTH

Although *Alistipes* can be found commonly in the intestinal tract, it has been shown to have a significant effect on diseases with localization outside of the gut such depression, anxiety, chronic fatigue syndrome, autism, cirrhosis, and aging. Dysbiosis within the intestine can affect the gut-brain axis and be used to explain the relationship between the gut microbiota, depression, and other mood disorders such as anxiety.

In a study conducted with BALB/c mice placed in a stressful environment, induced by grid-floor housing, there was a significant increase in *Alistipes* abundance (17). Furthermore, *Alistipes* concentration was also found to be increased, almost 4-fold, in Norwegian patients suffering from chronic fatigue syndrome (51). These findings correlate with the evidence of an increase in *Alistipes* for patients suffering from depression, since patients with depression typically struggle with fatigue and stress (75). It is believed that this increase in *Alistipes* disrupts the gut-brain axis because *Alistipes* is an indole-positive organism, and, thus decreases serotonin availability. Tryptophan is a precursor for serotonin, and a decrease in serotonin is associated with depression (52). Moreover, *Alistipes* has been shown to express glutamate decarboxylase, an enzyme that metabolizes glutamate into γ-aminobutyric acid (GABA) in chickens (58). This increase in *Alistipes* abundance could also possibly be related to the increase in GABA. However, studies should be done to show if the GABA is being secreted into the gut lumen (58).

Additionally, there are associations between the brain and gut amongst patients suffering from autism spectrum disorder. It is often found that individuals suffering from autism have frequent GI symptoms, speculating that it could be due to a dysbiosis within the microbiota. Strati et al. (53) found that there was a decrease in *Alistipes* in patients with autism spectrum disorder. However, another study done on a different form of autism, PDD-NOS, showed a significant abundance of *Alistipes* in children (54). It has been speculated that this could be from the production of propionic acid, which has shown to have neurobiological effects in rats (76). There is need for more studies on *Alistipes* and its effects on the gut-brain axis, since there is contradictory evidence regarding its protective/pathogenic role in both systems.

SULFONOLIPIDS AND BIOCHEMICAL MARKERS

Alistipes is a genus of bacteria with numerous immunological and biochemical pathways that are associated with the diseases mentioned above. One important implication is the promotion of CRC by *Alistipes* via IL-6/STAT 3 pathway. Thus, future studies could consider the use of *Alistipes* species as potential biomarkers for CRC, using our understanding based on microbiome DNA based data and the integration of biochemical concepts on disease pathogenesis. A potential method to accomplish this would be to look for sulfonolipids, a unique class of sphingolipids with a sulfonic acid group in the sphingoid base (77). Walker et al. (78) showed that when C57BL/6N mice are fed high fat diets with either safflower oil or lard fat for 3 weeks there is an increase in sulfonolipids, as well as, body weight when compared to mice fed the normal chow diet. A metagenome analysis was performed and screened for bacterial genes involved in sulfonolipid biosynthesis in the cecum of these mice. All species of *Alistipes* were found to produce sulfonolipids except *A. inops* (information on the most recent species A. *megaguti*, *A. provencensis*, and sulfonolipid production remain unknown). To further prove that sulfonolipids are a product of bacteria and a marker of *Alistipes*, scientists performed a mono-colonization study of germ-free (GF) mice with *Alistipes* spp. and detected a significant emergence of sulfonolipids in the cecum of the mono-colonized mice that was previously absent in the GF mice. Therefore, with common risk factors of CRC being high fat diets, obesity, and age (79), in addition to the increased abundance of *Alistipes* in these colonic conditions, there is the intriguing proposition for the potential of using sulfonolipids as markers for patients at risk for developing CRC, particularly within ethnicities, such as African-Americans with family histories of CRC. Additionally, studies should be conducted to verify if *Alistipes* abundance is increased in polyps, pre-cancerous vs. cancerous, being polyps another risk factor for CRC.

Moreover, *Alistipes* has the highest number of putrefaction pathways amongst commensal bacteria. Putrefaction is the fermentation of undigested proteins in the GI tract by the gut microbiota typically leading to bacterial production of harmful metabolites (80). These products have been reported as deleterious and associated with CRC (81). Such products include ammonia, H_2S, cresol, indole, and phenol (82). In a study done to identify the main putrefaction pathways used by the gut bacteria, Kaur et al. (18), found that *Alistipes* contributed to histidine degradation/THF production, indole production, and phenol production. Histidine degradation/THF production have been found to release excess ammonia, which when absorbed, damages the colonic cells (83). Ammonia has also been found to increase intestinal cell proliferation and assist in the growth of cancer cells in CRC (84). Findings of excess ammonia and other *Alistipes* produced putrefaction products could be of use to clinicians when patients are at risk for developing CRC.

CONCLUSION, LIMITATIONS, AND FUTURE DIRECTIONS

Alistipes is a relatively new genus of bacteria isolated from clinical samples, although at a low rate compared to others within the *Bacteroidetes* phylum. At the protein level, a genome-wide protein phylogenetic analysis shown in **Figure 2** illustrates that this genus may have unique functional properties that may enable them to have unique physiological roles, compared to other members within the *Bacteroidetes*, and/or also affect our ability to isolate these species *in vitro*. Therein, it is possible that the identification of this genus in clinical samples may be underrepresented as novel MS-TOF methods may not be fully capable to discriminate distinct species as separate. Immunologically, *Alistipes* has been seen to contribute to disease in both clinical and preclinical studies. Intriguingly, other studies have shown their presence is correlated with the promotion of healthy phenotypes such as *Alistipes* protective roles in diseases such as colitis, autism spectrum disorder, and various liver and cardiovascular fibrotic disorders. Despite *Alistipes* role in healthy phenotypes, *Alistipes* contrastingly has been shown to have a pathogenic role in diseases such as anxiety, myalgic encephalomyelitis/chronic fatigue syndrome, depression, PDD-NOS, and CRC.

Collectively, this review represents a summary of studies where *Alistipes* has been experimentally tested after inoculation into animal models, or where *Alistipes* has been found among other abnormally present species in human or animal microbiome studies. Thus, the perspective here presented, indicates that the genus, depending on the study discussed, could

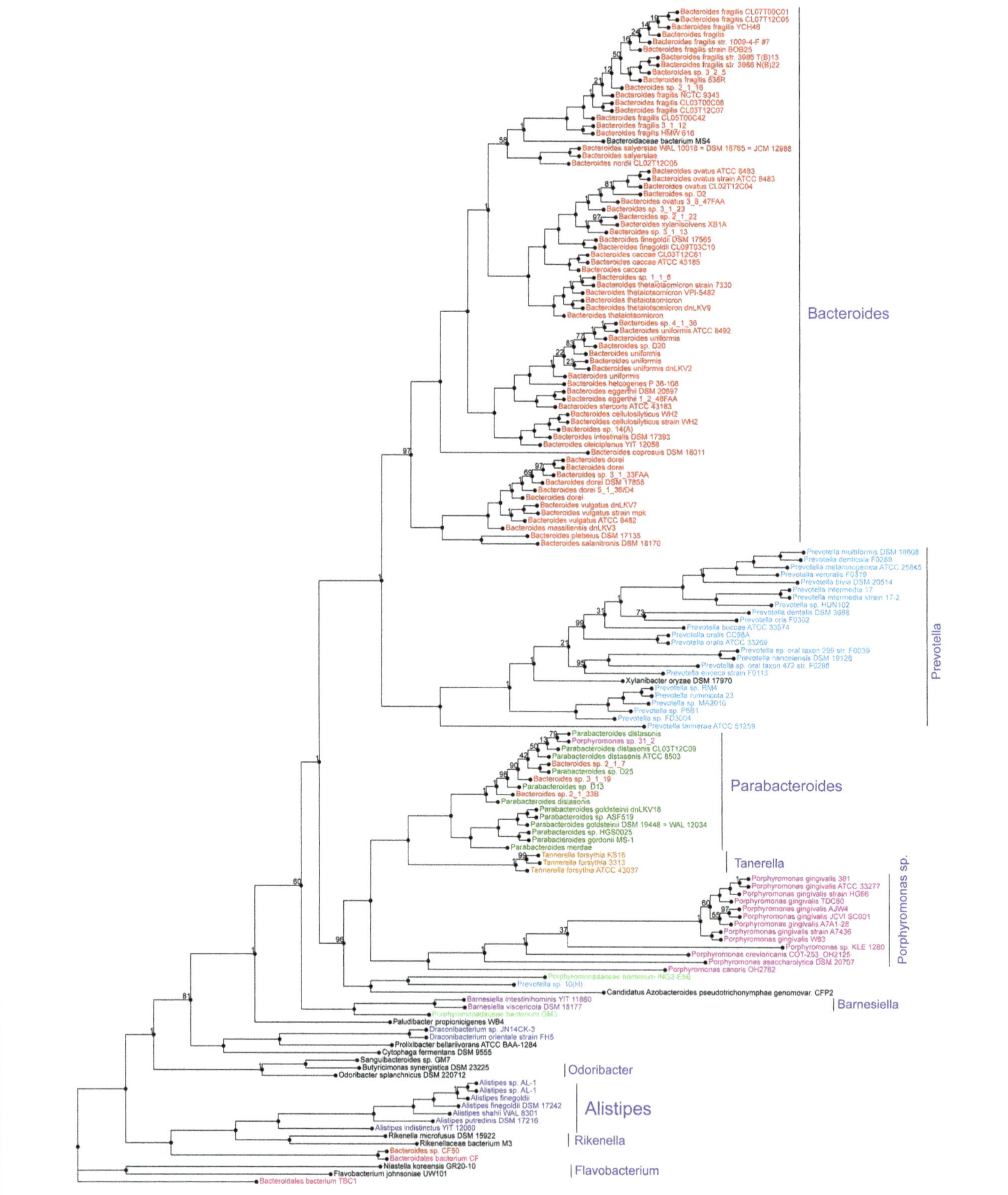

FIGURE 2 | Protein phylogram of 155 complete genomes of the *Bacteroidetes* phylum to illustrate the potential functional distinction of the genus *Alistipes* within the group. The pipeline for genomic phylograms is described in detail as follow by PATRIC, the Pathosystems Resource Integration Center, https://docs.patricbrc.org. In short, the order-level pre-built trees in PATRIC are constructed by an automated pipeline that begins with amino acid sequence files for each genome. For each order-level tree the genomes from that order are used along with a small set of potential outgroup genomes. Branch values are not bootstrap values, which can be overly optimistic for long genomes. Instead, trees are built from random samples of 50% of the homology groups used for the main tree (gene-wise jackknifing). One hundred of these 50% gene-wise jackknife trees are made using FastTree, and the support values shown indicate the number of times a particular branch was observed in the support trees. As of May 19, 2020, there were 140 Alistipes genomes available (11287 unique contigs), of which 10 are complete.

have a leading role in the modulation of diseases, or alternatively could just have either a bystander role, or a co-inducer role (with other gut microbes) of the observed clinical phenotypes. Animal studies will be further needed to decipher the mechanisms that may explain disease modulation alone and as symbiont by this genus across a multitude of complex multimodal diseases, which will benefit from the targeted study of subtype phenotypes, as we have analytically illustrated (9).

The use of germ-free animals and models will be beneficial to understand the role of this genus in disease and health and the interaction with the host immune defense tolerance, such as there should be studies investigating the roles on the SCFAs produced by *Alistipes* and their effect on the various liver diseases and *Alistipes* direct role on T-cell differentiation.

AUTHOR CONTRIBUTIONS

BP, PW, AV, and AR-P conceived the performed review and wrote the manuscript. All authors discussed and edited the manuscript and approved its final version.

FUNDING

This project was primarily supported by NIH grant R21 DK118373 to AR-P, entitled Identification of pathogenic bacteria in Crohn's disease. We acknowledge the Biorepository Core of the NIH Silvio O. Conte Cleveland Digestive Disease Research Core Center (P30DK097948) for supporting the above-mentioned R21 project. Partial support also originated for AR-P from a career development award from the Crohn's and Colitis Foundation and National Institutes of Health award 2P01DK091222-06 (Germ-Free and Gut Microbiome Core to Dr. Fabio Cominelli, Case Western Reserve University and AR-P).

ACKNOWLEDGMENTS

BP was especially grateful to the Department of Pathology for the scientific and academic opportunities, their mentoring, and their support during the preparation of this manuscript. This project was part of a Master's of Science program in Pathology at Case Western Reserve University and she is currently admitted to the medical school at Wayne State University School of Medicine.

REFERENCES

Goodrich JK, Davenport ER, Clark AG, Ley RE. The relationship between the human genome and microbiome comes into view. *Annu Rev Genet.* (2017) 51:413–33. doi: 10.1146/annurev-genet-110711-155532

Lynch SV, Pedersen O. The human intestinal microbiome in health and disease. *N Engl J Med.* (2016) 375:2369–79. doi: 10.1056/NEJMra1600266

Vivarelli S, Salemi R, Candido S, Falzone L, Santagati M, Stefani S, et al. Gut microbiota and cancer: from pathogenesis to therapy. *Cancers.* (2019) 11:38. doi: 10.3390/cancers11010038

Halfvarson J, Brislawn CJ, Lamendella R, Vázquez-Baeza Y, Walters WA, Bramer LM, et al. Dynamics of the human gut microbiome in inflammatory bowel disease. *Nat Microbiol.* (2017) 2:17004. doi: 10.1038/nmicrobiol.2017.4

Yoshida N, Yamashita T, Hirata KI. Gut microbiome and cardiovascular diseases. *Diseases.* (2018) 6:56. doi: 10.3390/diseases6030056

Petra AI, Panagiotidou S, Hatziagelaki E, Stewart JM., Conti P, Theoharides TC. Gut-microbiota-brain axis and its effect on neuropsychiatric disorders with suspected immune dysregulation. *Clin Ther.* (2015) 37:984–95. doi: 10.1016/j.clinthera.2015.04.002

Rautio M, Eerola E, Väisänen-Tunkelrott ML, Molitoris D, Lawson P, Collins MD, et al. Reclassification of *Bacteroides putredinis* (Weinberg et al., 1937) in a new genus *Alistipes* gen. nov., as *Alistipes putredinis* comb. nov., and description of *Alistipes finegoldii* sp. nov., from human sources. *Syst Appl Microbiol.* (2003) 26:182–8. doi: 10.1078/072320203322346029

Shkoporov AN, Chaplin AV, Khokhlova EV, Shcherbakova VA, Motuzova OV, Bozhenko VK, et al. *Alistipes inops* sp. nov. and *Coprobacter secundus* sp. nov., isolated from human faeces. *Int J Syst Evol Microbiol.* (2015) 65:4580– 8. doi: 10.1099/ijsem.0.000617

Basson AR, Cominelli F, Rodriguez-Palacios A. Patterns of 'analytical irreproducibility' in multimodal diseases. *bioRxiv [preprint]*:bioRxiv 2020.03.22.002469. (2020). doi: 10.1101/2020.03.22.002469

Sakamoto M, Ikeyama N, Ogata Y, Suda W, Iino T, Hattori M, et al. *Alistipes communis* sp. nov., *Alistipes dispar* sp. nov. and *Alistipes onderdonkii* subsp. *vulgaris* subsp. nov., isolated from human faeces, and creation of *Alistipes onderdonkii* subsp. *onderdonkii* subsp. nov. *Int J Syst Evol Microbiol.* (2020) 70:473–80. doi: 10.1099/ijsem.0.003778

In Memoriam: Sydney "Sid" Finegold, MD, FIDSA 1921–2018. Infectious Disease Society of America News Archives (2018).

Sydney M. Finegold. Biographical Feature: Sydney M. Finegold. *J Clin Microbiol.* (2012) 50:2546–7. doi: 10.1128/JCM.01295-12

Abbreviated Curriculum Vitae: Sydney M. Finegold MD. *Clin Infect. Dis.* (2002) 35:287. doi: 10.1086/341912

Rau M, Rehman A, Dittrich M, Groen AK, Hermanns HM, Seyfried F, et al. Fecal SCFAs and SCFA-producing bacteria in gut microbiome of human NAFLD as a putative link to systemic T-cell activation and advanced disease. *United Euro. Gastroenterol J.* (2018) 6:1496– 1507. doi: 10.1177/2050640618804444

Moschen AR, Gerner RR, Wang J, Klepsch V, Adolph TE, Reider SJ, et al. Lipocalin 2 protects from inflammation and tumorigenesis associated with gut microbiota alterations. *Cell Host Microbe.* (2016) 19:455– 69. doi: 10.1016/j.chom.2016.03.007

Zuo K, Li J, Li K, Hu C, Gao Y, Chen M, et al. Disordered gut microbiota and alterations in metabolic patterns are associated with atrial fibrillation. *Gigascience.* (2019) 8:giz058. doi: 10.1093/gigascience/giz058

Bangsgaard Bendtsen KM, Krych L, Sørensen DB, Pang W, Nielsen DS, Josefsen K, et al. Gut microbiota composition is correlated to grid floor induced stress and behavior in the BALB/c mouse. *PLoS ONE.* (2012) 7:e46231. doi: 10.1371/journal.pone.0046231

Kaur H, Das C, Mande SS. Analysis of putrefaction pathways in bacteria and its implication in colorectal cancer. *Front Microbiol.* (2017) 8:2166. doi: 10.3389/fmicb.2017.02166

Jousimies-Somer H. *Wadsworth-KTL Anaerobic Bacteriology Manual.* Star Pub. (2002).

Wexler HM. Bacteroides: the good, the bad, and the nitty-gritty. *Clin Microbiol Rev.* (2007) 20:593–621. doi: 10.1128/CMR.00008-07

Mishra AK, Gimenez G, Lagier JC, Robert C, Raoult D, Fournier PE. Genome sequence and description of *Alistipes senegalensis* sp. nov. *Stand Genomic Sci.* (2012) 6:1–16. doi: 10.4056/sigs.3076460

Urdaneta V, Casadesús J. Interactions between bacteria and bile salts in the gastrointestinal and hepatobiliary tracts. *Front Med.* (2017) 4:163. doi: 10.3389/fmed.2017.00163

Cao W, Kayama H, Chen ML, Delmas A, Sun A, Kim SY, et al. The xenobiotic transporter Mdr1 enforces T cell homeostasis in the presence of intestinal bile acids. *Immunity.* (2017) 47:1182–96.e10. doi: 10.1016/j.immuni. 2017.11.012

Song Y, Könönen E, Rautio M, Liu C, Bryk A, Eerola E, et al. *Alistipes onderdonkii* sp. nov. and *Alistipes shahii* sp. nov., of human origin. *Int J Syst Evol Microbiol.* (2006) 56:1985–90. doi: 10.1099/ijs.0.64318-0

Nagai F, Morotomi M, Watanabe Y, Sakon H, Tanaka, R. *Alistipes indistinctus* sp. nov. and *Odoribacter laneus* sp. nov., common members of the human intestinal microbiota isolated from faeces. *Int J Syst Evol Microbiol.* (2010) 60:1296–302. doi: 10.1099/ijs.0.014571-0

Lagier JC, Armougom F, Mishra AK, Nguyen TT, Raoult D, Fournier PE. Non-contiguous finished genome sequence and description of *Alistipes timonensis* sp. nov. *Stand Genomic Sci.* (2012) 6:315–24. doi: 10.4056/sigs.2685971

Hugon P, Ramasamy D, Lagier JC, Rivet R, Couderc C, Raoult D, et al. Non contiguous-finished genome sequence and description of *Alistipes obesi* sp. nov. *Stand Genomic Sci.* (2013) 7:427–39. doi: 10.4056/sigs.3336746

Pfleiderer A, Mishra AK, Lagier JC, Robert C, Caputo A, Raoult D. et al. Non-contiguous finished genome sequence and description of *Alistipes ihumii* sp. nov. *Stand Genomic Sci.* (2014) 9:1221–35. doi: 10.4056/sigs.4698398

Bellali S, Naud S, Ndongo S, Lo CI, Anani H, Raoult D, *Corynebacterium pacaense* sp. nov., *Alistipes megaguti* sp. nov., *Alistipes provencensis* sp. nov., 3 new bacteria isolated from fresh human stool specimens. *New Microbes New Infect.* (2019) 32:100593. doi: 10.1016/j.nmni.2019.100593

Fenner L, Roux V, Ananian P, Raoult D. *Alistipes finegoldii* in blood cultures from colon cancer patients. *Emerg Infect Dis.* (2007) 13:1260– 2. doi: 10.3201/eid1308.060662

Paster BJ, Dewhirst FE, Olsen I, Fraser GJ. Phylogeny of *Bacteroides*, *Prevotella*, and *Porphyromonas* spp. and related bacteria. *J Bacteriol.* (1994) 176:725–32. doi: 10.1128/JB.176.3.725-732.1994

Lagier JC, Armougom F, Million M, Hugon P, Pagnier I, Robert C, et al. Microbial culturomics: paradigm shift in the human gut microbiome study. *Clin Microbiol Infect.* (2012) 18:1185–93. doi: 10.1111/1469-0691.12023

Hardham JM, King KW, Dreier K, Wong J, Strietzel C, Eversole RR, et al. Transfer of *Bacteroides splanchnicus* to Odoribacter gen. nov. as *Odoribacter splanchnicus* comb. nov., and description of *Odoribacter denticanis* sp. nov., isolated from the crevicular spaces of canine periodontitis patients. *Int J Syst Evol Microbiol.* (2008) 58:103–9. doi: 10.1099/ijs.0.63458-0

Werner H, Rintelen G, Kunstek-Santos H. A new butyric acid-producing bacteroides species: B. splanchnicus n. sp. (author's transl). *Zentralbl Bakteriol Orig A.* (1975) 231:133–44.

Downes J, Tanner AC, Dewhirst FE, Wade WG. Prevotella saccharolytica sp. nov., isolated from the human oral cavity. *Int J Syst Evol Microbiol.* (2010) 60:2458–61. doi: 10.1099/ijs.0.014720-0

van Winkelhoff AJ, van Steenbergen TJ, de Graaff J. Porphyromonas (Bacteroides) endodontalis: its role in endodontal infections. *J Endod.* (1992) 18:431–4. doi: 10.1016/S0099-2399(06)80843-5

Weisburg WG, Barns SM, Pelletier DA, Lane DJ. 16S ribosomal DNA amplification for phylogenetic study. *J Bacteriol.* (1991) 173:697–703. doi: 10.1128/JB.173.2.697-703.1991

Veloo ACM, Jean-Pierre H, Justesen US, Morris T, Urban E, Wybo I, et al. Validation of MALDI-TOF MS Biotyper database optimized for anaerobic bacteria: The ENRIA project. *Anaerobe.* (2018) 54:224– 230. doi: 10.1016/j.anaerobe.2018.03.007

Kulagina EV, Efimov BA, Maximov PY, Kafarskaia LI, Chaplin AV, Shkoporov AN. Species composition of Bacteroidales order bacteria in the feces of healthy people of various ages. *Biosci Biotechnol Biochem.* (2012) 76:169– 71. doi: 10.1271/bbb.110434

Torok VA, Hughes RJ, Mikkelsen LL, Perez-Maldonado R, Balding K, MacAlpine R, et al. Identification and characterization of potential performance-related gut microbiotas in broiler chickens across various feeding trials. *Appl Environ Microbiol.* (2011) 77:5868–78. doi: 10.1128/AEM.00165-11

Li F, Hullar MA, Schwarz Y, Lampe JW. Human gut bacterial communities are altered by addition of cruciferous vegetables to a controlled fruit- and vegetable-free diet. *J Nutr.* (2009) 139:1685–91. doi: 10.3945/jn.109.108191

Dziarski R, Park SY, Kashyap DR, Dowd SE, Gupta, D. Pglyrp-regulated gut microflora *Prevotella falsenii*, *Parabacteroides distasonis* and *Bacteroides eggerthii* enhance and *Alistipes finegoldii* attenuates colitis in mice. *PLoS ONE.* (2016) 11:e0146162. doi: 10.1371/journal.pone.0146162

Shao L, Ling Z, Chen D, Liu Y, Yang F, Li, L. Disorganized gut microbiome contributed to liver cirrhosis progression: a meta-omics-based study. *Front Microbiol.* (2018) 9:3166. doi: 10.3389/fmicb.2018.03166

Sung CM, Lin YF, Chen KF, Ke HM, Huang HY, Gong YN, et al. Predicting clinical outcomes of cirrhosis patients with hepatic encephalopathy from the fecal microbiome. *Cell Mol Gastroenterol Hepatol.* (2019) 8:301– 18.e2. doi: 10.1016/j.jcmgh.2019.04.008

Li J, Sung CY, Lee N, Ni Y, Pihlajamäki J, Panagiotou G, et al. Probiotics modulated gut microbiota suppresses hepatocellular carcinoma growth in mice. *Proc Natl Acad Sci USA.* (2016) 113:E1306–15. doi: 10.1073/pnas.1518189113

Feng Q, Liang S, Jia H, Stadlmayr A, Tang L, Lan Z, et al. Gut microbiome development along the colorectal adenoma-carcinoma sequence. *Nat Commun.* (2015) 6:6528. doi: 10.1038/ncomms7528

Jama HA, Beale A, Shihata WA, Marques FZ. The effect of diet on hypertensive pathology: is there a link via gut microbiota-driven immunometabolism? *Cardiovasc Res.* (2019) 115:1435–47. doi: 10.1093/cvr/cvz091

Kim S, Goel R, Kumar A, Qi Y, Lobaton G, Hosaka K, et al. Imbalance of gut microbiome and intestinal epithelial barrier dysfunction in patients with high blood pressure. *Clin Sci.* (2018) 132:701–18. doi: 10.1042/CS20180087

Cui X, Ye L, Li J, Jin L, Wang W, Li S, et al. Metagenomic and metabolomic analyses unveil dysbiosis of gut microbiota in chronic heart failure patients. *Sci Rep.* (2018) 8:635. doi: 10.1038/s41598-017-18756-2

Jie Z, Xia H, Zhong SL, Feng Q, Li S, Liang S, et al. The gut microbiome in atherosclerotic cardiovascular disease. *Nat Commun.* (2017) 8:845. doi: 10.1038/s41467-017-00900-1

Frémont M, Coomans D, Massart S, De Meirleir, K. High-throughput 16S rRNA gene sequencing reveals alterations of intestinal microbiota in myalgic encephalomyelitis/chronic fatigue syndrome patients. *Anaerobe.* (2013) 22:50–6. doi: 10.1016/j.anaerobe.2013.06.002

Jiang H, Ling Z, Zhang Y, Mao H, Ma Z, Yin Y, et al. Altered fecal microbiota composition in patients with major depressive disorder. *Brain Behav Immun.* (2015) 48:186–94. doi: 10.1016/j.bbi.2015.03.016

Strati F, Cavalieri D, Albanese D, De Felice C, Donati C, Hayek J, et al. New evidences on the altered gut microbiota in autism spectrum disorders. *Microbiome.* (2017) 5:24. doi: 10.1186/s40168-017-0242-1

De Angelis M, Piccolo M, Vannini L, Siragusa S, De Giacomo A, Serrazzanetti DI, et al. Fecal microbiota and metabolome of children with autism and pervasive developmental disorder not otherwise specified. *PLoS ONE.* (2013) 8:e76993. doi: 10.1371/journal.pone.0076993

Tang A, Hallouch O, Chernyak V, Kamaya A, Sirlin CB. Epidemiology of hepatocellular carcinoma: target population for surveillance and diagnosis. *Abdom Radiol.* (2018) 43:13–25. doi: 10.1007/s00261-017-1209-1

Campion D, Giovo I, Ponzo P, Saracco GM, Balzola F, Alessandria, C. Dietary approach and gut microbiota modulation for chronic hepatic encephalopathy in cirrhosis. *World J Hepatol.* (2019) 11:489–512. doi: 10.4254/wjh.v11.i6.489

Iebba V, Guerrieri F, Di Gregorio V, Levrero M, Gagliardi A, Santangelo F, et al. Combining amplicon sequencing and metabolomics in cirrhotic patients highlights distinctive microbiota features involved in bacterial translocation, systemic inflammation and hepatic encephalopathy. *Sci Rep.* (2018) 8:8210. doi: 10.1038/s41598-018- 26509-y

Polansky O, Sekelova Z, Faldynova M, Sebkova A, Sisak F, Rychlik, Important metabolic pathways and biological processes expressed by chicken cecal microbiota. *Appl Environ Microbiol.* (2015) 82:1569– 76. doi: 10.1128/AEM.03473-15

Oliphant K, Allen-Vercoe E. Macronutrient metabolism by the human gut microbiome: major fermentation by-products and their impact on host health. *Microbiome.* (2019) 7:91. doi: 10.1186/s40168-019-0704-8

Brown CT, Davis-Richardson AG, Giongo A, Gano KA, Crabb DB, Mukherjee N, et al. Gut microbiome metagenomics analysis suggests a functional model for the development of autoimmunity for type 1 diabetes. *PLoS ONE.* (2011) 6:e25792. doi: 10.1371/journal.pone.0025792

Iida N, Dzutsev A, Stewart CA, Smith L, Bouladoux N, Weingarten RA, et al. Commensal bacteria control cancer response to therapy by modulating the tumor microenvironment. *Science.* (2013) 342:967– 70. doi: 10.1126/science.1240527

Bindels LB, Porporato P, Dewulf EM, Verrax J, Neyrinck AM, Martin JC, et al. Gut microbiota-derived propionate reduces cancer cell proliferation in the liver. *Br J Cancer.* (2012) 107:1337–44. doi: 10.1038/bjc.2012.409

Oldgren J, Healey JS, Ezekowitz M, Commerford P, Avezum A, Pais P, et al. Variations in cause and management of atrial fibrillation in a prospective registry of 15,400 emergency department patients in 46 countries: the RE-LY Atrial Fibrillation Registry. *Circulation.* (2014) 129:1568– 76. doi: 10.1161/CIRCULATIONAHA.113.005451

Kirchhof P, Benussi S, Kotecha D, Ahlsson A, Atar D, Casadei B, et al. 2016 ESC Guidelines for the management of atrial fibrillation developed in collaboration with EACTS. *Eur J Cardiothorac Surg.* (2016) 50:e1– e88. doi: 10.5603/KP.2016.0172

Rodriguez-Palacios A, Kodani T, Kaydo L, Pietropaoli D, Corridoni D, Howell S, et al. Stereomicroscopic 3d-pattern profiling of murine and human intestinal inflammation reveals unique structural phenotypes. *Nat Commun.* (2015) 6:7577.

Rodriguez-Palacios A, Conger M, Hopperton A, Ezeji JC, Erkkila HL, Fiocchi C, et al. Identification of pathogenic bacteria in severe Crohn's disease. *Inflamm Bowel Dis.* (2019) 25(Suppl 1):S70. doi: 10.1093/ibd/izy393.175

Yang F, Kumar A, Davenport KW, Kelliher JM, Ezeji JC, Good CE, et al. Complete genome sequence of a parabacteroides distasonis strain (CavFT hAR46) isolated from a gut wall-cavitating microlesion in a patient with severe Crohn's disease. *Microbiology Resource Announcements.* (2019) 8:e00585-19. doi: 10.1128/MRA.00585-19

Butera A, Di Paola M, Pavarini L, Strati F, Pindo M, Sanchez M, et al. Nod2 Deficiency in mice is associated with microbiota variation favouring the expansion of mucosal CD4+ LAP+ regulatory cells. *Sci Rep.* (2018) 8:14241. doi: 10.1038/s41598-018-32583-z

Shen L, Liu L, Ji HF. Regulative effects of curcumin spice administration on gut microbiota and its pharmacological implications. *Food Nutr Res.* (2017) 61:1361780. doi: 10.1080/16546628.2017.1361780

Frank DN, St Amand AL, Feldman RA, Boedeker EC, Harpaz N, Pace NR. Molecular-phylogenetic characterization of microbial community imbalances in human inflammatory bowel diseases. *Proc Natl Acad Sci USA.* (2007) 104:13780–5. doi: 10.1073/pnas.0706625104

Rodriguez-Palacios AAN, Cominelli F. "Stereomicroscopy and 3d- Target myeloperoxidase intestinal phenotyping following a fecal flora homogenization protocol," In: *Protocol Exchange.* (2015). doi: 10.1038/protex.2015.065

Rodriguez-Palacios A, Harding A, Menghini P, Himmelman C, Retuerto M, Nickerson KP, et al. The artificial sweetener splenda promotes gut proteobacteria, dysbiosis, and myeloperoxidase reactivity in Crohn's disease-like ileitis. *Inflamm Bowel Dis.* (2018) 24:1005–20. doi: 10.1093/ibd/izy060

Goetz DH, Holmes MA, Borregaard N, Bluhm ME, Raymond KN, Strong RK. The neutrophil lipocalin NGAL is a bacteriostatic agent that interferes with siderophore-mediated iron acquisition. *Mol Cell.* (2002) 10:1033– 43. doi: 10.1016/S1097-2765(02)00708-6

Jin Y, Dong H, Xia L, Yang Y, Zhu Y, Shen Y, et al. The diversity of gut microbiome is associated with favorable responses to anti-PD-1 immunotherapy in Chinese non-small cell lung cancer patients. *J Thorac Oncol.* (2019) 14:1378–89. doi: 10.1016/j.jtho.2019.04.007

Naseribafrouei A, Hestad K, Avershina E, Sekelja M, Linløkken A, Wilson R, et al. Correlation between the human fecal microbiota and depression. *Neurogastroenterol Motil.* (2014) 26:1155–62. doi: 10.1111/ nmo.12378

MacFabe DF, Cain NE, Boon F, Ossenkopp KP, Cain DP. Effects of the enteric bacterial metabolic product propionic acid on object-directed behavior, social behavior, cognition, and neuroinflammation in adolescent rats: relevance to autism spectrum disorder. *Behav Brain Res.* (2011) 217:47– 54. doi: 10.1016/j.bbr.2010.10.005

Merrill AH. Sphingolipid and glycosphingolipid metabolic pathways in the era of sphingolipidomics. *Chem Rev.* (2011) 111:6387–422. doi: 10.1021/cr2002917

Walker A, Pfitzner B, Harir M, Schaubeck M, Calasan J, Heinzmann SS, et al. Sulfonolipids as novel metabolite markers of *Alistipes* and *Odoribacter* affected by high-fat diets. *Sci Rep.* (2017) 7:11047. doi: 10.1038/s41598-017- 10369-z

Thanikachalam K, Khan G. Colorectal cancer and nutrition. *Nutrients.* (2019) 11:164. doi: 10.3390/nu11010164

Windey K, De Preter V, Verbeke K. Relevance of protein fermentation to gut health. *Mol Nutr Food Res.* (2012) 56:184–96. doi: 10.1002/mnfr.201100542

Hughes R, Magee EA, Bingham S. Protein degradation in the large intestine: relevance to colorectal cancer. *Curr Issues Intest Microbiol.* (2000) 1:51–8.

Yao CK, Muir JG, Gibson PR. Review article: insights into colonic protein fermentation, its modulation and potential health implications. *Aliment Pharmacol Ther.* (2016) 43:181–96. doi: 10.1111/apt.13456

Fung KY, Ooi CC, Zucker MH, Lockett T, Williams DB, Cosgrove LJ, et al. Colorectal carcinogenesis: a cellular response to sustained risk environment. *Int J Mol Sci.* (2013) 14:13525–41. doi: 10.3390/ijms1407 13525

Lin HC, Visek WJ. Colon mucosal cell damage by ammonia in rats. *J Nutr.* (1991) 121:887–93. doi: 10.1093/jn/121.6.887

10

Targeting Gremlin 1 Prevents Intestinal Fibrosis Progression by Inhibiting the Fatty Acid Oxidation of Fibroblast Cells

Yang Yang[1,2,3], *Qi-Shan Zeng*[1,2], *Min Zou*[1,2], *Jian Zeng*[4], *Jiao Nie*[2,5], *DongFeng Chen*[3] *and Hua-Tian Gan*[1,2,5]*

[1]Department of Gastroenterology and the Center of Inflammatory Bowel Disease, West China Hospital, Sichuan University, Chengdu, China, [2]Lab of Inflammatory Bowel Disease, Clinical Institute of Inflammation and Immunology, Frontiers Science Center for Disease-related Molecular Network, West China Hospital, Sichuan University, Chengdu, China, [3]Department of Gastroenterology, Daping Hospital, Army Medical University, Chongqing, China, [4]Department of Gastroenterology, Chongqing Traditional Chinese Medicine Hospital, Chongqing, China, [5]Department of Geriatrics and National Clinical Research Center for Geriatric, West China Hospital, Sichuan University, Chengdu, China

***Correspondence:**
Hua-Tian Gan
ght_2021@163.com*

Intestinal fibrosis is a consequence of continuous inflammatory responses that negatively affect the quality of life of patients. By screening altered proteomic profiles of mouse fibrotic colon tissues, we identified that GREM1 was dramatically upregulated in comparison to that in normal tissues. Functional experiments revealed that GREM1 promoted the proliferation and activation of intestinal fibroblast cells by enhancing fatty acid oxidation. Blocking GREM1 prevented the progression of intestinal fibrosis *in vivo*. Mechanistic research revealed that GREM1 acted as a ligand for VEGFR2 and triggered downstream MAPK signaling. This facilitated the expression of FAO-related genes, consequently enhancing fatty acid oxidation. Taken together, our data indicated that targeting GREM1 could represent a promising therapeutic approach for the treatment of intestinal fibrosis.

Keywords: intestinal fibrosis, gremlin 1, fibroblast cell, fatty acid oxidation, VEGFR2

INTRODUCTION

Intestinal fibrosis, a common complication of inflammatory bowel disease (IBD) (Leake, 2015), is characterized by exaggerated scar tissue formation in the colon mucosa (Rieder and Fiocchi, 2009) resulting from intestinal damage induced by chronic inflammation (Lawrance et al., 2017). Despite great progress in the treatment of IBD, the incidence of intestinal fibrosis has not markedly reduced (Su et al., 2016; Vítek and Tiribelli, 2020), indicating that the development of new targeted therapies or effective interventions for intestinal fibrosis are urgently needed.

Intestinal fibroblasts, the major effector cells of gastrointestinal fibrosis (Weder et al., 2018), mainly account for the synthesis of several extracellular matrix proteins. This includes collagens, vimentin, and fibronectin (Hagenlocher et al., 2017). During chronic inflammation processes, local gut mesenchymal cells are activated and proliferated. This leads to enhanced deposition of extracellular-matrix proteins. Previous studies reported that resident fibroblasts can be activated by inflammation-related proteins (Lawrance et al., 2001), including the growth factors IGF-I, FGF, and PDGF, and the pro-inflammatory cytokines IL-1β and TNF-α (Simmons et al., 2002). This results in expansion of fibroblast cell numbers and fibroblast differentiation. In addition, colonic transforming growth factor (TGF)-β1 overexpression results in fibroblast accumulation and bowel wall thickening (Vallance et al., 2005). Apart from cytokines, growth factors, and chemokines, local fibroblasts resident in the colon can also respond to other biological mediators (Fichtner-Feigl et al., 2007; Burke et al., 2008). Thus, screening new biological mediators may provide potential therapeutic targets.

GREM1, encoded by the *GREM1* gene (Mezzano et al., 2018), is an important protein secreted in development, including organ formation, physique development, and tissue differentiation. GREM1 is considered to be an antagonist of the bone morphogenetic protein (BMP) family members and binds to BMP2 to regulate the BMP signaling pathway (Hsu et al., 1998). Later studies revealed that GREM1 can act as a vascular endothelial growth factor receptor 2 (VEGFR2) ligand in vascular endothelial cells to regulate angiogenesis (Mitola et al., 2010). Additionally, GREM1 has been reported to be both tumor promotive and suppressive in cancer. Elevated GREM1 expression is associated with favorable outcomes in several malignancies, including colon adenocarcinoma (Nyqvist et al., 2017) and gastric cancer (Honma et al., 2018). On the other hand, increased GREM1 expression facilitates the proliferation of cancer cells in lung adenocarcinoma and glioma. However, the role of GREM1 in intestinal fibrosis remains unknown.

In this study, we found that protein levels of GREM1 were dramatically increased in fibrotic colon. The loss and gain of function experiments revealed that GREM1 promoted intestinal fibroblast cell proliferation by enhancing fatty acid oxidation. Further mechanistic studies revealed that GREM1 could activate VEGFR2 and trigger downstream MAPK signaling. This facilitates FAO-related gene expression, consequently enhancing fatty acid oxidation and results in fibroblast cell proliferation and activation. Taken together, these results provide evidence that GREM1 could be a potential target for intestinal fibrosis therapy.

MATERIALS AND METHODS

Animal Experiments

All animal experiments were approved by the Institutional Animal Care and Use Committee (IACUC) of the Army Medical University, and were authorized by the Institutional Animal Care and Use Committee of the Laboratory Animal Center of Daping Hospital, Army Medical University. Mouse intestinal fibrosis was induced by the administration of 2.5% dextran sulfate sodium (DSS) in tap water for 5 days followed by 1°week of normal drinking water for three cycles (Speca et al., 2016). The mice were sacrificed at nine weeks after DSS treatment. Intestinal tissues were formalin-fixed and embedded in paraffin for further analysis.

Cell Lines

Human intestinal fibroblast cell lines CCD-18Co and CCD-112Co were maintained at the Daping Hospital, Army Medical University. Cells were cultured in Dulbecco's modified Eagle's medium (DMEM) supplemented with 10% fetal bovine serum (FBS, Gibco), 100°U/ml penicillin and 100 μg/ml streptomycin at 37°C in a 5% CO_2 atmosphere. Exogenous GREM1, used for cell treatment, purchased from R&D system (cat#:5190-GR-050). STR identification was conducted to exclude exogenic cell contamination.

Cell Proliferation Assays

Enumeration of fibroblasts was performed using Cell Counting Kit-8 (CCK8, NCM), according to the manufacturer's instructions. Cells were cultured in 96-well plates at 3,000 cells/well. Serum conditions included no serum added to the culture medium, and other components were consistent with full medium. At the indicated time points, the cell culture medium was changed to a CCK8 buffer, and after 90 min incubation at 37°C, under 5% CO_2, OD_{450} values were measured to determine cell viability.

Transfection and RNA Interference

siRNA transfection was conducted using Lipofectamine® 2000 (Invitrogen) according to the manufacturer's instructions. siRNA was purchased from GenePharma and Shanghai BioTend Biotech Co. Total cellular RNA was extracted after 48 h of transfection. SiRNA sequences are presented in **Supplementary Material**.

RNA Isolation and Q-PCR

Total RNA was isolated using Trizol reagent (Takara, 9109) and reverse transcription was performed using PrimeScript kits (Takara, RR037A). To detect gene expression, RT-qPCR assays were performed using SYBR Premix Ex Taq (Roche) using the recommended thermal settings. Relative mRNA expression was analyzed using the 2 (-ΔΔCt) method and normalized to that of 18S ribosomal RNA. PCR primer sequences are presented in Supplementary materials.

Immunoblotting

Whole cell lysates were prepared with RIPA lysis buffer (share-bio Tech) and membrane proteins were extracted using a Membrane and Cytosol Protein Extraction Kit (Beyotime). Quantification of protein concentrations was performed using a BCA protein assay kit (Thermo Fisher Scientific Proteins were resolved by 4–20% SDS-PAGE and transferred to NC membranes (Whatman), then antibody and ECL methods were employed to measure protein expression levels. Primary antibodies used were as follows: anti-GREM1 (R&D Systems, AF956, 1:1,000), anti-phospho-VEGF Receptor 2 (Tyr1175) (CST, #3770, 1:1,000), anti-VEGF receptor 2 (CST, #2479, 1:1,000), anti-phospho-MEK1/2 (Ser217/221) (CST, #3958, 1:1,000), anti-MEK1/2 (CST, #4694, 1:1,000), anti-phospho-p44/42 MAPK (Erk1/2) (Thr202/Tyr204) (CST, #9101,1:1,000), and anti-p44/42 MAPK (Erk1/2) (CST, #4695, 1:1,000). The secondary antibodies were anti-rabbit (share-bio, SB-AB0101, Abways Technology, AB0151), anti-mouse (share-bio, SB-AB0102, Yeasen Biotech Co., 33206ES60), and anti-goat (Immunoway Biotech Co., RS2123; Abcam, ab175776).

Sample Preparation and Proteomic Analyses

The fibrosis colon and control group samples were grinded by liquid nitrogen into cell powder and then transferred to a 5-ml centrifuge tube. After that, four volumes of lysis buffer (8 M urea, 1% protease Inhibitor Cocktail) was added to the cell powder, followed by sonication three times on ice using a high intensity ultrasonic processor (Scientz). The remaining debris was removed by centrifugation at 12,000 g at 4°C for 10 min. As for proteomic analyses, trypsin was added into the protein solution at 1:50 trypsin-to-protein mass ratio for the first digestion overnight and 1:100 trypsin-to-protein mass ratio for a second 4 h-digestion. Then, the tryptic peptides were dissolved in 0.1% formic acid (solvent A), directly loaded onto a home-made reversed-phase analytical column (15-cm length, 75 μm i. d.). The gradient was comprised of an increase from 6 to 23% solvent B (0.1% formic acid in 98% acetonitrile) over 26 min, 23–35% in 8 min and climbing to 80% in 3 min then holding at 80% for the last 3 min, all at a constant flow rate of 400 nL/min on an EASY-nLC 1000 UPLC system.

The peptides were subjected to NSI source followed by tandem mass spectrometry (MS/MS) in Q ExactiveTM Plus (Thermo) coupled online to the UPLC. The electrospray voltage applied was 2.0 kV. The m/z scan range was 350–1800 for full scan, and intact peptides were detected in the Orbitrap at a resolution of 70,000. Peptides were then selected for MS/MS using NCE setting as 28 and the fragments were detected in the Orbitrap at a resolution of 17,500. A data-dependent procedure that alternated between one MS scan followed by 20 MS/MS scans with 15.0 s dynamic exclusion. Automatic gain control (AGC) was set at 5E4. Fixed first mass was set as 100 m/z. The resulting MS/MS data were processed using Maxquant search engine (v.1.5.2.8). Tandem mass spectra were searched against human uniprot database concatenated with reverse decoy database. Trypsin/*P* was specified as cleavage enzyme allowing up to four missing cleavages. The mass tolerance for precursor ions was set as 20 ppm in First search and 5 ppm in Main search, and the mass tolerance for fragment ions was set as 0.02 Da. Carbamidomethyl on Cys was specified as fixed modification and acetylation modification and oxidation on Met were specified as variable modifications. FDR was adjusted to <1% and minimum score for modified peptides was set >40.

Histology Score

We scored all histological sections of the colonic samples in double-blind, according to the presence of ulcerations (0 = absent, 1 = small ulcers, 2 = big ulcers), degree of inflammation (0 = absent, 1 = mild, 2 = moderate, and 3 = severe), depth of the lesions (0 = absent, 1 = lesions extending in the submucosa, 2 = lesions in the muscularis propria, and 3 = lesions in the serosa), and degree of fibrosis (0 = absent; 1 = mild, 2 = moderate, and 3 = severe). The sum of these scores was expressed as total microscopic score.

Immunofluorescence and Immunohistochemistry

Cells cultured on Millicell® EZ SLIDE (MILLIPORE) were fixed with 4% paraformaldehyde for 15 min and permeabilized with 0.1% Triton X-100 for 1 min at room temperature. After blocking with BSA (Sangon Biotech), samples were incubated with the primary antibody (1:200) overnight at 4°C, and the secondary antibody–labeled with fluorescein (1: 200)–for 1 h at room temperature. Finally, DAPI was used to counterstain nuclei and the sample images were captured using a confocal microscope. For immunofluorescent staining of living cells to locate membrane proteins, cells were rinsed with cold PBS, followed by incubation with primary and secondary antibodies (1:500) for 1 h at 4°C. Next, the cells were fixed with 4% paraformaldehyde and stained with DAPI. For immunohistochemistry, slides were deparaffinized in xylene, and then antigen retrieval was performed using a citrate antigen retrieval solution. Endogenous peroxidase activity was blocked through the addition of hydrogen peroxide. After blocking with 10% BSA at room temperature, slides were incubated with primary antibodies at 4°C overnight. Following 1 h incubation with HPR-conjugated secondary antibody (anti-mouse, 1:500, Jackson ImmunoResearch, 115–035–003 or rabbit secondary antibodies 1:500 Jackson ImmunoResearch, 111–035–003), slides were developed in DAB (CST, 8059) and counterstained with hematoxylin.

BODIPY Staining

BODIPY staining was conducted according to standard procedures. Briefly, control and GREM1 treated fibroblasts were incubated with the BODIPY dye solution (Servicebio, GP1104) at room temperature in the dark for 1 h, followed by nuclear staining with DAPI and examination by confocal microscopy. Cells in five images of each sample were counted using ImageJ software.

Lipid Lysis Product Analysis

The amounts of acylcarnitine and acetyl-CoA were measured according to a previously reported method (Cheng et al., 2020). Briefly, serum-free cultured fibroblasts were treated with GREM1 and were collected and homogenized. They were then suspended in chloroform/methanol (1:1), and analyzed by mass spectrometry. The amounts of acylcarnitine and acetyl-CoA were normalized to the total protein content of fibroblast cells.

Public Dataset Bioinformatic Analysis

SRA datasets (SRP077046 and SRP100787) containing data for tissues from both healthy controls and CD and UC patients. The mRNA expression level of *GREM1* was compared in both healthy controls and CD and UC patients.

Seahorse Assays

The extracellular acidification rate (ECAR) and oxygen consumption rate (OCR) were determined using standard methods. Briefly, cells were seeded in XF96-well plates at a density of 2×10^4/well. For glycolytic stress testing (Seahorse Bioscience, catalog no. 103020–100), 10 mmol/L glucose, 1 mmol/L oligomycin, and 50 mmol/L 2-deoxyglucose (2-DG) were used. For mitochondrial stress tests (Seahorse Bioscience, catalog no. 103015–100), 1 mmol/L oligomycin, 1 mmol/L FCCP, 0.5 mmol/L rotenone, and 0.5 mmol/L actinomycin A were used. Total cellular protein was used to normalize the measurements.

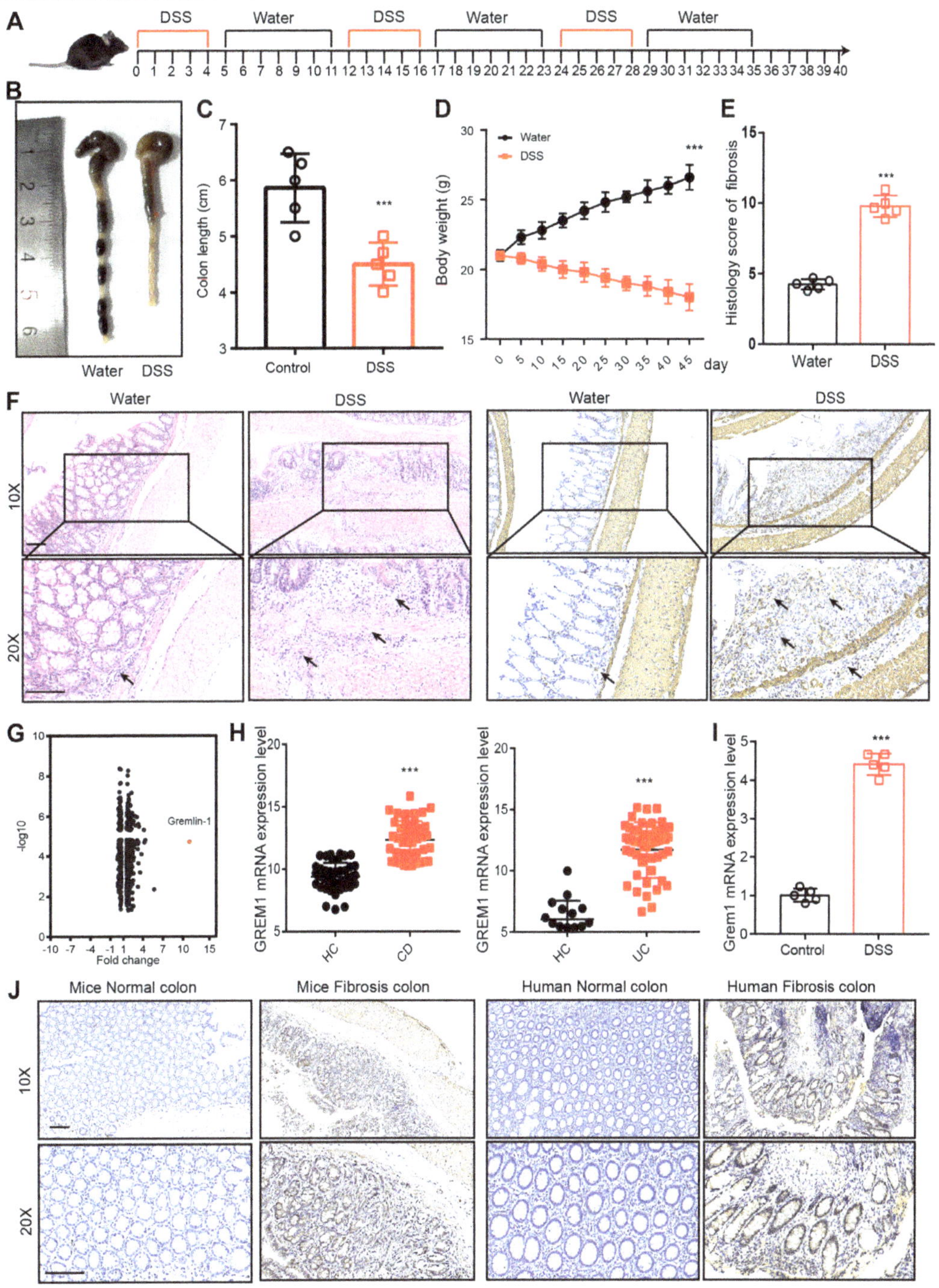

FIGURE 1 | GREM1 expression increased in intestinal fibrosis. **(A)**. C57BL/6J mice were subjected to three cycles of 2.5% DSS for 5°days followed by 1 week of recuperation to establish mice intestinal fibrosis model. **(B)**. The appearance of the colons from the mice in control or DSS treated groups. **(C)**. The colon length statical results of mice from control or DSS treated group ($n = 5$). **(D)**. The body weight curve of mice received control or DSS treatment ($n = 5$), p values are derived from one-way ANOVA analysis. **(E)**. The histology score of intestinal fibrosis mice with different treatment. Fibrosis was quantified using a combined score of fibrosis severity, circularity and the extent of fibrosis ($n = 5$). **(F)**. The hematoxylin and eosin staining **(left panel)** and α SMA IHC staining **(right panel)** of distal colon sections from control and DSS treated mice. scale bar 200 μm. **(G)**. The different expressed protein in DSS treatment mice and control mice that derived from proteomics analysis. **(H)**. The mRNA expression of GREM1 (human) in healthy control (HC) and IBD patient's data from SRP077046 and SRP100787. **(I)**. The mRNA expression of *Grem1* in control and intestinal fibrosis mice ($n = 5$). **(J)**. IHC staining of GREM1 in both mice and human in intestinal fibrosis tissues. scale bar 200 μm. p values are derived from two-sided Student's t test. $^{**}p \le 0.01$; $^{***}p \le 0.001$.

Statistical Analysis

All statistical analyses were carried out using GraphPad Prism v.7.0. D'Agostino and Pearson omnibus normality test to determine whether the data are normally distributed. For two-group comparisons, two-tailed Student's *t*-test was used for statistical analysis. After testing for normal distribution, statistical analysis was performed using ANOVA when more than two groups were compared. All data are presented as means ± SD (n.s., $p > 0.05$; $^*p \leq 0.05$; $^{**}p \leq 0.01$; $^{***},p \leq 0.001$).

RESULTS

Increased GREM1 Expression in Intestinal Fibrosis

To screen for potential therapeutic targets for intestinal fibrosis, we established an intestinal fibrosis mouse model by oral administration of three 2.5% DSS cycles to C57BL/6J mice (**Figure 1A**). The results showed that all DSS-treated mice developed serious colitis, and colon length and body weight were significantly lower in DSS-treated mice (**Figures 1B–E**). Further, intestinal tissue sections were subjected to hematoxylin-eosin (H&E) and anti-α-SMA immunohistochemical (IHC) staining. Pathological examination revealed that mice that received DSS treatment developed intestinal fibrosis, with fibroblast proliferation and ECM deposition (**Figure 1F**). Proteomic analysis of intestinal tissues indicated that GREM1 protein levels were dramatically elevated in fibrosed colon compared to that in normal colon tissue (**Figure 1G**). To confirm this in humans, we first compared *GREM1* mRNA expression using SRA datasets (SRP077046 and SRP100787) containing data for tissues from both healthy controls and CD and UC patients. The results showed that *GREM1* mRNA levels were significantly increased in human intestinal colitis samples (**Figure 1H**). Furthermore, we detected *GREM1* mRNA expression in intestinal fibrosis tissue and found that *GREM1* mRNA expression was also upregulated in fibrosed colon (**Figure 1I**). In line with this, IHC staining results revealed that GREM1 protein levels were greatly elevated in both murine and human intestinal fibrosis sections (**Figure 1J**). Collectively, these results suggested that GREM1 abundance was significantly increased in fibrosed colon tissues.

GREM1 Promotes Intestinal Fibroblast Proliferation and Activation

Next, we aimed to investigate the functional roles of GREM1 in the process of intestinal fibrosis development. Given that fibroblasts are the dominant effector cells in the development of intestinal fibrosis, we postulated whether GREM1 could promote proliferation and activation of intestinal fibroblasts. Two human intestinal fibroblast cell lines, CCD-18Co and CCD-112Co, were treated with different doses of the GREM1 protein in a serum-free culture medium. The results showed that GREM1 promoted fibroblast cell growth in a dose-dependent manner (**Figure 2A**). Further, to reveal whether GREM1 could facilitate the activation of fibroblasts, RT-qPCR was performed to detect altered expression of several typical fibroblast activation related genes, including *ACTA2, COL1A1, COL4A1*, and *VIM* in fibroblast cells upon administration of GREM1. Consistently, GREM1 treatment significantly increased the expression of these genes (**Figures 2B–E**). Given that activated fibroblasts could facilitate the progression of intestinal fibrosis by secreting cytokines, ELISA was performed to detect protein levels of IL-6, IL-1β, MCP1, and TNF. Levels of these cytokines were greatly increased after GREM1 treatment (**Figure 2F**). To further confirm this, intestinal fibroblast cell lines derived from patients with colon fibrosis were established following GREM1 ectopic expression or knockdown (**Supplementary Figure S1**). The results showed that additional GREM1 treatment significantly promoted the proliferation and activation of fibroblasts (**Figure 2G**). Conversely, the silencing of *GREM1* in fibroblasts delayed the fibrotic process (**Figure 2H**). Taken together, these data indicated that GREM1 could promote intestinal fibroblast proliferation and activation.

GREM1 Promotes Intestinal Fibroblast Proliferation by Enhancing Fatty Acid Oxidation

After stimulation with inflammatory effectors, fibroblasts start to proliferate and undergo trans-differentiation into contractile myofibroblasts, accompanied by energy status switching from quiescent to activated. In the kidney fibroblasts, Dario reported that Interleukin-1β activates a MYC-dependent metabolic switch in kidney stromal cells necessary for progressive tubulointerstitial fibrosis (Lemos et al., 2018). In addition, proceeding study reported that lipid metabolism in activated hepatic stellate cells is enhanced during liver fibrosis (Khomich et al., 2019); thus, we measured the lipid droplet content in GREM1-treated fibroblasts. BODIPY staining results showed that the abundance of lipid droplets was significantly decreased in GREM1 treated fibroblasts (**Figure 3A**). Next, the two major fatty acid oxidation products were measured in fibroblast cells treated with GREM1 or not. The results showed that acylcarnitine, derived from fatty acid oxidation by carnitine palmitoyl-transferase 1, (Schreurs et al., 2010; Qu et al., 2016), was significantly increased (**Figure 3B**). In line with this, the amounts of acetyl-CoA and fatty acid β-oxidation breakdown products were greatly elevated (**Figure 3C**). Furthermore, the OCR of GREM1-treated fibroblast cells was detected using a Seahorse. The data showed that GREM1 treatment markedly enhanced OCRs in fibroblast cells (**Figure 3D, Supplementary Figure S2A**). Moreover, GREM1 treatment did not affect the ECAR (**Supplementary Figure S2B**). Given that fatty acid oxidation produced much amount of energy, which could support the activation and proliferation of fibroblast. Furthermore, we aim to identify whether the promoting effects of GREM1 depended on enhanced FAO

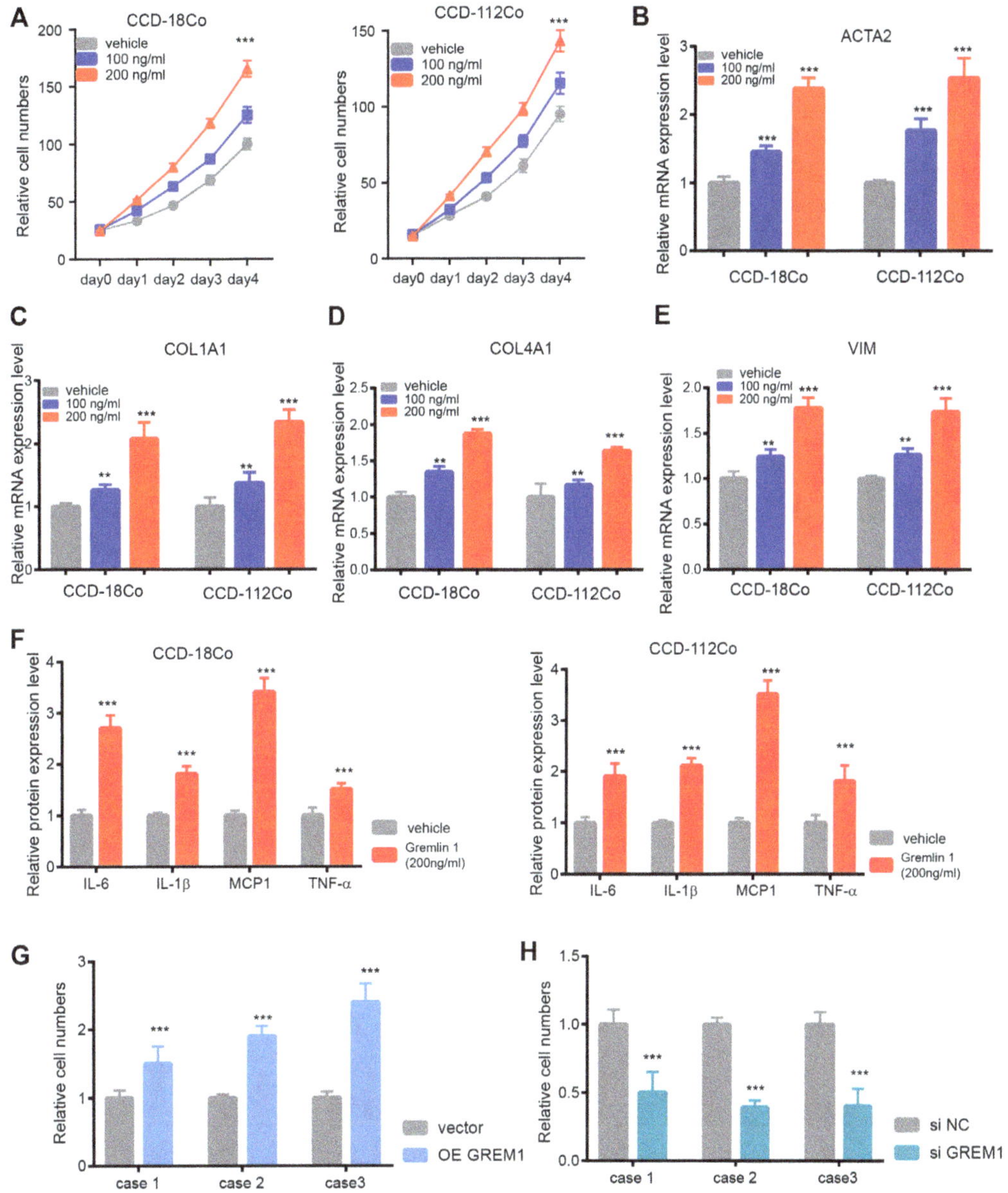

FIGURE 2 | Gremlin 1 promotes the proliferation and activation of intestinal fibroblast. **(A)**. Cell viability assay of human intestinal fibroblast cells CCD-18Co and CCD-112Co upon different dose of Gremlin 1 (100 and 200 ng/ml) treatment. **(B–E)**. The Q-PCR results of ACTA2 **(B)**, COL1A1 **(C)**, COL4A1 **(D)** and VIM **(E)**, intestinal fibroblast cells CCD-18Co and CCD-112Co upon 100 and 200 ng/ml of Gremlin 1 treatment for 24 h. **(F)**. The foldchanges of inflammation cytokines in human fibroblast cells CCD-18Co and CCD-112Co upon 200 ng/ml Gremlin 1 treatment for 24 h. **(G)**. The system of fibroblast and intestinal organoid culture system. **(H–I)**. The relative IL-1β level in the culture medium of the human intestinal organoid upon co-cultured with GREM1 gene overexpressed fibroblast cell **(H)** or GREM1 gene knockdown fibroblast cell **(I)** for 48 h. These experiments were repeated twice. p values are derived from one-way ANOVA analysis. Dunnett's test was used to analysis the difference between control group to the other groups. $^{**}p \leq 0.01$; $^{***}p \leq 0.001$.

in fibroblasts. We firstly detected the expression of FAO related genes in fibroblast cells upon GREM1 treatment. The results showed that *CPT1A, ACADM, ACADS ECI2 ACAT2,* and *ACAA2* expression significantly increased upon GREM1 treatment (**Figure 3E**). Further, we blocked the FAO in mitochondria using Etomoxir, an inhibitor of FAO. As expected, the indicated that Etomoxir usage impeded the proliferation and activation of fibroblasts otherwise mediated by GREM1 treatment (**Supplementary Figure S3**). Collectively, GREM1 promoted intestinal fibroblast proliferation by enhancing fatty acid oxidation.

GREM1 Activated VEGFR-2 Receptor in Fibroblasts

Next, we aimed to identify the receptor that senses GREM1 stimulation. Given that GREM1 is reported to be a BMP2 antagonist and ligand of VEGFR-2, we detected fibroblast cell

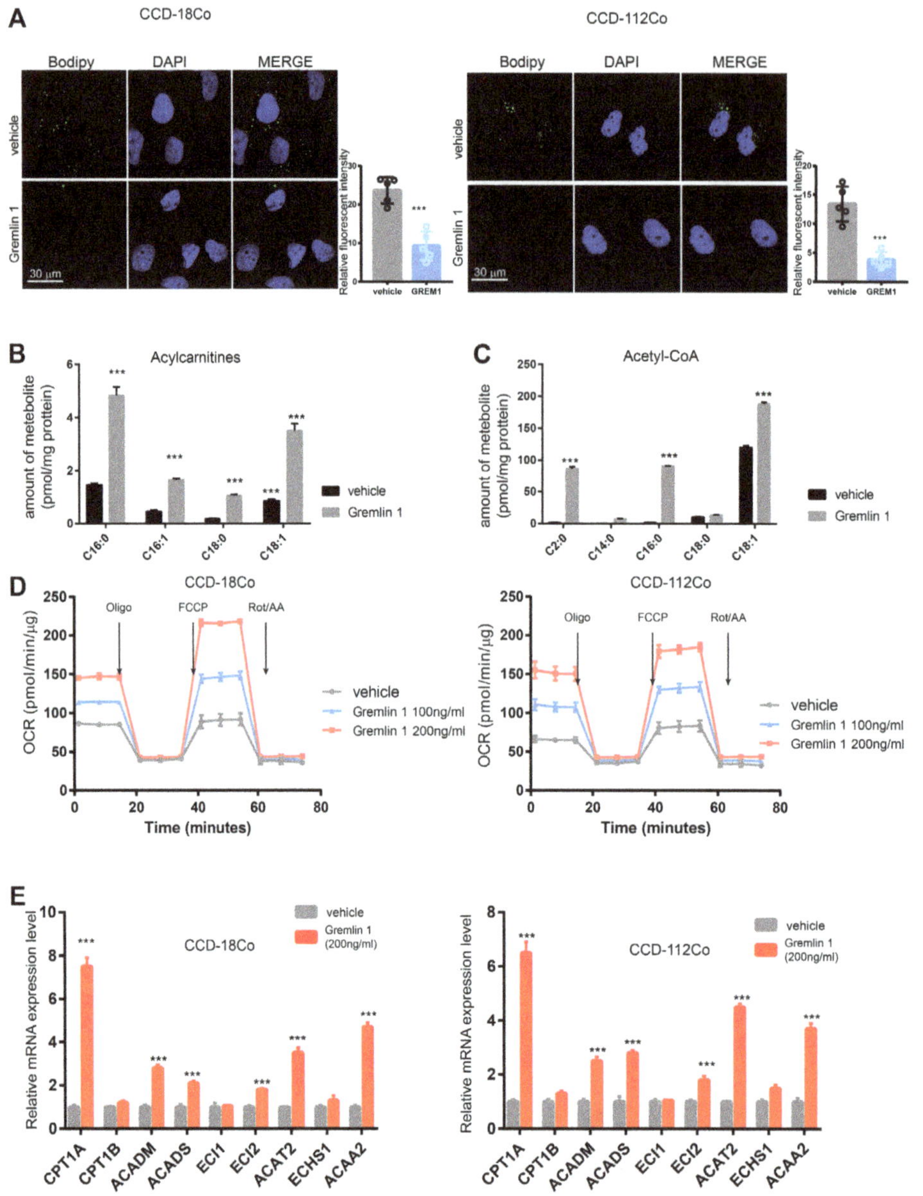

FIGURE 3 | Gremlin 1 facility the FAO of intestinal fibroblast cell. **(A)**. Bodipy assay of human intestinal fibroblast cells CCD-18Co and CCD-112Co cells that treated with 200 ng/ml Gremlin 1 for 24 h or not. Relative fluorescent intensity was calculated of five random fields of slides **(B, C)**. The amount of representative individual lipid species, lipid droplets degraded production, Acylcarnitines **(B)** and Acetyl-CoA **(C)** in human intestinal fibroblast cells CCD-18Co and CCD-112Co cells treated with 200 ng/ml Gremlin 1 for 24 h or not. The amounts of acylcarnitine and acetyl-CoA (were normalized to the total protein of fibroblast cells. **(D)**. The measurement of OCR in human intestinal fibroblast cells CCD-18Co and CCD-112Co cells treated with 200 ng/ml Gremlin 1 for 24 h or not. **(E)**. Q-PCR results of the FAO related genes expression in human intestinal fibroblast cells CCD-18Co and CCD-112Co cells treated with 200 ng/ml Gremlin 1 for 24 h or not. These experiments were repeated twice p values are derived from two-sided Student's t test. $^{**}p \leq 0.01$; $^{***}p \leq 0.001$.

proliferation upon knockdown of BMP2 or VEGFR-2 using siRNA (**Figures 4A,B**). The data showed that silencing VEGFR-2 expression dramatically diminished the growth-promoting effects of GREM1 in fibroblast cells, which was not observed in BMP2-silenced fibroblast cells, indicating that VEGFR-2 may act as a GREM1 receptor in intestinal fibroblasts. To further confirm this, VEGFR-2 was inhibited using the specific inhibitor SU5408. As anticipated, SU5408 also blocked the growth-promoting effects of GREM1 in fibroblasts (**Supplementary Figure S4**). Next, we measured OCRs to determine whether VEGFR-2 inhibition could block the enhanced FAO in fibroblasts. The data showed that both genetic and pharmacological VEGFR-2 inhibition could decrease the enhanced FAO mediated by GREM1 treatment (**Figures 4C,D**). Additionally, FAO-related mRNAs were also measured, and the results showed that expression of such genes decreased with VEGFR-2 inhibition (**Figure 4E**).

Taken together, GREM1 promoted intestinal fibroblast proliferation by activating VEGFR-2 receptor.

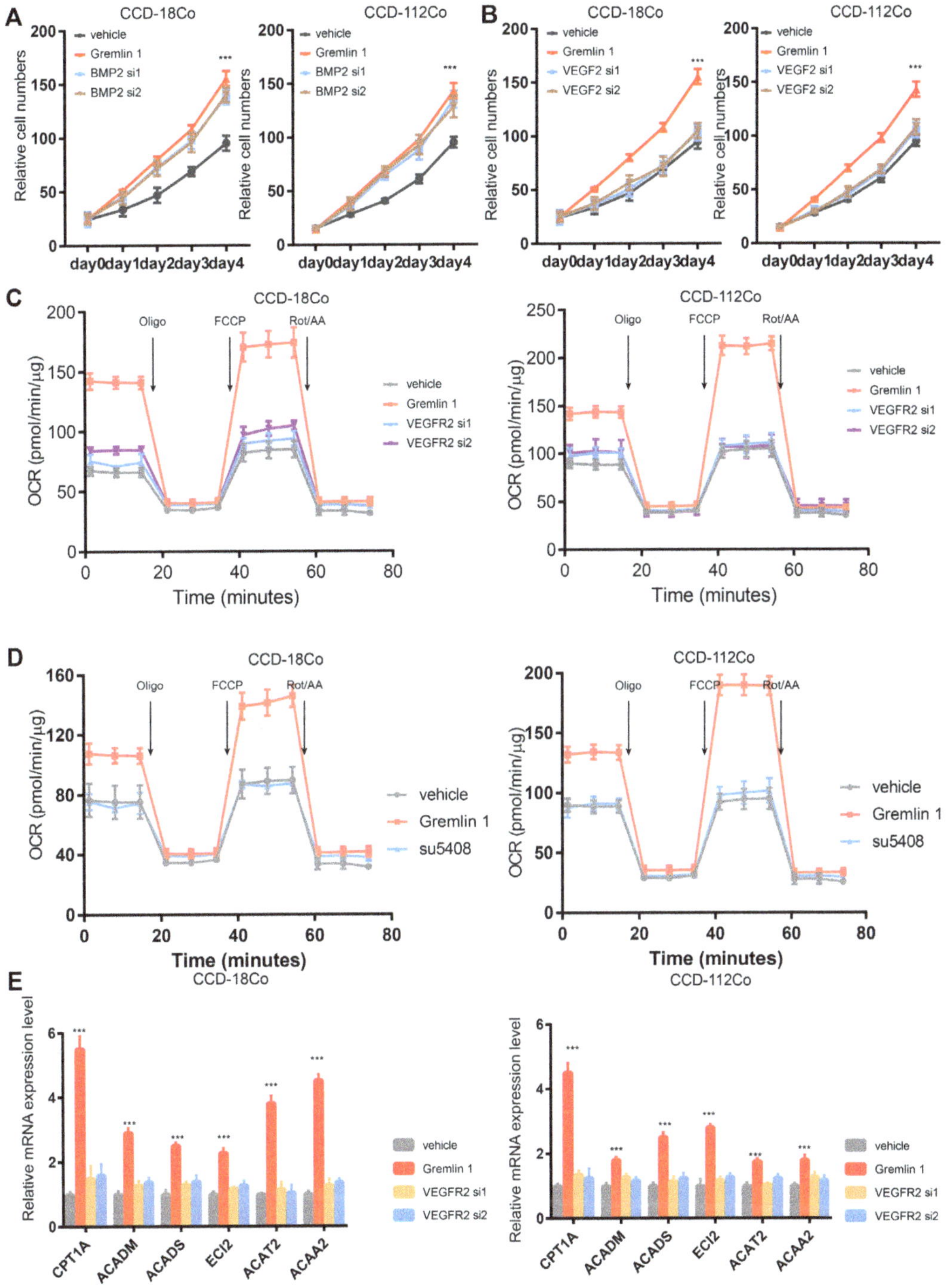

FIGURE 4 | Gremlin 1 activated VEGFR-2 to enhance the FAO of fibroblast. **(A)**. Cell viability assay of human intestinal fibroblast cells CCD-18Co and CCD-112Co treated with 200 ng/ml Gremlin 1 with or with not silencing BMP2 with siRNA. **(B)**. Cell viability assay of human intestinal fibroblast cells CCD-18Co and CCD-112Co treated with 200 ng/ml Gremlin 1 with or with not silencing VEGFR-2 with siRNA. **(C)**. The OCR results of CCD-18Co and CCD-112Co cells treated with 200 ng/ml Gremlin 1 for 24 h, following silencing VEGFR-2 with siRNA or not. **(D)**. The OCR results of human intestinal fibroblast cells CCD-18Co and CCD-112Co cells treated with 200 ng/ml Gremlin 1, following VEGFR-2 inhibitor SU5408 (100 nM) treatment for 24 h. **(E)**. Q-PCR results of genes related with FAO metabolism in the human intestinal fibroblast cells CCD-18Co and CCD-112Co cells. *p* values are derived from two-sided Student's *t* test. $^{**}p \leq 0.01$; $^{***}p \leq 0.001$.

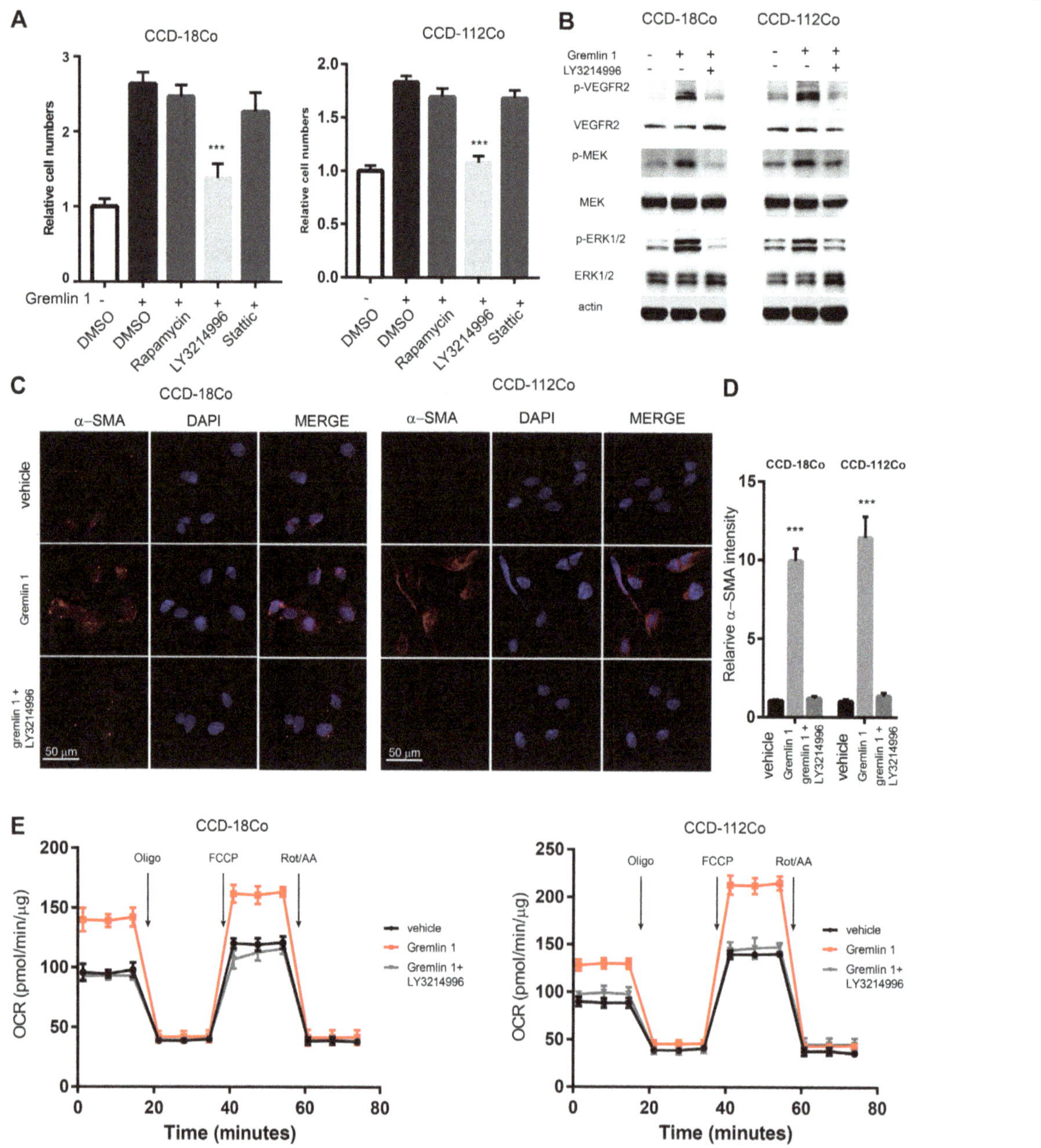

FIGURE 5 | VEGFR2-MEK-ERK axis mediated the enhancement of FAO from Gremlin 1. **(A)**. Cell viability assay of human intestinal fibroblast cells CCD-18Co and CCD-112Co cells treated with 200 ng/ml Gremlin 1 and Rapamycin (10 nM), LY3214996 (10 nM) or stattic (10 μM) for 24 h. **(B)**. Immunoblotting analysis of VEGFR2-MEK-ERK signaling in human intestinal fibroblast cells CCD-18Co and CCD-112Co cells treated with 200 ng/ml Gremlin 1 and LY3214996 (10 nM) for 24 h. Actin acted as loading control and re-used for illustrative purposes. **(C)**. Immunofluorescence staining of a-SMA in human intestinal fibroblast cells CCD-18Co and CCD-112Co cells treated with 200 ng/ml Gremlin 1 and LY3214996 (10 nM). **(D)**. The intensity statistical results of a-SMA immunofluorescence staining from five random fields of slides. E. OCR measurement of CCD-18Co and CCD-112Co cells treated with 200 ng/ml Gremlin 1 and LY3214996 (10 nM) for 24 h. *p* values are derived from one-way ANOVA analysis. Dunnett's test was used to analysis the difference between control group to the other groups. $^{**}p \leq 0.01$; $^{***}p \leq 0.001$.

GREM1 Activates MAPK Pathway to Enhance Fatty Acid Oxidation

In order to uncover the underlying signaling mechanisms leading to FAO enhancement, the reported VEGFR-2 downstream signaling pathways (including the PI3K-mTOR, MAPK, and STAT3 pathways) were inhibited with the specific inhibitors Rapamycin, LY3214996, and Stattic, respectively, (**Figure 5A**). Cell viability assays showed that only the MAPK signaling inhibitor LY3214996 could diminish the otherwise increased proliferation mediated by GREM1. Western blot analysis showed that treatment with GREM1 strongly increased the phosphorylation levels of p-VEGFR-2, its downstream signaling p-MEK, and p-ERK1/2,

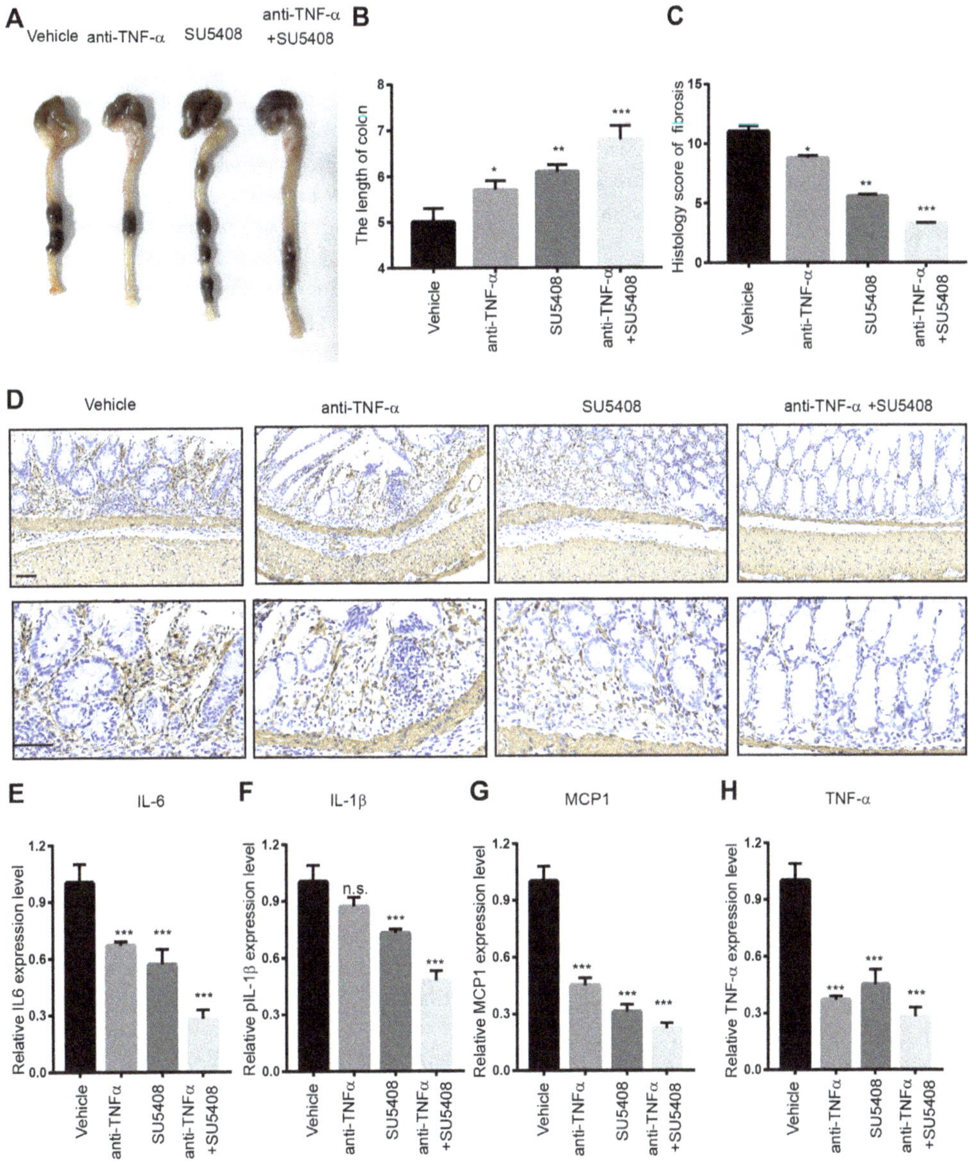

FIGURE 6 | Gremlin 1-VEGFR2 axis disruption impeded the progression of intestinal fibrosis. **(A)**. The appearance of the colons from the mice with intestinal fibrosis treated with vehicle, anti-TNF-α monotherapy (100 μg), SU5408 (5 mg/kg), or anti-TNF-α therapy combined with SU5408 treatment. **(B)**. The statistical results of colon length in mice with vehicle, anti-TNF-α monotherapy (100 μg), SU5408 (5 mg/kg), or anti-TNF-α therapy combined with SU5408 treatment ($n = 5$). **(C)**. The histology score of intestinal fibrosis mice with different treatment. Fibrosis was quantified using a combined score of fibrosis severity, circularity and the extent of fibrosis ($n = 5$). **(D)**. α-SMA IHC staining of intestinal sections from intestinal fibrosis mice with different treatment. scale bar 100 μm **(E–H)**. The protein expression level of IL-6, IL-1β, MCP1, and TNF-α in the colon of different group mice treated with vehicle, anti-TNF-α monotherapy (100 μg), SU5408 (5 mg/kg), or anti-TNF-α therapy combined with SU5408 treatment ($n = 5$). p values are derived from one-way ANOVA analysis. Dunnett's test was used to analysis the difference between control group to the other groups. n. s., $p > 0.05$; $^{*}p \le 0.05$; $^{**}p \le 0.01$; $^{***}p \le 0.001$.

which were inhibited by LY3214996 treatment (**Figure 5B**). Immunofluorescent imaging also revealed that MAPK signaling inhibition blocked increased α-SMA expression in intestinal fibroblasts (**Figures 5C,D**). Furthermore, we measured OCR levels in intestinal fibroblasts. Accordingly, the elevated OCRs were abolished by LY3214996 treatment (**Figure 5E**). In line with this, the increased acylcarnitine and acetyl-CoA levels decreased upon LY3214996 treatment (**Supplementary Figure S5**). Together, these data sets suggested that GREM1 activated the MAPK pathway to enhance fatty acid oxidation in intestinal fibroblasts.

Blocking GREM1-VEGFR2 Axis Impedes Intestinal Fibrosis Progression *in vivo*

Next, we evaluated whether GREM1-VEGFR2 axis downstream signaling blockage by a VEGFR2-specific inhibitor could prevent intestinal fibrosis progression upon DSS challenge. Anti-TNFα therapy is one of standard treatment strategies for intestinal fibrosis. We aim to determine whether combine SU5408 with Anti-TNF therapy could provide more benefits for intestinal fibrosis patients. For this purpose, either VEGFR2-specific inhibitor SU5408 or SU5408 plus anti-TNF-α therapy was applied to the intestinal fibrosis mouse model (**Figure 6A**). The results showed that SU5408 usage could restore the duration of colon reduction mediated by DSS challenge, while anti-TNF-α monotherapy was associated with a slight improvement in colonic length. Of note, combining anti-TNF-α antibody with SU5408 significantly restored colonic length (**Figures 6B,C**). Furthermore, the deposition of ECM was found to be dramatically reduced in both groups of mice treated with SU5408 alone or in combination with anti-TNF-α therapy. In addition, α-SMA IHC staining intensity was much weaker in colon sections derived from SU5048-treated mice than in mice in the control group, suggesting a reduction in the proportion of fibroblasts (**Figure 6D**). Additionally, we measured *Col1a1* and *Vim* mRNA expression levels in colon. GREM1-VEGFR2 axis blockage treatment greatly inhibited the expression of *Col1a1* and *Vim* (**Supplementary Figure 6**). Moreover, VEGFR2 inhibition significantly attenuated the levels of the inflammation-related cytokines TNF-α, MCP1, IL-6, and IL-1β (**Figures 6E–H**). Together, these data sets indicated that GREM1-VEGFR2 axis disruption could diminish the proliferation and function of fibroblasts in the colon of mice with intestinal fibrosis.

DISCUSSION

In this study, we found that GREM1 levels were greatly increased in both human and murine fibrosed colon. Functional experiments revealed that GREM1 promoted intestinal fibroblast cell proliferation by enhancing fatty acid oxidation. Further mechanistic studies revealed that GREM1 could activate VEGFR2 and trigger downstream MAPK signaling, which facilitated the expression of FAO-related genes, consequently enhancing fatty acid oxidation.

Intestinal fibrosis is a common finding in patients with IBD (Latella et al., 2014). Current studies indicate that only anti-inflammatory therapy does not impede the development of fibrosis (Latella and Papi, 2012). Fibroblast expansion and activation are major factors that facilitate the progression of intestinal fibrosis. Rapid growth and ECM deposition require a huge amount of energy. Previous studies reported that fibroblasts could reprogram their metabolism by enhancing glycolysis and FAO to sustain cell proliferation and activation (Schreurs et al., 2010; Latella and Papi, 2012; Latella et al., 2014; Qu et al., 2016; Khomich et al., 2019; Chen et al., 2020). In kidney stromal cells, Interleukin-1β induced glycolysis enhancement is necessary for progressive tubulointerstitial fibrosis (Lemos et al., 2018). Additionally, hepatic stellate cell activation results in decrease of lipid droplet abundance and increased levels of polyunsaturated fatty acids (Tuohetahuntila et al., 2015). We consistently observed significant numbers of lipid droplets and enhanced FAO in intestinal fibroblast cells upon GREM1 treatment. On the other hand, Chung et al. (Chen et al., 2020) reported that the expression of FAO-associated enzymes in renal tubule epithelium is reduced in aged rat kidneys. This facilitates the progression of renal fibrosis indicating that FAO alterations in fibroblast and epithelial cells affect the progression of fibrosis differently.

Recent studies have shown that GREM1 is mainly secreted by fibroblast cells, including cancer-associated fibroblasts (Worthley et al., 2015) which can promote the proliferation of cancer cells (Sneddon et al., 2006). High GREM1 expression is related to poorer outcomes in CRC and breast cancer patients (Dutton et al., 2019; Neckmann et al., 2019; Ren et al., 2019). GREM1 also regulates differentiation of glioma cells (Yan et al., 2014). In the current study, we found that GREM1 could activate VEGFR 2, but is not involved in BMP signaling, which further activated downstream MAPK signaling, resulting in FAO enhancement. Recently, GREM1 was reported to activate STAT3 signaling in breast cancer cells (Sung et al., 2020). However, our data suggested that STAT3 was not involved in GREM1-mediated fibroblast cell proliferation and activation, indicating that the signaling regulated by GREM1 is largely context-dependent.

Our *in vivo* experimental results showed that disruption to the GREM1-VEGFR2 axis downstream signaling using SU5408 could delay the progression of intestinal fibrosis. Recently, Kobayashi and colleagues reported that a GREM1-neutralizing antibody could prevent colorectal carcinogenesis (Kobayashi et al., 2020). We realized that a GREM1-neutralizing antibody might be a superior option for our animal studies. However, such a neutralizing antibody is commercially inaccessible. In addition, after carefully checking the patent, such a GREM1-neutralizing antibody was designed to block interactions involving GREM1 and BMP proteins, indicating that this antibody is not the best choice for blocking the GREM1 and VEGFR2 axis. Thus, further efforts are needed to develop neutralizing antibodies or peptides that block interactions between GREM1 and VEGFR2. In addition, our current data showed that blocking the GREM1–VEGFR2 axis combined with anti-TNF-α therapy could provide benefits in mice suffering from intestinal fibrosis, indicating that the combine therapy of anti-TNF-α and GREM1–VEGFR2 blockage could be a potential strategy for intestinal fibrosis patients.

In conclusion, our data revealed that GREM1 promoted the proliferation and activation of fibroblasts by activating VEGFR-2, leading to FAO enhancement. Inhibition of the GREM1-VEGFR2 axis impeded progression in the murine intestinal fibrosis model, indicating that GREM1 could represent a potential target for anti-fibrotic therapy.

ETHICS STATEMENT

The studies involving human participants were reviewed and approved by Institutional Animal Care and Use Committee of

Laboratory Animal Center of Daping Hospital, Army Medical University. The patients/participants provided their written informed consent to participate in this study. The animal study was reviewed and approved by Institutional Animal Care and Use Committee of Laboratory Animal Center of Daping Hospital, Army Medical University.

AUTHOR CONTRIBUTIONS

H-TG and YY were responsible for the study concept and design. YY and QSZ performed all the experiments with help from JZ and MZ. JN, and DC provided human samples. H-TG, YY, and DC analyzed and all authors helped to interpret the data. All authors revised the manuscript.

81470826 to H-TG), Foundation and Frontier Projects of Chongqing Science and Technology Commission (No. cstc2016jcyjA0079 to YY), the Science Foundation from Science and Technology Department of Sichuan Province (No. 2019YFS0262 to H-TG) and 1.3.5 Project for Disciplines of Excellence, West China Hospital, Sichuan University (No. ZYGD18023 to H-TG).

ACKNOWLEDGMENTS

We would like to thank editage (www.editage.cn) for English language editing.

REFERENCES

Burke, J. P., Ferrante, M., Dejaegher, K., Watson, R. W. G., Docherty, N. G., De Hertogh, G., et al. (2008). Transcriptomic Analysis of Intestinal Fibrosis-Associated Gene Expression in Response to Medical Therapy in Crohn's Disease. *Inflamm. Bowel Dis.* 14 (9), 1197–1204. doi:10.1002/ibd.20482

Chen, Y., Yan, Q., Lv, M., Song, K., Dai, Y., Huang, Y., et al. (2020). Involvement of FATP2-Mediated Tubular Lipid Metabolic Reprogramming in Renal Fibrogenesis. *Cell Death Dis.* 11 (11), 994. doi:10.1038/s41419-020-03199-x

Cheng, X., Geng, F., Pan, M., Wu, X., Zhong, Y., Wang, C., et al. (2020). Targeting DGAT1 Ameliorates Glioblastoma by Increasing Fat Catabolism and Oxidative Stress. *Cel Metab.* 32 (2), 229–242. doi:10.1016/j.cmet.2020.06.002

Dutton, L. R., Hoare, O. P., McCorry, A. M. B., Redmond, K. L., Adam, N. E., Canamara, S., et al. (2019). Fibroblast-derived Gremlin1 Localises to Epithelial Cells at the Base of the Intestinal Crypt. *Oncotarget* 10 (45), 4630–4639. doi:10.18632/oncotarget.27050

Fichtner-Feigl, S., Fuss, I. J., Young, C. A., Watanabe, T., Geissler, E. K., Schlitt, H.-J., et al. (2007). Induction of IL-13 Triggers TGF-β1-dependent Tissue Fibrosis in Chronic 2,4,6-Trinitrobenzene Sulfonic Acid Colitis. *J. Immunol.* 178, 5859–5870. doi:10.4049/jimmunol.178.9.5859

Hagenlocher, Y., Satzinger, S., Civelek, M., Feilhauer, K., Köninger, J., Bischoff, S. C., et al. (2017). Cinnamon Reduces Inflammatory Response in Intestinal Fibroblasts In Vitro and in Colitis In Vivo Leading to Decreased Fibrosis. *Mol. Nutr. Food Res.* 61 (9), 1601085. doi:10.1002/mnfr.201601085

Honma, R., Sakamoto, N., Ishikawa, A., Taniyama, D., Fukada, K., Hattori, T., et al. (2018). Clinicopathological and Prognostic Significance of Epithelial Gremlin1 Expression in Gastric *Cancer. Anticancer Res.* 38 (3), 1419–1425. doi:10.21873/anticanres.12366

Hsu, D. R., Economides, A. N., Wang, X., Eimon, P. M., and Harland, R. M. (1998). The *Xenopus* Dorsalizing Factor Gremlin Identifies a Novel Family of Secreted Proteins that Antagonize BMP Activities. *Mol. Cel.* 1 (5), 673–683. doi:10.1016/s1097-2765(00)80067-2

Khomich, O., Ivanov, A. V., and Bartosch, B. (2019). Metabolic Hallmarks of Hepatic Stellate Cells in Liver Fibrosis. *Cells* 9 (1), 24. doi:10.3390/cells9010024

Kobayashi, H., Gieniec, K., Wright, J., Wang, T., Asai, N., Mizutani, Y., et al. (2020). The Balance of Stromal BMP Signaling Mediated by GREM1 and ISLR Drives Colorectal Carcinogenesis. *Gastroenterology* 160, 1224-1239. doi:10.1053/j.gastro.2020.11.011

Latella, G., and Papi, C. (2012). Crucial Steps in the Natural History of Inflammatory Bowel Disease. *Wjg* 18 (29), 3790–3799. doi:10.3748/wjg.v18.i29.3790

Latella, G., Rogler, G., Bamias, G., Breynaert, C., Florholmen, J., Pellino, G., et al. (2014). Results of the 4th Scientific Workshop of the ECCO (I): Pathophysiology of Intestinal Fibrosis in IBD. *J. Crohn's Colitis* 8 (10), 1147–1165. doi:10.1016/j.crohns.2014.03.008

Lawrance, I. C., Maxwell, L., and Doe, W. (2001). Altered Response of Intestinal Mucosal Fibroblasts to Profibrogenic Cytokines in Inflammatory Bowel Disease. *Inflamm. Bowel Dis.* 7 (3), 226–236. doi:10.1097/00054725-200108000-00008

Lawrance, I. C., Rogler, G., Bamias, G., Breynaert, C., Florholmen, J., Pellino, G., et al. (2017). Cellular and Molecular Mediators of Intestinal Fibrosis. *Eccojc* 11 (12), j.crohns.2014.09.008–503. doi:10.1016/j.crohns.2014.09.008

Leake, I. (2015). Cathelicidin Can Reverse Intestinal Fibrosis in Models of Colitis. *Nat. Rev. Gastroenterol. Hepatol.* 12 (1), 3. doi:10.1038/nrgastro.2014.214

Lemos, D. R., McMurdo, M., Karaca, G., Wilflingseder, J., Leaf, I. A., Gupta, N., et al. (2018). Interleukin-1β Activates a MYC-dependent Metabolic Switch in Kidney Stromal Cells Necessary for Progressive Tubulointerstitial Fibrosis. *Jasn* 29 (6), 1690–1705. doi:10.1681/asn.2017121283

Mezzano, S., Droguett, A., Lavoz, C., Krall, P., Egido, J., and Ruiz-Ortega, M. (2018). Gremlin and Renal Diseases: Ready to Jump the Fence to Clinical Utility?. *Nephrol. Dial. Transplant.*, 33, 735–741. doi:10.1093/ndt/gfx194

Mitola, S., Ravelli, C., Moroni, E., Salvi, V., Leali, D., Ballmer-Hofer, K., et al. (2010). Gremlin Is a Novel Agonist of the Major Proangiogenic Receptor VEGFR2. *Blood* 116 (18), 3677–3680. doi:10.1182/blood-2010-06-291930

Neckmann, U., Wolowczyk, C., Hall, M., Almaas, E., Ren, J., Zhao, S., et al. (2019). GREM1 Is Associated with Metastasis and Predicts Poor Prognosis in ER-Negative Breast Cancer Patients. *Cell Commun Signal* 17 (1), 140. doi:10.1186/s12964-019-0467-7

Nyqvist, J., Persson, F., Parris, T. Z., Helou, K., Kenne Sarenmalm, E., Einbeigi, Z., et al. (2017). Metachronous and Synchronous Occurrence of 5 Primary Malignancies in a Female Patient between 1997 and 2013: A Case Report with Germline and Somatic Genetic Analysis. *Case Rep. Oncol.* 10 (3), 1006–1012. doi:10.1159/000484403

Qu, Q., Zeng, F., Liu, X., Wang, Q. J., and Deng, F. (2016). Fatty Acid Oxidation and Carnitine Palmitoyltransferase I: Emerging Therapeutic Targets in Cancer. *Cel Death Dis.* 7 (5), e2226. doi:10.1038/cddis.2016.132

Ren, J., Smid, M., Iaria, J., Salvatori, D. C. F., van Dam, H., Zhu, H. J., et al. (2019). Cancer-associated Fibroblast-Derived Gremlin 1 Promotes Breast Cancer Progression. *Breast Cancer Res.* 21 (1), 109. doi:10.1186/s13058-019-1194-0

Rieder, F., and Fiocchi, C. (2009). Intestinal Fibrosis in IBD-A Dynamic, Multifactorial Process. *Nat. Rev. Gastroenterol. Hepatol.* 6 (4), 228–235. doi:10.1038/nrgastro.2009.31

Schreurs, M., Kuipers, F., and van der Leij, F. R. (2010). Regulatory Enzymes of Mitochondrial β-oxidation as Targets for Treatment of the Metabolic Syndrome. *Obes. Rev. : official J. Int. Assoc. Study Obes.* 11 (5), 380–388. doi:10.1111/j.1467-789X.2009.00642.x

Simmons, J. G., Pucilowska, J. B., Keku, T. O., and Lund, P. K. (2002). IGF-I and TGF-B1 Have Distinct Effects on Phenotype and Proliferation of Intestinal Fibroblasts. *Am. J. Physiology-Gastrointestinal Liver Physiol.* 283 (3), G809–G818. doi:10.1152/ajpgi.00057.2002

Sneddon, J. B., Zhen, H. H., Montgomery, K., van de Rijn, M., Tward, A. D., West, R., et al. (2006). Bone Morphogenetic Protein Antagonist Gremlin 1 Is Widely Expressed by Cancer-Associated Stromal Cells and Can Promote Tumor Cell Proliferation. *Proc. Natl. Acad. Sci.* 103 (40), 14842–14847. doi:10.1073/pnas.0606857103

Speca, S., Rousseaux, C., Dubuquoy, C., Rieder, F., Vetuschi, A., Sferra, R., et al. (2016). Novel PPARγ Modulator GED-0507-34 Levo Ameliorates Inflammation-Driven Intestinal Fibrosis. *Inflamm. Bowel Dis.* 22 (2), 279–292. doi:10.1097/mib.0000000000000618

Su, H. Y., Gupta, V., Day, A. S., and Gearry, R. B. (2016). Rising Incidence of Inflammatory Bowel Disease in Canterbury, New Zealand. *Inflamm. Bowel Dis.* 22 (9), 2238–2244. doi:10.1097/mib.0000000000000829

Sung, N. J., Kim, N. H., Surh, Y.-J., and Park, S.-A. (2020). Gremlin-1 Promotes Metastasis of Breast *Cancer* Cells by Activating STAT3-MMP13 Signaling Pathway. *Ijms* 21 (23), 9227. doi:10.3390/ijms21239227

Tuohetahuntila, M., Spee, B., Kruitwagen, H. S., Wubbolts, R., Brouwers, J. F., van de Lest, C. H., et al. (2015). Role of Long-Chain Acyl-CoA Synthetase 4 in Formation of Polyunsaturated Lipid Species in Hepatic Stellate Cells. *Biochim. Biophys. Acta (Bba) - Mol. Cel Biol. Lipids* 1851 (2), 220–230. doi:10.1016/j.bbalip.2014.12.003

Vallance, B. A., Gunawan, M. I., Hewlett, B., Bercik, P., Van Kampen, C., Galeazzi, F., et al. (2005). TGF-β1 Gene Transfer to the Mouse Colon Leads to Intestinal Fibrosis. *Am. J. Physiology-Gastrointestinal Liver Physiol.* 289 (1), G116–G128. doi:10.1152/ajpgi.00051.2005

Vítek, L., and Tiribelli, C. (2020). Bilirubin, Intestinal Integrity, the Microbiome, and Inflammation. *N. Engl. J. Med.* 383 (7), 684–686. doi:10.1056/NEJMcibr2013250

Weder, B., Mamie, C., Rogler, G., Clarke, S., McRae, B., Ruiz, P. A., et al. (2018). BCL2 Regulates Differentiation of Intestinal Fibroblasts. *Inflamm. Bowel Dis.* 24 (9), 1953–1966. doi:10.1093/ibd/izy147

Worthley, D. L., Churchill, M., Compton, J. T., Tailor, Y., Rao, M., Si, Y., et al. (2015). Gremlin 1 Identifies a Skeletal Stem Cell with Bone, Cartilage, and Reticular Stromal Potential. *Cell* 160, 269–284. doi:10.1016/j.cell.2014.11.042

Yan, K., Wu, Q., Yan, D. H., Lee, C. H., Rahim, N., Tritschler, I., et al. (2014). Glioma Cancer Stem Cells Secrete Gremlin1 to Promote Their Maintenance within the Tumor Hierarchy. *Genes Development* 28 (10), 1085–1100. doi:10.1101/gad.235515.113

11

A Retinoid X Receptor Agonist Directed to the Large Intestine Ameliorates T-Cell-Mediated Colitis in Mice

Ryohtaroh Matsumoto[1], Daisuke Takahashi[1], Masaki Watanabe[2], Shunsuke Nakatani[2], Yuta Takamura[2], Yuji Kurosaki[2], Hiroki Kakuta[2] and Koji Hase[1,3]**

[1]*Division of Biochemistry, Graduate School of Pharmaceutical Science and Faculty of Pharmacy, Keio University, Tokyo, Japan,* [2]*Division of Pharmaceutical Sciences, Graduate School of Medicine Dentistry and Pharmaceutical Sciences, Okayama University, Okayama, Japan,* [3]*International Research and Development Center for Mucosal Vaccines, The Institute of Medical Science, The University of Tokyo (IMSUT), Tokyo, Japan*

***Correspondence:**
Hiroki Kakuta
kakuta-h@okayama-u.ac.jp
Koji Hase
hase-kj@pha.keio.ac.jp

Retinoid X receptor (RXR) is a nuclear receptor that heterodimerizes with several nuclear receptors, integrating ligand-mediated signals across the heterodimers. Synthetic RXR agonists have been developed to cure certain inflammatory diseases, including inflammatory bowel diseases (IBDs). However, pre-existing RXR agonists, which are lipophilic and readily absorbed in the upper intestine, cause considerable adverse effects such as hepatomegaly, hyperlipidemia, and hypothyroidism. To minimize these adverse effects, we have developed an RXR agonist, NEt-3IB, which has lipophilic and thus poorly absorptive properties. In this study, we evaluated the effects of NEt-3IB in an experimental murine colitis model induced through the adoptive transfer of CD45RB^{high}CD4^{+} T cells. Pharmacokinetic studies demonstrated that the major portion of NEt-3IB was successfully delivered to the large intestine after oral administration. Notably, NEt-3IB treatment suppressed the development of T cell-mediated chronic colitis, as indicated by improvement of wasting symptoms, inflammatory infiltration, and mucosal hyperplasia. The protective effect of NEt-3IB was mediated by the suppression of IFN-γ-producing Th1 cell expansion in the colon. In conclusion, NEt-3IB, a large intestine-directed RXR agonist, is a promising drug candidate for IBDs.

Keywords: RXR, NEt-3IB, inflammatory bowel disease, colitis, Th1 cells

INTRODUCTION

Crohn's disease (CD) is an inflammatory bowel disease (IBD) that is characterized by intermittent abdominal pain, diarrhea, bodyweight loss, and hematochezia (bloody stools) (Ho and Khalil, 2015). Although the exact etiology of CD is unknown, genetic variations and immune dysregulation have been implicated in CD development (De Souza and Fiocchi, 2016). In the gastrointestinal mucosal of patients with CD, inflammation is prolonged by excessive activation of immune cells such as effector T cells and inflammatory macrophages (De Souza and Fiocchi, 2016). For decades, steroids have been used to cure CD, although long-term treatment with these agents causes considerable adverse effects such as edema and sleep disturbance (Carter et al., 2004). More recently, biological agents such as anti-TNF-α antibodies were developed to potently suppress the inflammatory response in CD.

However, the cost of biological agents is much higher than that of the classical chemical drugs, and approximately 30% of CD patients fail to respond to therapy using anti-TNF-α antibodies (Adegbola et al., 2018). Moreover, half of the primary responders lose their therapeutic response over time, thereby facing an increased dosage or a revised therapeutic strategy (Adegbola et al., 2018). These facts emphasize the medical need for the development of first-in-class medicines with high efficacy, low cost, and minimal adverse effects.

Retinoid X receptor (RXR) is a nuclear receptor that heterodimerizes with other nuclear receptors such as peroxisome proliferator-activated receptor (PPAR), liver X receptor (LXR), pregnane X receptor (PXR), and NR4A1 (Nur77) (Evans and Mangelsdorf, 2014). Treatment with an RXR agonist can activate these partner nuclear receptors without their own ligand stimulation (Takeuchi et al., 2013; Evans and Mangelsdorf, 2014), a phenomenon termed the "permissive effect." Activation of these nuclear receptors shows an anti-inflammatory effect, at least partly through mitigating the proliferation and differentiation of inflammatory macrophages and effector T cells (Onuki et al., 2018). In particular, activation of PPARγ by agonist treatment inhibits the differentiation of IFN-γ-producing type 1 helper T (Th1) cells by blocking the JAK–STAT signaling pathway (Natarajan and Bright, 2002; Kanakasabai et al., 2010; Solt et al., 2012). Similarly, activation of LXR inhibits the proliferation of T cells by controlling sterol metabolism via induction of ATP-binding cassette transporter G1 (ABCG1), which is involved in the transmembrane transport of sterols (Bensinger et al., 2008). NR4A1 deficiency is reported to expand the Th1 response because activation of NR4A1 also limits the proliferation of $CD4^+$ T cells by controlling oxidative phosphorylation and aerobic glycolysis (Liebmann et al., 2018). Furthermore, treatment with a PXR agonist prevents the expansion of Th1 cells (Dubrac et al., 2010).

RXR agonists can activate these partner receptors simultaneously, and therefore RXR was considered a promising molecular target for inflammatory disorders. Nonetheless, pre-existing RXR agonists have been reported to induce various adverse effects, such as excess bodyweight gain, hepatomegaly, hypothyroidism, and hypertriglyceridemia (Standeven et al., 1997; Liu et al., 2002; de Vries-Van der Weij et al., 2009). To address this issue, we recently developed NEt-3IB, an RXR full agonist with lower lipophilicity compared with pre-existing RXR agonists such as bexarotene (**Figure 1A**) (Kobayashi et al., 2015). We demonstrated that NEt-3IB induces a low blood concentration after oral administration. Furthermore, using PET/CT imaging, we also observed that NEt-3IB exhibited enterohepatic circulation upon intestinal absorption and was delivered to the lower digestive tract (Kobayashi et al., 2015). These pharmacokinetic properties of NEt-3IB may be beneficial in avoiding systemic adverse effects and delivering the drug to the lower intestine (Kakuta et al., 2012). In this study, we evaluated the anti-inflammatory effects of NEt-3IB in an experimental CD model induced by adoptive transfer of $CD45RB^{high}CD4^+$ T cells (Powrie et al., 1993). We report that NEt-3IB was persistent in the intestinal lumen after oral administration and ameliorated the wasting and colitis. This effect was attributed to the reduced accumulation of Th1 cells in the colon.

MATERIALS AND METHODS

Chemical Reagents

Bexarotene and NEt-3IB were synthesized as described previously (Boehm et al., 1994; Takamatsu et al., 2008).

Animals

ICR mice were purchased from Charles River Laboratories Japan (Yokohama, Japan) and maintained under specific pathogen-free (SPF) conditions at Okayama University, Okayama, Japan. C.B-17-*scid/scid* and C.B-$17^{+/+}$ mice were purchased from CLEA Japan (Tokyo, Japan) and maintained under SPF conditions at Keio University, Tokyo, Japan. $Rag1^{-/-}$ mice were bred and maintained under SPF conditions at Keio University. C.B-17-scid/scid and $Rag1^{-/-}$ mice were fed with CE-2 diet (CLEA Japan) before T cell transfer and with MF diet (Oriental Yeast, Tokyo, Japan) containing 0.015% NEt-3IB or regular MF after transfer. Foxp3-hCD2 knock-in mice were bred and maintained under SPF conditions at Keio University. C57BL6/J mice were purchased from CLEA Japan. Foxp3-hCD2 knock-in mice and C57BL6/J mice were fed with AIN-93G diet (Research Diet, New Brunswick, NJ, United States) until their use in experiments at 6–12 weeks old. All animal experiments except for pharmacokinetic studies were approved by the Animal Studies Committees of Keio University.

Pharmacokinetic Studies

This experiment was conducted in accordance with the Guidelines for Animal Experiments at Department of Animal Resources, Advanced Science Research Center, Okayama University, and all procedures were approved by the Animal Care and Use Committee, Okayama University. The test compounds were administered to 6-week-old ICR male mice (n = 5 per group). In the oral administration study, the test compounds (10 mg/10 ml/kg) were suspended in 1% ethanol and 0.5% carboxymethyl cellulose (CMC) in distilled water and administered by oral gavage. In the intravenous administration study, the test compounds (1 mg/5 ml/kg) were dissolved in saline containing 20% WellSolve (Celeste Corporation, Tokyo, Japan) and administered via the tail vein. Blood samples (approximately 0.6–1.0 ml each) were taken from the inferior vena cava under isoflurane anesthesia at 0.5, 1, 3, 6, and 24 h after administration. Then the animals were killed by cervical dislocation. Brain, liver, kidney, bile, and large-intestinal contents were immediately extirpated. Blood treated with heparin in a centrifuge tube was centrifuged at 1,900 × g at room temperature for 5 min. To 100 μl of the resulting plasma, 100 μl ice-cold 5.0 mM ammonium acetate solution (adjusted with acetic acid to pH 5.0) and 1.0 ml ice-cold EtOAc were added. The resulting mixture was vortexed for 30 s, kept at room temperature for 10 min, and centrifuged at 1,900 ×g at room temperature for 30 s. An 800 μl aliquot of the EtOAc phase was removed and concentrated to dryness in a centrifugal evaporator.

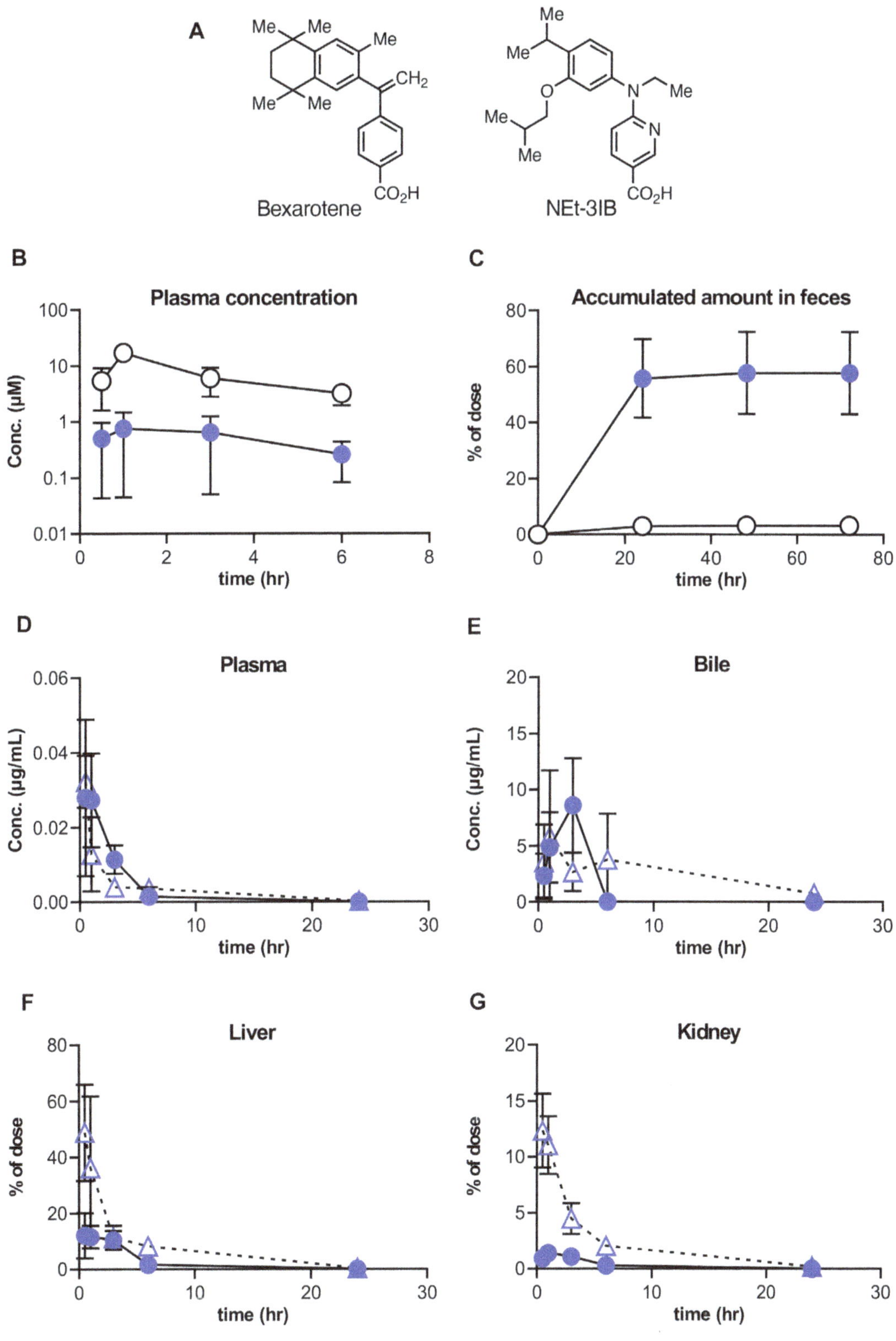

FIGURE 1 | Distribution of NEt-3IB after a single dosage to male mice. **(A, B)** Concentration of bexarotene or NEt-3IB in plasma and feces, respectively. Each compound was orally administered at **(A)** 30 mg/kg and **(B)** 10 mg/kg. **(C–F)** Plasma, bile, liver, and kidney distribution of NEt-3IB after single administration at 1 mg/kg (*i.v.*) and 10 mg/kg (p.o.). Circles and triangles show p.o. and i,v. data, respectively. Data shown are mean [*n* = 5 **(A, C–F)** or 3 **(B)**] ± SD.

The resulting residue was added to 100 µl acetonitrile. Brain, liver, and kidney samples were homogenized in ice-cold EtOAc (500 µL/100 mg tissue) using a Cell Destroyer PS1000 (BMS, Tokyo, Japan) and steel beads (for 5 mm) at 4,260 rpm for 60 s. Bile was collected by washing out the gallbladder with 500 µl EtOAc. The extract was vortexed for 30 s, kept under ultrasonic irradiation at room temperature for 5 min, and centrifuged at 12,000 ×*g* at 4°C for 10 min. A 200 µl aliquot of the EtOAc phase was collected and concentrated to dryness in a centrifugal evaporator. The resulting residue was dissolved by adding 100 µl acetonitrile. Each solution was directly subjected to LC-MS/MS analysis, and the concentration of each compound was determined from the peak area of the sample with reference to a calibration plot obtained with the authentic compound. All contents in the large intestine were collected, and MeOH (1 ml) was added under ultrasonic irradiation at room temperature for 20 min. The resultant suspension was centrifuged at 1,500 ×*g* at 4°C for 20 min. An 800 µl aliquot of the MeOH phase was diluted 10-fold with methanol. Each solution was directly subjected to High Performance Liquid Chromatography (HPLC) analysis, and the concentration of NEt-3IB was determined from the peak area of the sample with reference to a calibration plot obtained with the authentic compound.

Liquid Chromatography With Tandem Mass Spectrometry

The API4000 LC-MS/MS system (Applied Biosystems, Toronto, Canada) was used, consisting of an LC-20AD pump, an SPD-20AV UV-Vis spectrophotometric detector, and a CTO-20AC column oven (SHIMADZU, Kyoto, Japan) operating at 40°C. A TSKgel ODS-100V column (2.0 i.d. × 50 mm, 3 µm; TOSOH, Tokyo, Japan) was used. The mobile phase was acetonitrile/H_2O = 65/35 containing 0.1% formic acid, v/v, and the flow rate was set at 0.2 ml/min.

High-Performance Liquid Chromatography

A Shimadzu liquid chromatographic system (Kyoto, Japan) consisting of an LC-10AD pump, an SPD-10AV UV–vis spectrophotometric detector, a CTO-10AS column oven, and a C-R5A Chromatopac was used. An Inertsil ODS-3 column (4.6 mm i.d. × 100 mm, 5 µm, GL Sciences, Tokyo, Japan) with a guard column of Inertsil ODS-3 (4.6 mm i.d. × 10 mm, 5 µm, GL Sciences) was operated at 40°C. The mobile phase was methanol/H_2O = 85/15 containing 0.1% formic acid, v/v. The flow rate was set at 0.7 ml/min and the absorbance at 260 nm was monitored.

Induction of Colitis by Adoptive Transfer of $CD4^+$ $CD45RB^{high}$ T Cells

Colitis was induced in C.B-17-scid/scid mice by adoptive transfer of $CD45RB^{high}$ T cells. Mojosort Mouse CD 4 T Cell Isolation Kit (BioLegend, San Diego, CA, United States) and biotin-conjugated anti-mouse TER-119 (TER-119; BioLegend) were used to negatively select $CD4^+$ T cells of splenocytes from $C.B\text{-}17^{+/+}$ mice. Negatively selected $CD4^+$ T cells were labeled with Alexa Fluor 647-conjugated anti-mouse CD4 (RM-4-5; BioLegend), BV510-conjugated anti-mouse CD45 (30-F11; BioLegend), and BV421-conjugated anti-mouse CD45RB (16A; BD Horizon, San Jose, CA, United States). Dead cells were labeled with 7-aminoactinomycin D (7-AAD) (BioLegend). $CD45^+CD4^+CD45RB^{high}$ live T cells were isolated by FACS Aria III (BD Biosciences San Jose, CA, United States). The C.B-17-scid/scid recipients were each injected with 2×10^5 cells via the tail vein and transferred to conventional conditions in the animal facilities at Keio University. Mice were fed with 0.015% NEt-3IB-containing MF diet or control MF diet for 7 weeks. The body weights of the mice were measured every week, and the fecal diarrhea score was also measured from week 4. The diarrhea score were assessed as follows: normal stool (0), slightly soft (1), soft but formed (2), not formed (3), and liquid stool (4) (Kjellev et al., 2006). The mice were humanely killed at week 7.

Cell Preparation

Colonic lamina propria (LP) lymphocytes were obtained as follows. Colon tissues were treated with 1 mM dithiothreitol and 20 mM EDTA containing Hank's Balanced Salt Solutions (all from Nacalai-Tesque, Kyoto, Japan) for 20 min in a shaking incubator (37°C, 200 rpm) to remove epithelial cells. After the tissues were treated once more with 20 mM EDTA containing Hank's Balanced Salt Solution for 20 min, the tissues were then minced and dissociated with Liberase solution containing 26 units/ml Liberase TM (Roche, Basel, Switzerland), 5 mg/ml DNase I (Sigma Aldrich, St Louis, MO), 2% newborn calf serum (Thermo Fisher Scientific, Waltham, MA, United States), 100 µg/ml penicillin and streptomycin, and 20 mM HEPES in RPMI 1640 medium (all from Nacalai Tesque) at 37°C for 30 min. The cell suspensions were then filtered to obtain single-cell suspensions. Single-cell suspensions from mesenteric lymph nodes (MLNs) was prepared by mechanically crushing MLNs through 100 µm cell strainers (Greiner Bio-One) in RPMI 1640 medium containing 2% newborn calf serum (Thermo Fisher Scientific).

For cell counts, cells were mixed with Precision Count Beads (BioLegend), anti-mouse CD16/32 (93; BioLegend), eFluor 450-conjugated anti-mouse CD45 (30-F11; Thermo Fisher Scientific), and 7-aminoactinomycin D (7-AAD) (BioLegend) and were analyzed by FACS Celesta and FlowJo software version 10 (BD Biosciences).

Histology

Colonic tissue samples were fixed in Mildform (10% formalin; Wako Pure Chemical Industries, Osaka, Japan) overnight. After fixation, the samples were embedded in paraffin using a Leica EG1160. Samples were cut into 5 µm sections, deparaffinized and rehydrated, and then stained with hematoxylin (Agilent Technologies, Inc., Santa Clara, CA, United States) and eosin (Wako Pure Chemical Industries, Osaka, Japan). Histological colitis scores were reviewed by DT, who was blinded to each experiment. The sections were scored for the presence of crypt abscesses (0–1), the degree of thickness (0–3), and the degree of inflammatory infiltrate (0–3). The maximum score of the histological index was 7.

Flow Cytometry

For inflammatory T cell analysis of the colitis model, the following monoclonal antibodies were used: BV510-conjugated anti-mouse CD45 (30-F11; BioLegend), redFluor 710-conjugated anti-mouse CD4 (RM4-5; Tonbo Bioscience), BV605-conjugated anti-mouse TCRβ (H57-597; BD Biosciences), BV650-conjugated anti-mouse IFN-γ (XMG1.2; BD Horizon), and BV786-conjugated anti-mouse IL-17A (TC11-18H10.1; BD Horizon). For Treg cell analysis of the colitis model, the following monoclonal antibodies were used: BV510-conjugated anti-mouse CD45 (30-F11; BioLegend), redFluor-710-conjugated anti-mouse CD4 (RM4-5; Tonbo Biosciences, San Diego, CA, United States), FITC-conjugated anti-mouse TCRβ (H57-597; BD Biosciences), and eFluor 660-conjugated anti-mouse Foxp3 (FJK-16s; ThermoFisher Scientific). For macrophage analysis of the colitis model, the following monoclonal antibodies were used: BV510-conjugated anti-mouse CD45 (30-F11; BioLegend), Alexa Fluor 594-conjugated anti-mouse CD3 (17A2; BioLegend), redFluor 710-conjugated anti-mouse B220 (RA3-6B2; Tonbo Biosciences), APC-conjugated anti-mouse Ly-6C (AL-21; BD Pharmagen, San Jose, CA, United States), Alexa Fluor 488-conjugated anti-mouse Ly-6G/Ly-6C (Gr-1; BioLegend), BUV737-conjugated anti-mouse CD11b (M1/70; BD Horizon), BUV 395-conjugated anti-mouse CD11c (HL3; BD Horizon), and PerCP-Cy5.5-conjugated anti-mouse I-A/I-E (M5/114.15.2; BioLegend). For *in vitro* T cell analysis, the following monoclonal antibodies were used: BV510-conjugated anti-mouse CD45 (30-F11; BioLegend), redFluor 710-conjugated anti-mouse CD4 (RM4-5; Tonbo Biosciences), BUV737-conjugated anti-mouse TCRβ (H57-597; BD Horizon), PerCP-Cy5.5-conjugated anti-mouse IFN-γ (XMG1.2; BioLegend), PE-conjugated anti-mouse/human T-bet (O4-46; BD Pharmagen), and eFluor 660-conjugated anti-mouse Foxp3 (FJK-16s; Thermo Fisher Scientific). Dead cells were labeled with Fixable Viability Stain 780 (BD Biosciences). For intracellular cytokine and transcription factor staining, LP lymphocytes and MLN lymphocytes were cultured for 4 h in complete medium (RPMI containing 10% MP Biomedicals, Santa Ana, CA, United States: fetal bovine serum (FBS), Nacalai-Tesque 100 μg/ml penicillin and streptomycin, Thermo Fisher Scientific 55 μM mercaptoethanol, and Nacalai-Tesque 20 mM HEPES), and cultured T cells were cultured for 4 h in half-complete medium (RPMI containing 5% FBS, 100 μg/ml penicillin and streptomycin, 55 μM mercaptoethanol, and 20 mM HEPES), each supplemented with Cell Activation Cocktail (BioLegend) and Protein Transport Inhibitor Cocktail (Thermo Fisher Scientific). Lymphocytes and T cells were first blocked with anti-CD16/32 and then stained with the monoclonal antibodies described above. IC fixation buffer and permeabilization buffer (Thermo Fisher Scientific) were used for intracellular cytokine staining, and the Transcription Factor Buffer Set (BD Pharmagen) was used for transcription factor staining. For absolute cell counts, cells were mixed with Precision Count Beads (BioLegend) and anti-mouse CD16/32 (93; BioLegend) and stained with eFluor 450-conjugated anti-mouse CD45 (30-F11; Thermo Fisher Scientific) and 7-AAD. The stained samples were analyzed using an LSRII or a FACS Celesta (BD Biosciences), and FlowJo software version 10.

In vitro Cultures

$CD4^+$ T cells were enriched from splenocytes from C57BL6/J mice or *Foxp3-hCD2* knock-in mice by a negative selection method with the BD iMag cell separation system, using biotin-conjugated antibodies against mouse CD8α (53-6.7; Tonbo Biosciences), CD11b (M1/70; BioLegend), CD11c (N418; Thermo Fisher Scientific), B220 (RA3-6B2; BioLegend), Ly-6C/Ly6-G (Gr-1; BioLegend), TER-119 (TER-119; BioLegend), and Streptavidin Particle Plus (BD IMag). Negatively selected $CD4^+$ T cells were labeled with BV605-conjugated anti-mouse CD4 (RM4-5; BioLegend), BV510-conjugated anti-mouse CD44 (IM4; BD Horizon), redFluor 710-conjugated anti-mouse CD45 (30-F11; Tonbo Biosciences), PE-Cy7-conjugated anti-CD25 (PC61.5; Thermo Fisher Scientific), APC-eFluor 780-conjugated anti-mouse NK 1.1 (PK136; Thermo Fisher Scientific), eFluor450-conjugated anti-CD62L (MEL-14; Thermo Fisher Scientific), and APC-conjugated anti-human CD2 (RPA-2.10; BioLegend). Dead cells were labeled with 7-AAD (BioLegend). $CD45^+CD4^+CD62L^+CD44^-NK\ 1.1^-Foxp3^-(hCD2^-)$ live naive T cells were isolated by FACSAria III (BD Biosciences). In the experiments described in **Figure 4**, 1×10^5 of $CD4^+$ naive T cells were cultured in advanced RPMI containing 5% FBS in the presence or absence of NEt-3IB for 3–5 days. For the experiment using CellTrace Violet (Thermo Fisher Scientific), T cells were incubated at 37°C for 20 min with CellTrace Violet before culture. T cells were polarized to the Th1 subtype by the addition of 10 μg/ml anti-mouse IL-4 (Bio X Cell, Lebanon, NH, United States) and 20 ng/ml recombinant mouse IL-2 and IL-12 (BioLegend). The stained samples were analyzed using FACS LSR II (BD Biosciences) and Flowjo software version 10.

Statistical Analysis

Statistical significance between two groups was calculated by Student's t-test or Welch's t-test. In the *in vitro* study, statistical significance between the control group and other groups was calculated by Dunnet's multiple comparison test or Dunn's multiple comparison test. $p < 0.05$ indicated statistical significance. Data were output by Prism version 9 (GraphPad, San Diego, CA, United States).

RESULTS

NEt-3IB has Low Systemic Transferability and Reaches the Colon

To better understand the pharmacokinetics of NEt-3IB and bexarotene (**Figure 1A**), another RXR agonist clinically used for the treatment of cutaneous T cell lymphoma (Budgin et al., 2005), we initially measured their concentrations in plasma and feces after a single oral administration. The plasma concentrations of NEt-3IB were much lower than those of bexarotene at any timepoint (0.5–6 h post-administration) (**Figure 1B**). Correspondingly, the delivery of

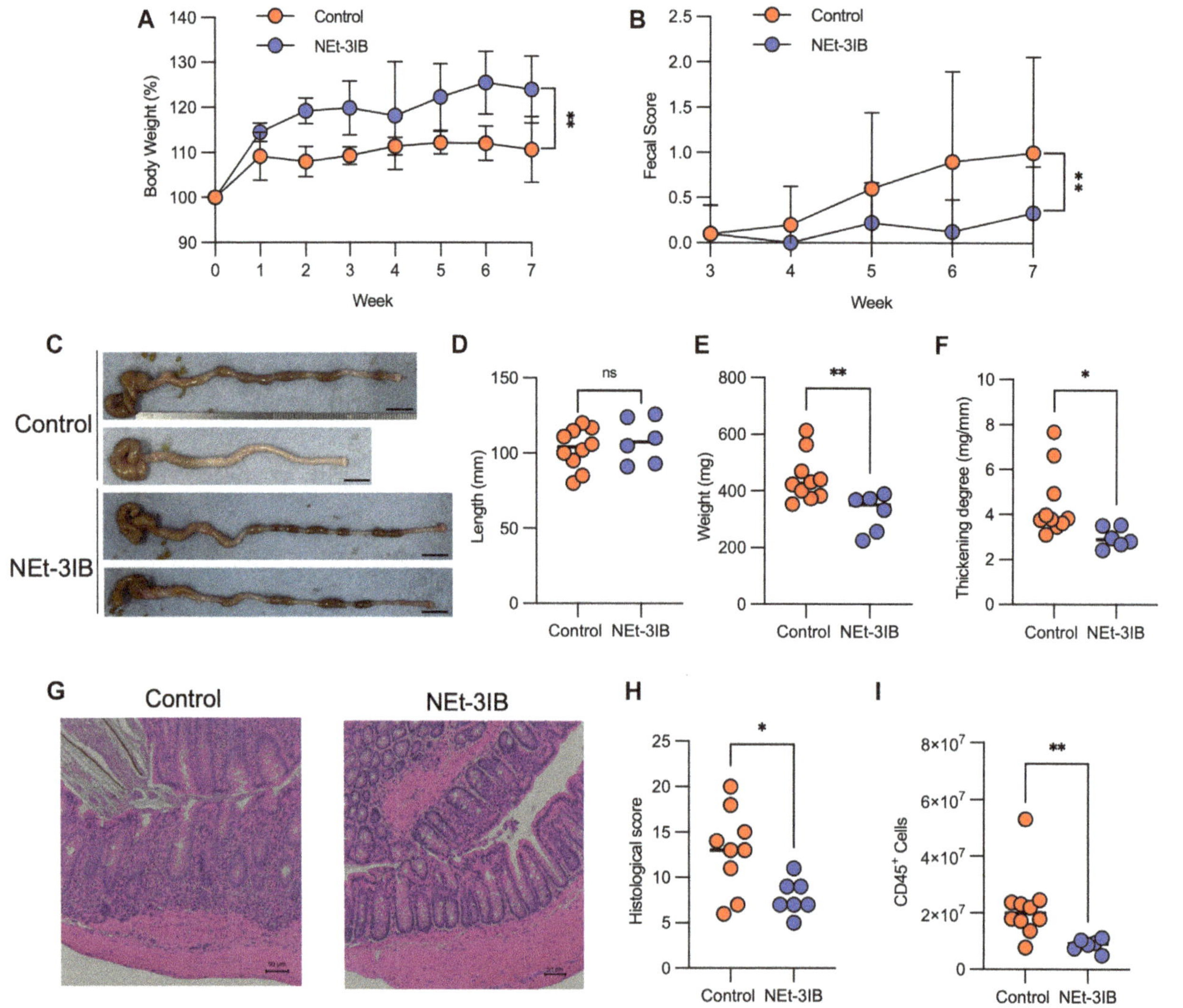

FIGURE 2 | NEt-3IB ameliorates T-cell-dependent experimental colitis. **(A–H)** Experimental colitis was induced by adoptive transfer of $CD4^+CD45RB^{high}$ T cells into C.B-17 scid/scid mice fed with control or NEt-3IB-containing diet for 7 weeks, and bodyweight loss **(A)** and diarrhea score **(B)** were observed. Data shown are the average. Area under the curve of bodyweight change and fecal score. **(C–F)** Colon length, colon weight, and colon thickening were observed and measured in week 7. Scale bar: 1 cm. **(G)** Colonic specimens were stained with hematoxylin and eosin (HE). **(H)** Histological scores of colonic specimens. **(I)** Total $CD45^+$ cells in the colon lamina propria of the $CD4^+$ $CD45RB^{high}$ T cell transfer model. $^*p < 0.05$, $^{**}p < 0.01$.

NEt-3IB to the feces accumulated to approximately 60% of the dosage, whereas that of bexarotene was less than 10% at 24 h post-administration (**Figure 1C**). These data confirm that orally administered NEt-3IB reaches the colon more efficiently compared with bexarotene due to its low systemic transferability.

To further examine the systemic pharmacokinetics of NEt-3IB, mice received intravenous (i.v.) injection (1 mg/kg) and oral administration (p.o.) (10 mg/kg) of NEt-3IB. The concentrations of NEt-3IB in plasma began to decline by 1 h after i.v. or 6 h after p.o. administration, and reciprocally, the concentrations in the bile increased at these time points (**Figures 1D,E**). On the basis of these observations, we assumed that the liver may excrete NEt-3IB to the intestinal tract via the bile duct. To test this assumption, we measured the concentration of NEt-3IB in the liver and the kidney. Although the concentration of NEt-3IB in the liver promptly decreased, that in the bile gradually increased after i.v. injection (**Figure 1F**). The hepatic concentration of NEt-3IB peaked immediately after p.o. administration and then gradually declined (**Figure 1F**). Conversely, NEt-3IB concentration in the kidney rapidly decreased after i.v. administration and remained consistently low after p.o. administration. Thus, NEt-3IB was excreted to the bile in the liver rather than the kidney (**Figure 1G**).

NEt-3IB Treatment Alleviates T Cell-dependent Colitis

We subsequently examined the anti-inflammatory effects of NEt-3IB in an experimental colitis model induced by transferring $CD4^+CD45RB^{high}$ T cells into C.B-17-scid/scid mice and treating with chow containing 0.015% NEt-3IB (approximately 30 mg/kg/

day) or with regular chow as a control. In the control group, bodyweight gain was suppressed from 1-week post-transfer onwards (**Figure 2A**). Meanwhile, the NEt-3IB-treated group gained weight gradually over the course of the experiment, suggesting that NEt-3IB alleviated wasting disease. Similarly, NEt-3IB administration ameliorated diarrhea associated with colitis, even though both groups exhibited only mild symptoms (**Figure 2B**). Likewise, the colon weight and degree of thickening (colon weight/length) were significantly lower in the NEt-3IB group than that in the control group at 7 weeks after cell transfer (**Figures 2C–F**). Histopathological examination also showed massive infiltration of mononuclear cells in the colon of the control group but not in the NEt-3IB group (**Figure 2G**). Furthermore, the control group exhibited more severe crypt loss and edema (**Figures 2G,H**). Flow cytometry confirmed the massive infiltration of leukocytes in the colon lamina propria (cLP) in the control group, whereas fewer inflammatory infiltrates were observed in the NEt-3IB group (**Figure 2I**).

To further confirm the pharmacological effects of NEt-3IB, we also evaluated the progressive bodyweight loss and diarrhea in a similar colitis model using *Rag1*$^{-/-}$ mice as a recipient. The control *Rag1*$^{-/-}$ recipients exhibited progressive body weight loss in association with severe diarrhea. However, the administration of NEt-3IB significantly mitigated the wasting disease (**Supplementary Figure S1A**). Furthermore, NEt-3IB improved colitis symptoms, namely, diarrhea, colon weight, colonic wall thickening, crypt loss, and edema (**Supplementary Figures S1B–G**). Collectively, these data revealed an anti-inflammatory effect of NEt-3IB in the T cell-dependent mouse colitis model.

NEt-3IB Suppressed the Accumulation of Th1 Cells in the cLP

In the CD4$^+$CD45RB^{high} T-cell-transferred colitis model, IFN-γ-producing effector T (T$_{eff}$) cells including conventional T helper 1 (Th1) cells and IFN-γ/IL-17-co-expressing T helper 17 (IFN-γ-producing Th17) cells are responsible for the pathogenesis (Powrie et al., 1993; Sujino et al., 2011). To determine whether NEt-3IB administration affects the development of these T$_{eff}$ cell subsets, we analyzed T cell profiles in the cLP and MLN of the colitis model at 7 weeks post-transfer by flow cytometry after intracellular cytokine staining. In the cLP, the numbers of Th1 cells, Th17 cells, and IFN-γ-producing Th17 cells in the NEt-3IB group were less than half that in the control group, although the frequencies of these cells were comparable between the two groups (**Supplementary Figure S2A** and **Figure 3A**). Moreover, Th1 and Th17 cells in the MLN were significantly decreased in the NEt-3IB group compared with the control group, and IFN-γ-producing Th17 cells also tended to be reduced. Of note, we also observed that the number of Foxp3$^+$ Treg cells was slightly but significantly decreased in both the cLP and MLN of the NEt-3IB group (**Supplementary Figure S2B** and **Figure 3C**). Colonic T$_{eff}$ cell-derived IFN-γ activates macrophages to produce pro-inflammatory cytokines that cause inflammation in the colon (Stout and Bottomly, 1989). Considering that NEt-3IB treatment reduced Th1 cells in the cLP in the colitis model, we analyzed the colonic macrophages at 7 weeks post-transfer. We observed that the total number of macrophages (CD11b$^+$ Ly6G$^-$Ly6C$^-$CD11c$^-$ MHC class II$^+$) was decreased significantly in the NEt-3IB-treated group compared with the control group (**Supplementary Figure S2C** and **Figure 3D**). These data illustrated that NEt-3IB diminishes colitis by inhibiting the accumulation of IFN-γ-producing T$_{eff}$ cells and inflammatory macrophages in the cLP and MLN.

NEt-3IB Inhibits the Differentiation and Proliferation of Th1 Cells

We further investigated whether NEt-3IB has a direct impact on the differentiation of Th cells using an *in vitro* culture system. Sorted naïve CD4$^+$ T cells were cultured under Th1-skewed conditions for 5 days with or without NEt-3IB treatment before flow cytometric analysis for the expression of Th1 markers (T-bet, IFN-γ), and a Treg marker (Foxp3). We found that the frequencies of the T-bet$^+$ and IFN-γ^+ cells decreased in the NEt-3IB-treated group in a dose-dependent manner (**Supplementary Figure S2D** and **Figure 4A**). Surprisingly, NEt-3IB treatment increased the proportion of Foxp3$^+$ T cells in a dose-dependent manner despite culture in Th1 conditions (**Supplementary Figure S2E** and **Figure 4B**).

We subsequently examined whether NEt-3IB affected the proliferation of Th1 cells *in vitro*. Fluorescent dye-labeled naïve CD4$^+$ T cells were cultured under Th1-differentiating conditions for 5 days with or without Net-3IB treatment, and then the dilution of CellTrace Violet was analyzed to detect proliferating cells. NEt-3IB treatment significantly reduced the frequency of proliferating cells in the T-bet$^+$IFN-γ^+ Th1 population when compared with the vehicle control (**Supplementary Figure S2F** and **Figure 4C**). Together, these data suggest that NEt-3IB directly inhibits both the differentiation and proliferation of Th1 cells.

DISCUSSION

In this study, we demonstrated that NEt-3IB attenuated the development of wasting disease and colitis in T cell-dependent experimental colitis models by inhibiting the accumulation of Th1 cells, which is the most dominant cell type contributing to the pathogenesis of CD. Furthermore, our *in vitro* data revealed that NEt-3IB directly inhibited the differentiation and expansion of Th1 cells. NEt-3IB was designed to have lower lipophilicity compared with conventional RXR agonists such as bexarotene (Takamatsu et al., 2008; Kobayashi et al., 2015). We confirmed that NEt-3IB exhibits a lower plasma concentration compared with bexarotene after oral administration. In the detailed pharmacokinetics analysis after i.v. administration, the distribution to the liver represented approximately 49% of the total dosage of NEt-3IB, while in the kidney there was only 12% of the total dosage. Considering that the concentration of NEt-3IB in bile rises after its peak in the liver, NEt-3IB is mostly likely to be excreted efficiently to the bile. Notably, we observed that 60% of

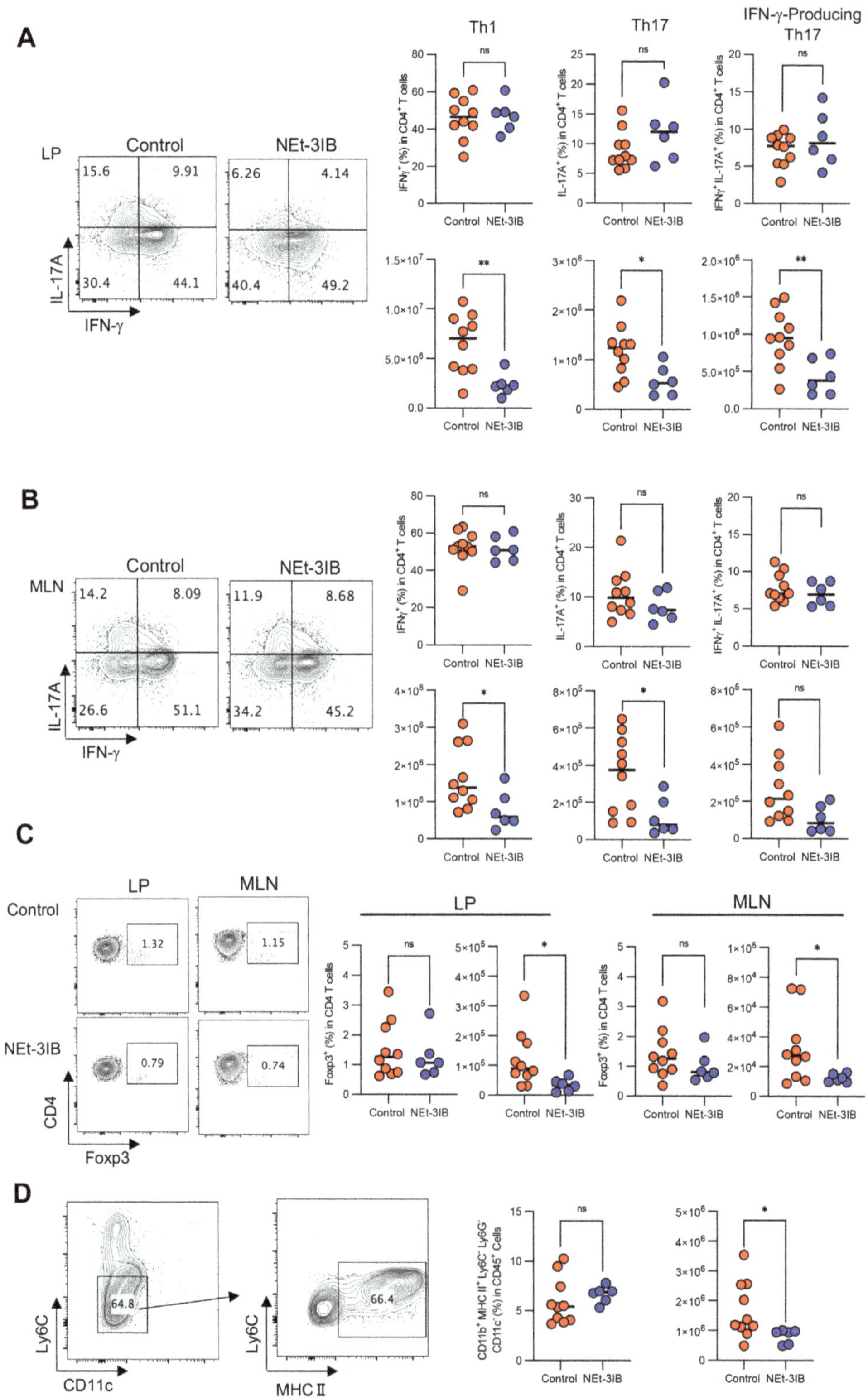

FIGURE 3 | NEt-3IB inhibits inflammatory T cells. **(A)** Frequency and cell number of IFN-γ-producing cells and IL-17A-producing cells in the colon lamina propria. **(B)** Frequency and cell number of Th1 transcription factor T-bet and Th17 transcription factor RORγt-presenting cells of the colon lamina propria and mesenteric lymph nodes. **(C)** Frequency and cell number of Foxp3$^+$ regulatory T cells in the colon lamina propria and mesenteric lymph node of T cell-transferred SCID mice. **(D)** Macrophages were gated as CD11b$^+$Ly6G$^-$Ly6C$^-$CD11c$^-$MHC2$^+$. The right-hand graphs show the frequency of macrophages in CD45$^+$ cells and the number of macrophages. **(A–D)** are from CD45RB^{high} T cell transfer model mice at 7 weeks post-transfer.

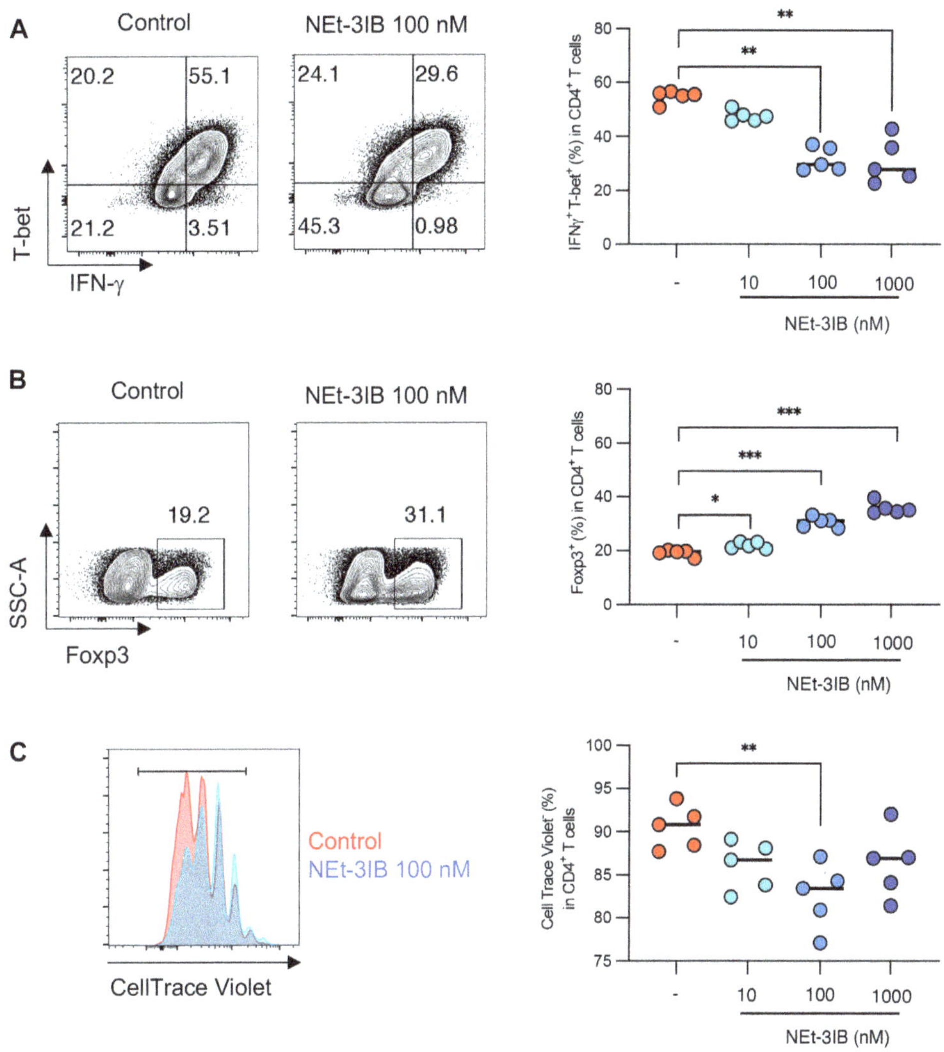

FIGURE 4 | NEt-3IB inhibits differentiation of inflammatory T cells and induces Foxp3⁺ cells in Th1 and Th17 conditions. **(A, B)** Naïve T cells were cultured in Th1 conditions, with or without NEt-3IB treatment for 5 days and analyzed for T-bet and IFN-γ expression **(A)**, and for Foxp3 expression in the CD4⁺ T cell population **(B)**. **(C)** Naïve T cells were labeled with CellTrace Violet and cultured in Th1 conditions with or without NEt-3IB treatment for 5 days. Cultured cells were analyzed for their degree of proliferation in the CD4⁺ T-bet⁺ IFN-γ⁺ population. $^{*}p < 0.05$, $^{**}p < 0.01$, $^{***}p < 0.005$.

the total dosage reached the colon within 24 h post-oral administration, after the bile concentration peaked at 4 h. These data support the enterohepatic circulation of NEt-3IB, consistent with our previous report (Kobayashi et al., 2015). In contrast, such enterohepatic circulation was not observed in bexarotene, which was readily absorbed in the upper intestine after oral administration with only a small portion delivered to the colon. Thus, NEt-3IB is efficiently delivered to the colonic lumen and should be translocated to the cLP under inflammatory conditions, which are often associated with mucosal barrier disruption.

Early studies showed that the activation and overexpression of certain nuclear receptors exert anti-inflammatory effects. For instance, PPAR agonists suppress the differentiation of Th1 cells *in vitro* by inhibiting the JAK–STAT signaling pathway (Natarajan and Bright, 2002). LXR agonists also display similar effects on the differentiation of Th1 cells (Solt et al., 2012). Moreover, PPARγ and LXR agonists both suppress the proliferation of T cells (Yang et al., 2000; Cunard et al., 2002; Diab et al., 2004; Bensinger et al., 2008; Solt et al., 2012). Given that these nuclear receptors heterodimerize with RXR, and RXR agonists can activate these partner nuclear receptors, the inhibitory effect of NEt-3IB on Th1 response may depend on the activation of LXR and PPAR signaling. Additionally, PPARγ agonists inhibit IL-12 production by macrophages, which is important for the differentiation and survival of Th1 cells (Natarajan and Bright, 2002). Thus, NEt-3IB may directly and indirectly suppress the Th1 response through the inhibition of IL-12 production by macrophages.

Our *in vitro* experiments demonstrated that Foxp3$^+$ cells arose in the NEt-3IB-treated group despite the Th1-differentiation conditions. Given that RXR agonists modulate Foxp3$^+$ Treg cell differentiation (Takeuchi et al., 2013), NEt-3IB may drive naïve CD4$^+$ T cells to upregulate Foxp3 regardless of the culture conditions. Because ectopic Foxp3 expression represses IFN-γ expression, it is possible that NEt-3IB reduced the number of Th1 cells *in vitro* by downregulating T-bet expression. Nevertheless, in the CD4$^+$CD45RB^{high} T-cell-transfer colitis model, no significant difference in the frequency of Treg cells was identified between the control and NEt-3B-treated groups. This observation implies that NEt-3IB may repress IFN-γ expression via an unknown mechanism other than upregulation of Foxp3. For instance, NEt-3IB may indirectly dampen Th1 cell expansion by diminishing Th17 cell differentiation. We observed a reduction in IFN-γ-producing Th17 cells in the cLP of the NEt-3IB-treated group. This transient cell population is generated from conventional Th17 cells and further differentiates into Th1 cells (Sujino et al., 2011; Basdeo et al., 2017). Therefore, the reduction in IFN-γ-producing Th17 cells in the cLP of the NEt-3IB group cells may lead to a decrease in Th1 cells. Notably, RXR and LXR agonists negatively regulate the differentiation of Th17 cells *in vitro* (Solt et al., 2012; Takeuchi et al., 2013). Thus, NEt-3IB possibly restricted the development of Th17 cells in the colitis model mice, resulting in the reduction of IFN-γ-producing Th17, and in turn, Th17 cell-derived Th1 cells.

NEt-3IB treatment also reduced the number of macrophages. NEt-3IB is likely to indirectly suppress the infiltration of macrophages by inhibiting the expansion of IFN-γ-producing Th17 and Th1 cells. Furthermore, NEt-3IB may directly diminish macrophage activation. In support of this, we previously found that a partial RXR agonist, CBT-PMN, downregulates the production of pro-inflammatory cytokines by bone marrow-derived macrophages (Onuki et al., 2018). Furthermore, other groups showed that FXR agonist treatment significantly downregulated IFN-γ-related gene expression (Renga et al., 2009), and that PPAR and LXR agonists also suppress the production of inflammatory cytokines from macrophages (Birrell et al., 2007; Paukkeri et al., 2013) Additionally, overexpression of NR4A1 and NR4A2 in human macrophages inhibits pro-inflammatory cytokines (Bonta et al., 2006). All these nuclear receptors form heterodimers with RXR and are activated by RXR agonists. These facts support the possibility that NEt-3IB directly inhibits the activation and cytokine production of macrophages by activating RXR partner nuclear receptors.

In conclusion, the present study demonstrated that NEt-3IB ameliorated colitis by inhibiting both the expansion of Th1 cells and the activation of inflammatory macrophages locally in the colon. Our results indicate that NEt-3IB is a promising candidate for IBD treatment as a small molecule inhibitor.

ETHICS STATEMENT

The animal studies were reviewed and approved by Animal Studies Committees of Keio University, and the Animal Care and Use Committee of Okayama University.

AUTHOR CONTRIBUTIONS

MW, SN, and YT synthesized NEt-3IB and bexarotene. MW, SN, and YK performed the pharmacokinetic experiments and analysis. RM and DT performed the colitis experiments, and RM performed the *in vitro* experiments. HK and KH designed the study. RM, MW, and DT wrote the manuscript. HK and KH revised the manuscript.

FUNDING

This study was supported by grants from the Japan Society for the Promotion of Science (20H00509, and 20H05876 to KH), JST Moonshot (21-201033024 to KH), AMED-Crest (18gm1010004h0103, 19gm1010004s0104, 20gm1010004h0105, and 20gm1310009h0001 to KH), The Science Research Promotion Fund, and The Promotion and Mutual Aid Corporation for Private Schools of Japan (KH). Furthermore, this study received funding from AIBIOS Co., Ltd. (HK and KH). The funder was not involved in the study design, collection, analysis, interpretation of data, the writing of this article or the decision to submit it for publication.

ACKNOWLEDGMENTS

We thank Yumiko Fujimura for assistance with the animal experiments. The authors are grateful to the Division of Instrumental Analysis, Okayama University for the NMR and MS measurements. We also thank H. Nikki March, from Edanz (https://jp.edanz.com/ac) for editing a draft of this manuscript.

REFERENCES

Adegbola, S. O., Sahnan, K., Warusavitarne, J., Hart, A., and Tozer, P. (2018). Anti-TNF Therapy in Crohn's Disease. *Ijms* 19, 2244–2321. doi:10.3390/ijms19082244

Basdeo, S. A., Cluxton, D., Sulaimani, J., Moran, B., Canavan, M., Orr, C., et al. (2017). Ex-Th17 (Nonclassical Th1) Cells Are Functionally Distinct from Classical Th1 and Th17 Cells and Are Not Constrained by Regulatory T Cells. *J.I.* 198, 2249–2259. doi:10.4049/jimmunol.1600737

Bensinger, S. J., Bradley, M. N., Joseph, S. B., Zelcer, N., Janssen, E. M., Hausner, M. A., et al. (2008). LXR Signaling Couples Sterol Metabolism to Proliferation in the Acquired Immune Response. *Cell* 134, 97–111. doi:10.1016/j.cell.2008.04.052

Birrell, M. A., Catley, M. C., Hardaker, E., Wong, S., Willson, T. M., McCluskie, K., et al. (2007). Novel Role for the Liver X Nuclear Receptor in the Suppression of Lung Inflammatory Responses. *J. Biol. Chem.* 282, 31882–31890. doi:10.1074/jbc.M703278200

Boehm, M. F., Zhang, L., Badea, B. A., White, S. K., Mais, D. E., Berger, E., et al. (1994). Synthesis and Structure-Activity Relationships of Novel Retinoid X Receptor-Selective Retinoids. *J. Med. Chem.* 37, 2930–2941. doi:10.1021/jm00044a014

Bonta, P. I., Van Tiel, C. M., Vos, M., Pols, T. W. H., Van Thienen, J. V., Ferreira, V., et al. (2006). Nuclear Receptors Nur77, Nurr1, and NOR-1 Expressed in Atherosclerotic Lesion Macrophages Reduce Lipid Loading and Inflammatory Responses. *Atvb* 26, 2288. doi:10.1161/01.ATV.0000238346.84458.5d

Budgin, J. B., Richardson, S. K., Newton, S. B., Wysocka, M., Zaki, M. H., Benoit, B., et al. (2005). Biological Effects of Bexarotene in Cutaneous T-Cell Lymphoma. *Arch. Dermatol.* 141, 315–320. doi:10.1001/archderm.141.3.315

Carter, M. J., Lobo, A. J., and Travis, S. P. L. (2004). Guidelines for the Management of Inflammatory Bowel Disease in Adults. *Gut* 53, v1–v16. doi:10.1136/gut.2004.043372

Cunard, R., Ricote, M., DiCampli, D., Archer, D. C., Kahn, D. A., Glass, C. K., et al. (2002). Regulation of Cytokine Expression by Ligands of Peroxisome Proliferator Activated Receptors. *J. Immunol.* 168, 2795–2802. doi:10.4049/jimmunol.168.6.2795

De Souza, H. S. P., and Fiocchi, C. (2016). Immunopathogenesis of IBD: Current State of the Art. *Nat. Rev. Gastroenterol. Hepatol.* 13, 13–27. doi:10.1038/nrgastro.2015.186

de Vries-van der Weij, J., De Haan, W., Hu, L., Kuif, M., Oei, H. L., Van Der Hoorn, J. W., et al. (2009). Bexarotene Induces Dyslipidemia by Increased Very Low-Density Lipoprotein Production and Cholesteryl Ester Transfer Protein-Mediated Reduction of High-Density Lipoprotein. *Endocrinology* 150, 2368–2375. doi:10.1210/en.2008-1540

Diab, A., Drew, P. D., Racke Judy Choy, M. K., Rocchini, A., Matthes, L., Amy E Lovett-Racke, J. A., et al. (2004). Peroxisome Proliferator-Activated Receptor Agonists as Therapy for Autoimmune Disease. *J. Immunol.* doi:10.4049/jimmunol.172.9.5790

Dubrac, S., Elentner, A., Ebner, S., Horejs-Hoeck, J., and Schmuth, M. (2010). Modulation of T Lymphocyte Function by the Pregnane X Receptor. *J.I.* 184, 2949–2957. doi:10.4049/jimmunol.0902151

Evans, R. M., and Mangelsdorf, D. J. (2014). Nuclear Receptors, RXR, and the Big Bang. *Cell* 157, 255–266. doi:10.1016/j.cell.2014.03.012

Ha, F., and Khalil, H. (2015). Crohn's Disease: a Clinical Update. *Therap. Adv. Gastroenterol.* 8, 352–359. doi:10.1177/1756283X15592585

Kakuta, H., Ohsawa, F., Yamada, S., Makishima, M., Tai, A., Yasui, H., et al. (2012). Feasibility of Structural Modification of Retinoid X Receptor Agonists to Separate Blood Glucose-Lowering Action from Adverse Effects: Studies in KKAy Type 2 Diabetes Model Mice. *Biol. Pharm. Bull.* 35, 629–633. doi:10.1248/bpb.35.629

Kanakasabai, S., Chearwae, W., Walline, C. C., Iams, W., Adams, S. M., and Bright, J. J. (2010). Peroxisome Proliferator-Activated Receptor δ Agonists Inhibit T Helper Type 1 (Th1) and Th17 Responses in Experimental Allergic Encephalomyelitis. *Immunology* 130, 572–588. doi:10.1111/j.1365-2567.2010.03261.x

Kjellev, S., Lundsgaard, D., Poulsen, S. S., and Markholst, H. (2006). Reconstitution of Scid Mice with CD4+CD25− T Cells Leads to Rapid Colitis: An Improved Model for Pharmacologic Testing. *Int. Immunopharmacology* 6, 1341–1354. doi:10.1016/j.intimp.2006.04.017

Kobayashi, T., Furusawa, Y., Yamada, S., Akehi, M., Takenaka, F., Sasaki, T., et al. (2015). Positron Emission Tomography to Elucidate Pharmacokinetic Differences of Regioisomeric Retinoid X Receptor Agonists. *ACS Med. Chem. Lett.* 6, 334–338. doi:10.1021/ml500511m

Liebmann, M., Hucke, S., Koch, K., Eschborn, M., Ghelman, J., Chasan, A. I., et al. (2018). Nur77 Serves as a Molecular Brake of the Metabolic Switch during T Cell Activation to Restrict Autoimmunity. *Proc. Natl. Acad. Sci. USA* 115, E8017–E8026. doi:10.1073/pnas.1721049115

Liu, S., Ogilvie, K. M., Klausing, K., Lawson, M. A., Jolley, D., Li, D., et al. (2002). Mechanism of Selective Retinoid X Receptor Agonist-Induced Hypothyroidism in the Rat. *Endocrinology* 143, 2880–2885. doi:10.1210/endo.143.8.8930

Natarajan, C., and Bright, J. J. (2002). Peroxisome Proliferator-Activated Receptor-Gamma Agonists Inhibit Experimental Allergic Encephalomyelitis by Blocking IL-12 Production, IL-12 Signaling and Th1 Differentiation. *Genes Immun.* 3, 59–70. doi:10.1038/sj.gene.6363832

Onuki, M., Watanabe, M., Ishihara, N., Suzuki, K., Takizawa, K., Hirota, M., et al. 2018). A Partial Agonist for Retinoid X Receptor Mitigates Experimental Colitis. *Int Immunol.* 31, 251–262. doi:10.1093/intimm/dxy089

Paukkeri, E.-L., Leppänen, T., Lindholm, M., Yam, M. F., Asmawi, M., Kolmonen, A., et al. (2013). Anti-inflammatory Properties of a Dual PPARgamma/alpha Agonist Muraglitazar in *In Vitro* and *In Vivo* Models. *Arthritis Res. Ther.* 15, R51. doi:10.1186/ar4211

Powrie, F., Leach, M. W., Mauze, S., Caddie, L. B., and Coffman, R. L. (1993). Phenotypically Distinct Subsets of CD4+ T Cells Induce or Protect from Chronic Intestinal Inflammation in C. B-17 Scid Mice. *Int. Immunol.* 5, 1461–1471. doi:10.1093/intimm/5.11.1461

Renga, B., Migliorati, M., Mencarelli, A., and Fiorucci, S. (2009). Reciprocal Regulation of the Bile Acid-Activated Receptor FXR and the Interferon-γ-STAT-1 Pathway in Macrophages. *Biochim. Biophys. Acta (Bba) - Mol. Basis Dis.* 1792, 564 573. doi:10.1016/j.bbadis.2009.04.004

Solt, L. A., Kamenecka, T. M., and Burris, T. P. (2012). LXR-mediated Inhibition of CD4+ T Helper Cells. *PLoS One* 7, e46615. doi:10.1371/journal.pone.0046615

Standeven, A. M., Escobar, M., Beard, R. L., Yuan, Y. D., and Chandraratna, R. A. S. (1997). Mitogenic Effect of Retinoid X Receptor Agonists in Rat Liver. *Biochem. Pharmacol.* doi:10.1016/S0006-2952(97)00209-8

Stout, R. D., and Bottomly, K. (1989). Antigen-specific Activation of Effector Macrophages by IFN-Gamma Producing (TH1) T Cell Clones. Failure of IL-4-producing (TH2) T Cell Clones to Activate Effector Function in Macrophages. *J. Immunol.* 142, 760–765. Available at: http://www.jimmunol.org/content/142/3/760.abstract.

Sujino, T., Kanai, T., Ono, Y., Mikami, Y., Hayashi, A., Doi, T., et al. (2011). Regulatory T Cells Suppress Development of Colitis, Blocking Differentiation of T-Helper 17 into Alternative T-Helper 1 Cells. *Gastroenterology* 141, 1014–1023. doi:10.1053/j.gastro.2011.05.052

Takamatsu, K., Takano, A., Yakushiji, N., Morohashi, K., Morishita, K.-i., Matsuura, N., et al. (2008). The First Potent Subtype-Selective Retinoid X Receptor (RXR) Agonist Possessing a 3-Isopropoxy-4-Isopropylphenylamino Moiety, NEt-3IP (RXRα/β-Dual Agonist). *ChemMedChem* 3, 780–787. doi:10.1002/cmdc.200700313

Takeuchi, H., Yokota-Nakatsuma, A., Ohoka, Y., Kagechika, H., Kato, C., Song, S.-Y., et al. (2013). Retinoid X Receptor Agonists Modulate Foxp3+ Regulatory T Cell and Th17 Cell Differentiation with Differential Dependence on Retinoic Acid Receptor Activation. *J.I.* 191, 3725–3733. doi:10.4049/jimmunol.1300032

Yang, X. Y., Wang, L. H., Chen, T., Hodge, D. R., Resau, J. H., DaSilva, L., et al. (2000). Activation of Human T Lymphocytes Is Inhibited by Peroxisome Proliferator-Activated Receptor γ (PPARγ) Agonists. *J. Biol. Chem.* 275, 4541–4544. doi:10.1074/jbc.275.7.4541

12

Noncanonical NF-κB Signaling Upregulation in Inflammatory Bowel Disease Patients is Associated with Loss of Response to Anti-TNF Agents

Vu Q. Nguyen[1†], *Kristin Eden*[2,3†], *Holly A. Morrison*[2†], *Megan B. Sammons*[2], *Kristin K. Knight*[1], *Siena Sorrentino*[2], *Rebecca M. Brock*[4], *Douglas J. Grider*[5], *Irving C. Allen*[2,3,4‡] and *Dario Sorrentino*[1,6*‡]

[1]*IBD Center, Division of Gastroenterology, Virginia Tech Carilion School of Medicine, Roanoke, VA, United States,* [2]*Department of Biomedical Sciences and Pathobiology, Virginia-Maryland College of Veterinary Medicine, Virginia Tech, Blacksburg, VA, United States,* [3]*Department of Basic Science Education, Virginia Tech Carilion School of Medicine, Roanoke, VA, United States,* [4]*Graduate Program in Translational Biology, Medicine, and Health, Virginia Tech, Blacksburg, VA, United States,* [5]*Department of Pathology, Virginia Tech Carilion School of Medicine, Roanoke, VA, United States,* [6]*Department of Clinical and Experimental Medical Sciences, University of Udine School of Medicine, Udine, Italy*

Correspondence:
Dario Sorrentino
drsorrentino@carilionclinic.org

†*These authors have contributed equally to this work*
‡*These authors share senior authorship*

Objectives: Targeting tumor necrosis factor (TNF) with biologic agents, such as infliximab and adalimumab, is a widely used and effective therapeutic strategy in inflammatory bowel disease (IBD). Unfortunately, a significant number of patients fail to respond or lose response over time to these agents. Previous studies have defined multiple complex roles for canonical NF-κB signaling in the pathogenesis of IBD. However, preliminary evidence suggests that the lesser defined noncanonical NF-κB signaling pathway also contributes to disease pathogenesis and response to anti-TNF agents. The objective of this study was to evaluate this hypothesis in Crohn's disease (CD) and ulcerative colitis (UC) patients.

Design: A total of 27 subjects with IBD (19 with CD and 8 with UC) and 15 control subjects were tested. Clinical criteria, patient history, and endoscopic disease activity were factors used to categorize patients and define therapeutic response. Biopsy specimens were collected during colonoscopy and expression was determined for 88 target genes known to be associated with noncanonical NF-κB signaling and IBD.

Results: Noncanonical NF-κB signaling was significantly upregulated in IBD patients and was associated with increased gastrointestinal inflammation, epithelial cell death, lymphocyte migration, and Nod-like receptor signaling. Furthermore, noncanonical NF-κB signaling was further upregulated in patients unresponsive to anti-TNF agents and was suppressed in responsive patients. *MAP3K14, NFKB2, CCL19, CXCL12*, and *CXCL13* were significantly dysregulated, as were genes that encode pathway regulators, such as *CYLD, NLRP12,* and *BIRC2/3*.

Conclusion: Our study identifies a previously uncharacterized role for the understudied noncanonical NF-κB signaling pathway in the pathogenesis of IBD and anti-TNF therapy responsiveness. The genes and pathways identified may ultimately prove useful in IBD management and could potentially be used as biomarkers of drug response.

Keywords: noncanonical NF-κB pathway, anti-TNF agents, inflammatory bowel disease, Crohn's disease, ulcerative colitis, alternative pathway, NIK, therapeutic response

INTRODUCTION

Inflammatory bowel diseases (IBD)–Crohn's disease (CD) and ulcerative colitis (UC)-are characterized by chronic inflammation of the gastrointestinal tract, driven by elements of both the innate and adaptive immune systems in genetically susceptible individuals. Together these diseases afflict approximately over 6 million people worldwide, which makes them a significant global health and economic burden (Ng et al., 2018). The nuclear factor kappa B (NF-κB) family of transcription factors are master regulators of inflammation and drive a diverse spectrum of biological processes (Rothschild et al., 2018). This signaling cascade is commonly found dysregulated in IBD patients, leading to dysfunctional cytokine and chemokine production in the gastrointestinal tract. NF-κB signaling occurs through two distinct pathways, defined as the canonical pathway and the noncanonical (or alternative) pathway.

In the context of IBD, the overwhelming majority of studies have focused on the canonical NF-κB signaling cascade. This cascade relies on the proteins RelA (p65) and p50 which form the heterodimer RelA/p50. Upon activation of this pathway, this heterodimer translocates into the nucleus, where it functions as a transcription factor. In this pathway, signaling is rapid and constitutive. Activation of the cascade results in the transcription of a wide range of well characterized inflammatory mediators such as IL-1β, TNF, and IL-6 (McDaniel et al., 2016). TNF in particular plays a central role in the pathogenesis of IBD (Billmeier et al., 2016) as shown by the clinical efficacy of anti-TNF medications such as infliximab (IFX) or adalimumab (ADA)-mainstay therapies for both CD and UC. These therapies have been shown to reduce the risk of hospitalization, surgery, and improve quality of life (Mao et al., 2017). In addition, they have been shown to prevent CD relapse after surgery (Sorrentino 2013). However, up to 40% of IBD patients do not respond to initial treatment with anti-TNF agents [primary nonresponse (PNR)], and a similar proportion of patients lose response over time [secondary loss of response (SLR)] after initially achieving clinical remission (Danese et al., 2011; Ben-Horin et al., 2014). The mechanism of PNR and SLR to anti-TNF agents is not completely understood and likely to be multifactorial. Several explanations have been suggested, including the immune system switch to an alternative inflammatory pathway, immunogenicity with production of drug neutralizing antibodies and medical unresposiveness due to advanced disease (Sorrentino 2008; Yarur et al., 2014; Biancheri et al., 2015; Brandse et al., 2016). While one mechanism does not exclude others and they might all play a role in different circumstances, the possibility of alternative pathways driving inflammation in IBD may provide insight into why medications targeting molecules different from TNF might be effective in SLR and PNR.

Unlike the canonical pathway, there is minimal data on the role of this signaling cascade in IBD. Noncanonical NF-κB signaling is highly regulated at the post-transcriptional and post-translational level, resulting in a slower, more controlled, and chronic signaling response. The noncanonical pathway relies on a heterodimer different from that of the canonical pathway and is comprised of RelB and 100, which is later cleaved into its active form of RelB and p52 (Sun 2011). In the noncanonical signaling cascade, NF-κB initiates the transcription of a limited repertoire of target genes, including those coding for the chemokines CXCL12, CXCL13, CCL19, and CCL21 (**Supplementary Figure S1**). Prior research from our group using a pre-clinical mouse model found that mice lacking negative regulators of noncanonical NF-κB signaling - such as the Nod-like receptor NLRP12-demonstrated increased noncanonical pathway activation and susceptibility to models of IBD and inflammation-driven colon tumorigenesis (Allen et al., 2012). These findings suggest a role of noncanonical NF-κB signaling in IBD pathogenesis. In this study, we examine the hypothesis that this pathway may be involved in anti-TNF agents response in IBD patients.

MATERIALS AND METHODS

Protection of Human Subjects

All studies were conducted following the regulations, policies, and guidelines set forth by the National Institutes of Health for research involving human subjects. All studies were conducted under the approval of the Institutional Review Board of Carilion Clinic and Virginia Tech Carilion School of Medicine.

Patient Selection

A total of 27 established IBD patients (19 with CD and 8 with UC) and 15 control subjects were prospectively recruited from the IBD Center at Carilion Clinic from 2015 to 2018. Patients were ≥ 18 years of age, without other gastrointestinal or systemic disorders, without recent NSAIDs use, and scheduled for colonoscopy for clinical indications. Pregnant patients were excluded.

Sample Collection

Tissue samples from each patient were obtained through biopsies of both visible lesions and non-affected areas in the colon and/or the terminal ileum. Tissue samples were stored in RNAlater at −80°C. Patients were separated into different groups based on diagnosis (CD or UC), type of medication use, and response to therapy. Tissue from controls was obtained from patients undergoing colonoscopy for reasons other than IBD (e.g., rectal bleeding) and included in the study only after endoscopy and histology proved to be normal.

Data Collection

Clinical data were abstracted from the patient medical charts. Demographics variables collected included age, gender, and smoking status. For IBD patients, disease diagnosis, and phenotype were determined at the time of study enrollment based on the Montreal disease classification (Satsangi et al., 2006). IBD medications and response to anti-TNF agents were recorded. Anti-TNF agents consisted of IFX and ADA in this patient cohort. Loss of response to anti-TNF therapy was classified as PNR or SLR. PNR was defined as complete lack of response to initiation of anti-TNF therapy whereas patients with SLR were those who initially responded to an anti-TNF agent - at least through the induction phase - but subsequently lost response. Clinical symptoms, inflammatory markers, imaging, and/or endoscopy findings were used to determine response.

Tissue Processing and Data Analysis

Biopsy samples were removed from RNAlater, finely minced, and homogenized in RLT buffer (Qiagen) with 2-mercaptoethanol. Tissues were processed using an AllPrep Kit (Qiagen) following the manufacturer's protocol. RNA was analyzed for quality and concentration using a NanoDrop™. Pools were made using equal concentrations of RNA from each patient sample for each experimental group. Patient samples were assigned to pools randomly and at least three pools were generated for each experimental group. The total amount of RNA used for each cDNA reaction was 600 ng and cDNA was generated using a First Strand Kit (Qiagen) following manufacturer's protocols. Following cDNA preparation, gene expression was evaluated using a custom Qiagen RT^2 Superarray following manufacturer's protocol. A list of 88 candidate genes for the custom Superarray platform is provided in **Supplementary Figure S2**. For each array, gene expression was determined utilizing the ΔΔCt method, using a panel of five housekeeping genes and internal controls provided on each array. Gene expression was determined using a 7,500 Fast Block Real-Time PCR System (ABI). Data was analyzed using SA Biosciences Data Analysis Center and Ingenuity Pathway Analysis (IPA). IPA images were then generated using BioRender.

In addition to the analysis of pooled samples, quantitative rtPCR was also performed in select genes of interest for each individual specimen. Complimentary DNA was generated from each specimen using an ABI High Capacity cDNA kit, in accordance with the manufacturer's protocol and 1 µg amplified using the Taqman-based rtPCR platform (ThermoFisher) on the ABI system. Gene expression was determined using the ΔΔCt method. All data were normalized to 18s and the fold change in gene expression was determined.

Statistical Analysis

For gene expression analysis, data was analyzed using GraphPad Prism, version 6 (GraphPad Software, Inc., San Diego, CA).

TABLE 1 | Patient characteristics.

	IBD	Controls
N	27	15
Age (years)	41 ± 15	55 ± 14
Female	12 (44%)	6 (40%)
Smoker	4 (15%)	2 (13%)
CD	19 (70%)	
CD extent		
L1 (ileal)	5 (26%)	
L2 (colonic)	7 (37%)	
L3 (ileocolonic)	7 (37%)	
UC extent		
E1 (rectum)	2 (25%)	
E2 (left sided)	2 (25%)	
E3 (extensive)	4 (50%)	
IBD medications		
Anti-TNF agents	15 (56%)	
Non-anti-TNF therapies	10 (37%)	
No therapy	2 (7%)	
Anti-TNF responsive	5/15 (33%)	

Age is reported as mean ± SD.

Student's two-tailed t test was used for comparison between experimental groups. Multiple comparisons were conducted using one-way and two-way ANOVA where appropriate followed by Tukey post-test for multiple pairwise examinations. Correlation was computed using GraphPad Prism. Changes were identified as statistically significant if *p*-value was less than 0.05. Mean values were reported together with the SEM. The number of patients were determined based on a power analysis conducted using findings from a retrospective metadata analysis of publicly accessible gene expression data from dataset GSE16879. Gene expression was determined for a single marker of noncanonical NF-κB signaling (CXCL13) and the average and standard deviation of expression for this gene was used to determine the number of patients to target in the clinical study presented here.

RESULTS

Noncanonical NF-κB is Upregulated in IBD

Tissues samples were obtained from 27 IBD patients and 15 controls. In the IBD group, 19 patients had CD and eight patients had UC (**Table 1**). The mean age of IBD patients was 41 years, 44% were females and 15% were active smokers. Of this patient pool, 33% of IBD patients were anti-TNF responders while 44% were not on medications or were taking medications other than anti-TNF agents. All anti-TNF non-responders in this study experienced SLR. The majority of CD and UC patients had ileocolonic and extensive colonic involvement respectively.

First, we examined the association of the noncanonical NF-κB pathway in IBD patients compared to controls. We found a

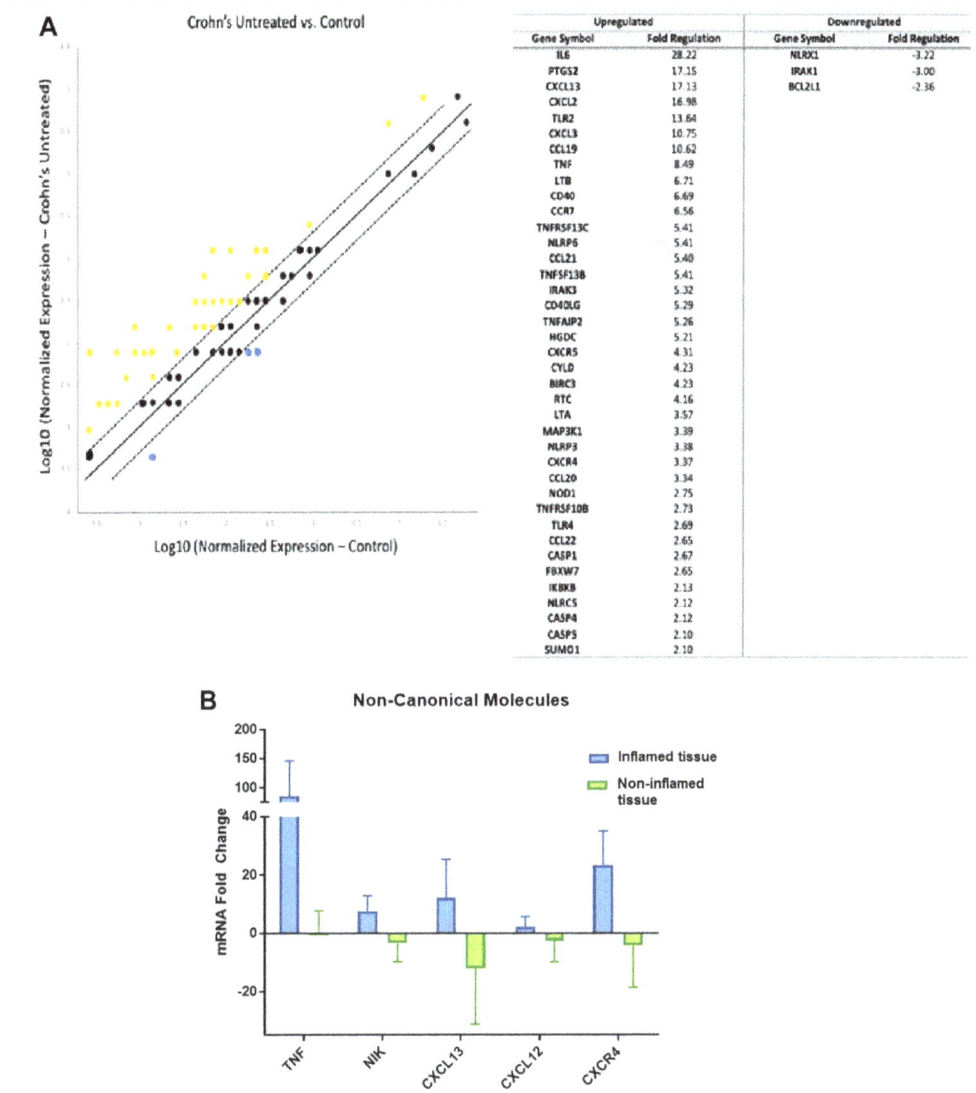

Upregulated		Downregulated	
Gene Symbol	Fold Regulation	Gene Symbol	Fold Regulation
IL6	28.22	NLRX1	-3.22
PTGS2	17.15	IRAK1	-3.00
CXCL13	17.13	BCL2L1	-2.36
CXCL2	16.98		
TLR2	13.64		
CXCL3	10.75		
CCL19	10.62		
TNF	8.49		
LTB	6.71		
CD40	6.69		
CCR7	6.56		
TNFRSF13C	5.41		
NLRP6	5.41		
CCL21	5.40		
TNFSF13B	5.41		
IRAK3	5.32		
CD40LG	5.29		
TNFAIP2	5.26		
HGDC	5.21		
CXCR5	4.31		
CYLD	4.23		
BIRC3	4.23		
RTC	4.16		
LTA	3.57		
MAP3K1	3.39		
NLRP3	3.38		
CXCR4	3.37		
CCL20	3.34		
NOD1	2.75		
TNFRSF10B	2.73		
TLR4	2.69		
CCL22	2.65		
CASP1	2.67		
FBXW7	2.65		
IKBKB	2.13		
NLRC5	2.12		
CASP4	2.12		
CASP5	2.10		
SUMO1	2.10		

FIGURE 1 | Noncanonical NF-κB Signaling is Upregulated in Inflammatory Bowel Disease Patients **(A)** Left: Compared to gene expression from intestinal tissues of controls (n = 15, 3 pools), 39 genes related to noncanonical NF-κB pathway were upregulated in intestinal tissues obtained from untreated CD patients (n = 2, 1 pool) with yellow indicating upregulation and blue indicating downregulation (lines represent 1, 0, and −1 fold change; genes outside of dashed lines are considered significantly dysregulated). Housekeeping genes used for normalization include *ACTB, B2M,* and *GADPH;* Right: list of 39 upregulated genes and three downregulated genes and fold change values. **(B)**. Using real-time PCR of individual patient samples, the main noncanonical NF-kB pathway components TNF, NIK, CXCL12, CXCL13, and CXCR4 were found to be upregulated in inflamed areas compared to non-inflamed areas obtained from the same individual patients (inflamed lesions n = 4; non-inflamed tissue n = 4).

significant upregulation of 39 genes and downregulation of three genes associated with noncanonical NF-κB signaling in the pooled untreated CD patients (**Figure 1A**). These dysregulated genes encode for proteins with crucial roles in the signaling cascade. We also conducted individual real-time PCR analysis on a selection of these genes to validate the findings of the gene expression arrays. Individual qPCR was conducted on five genes that were significantly dysregulated in the custom gene expression arrays and are critical points in the noncanonical NF-κB signaling pathway (**Supplementary Figure S1**). TNF is one of the activating molecules; NIK is a critical kinase required for perpetuation of this activating signal; and CXCL12, CXCL13, and CXCR4 are products of the signaling pathway. The individual gene expression was consistent with custom arrays: *TNF, MAP3K14* (NIK), *CXCL12, CXCL13,* and *CXCR4* genes were all significantly upregulated in biopsies collected from inflamed areas compared to biopsies collected from non-inflamed areas in the same individual patients (**Figure 1B**).

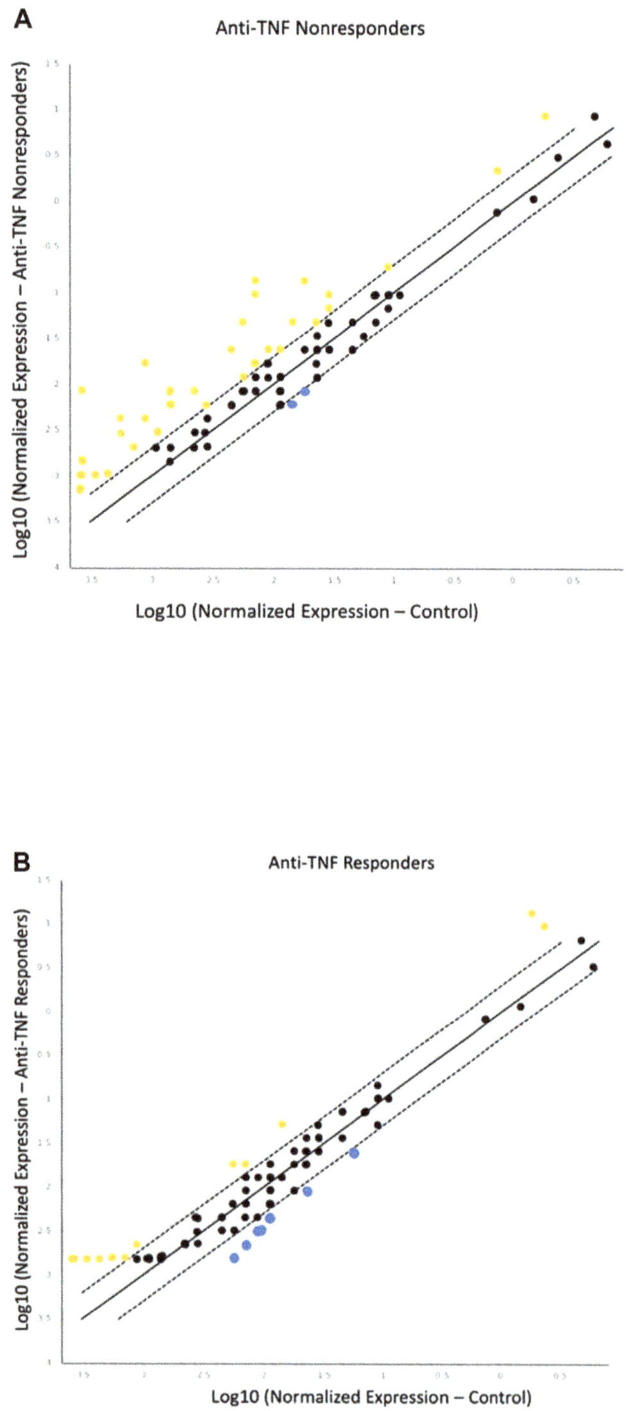

Anti-TNF Nonresponders			
Upregulated		**Downregulated**	
Gene Symbol	**Fold Regulation**	**Gene Symbol**	**Fold Regulation**
IL6	30.86	TLR3	-2.43
PTGS2	18.79	BCL2L1	-2.16
CXCL13	18.77		
CXCL2	13.13		
CXCL3	8.29		
TLR2	7.46		
CCL20	7.30		
CCL22	5.81		
NLRP6	5.75		
CD70	5.36		
LTB	5.20		
NLRC3	5.15		
NLRP3	5.02		
TNF	4.64		
RTC	4.59		
TNFSF13B	4.14		
IRAK3	4.06		
NOD2	3.78		
CD27	3.69		
CD40	3.68		
CASP5	3.27		
BIRC3	3.26		
HGDC	2.90		
TNFRSF13C	2.88		
CD40LG	2.81		
NLRP12	2.68		
IRAK2	2.60		
CXCR4	2.59		
PPC	2.59		
LTA	2.59		
TNFRSF8	2.59		
CCR7	2.58		
TNFRSF12A	2.35		
CXCR5	2.35		
CYLD	2.33		
CASP4	2.31		
RELA	2.07		
CASP1	2.07		
TNFAIP2	2.06		
FBXW7	2.06		
CCL19	2.06		
RELB	2.05		

Anti-TNF Responders			
Upregulated		**Downregulated**	
Gene Symbol	**Fold Regulation**	**Gene Symbol**	**Fold Regulation**
RTC	7.14	TNFAIP2	-3.70
NOD2	5.63	CXCL13	-3.25
TNFRSF8	5.63	TNFRSF1B	-2.94
NLRP12	5.63	CXCR4	-2.83
LTA	5.63	IRAK1	-2.54
PPC	5.63	TRAF2	-2.52
IL6	5.51	TNFRSF1A	-2.25
CD27	5.50		
CD70	5.49		
NLRC3	5.43		
TNFRSF13C	4.30		
RPLPO	3.99		
CASP5	3.56		
CXCR5	3.39		
CXCL3	3.18		
TLR2	2.76		
NLRP3	2.73		
CYLD	2.52		
TNF	2.44		
CD40LG	2.16		

FIGURE 2 | Noncanonical NF-κB is Downregulated in IBD Patients Responding To Anti-TNF Therapy. **(A)**: Inflamed tissues from anti-TNF nonresponders (n = 10, two pools, CD patients and UC patients) showed 39 upregulated genes related to the noncanonical NF-κB signaling, compared to only 19 genes in anti-TNF responders (n = 5, two pools) **(B)**, with yellow indicating upregulation and blue indicating downregulation (lines represent 1, 0, and −1 fold change; genes outside of dashed lines are considered significantly dysregulated). A list of the involved genes is provided next to each graph. Housekeeping genes used for normalization include *ACTB, B2M,* and *GADPH* **(C–F)**: Ingenuity Pathway Analysis revealed that noncanonical NF-κB was a significant signaling hub that was downregulated in patients responding to anti-TNF therapy. Expression levels of the main noncanonical genes *NIK (MAP3K14), CXCL12, CXCL13,* and *CCL21* were upregulated in both untreated patients (n = 2, one pool) **(C)** and patients treated with non-anti-TNF medications (n = 10, two pools) **(D)**. However, anti-TNF responders (n = 5, two pools) **(E)**, showed a distinct attenuation of expression of these genes. Meanwhile, anti-TNF non-responders showed upregulation of *CXCL12* and *CXCL13* and downregulation of *CCL21*. Note: green represents downregulation; red represents upregulation.

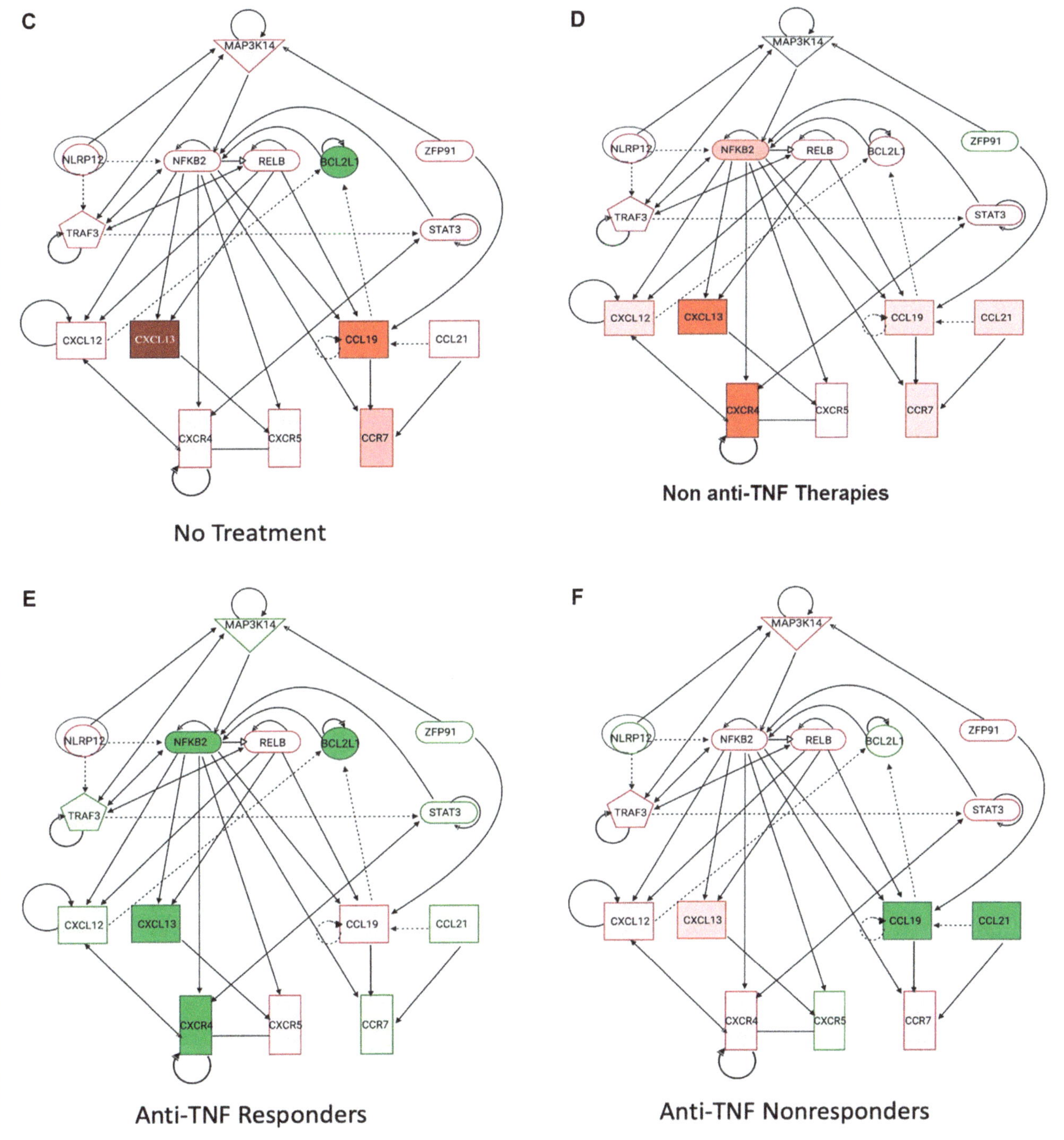

FIGURE 2 | (Continued).

Noncanonical NF-κB Signaling is Downregulated in Anti-TNF Responsive Patients

We then examined the role of the noncanonical NF-κB pathway in IBD patients in relation to their responsiveness to anti-TNF agents. Compared to controls, in IBD patients not responding to anti-TNF therapy, we identified 42 upregulated genes and only two downregulated genes (**Figure 2A**). Notably, CXCL13 was significantly upregulated (+18.77 fold) in nonresponders.

Conversely, in IBD patients responding to anti-TNF agents we identified 20 upregulated genes and seven downregulated genes involved in noncanonical NF-κB signaling (**Figure 2B**). Upregulated genes included *NLRP12*, a negative regulator of noncanonical signaling, while downregulated genes included

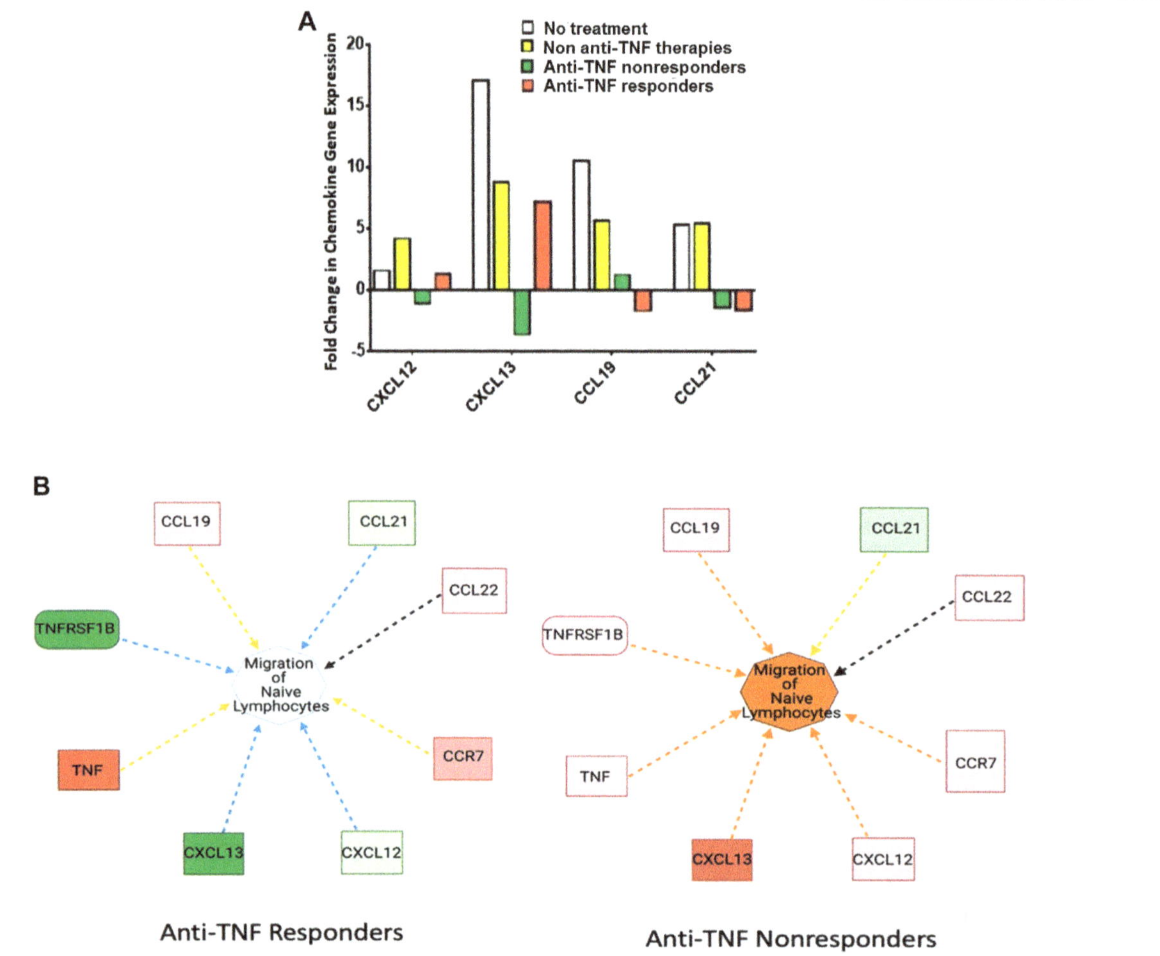

FIGURE 3 | CXCL12 and CXCL13 are Downregulated in IBD Patients Responding to Anti-TNFα Therapy. **(A)** CXCL12, CXCL13, CCL19, and CCL21 were significantly upregulated in both untreated IBD patients (n = 2, one pool) and IBD patients treated with non-anti-TNF medications (n = 10, two pools). CXCL12, CXCL13, and CCL19 displayed opposite expression profiles based on anti-TNF responsiveness, with upregulation in anti-TNF nonresponders (n = 10, two pools) and downregulation in responders (n = 5, two pools) for CXCL12 and CXCL13. CCL21 remained downregulated regardless of response to anti-TNF agents. **(B)** Predicted effect on the migration of naïve lymphocytes to inflamed tissue based on changes of the noncanonical chemokines which are involved in lymphocyte trafficking. In anti-TNF responders, lymphocyte trafficking is reduced. By contrast anti-TNF nonresponders demonstrate increased lymphocyte trafficking. In general, the increase in noncanonical signaling molecules results in a large increase in predicted lymphocyte migration. Note: Blue and orange dashed lines with arrows indicate indirect inhibition and activation, respectively. Yellow and black dashed lines with arrows depict inconsistent effects and no prediction, respectively.

noncanonical chemokine *CXCL13* and noncanonical receptor for *CXCR4*.

Pathway analysis revealed significant downregulation of noncanonical NF-κB signaling in IBD patients responsive to anti-TNFα therapy compared to untreated IBD patients and IBD patients treated with other (non-anti-TNF) medications (**Figures 2C–F**). This decreased expression was observed in several genes throughout the signaling pathway, and specifically included reduced expression of *MAP3K14, NFKB2, TRAF3, STAT3, CXCL12, CXCL13, CXCR4*, and *CCR7* that were not observed in the other IBD patient groups. Interestingly, in IBD patients unresponsive to anti-TNF therapy, noncanonical NF-κB signaling was upregulated compared to untreated IBD patients. In these patients, upregulation of noncanonical NF-κB signaling was strongly associated with the downregulation of *NLRP12* and upregulation of *MAP3K14, CXCL12*, and *CXCL13*. Together, these data demonstrate that noncanonical NF-κB signaling was significantly decreased in anti-TNF responders and increased in anti-TNF nonresponders.

CXCL12 and CXCL13 Expression is Correlated to Anti-TNF Responsiveness

Currently, only four major chemokines have been associated with the noncanonical NF-κB signaling cascade, CCL19, CCL21, CXCL12, and CXCL13. We examined these chemokine expression patterns in relation to anti-TNF responsiveness. In untreated IBD patients and in those treated with other (non-anti-TNF) therapies, *CCL19, CCL21, CXCL12, and CXCL13* expression were upregulated. IBD patients responding to anti-

TNF therapy demonstrated a significant decrease in *CXCL12*, *CXCL13*, and *CCL21* compared to those in the untreated IBD group (**Figure 3A**). By contrast, *CXCL12* and *CXCL13* were significantly upregulated in IBD patients not responding to anti-TNF therapy while *CCL19* and *CCL21* were downregulated in these patients. Both *CXCL12* and *CXCL13* were strongly correlated with anti-TNF responsiveness, whereas *CCL19* and *CCL21* only demonstrated a weak correlation. Based on the expression profile associated with these chemokines, it appears that migration of naïve lymphocytes was the signaling network most strongly altered in patients not responding to anti-TNF agents (**Figure 3B**). Hence, by contrast with nonresponders, in IBD patients responding to anti-TNF therapy, the downregulation of *CXCL12* and *CXCL13* could result in reduced migration of lymphocytes to inflamed tissues.

DISCUSSION

Anti-TNF therapy acting through the canonical NF-κB signaling pathway has been the cornerstone of IBD treatment for the past several years. Despite its success, a significant proportion of IBD patients may not respond or lose response over time to anti-TNF therapy. This population of anti-TNF nonresponders has an increased risk of disease complications but might respond to newer biologic medications such as ustekinumab or vedolizumab (Feagan et al., 2016 and Feagan et al.2017). The mechanisms of PNR and SLR to anti-TNF agents are poorly understood. One possible explanation is that the driving mechanism of inflammation in these IBD patients may have shifted to an alternative signaling pathway.

The noncanonical NF-κB pathway has been recognized as a key regulator and promoter of the adaptive immune system, particularly in the development of secondary lymphoid organs. Prior studies from our group have demonstrated the role of this signaling pathway in mouse models of colon inflammation and eosinophilic esophagitis (Allen et al., 2012; Eden et al., 2017).

In this study, we found significant upregulation of the genes involved in the noncanonical NF-κB pathway in IBD patients compared to healthy controls. Furthermore, the main chemokines in this pathway, namely CXCL12 and CXCL13, were significantly downregulated in IBD patients who responded to anti-TNF agents and were upregulated in nonresponders. These findings suggest that the activation of the noncanonical NF-κB signaling pathway may contribute to the mechanism underlying the lack/loss of response to anti-TNF therapy. The upregulated genes in the noncanonical NF-κB pathway involved in lack/loss of response to anti-TNF therapy may involve leukocyte migration to the affected tissue as predicted by IPA analysis.

The relatively small sample size and single center nature are limitations of our study. In addition, it is unclear how many of our anti-TNF nonresponders would respond to additional anti-TNF agents (Swaminath et al., 2009; Löfberg et al., 2012). Whether the expression pattern of the noncanonical genes differs in patients who respond to a second anti-TNF agent compared to those who do not respond to any anti-TNF medication remains unknown. Also, our study does not clarify the role of this pathway in PNR–since all of our patients experienced SLR.

In conclusion, this is the first study in humans that has explored the role of the noncanonical NF-κB signaling in the pathogenesis of IBD. More importantly, our findings provide a potential mechanistic insight into the lack/loss of response to anti-TNF agents in IBD. If our observations are confirmed, targeting the noncanonical NF-κB signaling pathway could significantly impact IBD management and therapy outcomes.

ETHICS STATEMENT

The studies involving human participants were reviewed and approved by IRB Carilion Clinic. The patients/participants provided their written informed consent to participate in this study.

AUTHOR CONTRIBUTIONS

VN was responsible for investigation and writing (review and editing); HM, KE, KK, SS, RB, and DG were responsible for investigation, DS and IA were responsible for conceptualization, investigation, methodology, formal analysis, supervision, and writing (initial draft, review and editing).

SUPPLEMENTARY MATERIAL

SUPPLEMENTARY FIGURE 1 | Schematic Illustration of Key Components of Noncanonical NF-κB Signaling Significantly Dysregulated in IBD Patients. Our data revealed a significant increase in chemokines associated with noncanonical NF-κB signaling, including CXCL12, CXCL13, CCL9, and CCL21. Additional pathway analysis revealed that these changes were associated with increased expression of genes encoding a variety of proteins that regulate the non-canonical NF-κB signaling pathway through modulation of NIK, including the up-regulation of cIAP1, cIAP2, CYLD, and NLRP12 and the down-regulation of BCL10, ZPF91, and A20. Created with BioRender.com.

SUPPLEMENTARY TABLE 1 | Custom Gene Array to Evaluate Noncanonical NF-κB Signaling in IBD Patients. The gene list for the custom superarray platform is provided with RefSeq Number and Gene Symbol. These 88 gene candidates serve a role in the noncanonical NF-κB pathway and dysregulated transcription levels may have implications on IBD pathogenesis and drug responsiveness. For each array, gene expression was determined utilizing the delta-deltaCt method, using a panel of five housekeeping genes and internal controls provided on each array.

REFERENCES

Allen, I. C., Wilson, J. E., Schneider, M., Lich, J. D., Roberts, R. A., Arthur, J. C., et al. (2012). NLRP12 Suppresses Colon Inflammation and Tumorigenesis through the Negative Regulation of Noncanonical NF-κB Signaling. *Immunity* 36, 742–754. doi:10.1016/j.immuni.2012.03.012

Ben-Horin, S., Kopylov, U., and Chowers, Y. (2014). Optimizing Anti-TNF Treatments in Inflammatory Bowel Disease. *Autoimmun. Rev.* 13, 24–30. doi:10.1016/j.autrev.2013.06.002

Biancheri, P., Brezski, R. J., Di Sabatino, A., Greenplate, A. R., Soring, K. L., Corazza, G. R., et al. (2015). Proteolytic Cleavage and Loss of Function of Biologic Agents that Neutralize Tumor Necrosis Factor in the Mucosa of Patients with Inflammatory Bowel Disease. *Gastroenterology* 149, 1564–1574. doi:10.1053/j.gastro.2015.07.002

Billmeier, U., Dieterich, W., Neurath, M. F., and Atreya, R. (2016). Molecular Mechanism of Action of Anti-tumor Necrosis Factor Antibodies in Inflammatory Bowel Diseases. *World J. Gastroenterol.* 22, 9300–9313. doi:10.3748/wjg.v22.i42.9300

Brandse, J. F., Mathôt, R. A., van der Kleij, D., Rispens, T., Ashruf, Y., Jansen, J. M., et al. (2016). Pharmacokinetic Features and Presence of Antidrug Antibodies Associate With Response to Infliximab Induction Therapy in Patients With Moderate to Severe Ulcerative Colitis. *Clin. Gastroenterol. Hepatol.* 14, 251–258. doi:10.1016/j.cgh.2015.10.029

Danese, S., Fiorino, G., and Reinisch, W. (2011). Review Article: Causative Factors and the Clinical Management of Patients with Crohn's Disease Who Lose Response to Anti-TNF-α Therapy. *Aliment. Pharmacol. Ther.* 34, 1–10. doi:10.1111/j.1365-2036.2011.04679.x

Eden, K., Rothschild, D. E., McDaniel, D. K., Heid, B., and Allen, I. C. (2017). Noncanonical NF-κB Signaling and the Essential Kinase NIK Modulate Crucial Features Associated with Eosinophilic Esophagitis Pathogenesis. *Dis. Model. Mech.* 10, 1517–1527. doi:10.1242/dmm.030767

Feagan, B. G., Rubin, D. T., Danese, S., Vermeire, S., Abhyankar, B., Sankoh, S., et al. (2017). Efficacy of Vedolizumab Induction and Maintenance Therapy in Patients With Ulcerative Colitis, Regardless of Prior Exposure to Tumor Necrosis Factor Antagonists. *Clin. Gastroenterol. Hepatol.* 15, 229–239. doi:10.1016/j.cgh.2016.08.044

Feagan, B. G., Sandborn, W. J., Gasink, C., Jacobstein, D., Lang, Y., Friedman, J. R., et al. (2016). Ustekinumab as Induction and Maintenance Therapy for Crohn's Disease. *N. Engl. J. Med.* 375, 1946–1960. doi:10.1056/NEJMoa1602773

Löfberg, R., Louis, E. V., Reinisch, W., Robinson, A. M., Kron, M., Camez, A., et al. (2012). Adalimumab Produces Clinical Remission and Reduces Extraintestinal Manifestations in Crohn's Disease: Results from CARE. *Inflamm. Bowel Dis.* 18, 1–9. doi:10.1002/ibd.21663

Mao, E. J., Hazlewood, G. S., Kaplan, G. G., Peyrin-Biroulet, L., and Ananthakrishnan, A. N. (2017). Systematic Review with Meta-Analysis: Comparative Efficacy of Immunosuppressants and Biologics for Reducing Hospitalisation and Surgery in Crohn's Disease and Ulcerative Colitis. *Aliment. Pharmacol. Ther.* 45, 3–13. doi:10.1111/apt.13847

McDaniel, D. K., Eden, K., Ringel, V. M., and Allen, I. C. (2016). Emerging Roles for -κB Signaling in the Modulation of Inflammatory Bowel Disease Pathobiology. *Inflamm. Bowel Dis.* 22, 2265–2279. doi:10.1097/MIB.0000000000000858

Ng, S. C., Shi, H. Y., Hamidi, N., Underwood, F. E., Tang, W., Benchimol, E. I., et al. (2018). Worldwide Incidence and Prevalence of Inflammatory Bowel Disease in the 21st century: a Systematic Review of Population-Based Studies. *Lancet* 390, 2769–2778. doi:10.1016/S0140-6736(17)32448-0

Rothschild, D. E., McDaniel, D. K., Ringel-Scaia, V. M., and Allen, I. C. (2018). Modulating Inflammation through the Negative Regulation of NF-κB Signaling. *J. Leukoc. Biol.* 103, 1131–1150. doi:10.1002/JLB.3MIR0817-346RRR

Satsangi, J., Silverberg, M. S., Vermeire, S., and Colombel, J.-F. (2006). The Montreal Classification of Inflammatory Bowel Disease: Controversies, Consensus, and Implications. *Gut* 55, 749–753. doi:10.1136/gut.2005.082909

Sorrentino, D. (2008). Role of Biologics and Other Therapies in Stricturing Crohn's Disease: what Have We Learnt So Far? *Digestion* 77, 38–47. doi:10.1159/000117306

Sorrentino, D. (2013). State-of-the-art Medical Prevention of Postoperative Recurrence of Crohn's Disease. *Nat. Rev. Gastroenterol. Hepatol.* 10, 413–422. doi:10.1038/nrgastro.2013.69

Sun, S.-C. (2011). Non-canonical NF-κB Signaling Pathway. *Cell Res.* 21, 71–85. doi:10.1038/cr.2010.177

Swaminath, A., Ullman, T., Rosen, M., Mayer, L., Lichtiger, S., and Abreu, M. T. (2009). Early Clinical Experience with Adalimumab in Treatment of Inflammatory Bowel Disease with Infliximab-Treated and Naïve Patients. *Aliment. Pharmacol. Ther.* 29, 273–278. doi:10.1111/j.1365-2036.2008.03878.x

Yarur, A. J., Abreu, M. T., Deshpande, A. R., Kerman, D. H., and Sussman, D. A. (2014). Therapeutic Drug Monitoring in Patients with Inflammatory Bowel Disease. *World J. Gastroenterol.* 20, 3475–3484. doi:10.3748/wjg.v20.i13.3475

13

Kaempferol Alleviates Steatosis and Inflammation During Early Non-Alcoholic Steatohepatitis Associated with Liver X Receptor α-Lysophosphatidylcholine Acyltransferase 3 Signaling Pathway

Hongjiao Xiang[1,2†], *Mingmei Shao*[1,2†], *Yifei Lu*[1,2], *Junmin Wang*[1,2], *Tao Wu*[1,2]* *and Guang Ji*[2]*

[1]*Institute of Interdisciplinary Integrative Medicine Research, Shanghai University of Traditional Chinese Medicine, Shanghai, China,* [2]*Institute of Digestive Disease, Longhua Hospital, Shanghai University of Traditional Chinese Medicine, Shanghai, China*

Correspondence:
Guang Ji
jiliver@vip.sina.com
Tao Wu
wutao001827@163.com

†*These authors have contributed equally to this work*

Background: Kaempferol (KP) has a variety of biological effects such as anti-inflammatory, anti-oxidant, anti-aging and cardiovascular protection. Whether KP has a therapeutic effect on non-alcoholic steatohepatitis (NASH), and the detailed mechanism is currently unclear. This study aims to explore the mechanism of KP in the treatment of NASH through *in vivo* and *in vitro* experiments.

Methods: 1) *In vivo* experiment: In the C57BL/6 NASH mice model induced by high fat diet (HFD), KP was administered by gavage at a dose of 20 mg/kg/day. 2) *In vitro* experiment: Palmitic acid/Oleic acid (PA/OA, 0.375/0.75 mM) was used to intervene HepG2 and AML12 cells to establish a steatosis cell model. Three concentrations of KP, low (20 μmol/L), medium (40 μmol/L) and high (60 μmol/L) were used *in vitro*. The mRNA and protein expression of related molecules involved in LXRα-LPCAT3-ERS pathway were detected using RT-qPCR and Western blot.

Results: In the NASH mouse model, KP can significantly reduce the expression of LXRα, LPCAT3 and ERS-related factors PERK, eIF2α, ATF6, ATF4, XBP1, CHOP, IRE1α and GRP78. In the PA/OA-induced cell model, KP could decrease the content of triglyceride and lipid droplets, and also decrease the expression of LXR α, LPCAT3 and ERS related factors PERK, eIF2α, ATF6, ATF4, XBP1, CHOP, IRE1α and GRP78.

Abbreviations: ABCA1, ATP binding cassette transporter A1; ALT, Alanine aminotransferase; ATF6, Activating transcription factor 6; BCA, Bicinchoninic acid; CCL5, C-C chemokine ligand 5; CCK8, Cell counting kit-8; CHOP, C/EBP homologous protein; CXCL10, C-X-C motif chemokine 10; eIF-2α, Eukaryotic translation initiation factor 2; ER, Endoplasmic reticulum; ERS, Endoplasmic reticulum stress; GPR78, Glucose-regulated protein 78; HFD, High-fat diet; HDL, High-density lipoprotein; IL6, Interleukin 6; IRE1, Inositol-requiring enzyme 1; KP, Kaempferol; LDL, Low density lipoprotein; LPCAT3, Lysophosphatidylcholine acyltransferase 3; LXRs, Liver X receptors; MAPK, Mitogen-activated protein kinase; MCP-1, Monocyte chemoattractant protein-1; NAFL, Non-alcoholic fatty liver; NAFLD, Non-alcoholic fatty liver disease; NASH, Non-alcoholic steatohepatitis; PA/OA, Palmitic acid/oleic acid; PERK, Protein kinase R-like ER kinase; PLs, Phospholipids; PPAR, Peroxisome proliferator-activated receptor; ROS, Reactive oxygen species; SREBP, Sterol regulatory element bingding proteins; TC, Total cholesterol; TG, Triglyceride; TNFα, Tumor necrosis factor α; UPR, Unfolded protein response; XBP1, X-box-binding protein 1.

Conclusion: KP may decrease the expression level of LXRα and LPCAT3, thus improve ERS and reduce hepatic steatosis and inflammation.

Keywords: kaempferol, NASH, LXR, LPCAT3, ERS

INTRODUCTION

Non-alcoholic fatty liver disease (NAFLD) is a clinical pathological syndrome, which includes simple steatosis, steatohepatitis (NASH), liver fibrosis and cirrhosis and their clinical consequences (Nobili et al., 2019). NASH is usually associated with more severer liver cirrhosis and liver cancer (Friedman et al., 2018). NAFLD is one of the leading cause of liver disease in the world, which is closely linked to the increased prevalence of obesity and metabolic diseases. NAFLD affects more than 20% of the population of the Europe and United States. NAFLD prevalence varies widely from the Asia-pacific region, ranging from about 5 to 32% (Younossi et al., 2018). Approximately one third of NAFLD patients will progress to NASH (Takahashi and Fukusato, 2014).

Phospholipids (PLs) is an important part of biological membranes and the precursors of many signal molecules (Vance, 2015). Liver X receptors (LXRs) are regulators of membrane phospholipid composition, important regulators for regulating cholesterol and fatty acid homeostasis, and effective inflammation inhibitors (Rong et al., 2013). Lysophosphatidylcholine acyltransferase 3 (LPCAT3) is a key enzyme that encodes the remodeling pathway to PLs, and is a direct target gene of mouse and human LXR (Demeure et al., 2011; Wang et al., 2016). LPCAT3 modulates the activation of inflammatory kinases by changing membrane components, and regulates inflammation by affecting the availability of substrates produced by inflammatory mediators (Singh and Liu, 2017b). Rong et al. stated that LXR activation increased the expression of LPCAT3 and reduced the saturation of the ER membrane. Acute knockout of LPCAT3 in the liver could aggravate endoplasmic reticulum stress (ERS). At the same time, the inflammation of the liver would increase because the activity of LPCAT3 was inhibited. It can be concluded that the LXR-LPCAT3 pathway is important to regulating ERS, and is involved in the progress of NASH.

Apoptosis is an active cell death process controlled by gene, which is mainly divided into endogenous pathway (mitochondrial pathway), exogenous pathway (death receptor pathway) and ERS induced apoptosis (Hu et al., 2018). The link between ERS and liver disease has been found in a growing number of studies, including NAFLD, alcoholic fatty liver, viral hepatitis, NASH, liver cancer, etc., (Brenner et al., 2013; Li F. et al., 2017). Endoplasmic reticulum (ER) is the main site for protein synthesis, lipid production and calcium ion storage in eukaryotic cells. When cells are stimulated externally, the ER produces a large number of unfolded or misfolded proteins, which leads to the unfolded protein response (UPR) (Chaudhari et al., 2014; Demirtas et al., 2016). In the early stage, UPR can relieve the pressure on the ER and promote the restoration of normal function of ER. However, sustained ERS induces apoptosis through UPR (Ozcan and Tabas, 2012). Cell signal transduction pathways induced by UPR include three pathways: protein kinase R-like ER kinase/eukaryotic translation initiation factor 2 (PERK/eIF-2α), activating transcription factor 6 (ATF6) pathway and inositol-requiring enzyme 1/X-box-binding protein 1 (IRE1/XBP1) (Wang and Kaufman, 2016). ERS activates sterol regulatory element binding protein (SREBP) through the ATF6, PERK and IRE1 signaling pathways to promote lipid accumulation in the liver (Zhang et al., 2012). It has been proved that ERS can activate the apoptotic pathway and induce apoptosis by activating downstream signal molecules (Iurlaro and Muñoz-Pinedo, 2016). Dasgupta et al. (2020) demonstrated that the destruction of IRE1A or inhibition of Ire1a in liver cells reduces the release of inflammatory extracellular vesicles (EVs), and reduces liver damaged and inflammation in the mice were fed a diet high in fat, fructose, and cholesterol. Bax inhibitor-1 (BI-1) is a negative regulator of the ER stress sensor IRE1α. Lebeaupin et al. (2018) treated BI-$1^{-/-}$ mice on a high-fat diet (HFD) with tunicamycin and developed liver failure of a short period of time. After IRE1α inhibitors were used to treat BI-$1^{-/-}$ mice, liver inflammation was significantly improved. Hernández-Alvarez et al. (2019) found that the lack of Mfn2 would promote ERS, leading to the progression of NASH to liver cancer. Therefore, regulating ERS can be considered as an important approach and new strategy for prevention and treatment of steatosis.

Kaempferol (KP) is a dietary bioflavonoid, which is widely present in various plants. It has a variety of biological effects such as anti-inflammatory, anti-oxidant, anti-aging and cardiovascular protection (Li and Pu, 2011; Lee B. et al., 2015; Suchal et al., 2017; Kouhestani et al., 2018). Lee B. et al. (2015) found that KP may bind to PPARα during adipocyte differentiation to stimulate fatty acid oxidation signals in adipocytes, thereby reducing cellular triglyceride (TG) accumulation. Lee Y.-J. et al. (2015) used zebrafish to verify the inhibitory effect of KP on lipid accumulation. KP inhibited lipid accumulation in zebrafish by inhibiting fat-related genes (Lee B. et al., 2015). Wang et al. (2019) found that KP can improve liver failure induced by lipopolysaccharide-galactosamine by reducing ERS. Other studies have shown that the regulation of KP on ERS was bidirectional, which can promote the apoptosis of tumor cells and inhibit the apoptosis of non-tumor cells (Ashrafizadeh et al., 2020). Our previous review summarized the application of KP in treating diseases and the underlying mechanisms that are currently being studied (Ren et al., 2019). In our previous study, it has been demonstrated that KP not only reduced serum alanine aminotransferase (ALT), low density lipoprotein (LDL), TG and total cholesterol (TC) content, but also reduced the accumulation of lipids in the liver (Lu et al., 2020). However, there are insufficient studies on the detailed mechanism of KP on improving NASH.

In this study, we revealed that the expression of LXR-LPCAT3-ERS pathway-related factors was remarkably increased to the liver of mice fed a HFD, and the similar results were observed in palmitic acid/oleic acid (PA/OA)-induced steatotic cells. After intervention with KP, either *in vitro* or *in vivo*, KP significantly reduced the expression of LXR-LPCAT3 pathway, inhibited the expression of molecules involved in ERS, and then improved HFD-related liver damage. Finally, we conclude that KP is a promising drug for the treatment of NASH.

MATERIALS AND METHODS

Animals and Treatment

Six-week-old male C57BL/6J mice were purchased from Shanghai SLAC Experimental Animal Co., Ltd. China. The experimental animals are kept in the specific pathogen free environment of the Experimental Animal Center of Shanghai University of Traditional Chinese Medicine. The temperature is about 20 ± 4°C, and the humidity is about 15–16%. C57BL/6J mice were randomly divided into normal control group (Control, NC group, N = 7), HFD (Calorie composition: fat 60%, protein 20%, carbohydrate 20%, D12492, Research Diets, United States) fed group (HFD model, HFD group, N = 8) and HFD fed with KP (HFD + KP, HFD + KP group, N = 8). The mice in group NC were fed normal diet, and the mice in group HFD and HFD + KP were fed HFD for 24 weeks. At the beginning of the 21st week, KP (4 mg/ml) was gavaged in the HFD + KP group at a dose of 0.5 ml/100 g on the basis of HFD feeding. At the same time, mice in NC and HFD groups received equal volume of normal saline (**Supplementary Figure S1**). The serum and liver tissue of mice was collected. All the experimental procedures were approved by the Institutional Animal Care and Use Committee at the Shanghai University of Traditional Chinese Medicine (SYXKhu 2014-0008).

Cell Lines

HepG2 and AML12 cells were obtained from the Cell bank of typical culture preservation Committee of Chinese Academy of Sciences. The cells were cultured in high glucose DMEM (containing 10% fetal bovine serum, 100 U/ml penicillin, 100 μg/ml streptomycin and 1‰ Amphotericin B) and was maintained at 37°C, 95% air humidity and 5% CO_2.

Establishment of Steatosis Cell Line

PA (P0500, Sigma, United States) was dissolved in methanol, and OA (0550, Sigma, United States) was dissolved in PBS. PA:OA was then added to the culture solution at a ratio of 1: 2. Final concentrations of PA/OA were as below: ①0 mM, ②0.25/0.5 mM, ③0.375/0.75 mM, ④0.5/1 mM, ⑤0.625/1.25 mM and ⑥0.75/1.5 mM. HepG2 and AML12 cells were cultured for 24 h to observe the morphological changes. Cells were detected with cell counting kit-8 (CCK8), TG kit and Oil-Red O staining.

Real-Time Quantitative PCR

Total RNA was extracted from mouse livers, HepG2 and AML12 cells using Trizol reagents (R0016, Beyotime Biotechnology, Shanghai, China). cDNA were transcribed according to the instructions in the reverse transcription kit (A5001, Promega, United States). The cDNA was using real-time quantitative polymerase chain reaction (RT-qPCR) performed with the SYBR Green PCR Master Mix (11201E03, YEASEN, Shanghai, China) and gene-specific primers. The results were normalized with β-actin as control RT-qPCR was performed using a CFX-96 Real Time System (Bio-Rad, United States). Polymerase chains reaction primers are listed in Supplementary Table S1.

Western Blot

Liver and cell sample were lysed with radio immunoprecipitation assay (RIPA) buffer (WB0102, Weiao, Shanghai, China) containing phenylmethylsulfonyl fluoride (PMSF) (WB0122, Weiao, Shanghai, China). The proteins were extracted after centrifugation, and subsequently a bicinchoninic acid (BCA) (B48110, YEASEN, Shanghai, China) protein quantitation kit was used to determine the concentrations. 30 μg of protein was subjected to 10% sodium dodecyl sulfate-polyacrylamide (SDS-PAGE) gel electrophoresis, then transferred to a polyvinylidene fluoride membrane, and then incubated with the corresponding primary antibody overnight at 4°C. Antibodies and dilution ratio were as below: 1:1,000 for rabbit anti-Actin (R1207, HUABIO, Hangzhou, China), 1:1,000 for rabbit anti-LXRα (ab176323, Abcam, Cambridge, MA), 1:500 for rabbit anti-LPCAT3 (HAPL0516, HUABIO, Hangzhou, China), 1:1,000 for rabbit anti-phospho-PERK (3,179, Cell Signaling Technology, MA), 1: 1,000 for rabbit anti-PERK (20582-1-AP, Proteintech Group, MA), 1:1,000 for rabbit anti-phospho-eIF2α (3398S, Cell Signaling Technology, MA), 1:1,000 for rabbit anti-eIF2α (3398S, Cell Signaling Technology, MA), 1:500 for rabbit anti-ATF4 (10835-1-AP, Proteintech Group, MA), 1:200 for rabbit anti-CHOP (15204-1-AP, Proteintech Group, MA), 1:500 for rabbit anti-ATF6 (ab203119, Abcam, Cambridge, MA), 1:1,000 for rabbit anti-GRP78 (3177S, Cell Signaling Technology, MA), 1:1,000 for rabbit anti-phospho-IRE1α (AF7150, Affbiotech, China), 1:1,000 for rabbit anti-IRE1α (3294S, Cell Signaling Technology, MA), 1: 1,000 for rabbit anti-XBP1 (ab220783, Abcam, Cambridge, MA), 1: 200 for rabbit anti-PPARα (ab215270, Abcam, Cambridge, MA), 1: 200 for rabbit anti-ABCA1 (ab18180, Abcam, Cambridge, MA). The membrane was then incubated with a secondary antibody (1: 5,000, Peroxidase-conjugated affinity goat anti-mice IgG, HA1001, HUABIO, China). ImageJsoftware (National Institutes of Health, Bethesda, MD) was used to scan and analyze the western blot band to obtain protein quantitative data.

Cell Proliferation Assay

The cells were planted in 96-well plates with a density of 1×10^4 cells per well. After the cells were cultured for 24 h, 10 μl of CCK8 solution was added to each well of the 96-well plate and mixed. After in a 37°C incubator for 3 h, the optical density was measured at 450 nm wavelength with a microplate reader (Infinite M200 PRO, TECAN, Switzerland).

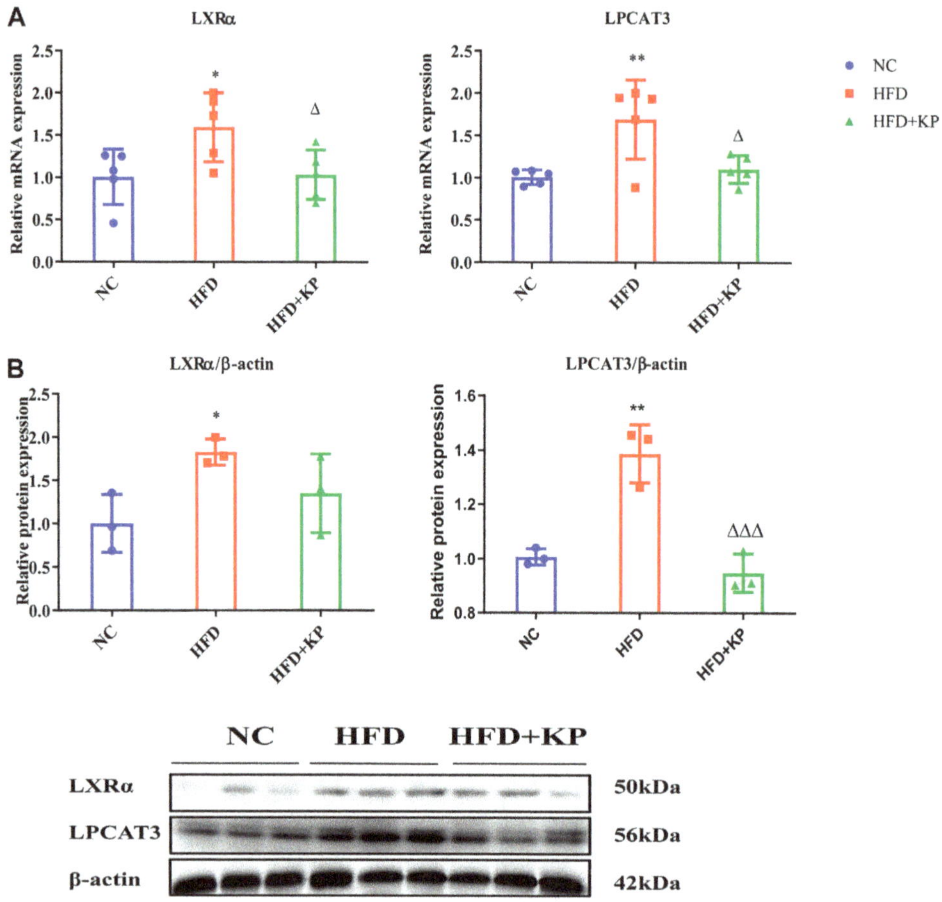

FIGURE 1 | KP regulated the mRNA and protein expression of LXRα and LPCAT3 *in vivo*. **(A)**: mRNA level expression of LXRα and LPCAT3 in liver samples; **(B)**: Protein level expression of LXRα and LPCAT3 in liver samples. NC: Normal control group, HFD: HFD group, HFD + KP: HFD + KP group. Quantification of mRNA and protein level expression was normalized to β-actin levels. Compared with group NC, *, $p < 0.05$, **, $p < 0.01$; Compared with group HFD, Δ, $p < 0.05$.

Triglyceride Detection

The cells were planted in 96-well plates with a density of 1×10^4 cells per well. After 24 h of incubation, the cell suspension was extracted, and TG was detected according to the instructions in the intracellular TG kit (A110-1, Jiancheng, Nanjing, China).

Oil Red O Staining

The cells were cultured in a 12-well plate with a cell density of 2×10^5 cells per well. After the cells were cultured for 24 h, the culture medium in the 12-well plate was discarded. The cells were washed twice with PBS and fixed with 4% paraformaldehyde for 30 min. The fixatives were removed in the 12-well plate and cells were washed twice with PBS. Oil Red O staining solution (G1262, Solarbio, Beijing, China) was added to the 12-well plate and incubate for 30 min. The cells were washed with 60% isopropanol and stained with hematoxylin for 30 s. Finally, the cells were rinsed three times with distilled water.

Statistical Analysis

All experimental data were analyzed using GraphPad Prism version 8.0, and all data are presented as the means ± SEM. One-way analysis of variance assessment with Tukey's test and Bonferroni's post hoc test was used to statistically analyze differences among groups. $p < 0.05$ was considered significant.

RESULTS

Kaempferol Significantly Reduced the Expression of Liver X Receptors α and Lysophosphatidylcholine Acyltransferase 3 in High-Fat Diet-Induced Non-Alcoholic Steatohepatitis Mouse Model

In order to study whether KP played a role in the LXRα-LPCAT3-ERS pathway, the mRNA and protein expression of LXRα and LPCAT3 levels in liver in the NASH mice model were first studied. Compared with group NC, the mRNA expression of LXRα and LPCAT3 in the liver in group HFD were significantly higher ($p < 0.05$ and $p < 0.01$, respectively) (**Figure 1A**). Compared with the HFD group, the expression of LXRα and LPCAT3 mRNA in the group HFD + KP was drastically

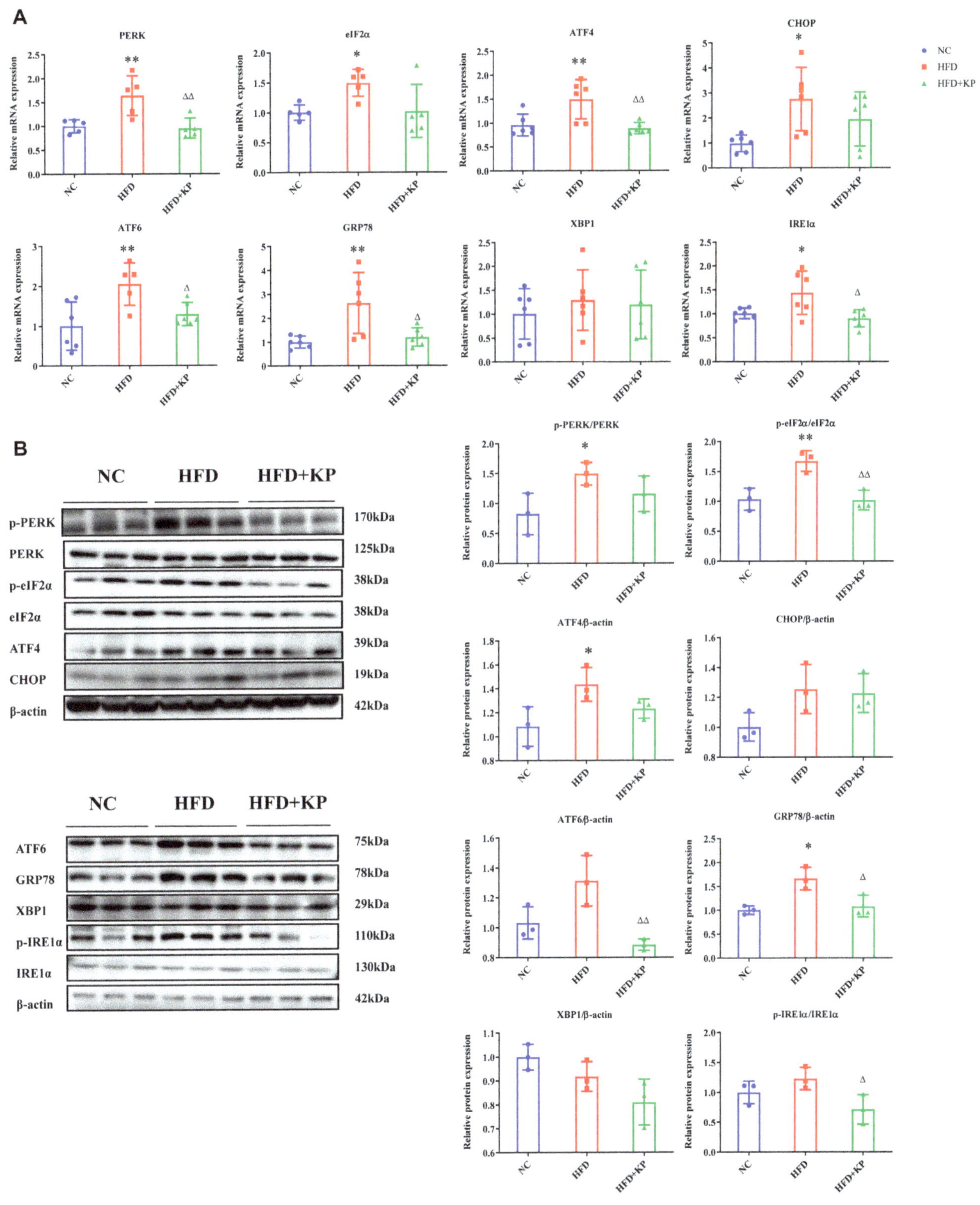

FIGURE 2 | KP regulated the mRNA and protein expression of factors related to ERS *in vivo*. **(A)**: mRNA expression in liver samples; **(B)**: protein expression in liver samples. NC: Normal control group, HFD: HFD group, HFD + KP: HFD + KP group. For **(A,B)**, Quantification of mRNA and protein level expression was normalized to β-actin levels, except protein phosphorylation level expression of PERK, eIF2α, IRE1α expression was normalized to their prototypes. Compared with group NC, *, $p < 0.05$, **, $p < 0.01$; Compared with group HFD, △, $p < 0.05$, △△, $p < 0.01$.

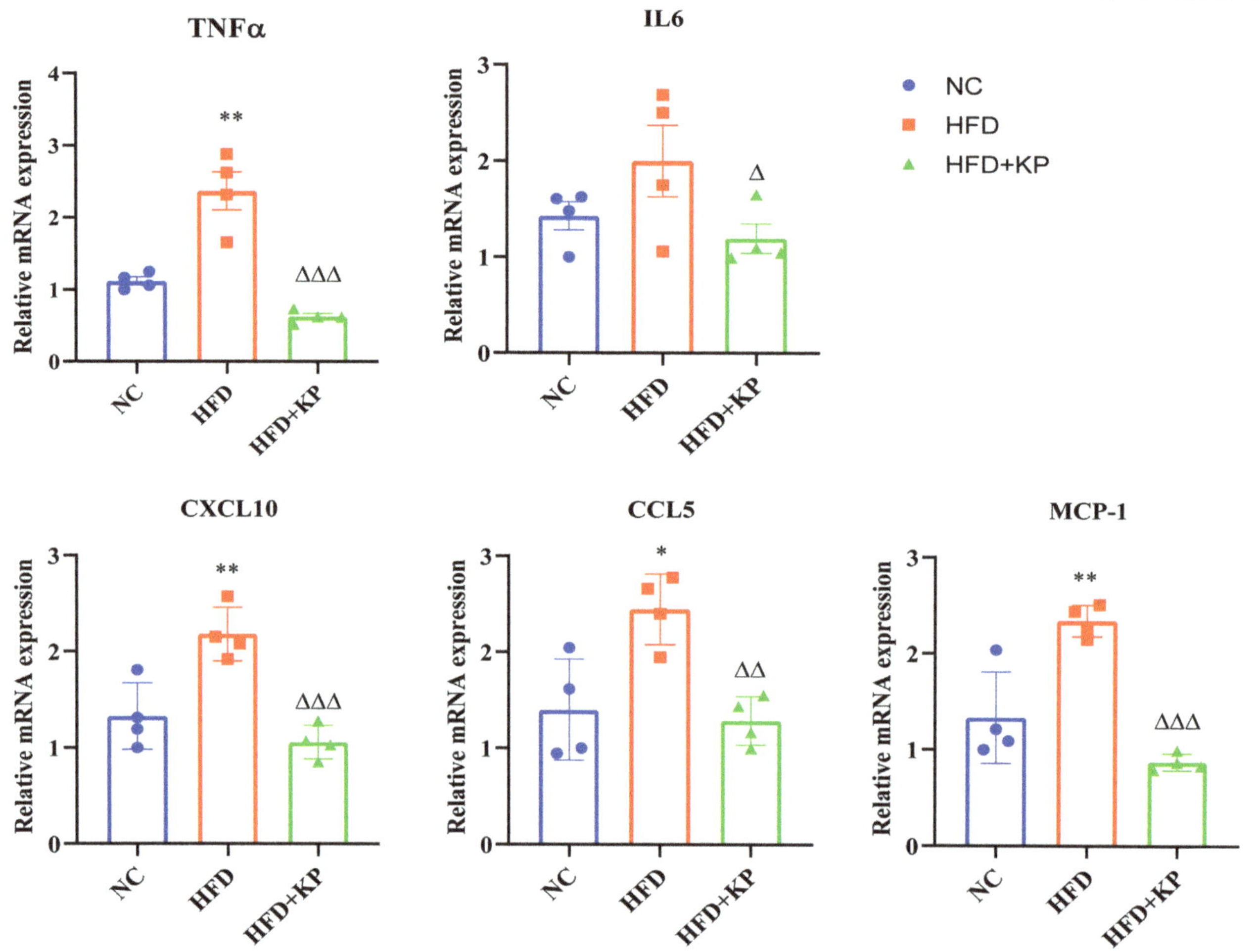

FIGURE 3 | KP reduced the mRNA expression of inflammatory factors *in vivo*. NC: Normal control group, HFD: HFD group, HFD + KP: HFD + KP group. Quantification of mRNA level expression was normalized to β-actin levels. Compared with group NC, *, $p < 0.05$, **, $p < 0.01$; Compared with group HFD, Δ, $p < 0.05$, ΔΔ, $p < 0.01$, ΔΔΔ, $p < 0.001$.

decreased ($p < 0.05$ and $p < 0.05$, respectively) (**Figure 1A**). The similar result was obtained at the protein level. However, though the protein expression of LXRα in group HFD + KP was lower than that in group M, there was no statistical difference (**Figure 1B**).

Kaempferol Regulated the Expression of Factors Related to the Endoplasmic Reticulum Stress Signaling Pathway in High-Fat Diet-Induced Non-Alcoholic Steatohepatitis Mouse Model

Next, we further analyzed the expression of related molecules in the following step involved in ERS. RT-qPCR results showed that the mRNA levels of PERK, eIF2α, ATF4, CHOP, ATF6, GRP78 and IRE1α in the liver in the HFD group were significantly increased than thoses in NC group. After KP intervention, the mRNA expressions of PERK, ATF4, ATF6, GRP78 and IRE1α were significantly reduced. However, there was no statistically significance of the mRNA levels of eIF2α, CHOP and XBP1 (**Figure 2A**).

At the protein level, compared with the NC group, the phosphorylation levels of PERK and eIF2α in the liver in the HFD group have been extensively multiplied ($p < 0.05$ and $p < 0.01$, respectively), and the protein expression of ATF4 and GRP78 also elevated notably ($p < 0.05$). However, the protein expression of ATF6, XBP1 and IRE1α in group HFD did not change appreciably compared with group NC. After KP intervention, the phosphorylation levels of eIF2α and IRE1α were significantly reduced, and the protein expression levels of eIF2α, ATF6 and GRP78 were also significantly reduced. The differences between PERK, ATF4, CHOP and XBP1 expression among groups were not statistically significant (**Figure 2B**). Collectively, these results indicate that KP can protect liver from ERS damage induced by HFD.

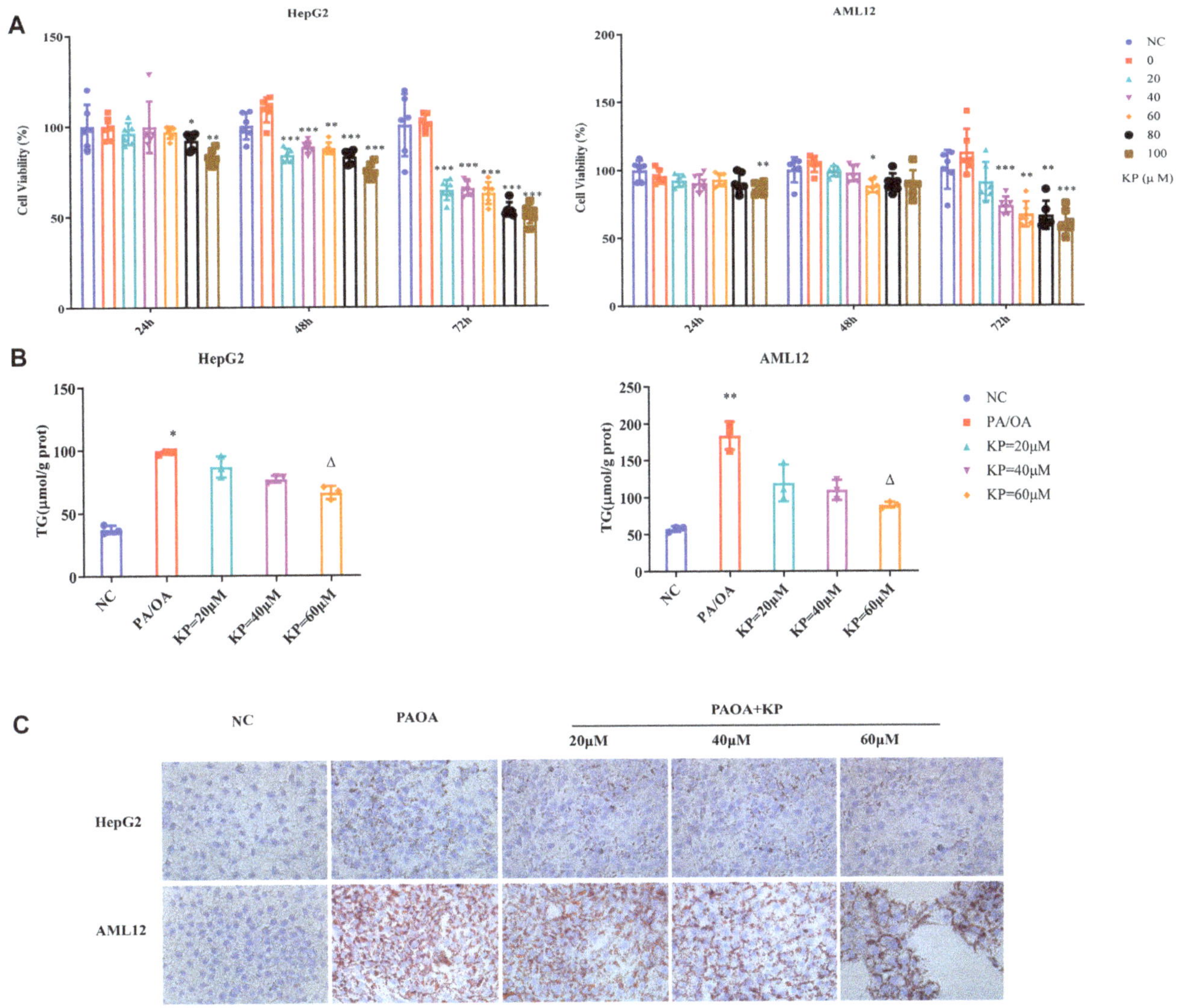

FIGURE 4 | KP reduced the deposition of lipid droplets in cells induced by PA/OA. **(A)**: The survival rate of HepG2 and AML12 cells after the intervention of KP in different concentration and time; **(B)**: The change of TG content after different concentration of KP in HepG2 and AML12 cells interfered with PA/OA (0.375/0.75 mM); **(C)**: The oil red O staining in HepG2 and AML12 cells interfered with PA/OA (0.375/0.75 mM) and/or KP with different concentrations (× 400). NC: Normal control group, PA/OA: PA/OA group, KP = 20 μM: KP low concentration group, KP = 40 μM: KP medium concentration group, KP = 60 μM: KP high concentration group. Compared with group NC, *, $p < 0.05$, **, $p < 0.01$, ***, $p < 0.001$; Compared with group PA/OA, Δ, $p < 0.05$.

Kaempferol Reduced the mRNA Expression of Inflammatory Factors in the High-Fat Diet-Induced Non-Alcoholic Steatohepatitis Mouse Model

In order to find out whether KP can improve the state of NASH, qRT-PCR was used to detect the mRNA expression of inflammation-related factors in liver tissues. Compared with the NC group, the expressions of tumor necrosis factor α (TNFα), C-X-C motif chemokine 10 (CXCL10), C-C chemokine ligand 5 (CCL5) and monocyte chemoattractant protein-1 (MCP-1) mRNA in the HFD group increased, and interleukin 6 (IL6) had a rising trend, but there was no statistical difference. After KP treatment, the mRNA expression levels of TNF-α, IL6, CXCL10, CCL5 and MCP-1 in the HFD + KP group were significantly reduced (**Figure 3**).

Kaempferol Reduced the Deposition of Lipid Droplets in Cells Induced by Palmitic Acid/Oleic Acid

In order to verify the efficacy of KP on NASH, we further established an *in vitro* steatosis model. First of all, the best simulation condition of PA/OA and the best intervention condition of KP in cells were selected. PA/OA was used to establish the model in HepG2 and AML12 cells. The three test results of CCK8 cell viability detection, oil red O staining method and cell TG content were comprehensively analyzed. We found

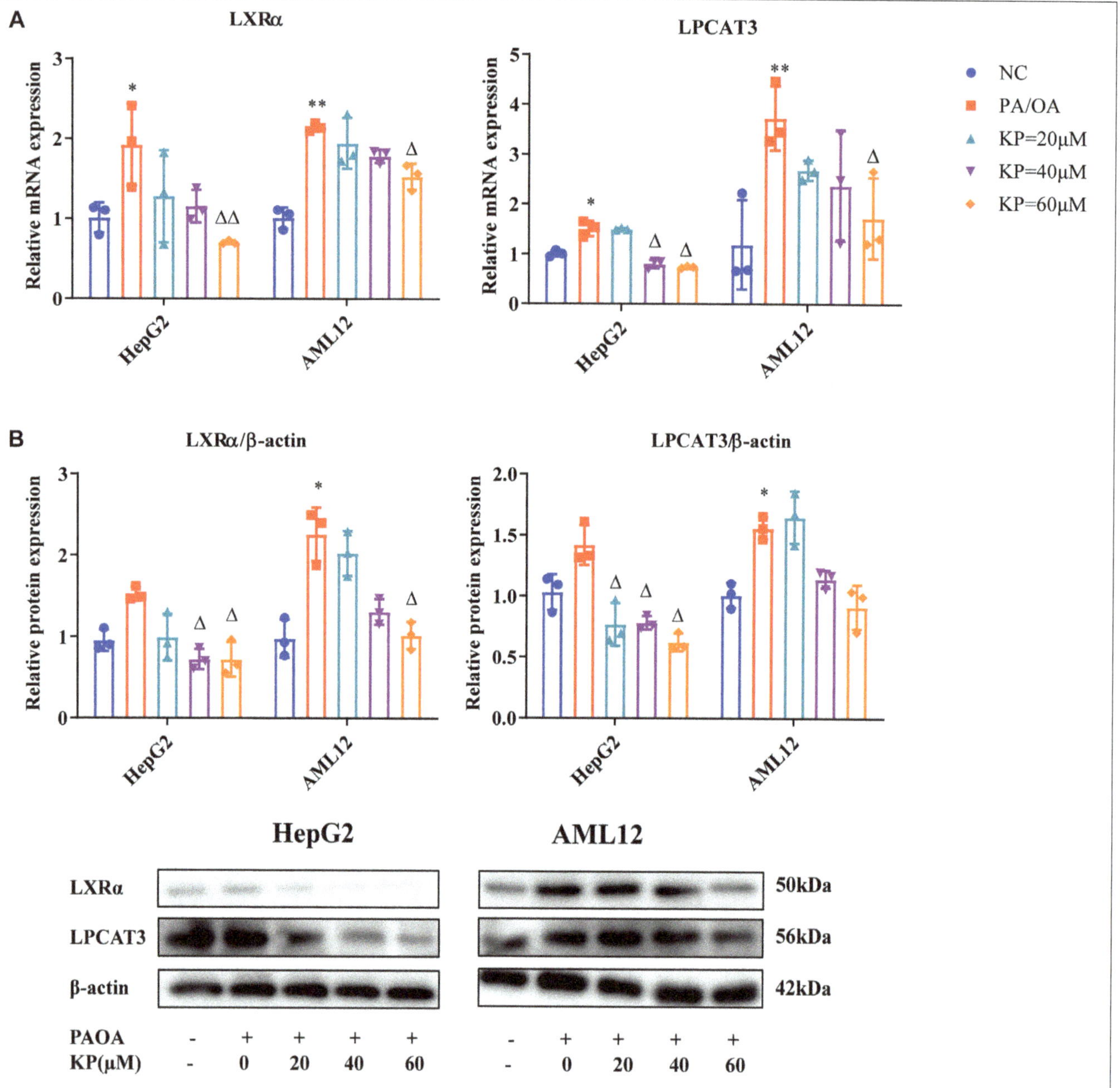

FIGURE 5 | KP regulated the mRNA and protein expression of LXRα and LPCAT3 *in vitro*. **(A)**: mRNA level expression of LXRα and LPCAT3 in HepG2 and AML12 cells; **(B)**: Protein level expression of LXRα and LPCAT3 in HepG2 and AML12 cells. NC: Normal control group, PA/OA: PA/OA group, KP = 20 μM: KP low concentration group, KP = 40 μM: KP medium concentration group, KP = 60 μM: KP high concentration group. Quantification of mRNA and protein level expression was normalized to β-actin levels. Compared with group NC, *, $p < 0.05$, **, $p < 0.01$; Compared with group PA/OA, Δ, $p < 0.05$, ΔΔ, $p < 0.01$.

that when the PA/OA concentration was 0.375/0.75 mM, the activity of HepG2 and AML12 cells was not significantly affected. At the same time, a large number of intracellular lipid droplets were formed, and the intracellular TG content was significantly higher than that of the normal control group (**Supplementary Figure S2**). Therefore, 0.375/0.75 mM PA/OA was selected as the best concentration for modeling. To evaluate the effect of KP on cell viability, KP at concentrations of 0, 20, 40, 60, 80, and 100 μM were added to HepG2 and AML12 cells, and then were cultured for 24, 48, and 72 h, respectively. It was finally found that when the concentration was not higher than 60 μM and within a 24 h time, KP was safe and non-toxic to HepG2 and AML12 cells. Therefore, this concentration range and time were selected as the intervention conditions for subsequent KP intervention experiments (**Figure 4A**).

Based on the above conditions, it was divided into normal control group (NC), PA/OA group (PA/OA 0.375/0.75 mM), KP low-dose group (PA/OA 0.375/0.75 mM + KP 20 μM), KP medium dose group (PA/OA 0.375/0.75 mM + KP 40 μM), KP high-dose group (PA/OA 0.375/0.75 mM + KP 60 μM) *in vitro*. In

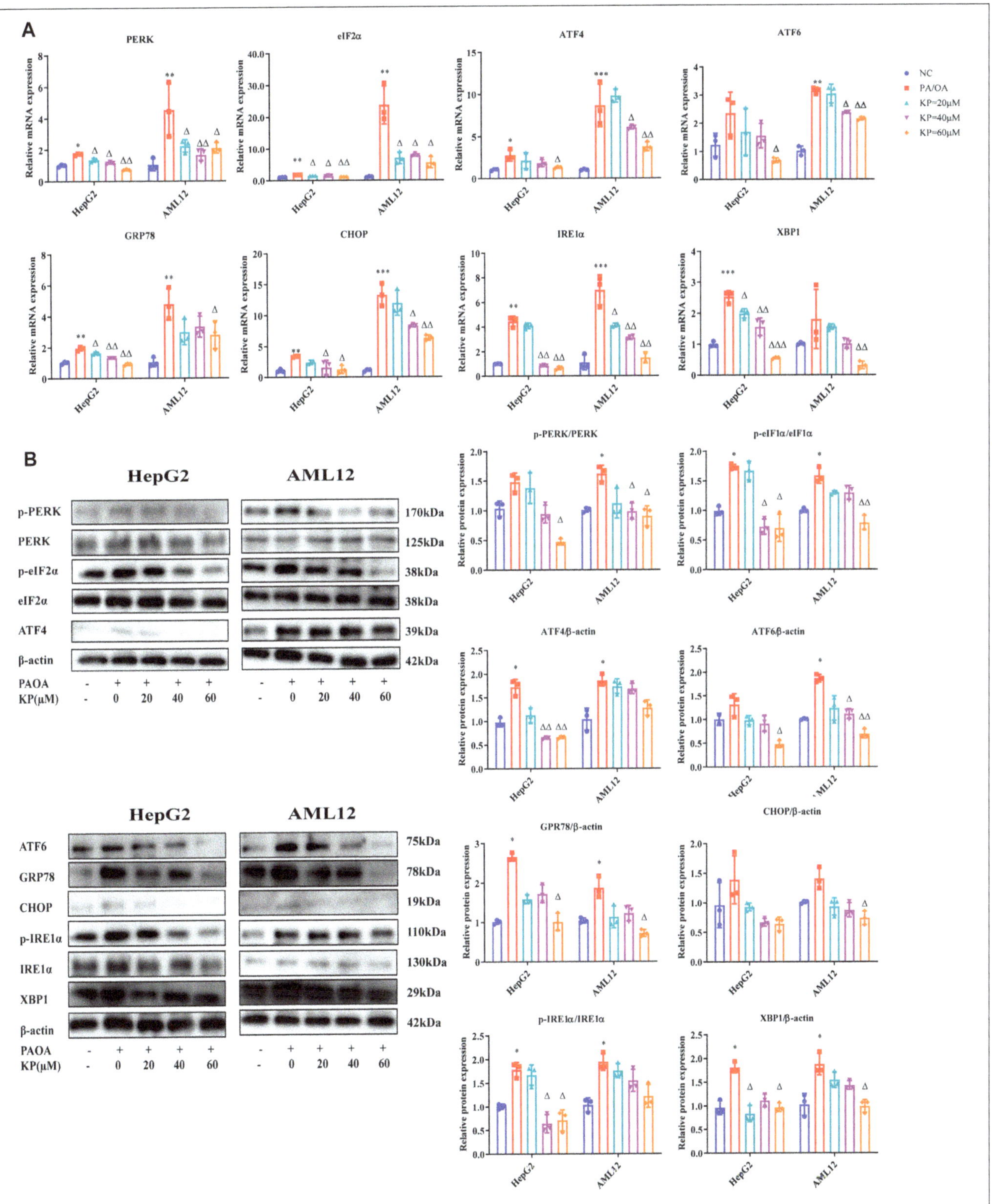

FIGURE 6 | KP regulated the mRNA and protein expression of factors related to ERS *in vitro*. **(A)**: mRNA Expression in HepG2 and AML12 cells; **(B)**: protein Expression in HepG2 and AML12 cells. NC: Normal control group, PA/OA: PA/OA group, KP = 20 μM: KP low concentration group, KP = 40 μM: KP medium concentration group, KP = 60 μM: KP high concentration group. Quantification of mRNA and protein level expression was normalized to β-actin levels, except protein phosphorylation level expression of PERK, eIF2α, IRE1α expression was normalized to their prototypes. Compared with group NC, *, $p < 0.05$, **, $p < 0.01$, ***, $p < 0.001$; Compared with group PA/OA, Δ, $p < 0.05$, ΔΔ, $p < 0.01$.

different dose groups of KP, PA/OA and KP were added to the medium at the same time and cultured for 24 h. The results confirmed that, in contrast with group NC, TG content in HepG2 cells and AML12 cells in group PA/OA were significantly increased ($p < 0.05$ and $p < 0.01$, respectively). After treatment with KP at three concentrations of 20, 40 and 60 μM, the TG content of HepG2 and AML12 cells decreased, and the concentration decreased notably at 60 μM ($p < 0.05$) (**Figure 4B**). Oil red O staining showed that the deposition of lipid droplets in HepG2 and AML12 cells in the PA/OA group increased compared with that in the NC group, and KP significantly reduced lipid deposition in both cells (**Figure 4C**).

Kaempferol Reduced the Expression of Liver X Receptors α and Lysophosphatidylcholine Acyltransferase 3 in Palmitic Acid/Oleic Acid-Induced Steatosis Model Cells

It has been validated that KP can reduce the expression of LXRα and LPCAT3 in liver tissue, and an *in vitro* model has been used to further verify this result.

The mRNA levels of LXRα and LPCAT3 in the PA/OA group were substantially up-regulated in both HepG2 and AML12 cells induced by PA/OA. After KP intervention, the mRNA transcription of LXRα and LPCAT3 were significantly down-regulated (**Figure 5A**).

Western blot results showed that the level of LXRα protein increased in the two cells in the PA/OA group, and it was more obvious in AML12 cells ($p < 0.05$). After the intervention of different concentrations of KP, the LXRα protein levels of the two cells were all down-regulated (**Figure 4B**). Compared with group NC, the protein level of LPCAT3 in each cell of group PA/OA was increased, while it was significantly increased in AML12 cells ($p < 0.05$) (**Figure 5B**). The protein level of LPCAT3 in the two cells decreased in a concentration-dependent manner when the KP concentration was 40 and 60 μM. It can be seen from the above results that KP can significantly reduce the expression of LXRα and LPCAT3 in the steatosis model.

Kaempferol Regulated the Expression of Factors Related to the Endoplasmic Reticulum Stress Signaling Pathway in Palmitic Acid/Oleic Acid-Induced Steatosis Model Cells

Subsequently, the mRNA expression and protein expression levels of the ERS-related factors of HepG2 and AML12 cells were detected.

Compared with group NC, the mRNA levels of PERK, eIF2α, ATF4, CHOP, ATF6, GRP78, XBP1 and IRE1α in group PA/OA were increased. The expression of PERK, eIF2α, ATF4, CHOP, ATF6, GRP78, XBP1 and IRE1α mRNA in the KP group were significantly reduced. After KP intervention, the down-regulation of eIF2α, ATF4, XBP1 and IRE1α mRNA in the two types of cells all showed concentration-dependent tolerance, whilst the down-regulation of PERK and CHOP mRNA was only concentration-dependent in HepG2 cells (**Figure 6A**).

The phosphorylation levels of PERK, eIF2α and IRE1α in the PA/OA group were higher than those in the NC group not only in HepG2 but also in AML12 cells, however the adjustments in the phosphorylation level of PERK in HepG2 cells were not statistically significant. The protein expressions of ATF4, CHOP, ATF6, GRP78 and XBP1 in the PA/OA group of the two cells also increased significantly. After the intervention of different concentrations of KP, the protein expression levels of these factors in the two cells were reduced, and the phosphorylation levels of PERK and eIF2α in the high-concentration group of KP decreased more significantly. In the two kinds of cells, the protein levels of ATF6, ATF4, CHOP, GRP78 and XBP1 were significantly reduced in the high concentration group. The phosphorylation level of IRE1α in the KP medium and high concentration groups of HepG2 cells extensively decreased, and the phosphorylation level of IRE1α in the KP intervention groups in AML12 cells showed a downward trend, but it was not obvious (**Figure 6B**).

Kaempferol Reduced the mRNA Expression of Inflammatory Factors in Palmitic Acid/Oleic Acid-Induced Steatosis Model Cells

We also examined the mRNA expression of inflammation-related factors in cells using qRT-PCR.

Compared with the NC group, the mRNA levels of TNFα, IL6, CXCL10, CCL5 and MCP-1 in the PA/OA group increased significantly in the two types of cells. In hepG2 cells, TNF-α, IL6, CCL5 and MCP-1 all showed a decrease in KP concentration dependent tolerance, and CXCL10 only decreased in the middle and high concentration groups of KP. In AML12 cells, the mRNA levels of IL6, CXCL10 and CCL5 were significantly down-regulated after KP intervention. TNFα did not decrease significantly when KP = 20 μM, but mRNA levels decreased significantly at KP = 40 and 60 μM. The expression of MCP-1 showed no obvious downward trend after KP intervention (**Figure 7**).

Kaempferol Regulated Lipid Metabolism Both *in vivo* and *in vitro*

Peroxisome proliferator-activated receptor-α (PPAR-α) belongs to the PPAR subfamily, which is a type of nuclear receptor highly expressed in the liver. PPARα will be activated to enhance the oxidation of fatty acids when fatty acids in the liver are elevated (Pawlak et al., 2015). It was found that when liver PPARα was specifically knocked out, liver steatosis would increase (Montagner et al., 2016a). ATP binding cassette transporter A1 (ABCA1) is a transport protein involved in high-density lipoprotein (HDL) biosynthesis and cellular cholesterol homeostasis. Phospholipids and free cholesterol can be transferred to apolipoprotein A1 by ABCA1, and then form new HDL particles (Phillips, 2018). Previous studies have shown that overexpression of ABCA1 can reduce liver lipid

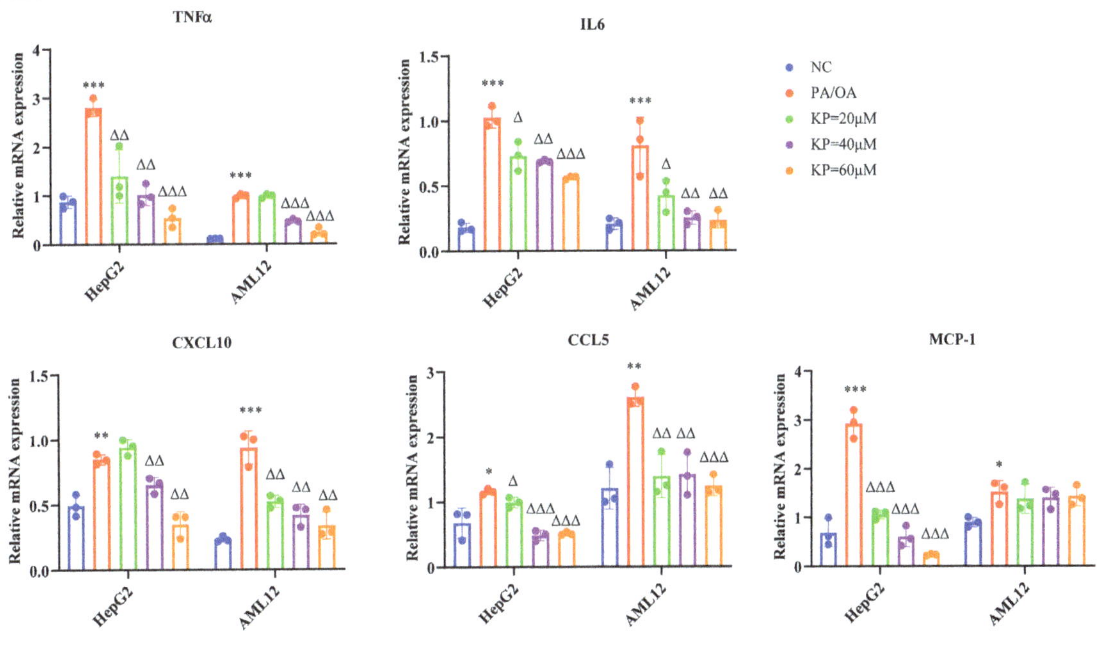

FIGURE 7 | KP reduced the mRNA expression of inflammatory factors *in vitro*. NC: Normal control group, PA/OA: PA/OA group, KP = 20 μM: KP low concentration group, KP = 40 μM: KP medium concentration group, KP = 60 μM: KP high concentration group. Quantification of mRNA expression was normalized to β-actin levels. Compared with group NC, *, $p < 0.05$, **, $p < 0.01$, ***, $p < 0.001$; Compared with group PA/OA, Δ, $p < 0.05$, ΔΔ, $p < 0.01$, ΔΔΔ, $p < 0.001$.

levels (Yang et al., 2010; Liu et al., 2014). In the present study, we found that the mRNA and protein expression of PPAR-α and ABCA1 decreased in the HFD-induced NASH model than the control group, and also in the PA/OA-induced steatosis cell model, while KP could increase their expression both *in vivo* and *in vitro* (**Supplementary Figure S3**). These results suggest that KP plays a role in regulating lipid metabolism.

DISCUSSION

NAFLD, as one of the common diseases affecting human life and health in the world, has attracted more and more attention to researchers (Fan et al., 2017; Younossi et al., 2018). It is expected that the incidence of NAFLD would increase to 314.58 million by 2030 in China. Compared with the number of cases in 2016 (246.33 million cases), the increase was 29.1% (Estes et al., 2018). NASH is a type of NAFLD, and approximately 20% of NASH patients will develop liver cirrhosis. Now, NASH has become the main cause of liver transplantation in American patients (Sheka et al., 2020).

Our former study has shown that KP was effective against improving liver injury in HFD-induced NASH mice model (Lu et al., 2020). In the present study, we further demonstrated that KP can modulate the mRNA or the protein expression of the molecules involved in LXRα-LPCAT3-ERS pathway in both HFD-induced mice model and PA/OA-induced steatosis cell model. To our best knowledge, it is the first time to illustrate the molecular mechanism of KP on improving NASH.

KP is a type of aglycone flavonoids existing in a variety of plants, which has antibacterial, anti-inflammatory, antioxidant, anti-tumor, heart protection, neuroprotective and anti-diabetes effects (Chen and Chen, 2013; Dabeek and Marra, 2019; Imran et al., 2019). In our previous studies, it has been proved that KP can alleviate liver injury in HFD-induced NASH mice model (Lu et al., 2020). In this study, in order to verify the efficacy of KP on NASH, HepG2 and AML12 cell lines were selected to establish an *in vitro* cell model of steatosis using PA/OA. As similiar as the results *in vivo*, the content of TG in the steatosis model group decreased after the intervention of KP (20, 40, and 60 μM), in particular in the high concentration group, suggesting that KP attenuates the TG storage of PA/OA-induced steatosis cell model. From the results of oil red O staining, KP can also substantially decrease lipid deposition in fatty degeneration cells. These data further verified that KP can improve PA/OA induced liver steatosis.

The LXRα-LPCAT3 pathway is an important regulator of PLs metabolism, metabolic stress response and inflammation. Till now, there are different points on the role of LPCAT3 in the lipogenesis. LXR activation promotes the entry of unsaturated fatty acids into PLs through LPCAT3, thereby reducing liver ERS and inflammation (Rong et al., 2013). Patrick et al. (Ferrara et al., 2021) found that mice with skeletal muscle-specific knockout of LPCAT3 (LPCAT3-MKO) exhibited greater muscle lyso-PC/PC, concomitant with improved skeletal muscle insulin sensitivity. Conversely, skeletal muscle-specific overexpression of LPCAT3 (LPCAT3-MKI) promoted glucose intolerance. Thibaut et al. (Bourgeois et al., 2020) found that deletion of

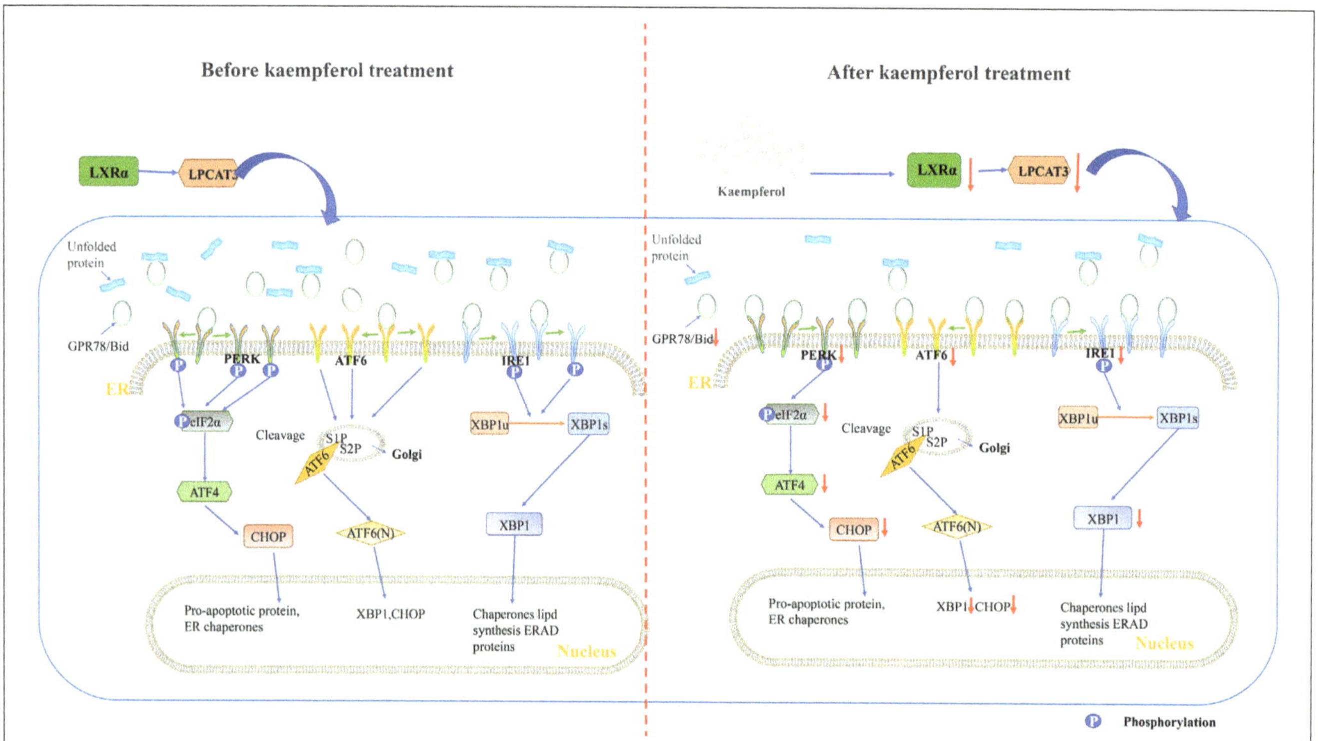

FIGURE 8 | Schematic diagram of the mechanism of KP regulating LXRα-LPCAT3 signaling pathway. KP intervention suppressed endoplasmic reticulum stress. The LXR-LPCAT3-ERS pathway is activated when induced by HFD or PA/OA. This allows unfolded proteins to accumulate in the ER. At the same time, GPR78 dissociates from PERK, IRE1, and ATF6, and then binds to the unfolded protein. The dissociated PERK, IRE1 and ATF6 were activated. CHOP-induced apoptosis occurs when PERK, IRE1, ATF6 and their downstream pathways are continuously activated. The expression of LXR and LPCAT3 decreased significantly when treated with KP, and then the unfolded protein decreased, PERK, IRE1 and ATF6 dissociated from GRP78 decreased. Abbreviations: HFD: high fat diet, PA/OA: Palmitic acid/Oleic acid, LPCAT3: lysophosphatidylcholine acyltransferase 3, LXR α: liver X receptor alpha, PERK: protein kinase R-like ER kinase, Eif-2α: eukaryotic translation initiation factor 2α, ATF6: activating transcription factor 6, IRE1: inositol-requiring enzyme 1, XBP1: X-box-binding protein 1, ATF4: activating transcription factor 4, CHOP: C/EBP homologous protein, ERAD: Endoplasmic reticulum-associated degradation.

LPCAT3 in myeloid cells worsened hepatic steatosis after a high-fat diet. Recent study has shown that LPCAT3 is a direct PPAR-δ target gene and has a novel function of PPAR-δ in regulation of phospholipid metabolism through LPCAT3 (Singh and Liu, 2017a).

In this study, after the intervention of KP, the mRNA levels and protein expression levels of LXR and LPCAT3 were decreased in the liver tissues of the NASH mice model. Our studies supported that LPCAT3 was highly expressed in NASH model by the involvement of lipogenesis. The above studies support that KP can improve lipid accumulation through LXR-LPCAT3.

Wang et al. (2013) showed that LPCAT3 regulated the formation of ERS and inflammation. ERS is considered to be one of the necessary mechanisms that purpose liver steatosis and inflammatory changes (Rong et al., 2013). After ERS stimulation, the PERK/elF2α, ATF6 and IRE1/XBP-1 signal pathways are activated, and the mRNA and protein expression of PERK, elF2α, ATF4, ATF6, IRE1α and GRP78 are considerably increased, which induces CHOP expression and promotes cell apoptosis (Wang and Kaufman, 2016). ERS will dissociate PERK from GPR78/bid, and then the downstream elF2α will be phosphorylated (Donnelly et al., 2013). Phosphorylated elF2α reduced the general translation rate, but activated the downstream translation of ATF4 and CHOP (Malhi and Kaufman, 2011; Luhr et al., 2019). The expression of the anti-apoptotic gene BCL-2 can be inhibited by CHOP, thereby accelerating cell death (Marciniak et al., 2004). ATF6 will transfer to the Golgi apparatus when it is activated. It becomes ATF6 (n) after being cleaved in the Golgi apparatus and regulates ERS together with XBP1s (Walter et al., 2018). The misfolded protein phosphorylates IRE1α and induces conformational changes in the RNase domain (Ghosh et al., 2014). Next, XBP1 is cut into XBP1s, which initiates the UPR gene expression program in response to ERS (Yoshida et al., 2001; Huang et al., 2019).

In our study, KP was used to interfere with NASH mouse model and PA/OA-induced steatosis model cells. It was found that after KP intervention, the expression of factors related to ERS decreased significantly from both mice and cells. First, the levels of PERK, eIF2α, ATF4 and CHOP in the PERK pathway were significantly decreased. Second, the expression of ATF6 in the ATF6 pathway also decreased. Third, the expression of IRE1α and XBP1 in the IRE1α pathway was also significantly inhibited. In addition, the expression of GPR78 was also suppressed, possibly because the dissociation of GPR78 from PERK, ATF6 and IRE1α became less. We concluded that KP regulates ERS status by reducing the expression of LXR-LPACT3, thereby improving lipid degeneration (**Figure 8**).

Cytokines are the main mediators required for the comprehensive response to various stimuli in the immune and inflammatory process. It includes interleukin, tumor necrosis factor, chemokine family, etc. These factors are key regulators that initiate and drive inflammatory diseases (Borish and Steinke, 2003). TNFα and IL6 are up-regulated in many inflammatory diseases, such as rheumatoid arthritis (van Schouwenburg et al., 2013; Pandolfi et al., 2020), inflammatory lung diseases (Malaviya et al., 2017) and tumors (Balkwill, 2006; Jones and Jenkins, 2018). Malaviya et al. (2017) showed that TNFα antagonists showed a good effect on inflammatory lung disease. Nakagawa et al. (2014) found that inflammatory macrophages activated by ERS promote the release of inflammatory mediators such as TNFα and IL6. In the liver, CCL5 and CXCL10 can regulate the cytopathic and antiviral immune response of T cells and natural killer cells. MCP-1 can promote the accumulation of macrophages, steatosis and inflammation (Marra and Tacke, 2014). Fan et al. (2020) found that CXCL10 promoted the recruitment of natural killer cells to the liver in the NASH model induced by the methionine-and choline-deficient diet (MCD). CCL5 was significantly up-regulated in HFD-induced liver fibrosis model (Li B.-H. et al., 2017). Baeck et al. (2012) found that blocking MCP-1 can reduced macrophage infiltration and reduced the release of pro-inflammatory factors TNFα, interferon g and IL6. Our results showed that KP can regulate the release of inflammatory factors in the NASH mouse model and cell model by improving ERS, and ultimately reduce liver inflammation.

However, there are still several limitations in the present study. For example, LPCAT3 gene knockout animal models or siRNA interference techniques have not been used to further confirm the role of LPCAT3 in the mechanism of KP on improving NASH. Primary cells have not been used to build cell models. In a bioinformatics analysis study on NAFLD, it is mentioned that the occurrence of NAFLD is also related to insulin signaling pathway, PPAR signaling pathway, p53 signaling pathway and mitogen-activated protein kinase (MAPK) signaling pathway (Liu et al., 2020). The study found that giving p53 knockout mice a high-fat diet reduced the occurrence of NAFLD. Moreover, knocking out P53 in the cell also reduced the accumulation of lipids in the cell (Zhang et al., 2020). Tomita et al. (2012) showed that the expression of p53 and p66Shc was up-regulated in the liver tissue of the NASH mouse model. Montagner et al. (2016a) found that lack of PPARα in hepatocytes leads to susceptibility to steatosis, which may be related to the damage of fatty acid catabolism. Inhibition of MAPK signaling pathway also showed the effect of reducing liver lipid deposition and liver fibrosis in rats (Shen et al., 2019). It has been discovered that KP intervention affects the expression of PPARα and ABCA1, but the specific mechanism is still unclear. The role of the above pathways in the occurrence of NAFLD and NASH, and whether KP also plays a therapeutic role through these pathways will be the direction of our further research.

CONCLUSION

In summary, this study has confirmed that KP can improve liver damage by regulating LXRα-LPCAT3 and inhibiting ERS from both *in vivo* and *in vitro*. At the same time, the expression of inflammatory factors is reduced. The role of KP provides a new direction for the treatment of NASH. LPCAT3 can also be used as a potential target for NASH treatment.

ETHICS STATEMENT

The animal study was reviewed and approved by the Shanghai University of Traditional Chinese Medicine. Written informed consent was obtained from the owners for the participation of their animals in this study.

AUTHOR CONTRIBUTIONS

TW and GJ, study design and conceptualization; HX, MS, and YL, Animal feeding and sample collection; HX, YL, and JW, data analysis; HX, MS, and TW, drafting the manuscript; TW and GJ, revising the manuscript and obtaining the funding. All authors have approved the final draft submitted.

REFERENCES

Ashrafizadeh, M., Tavakol, S., Ahmadi, Z., Roomiani, S., Mohammadinejad, R., and Samarghandian, S. (2020). Therapeutic Effects of Kaempferol Affecting Autophagy and Endoplasmic Reticulum Stress. *Phytother Res.* 34, 911–923. doi:10.1002/ptr.6577

Baeck, C., Wehr, A., Karlmark, K. R., Heymann, F., Vucur, M., Gassler, N., et al. (2012). Pharmacological Inhibition of the Chemokine CCL2 (MCP-1) Diminishes Liver Macrophage Infiltration and Steatohepatitis in Chronic Hepatic Injury. *Gut* 61, 416–426. doi:10.1136/gutjnl-2011-300304

Balkwill, F. (2006). TNF-alpha in Promotion and Progression of Cancer. *Cancer Metastasis Rev.* 25, 409–416. doi:10.1007/s10555-006-9005-3

Borish, L. C., and Steinke, J. W. (2003). 2. Cytokines and Chemokines. *J. Allergy Clin. Immunol.* 111, S460–S475. doi:10.1067/mai.2003.108

Bourgeois, T., Jalil, A., Thomas, C., Magnani, C., Le Guern, N., Gautier, T., et al. (2020). Deletion of Lysophosphatidylcholine Acyltransferase 3 in Myeloid Cells Worsens Hepatic Steatosis after a High-Fat Diet. *J. Lipid Res.* 62, 100013. doi:10.1194/jlr.RA120000737

Brenner, C., Galluzzi, L., Kepp, O., and Kroemer, G. (2013). Decoding Cell Death Signals in Liver Inflammation. *J. Hepatol.* 59, 583–594. doi:10.1016/j.jhep.2013.03.033

Chaudhari, N., Talwar, P., Parimisetty, A., Lefebvre D'hellencourt, C., and Ravanan, P. (2014). A Molecular Web: Endoplasmic Reticulum Stress, Inflammation, and Oxidative Stress. *Front Cel Neurosci* 8, 213. doi:10.3389/fncel.2014.00213

Chen, A. Y., and Chen, Y. C. (2013). A Review of the Dietary Flavonoid, Kaempferol on Human Health and Cancer Chemoprevention. *Food Chem.* 138, 2099–2107. doi:10.1016/j.foodchem.2012.11.139

Dabeek, W. M., and Marra, M. V. (2019). Dietary Quercetin and Kaempferol: Bioavailability and Potential Cardiovascular-Related Bioactivity in Humans. *Nutrients* 11. doi:10.3390/nu11102288

Dasgupta, D., Nakao, Y., Mauer, A. S., Thompson, J. M., Sehrawat, T. S., Liao, C. Y., et al. (2020). IRE1A Stimulates Hepatocyte-Derived Extracellular Vesicles that Promote Inflammation in Mice with Steatohepatitis. *Gastroenterology* 159, 1487–e17. doi:10.1053/j.gastro.2020.06.031

Demeure, O., Lecerf, F., Duby, C., Desert, C., Ducheix, S., Guillou, H., et al. (2011). Regulation of LPCAT3 by LXR. *Gene* 470, 7–11. doi:10.1016/j.gene.2010.09.002

Demirtas, L., Guclu, A., Erdur, F. M., Akbas, E. M., Ozcicek, A., Onk, D., et al. (2016). Apoptosis, Autophagy & Endoplasmic Reticulum Stress in Diabetes Mellitus. *Indian J. Med. Res.* 144, 515–524. doi:10.4103/0971-5916.200887

Donnelly, N., Gorman, A. M., Gupta, S., and Samali, A. (2013). The eIF2α Kinases: Their Structures and Functions. *Cell Mol Life Sci* 70, 3493–3511. doi:10.1007/s00018-012-1252-6

Estes, C., Anstee, Q. M., Arias-Loste, M. T., Bantel, H., Bellentani, S., Caballeria, J., et al. (2018). Modeling NAFLD Disease burden in China, France, Germany, Italy, Japan, Spain, United Kingdom, and United States for the Period 2016-2030. *J. Hepatol.* 69, 896–904. doi:10.1016/j.jhep.2018.05.036

Fan, J. G., Kim, S. U., and Wong, V. W. (2017). New Trends on Obesity and NAFLD in Asia. *J. Hepatol.* 67, 862–873. doi:10.1016/j.jhep.2017.06.003

Fan, Y., Zhang, W., Wei, H., Sun, R., Tian, Z., and Chen, Y. (2020). Hepatic NK Cells Attenuate Fibrosis Progression of Non-alcoholic Steatohepatitis in Dependent of CXCL10-mediated Recruitment. *Liver Int.* 40, 598–608. doi:10.1111/liv.14307

Ferrara, P. J., Rong, X., Maschek, J. A., Verkerke, A. R., Siripoksup, P., Song, H., et al. (2021). Lysophospholipid Acylation Modulates Plasma Membrane Lipid Organization and Insulin Sensitivity in Skeletal Muscle. *J. Clin. Invest.* 131, 135963. doi:10.1172/JCI135963

Friedman, S. L., Neuschwander-Tetri, B. A., Rinella, M., and Sanyal, A. J. (2018). Mechanisms of NAFLD Development and Therapeutic Strategies. *Nat. Med.* 24, 908–922. doi:10.1038/s41591-018-0104-9

Ghosh, R., Wang, L., Wang, E. S., Perera, B. G., Igbaria, A., Morita, S., et al. (2014). Allosteric Inhibition of the IRE1α RNase Preserves Cell Viability and Function during Endoplasmic Reticulum Stress. *Cell* 158, 534–548. doi:10.1016/j.cell.2014.07.002

Hernández-Alvarez, M. I., Sebastián, D., Vives, S., Ivanova, S., Bartoccioni, P., Kakimoto, P., et al. (2019). Deficient Endoplasmic Reticulum-Mitochondrial Phosphatidylserine Transfer Causes Liver Disease. *Cell* 177, 881–e17. doi:10.1016/j.cell.2019.04.010

Hu, H., Tian, M., Ding, C., and Yu, S. (2018). The C/EBP Homologous Protein (CHOP) Transcription Factor Functions in Endoplasmic Reticulum Stress-Induced Apoptosis and Microbial Infection. *Front. Immunol.* 9, 3083. doi:10.3389/fimmu.2018.03083

Huang, S., Xing, Y., and Liu, Y. (2019). Emerging Roles for the ER Stress Sensor IRE1α in Metabolic Regulation and Disease. *J. Biol. Chem.* 294, 18726–18741. doi:10.1074/jbc.REV119.007036

Imran, M., Salehi, B., Sharifi-Rad, J., Aslam Gondal, T., Saeed, F., Imran, A., et al. (2019). Kaempferol: A Key Emphasis to its Anticancer Potential. *Molecules* 24. doi:10.3390/molecules24122277

Iurlaro, R., and Muñoz-Pinedo, C. (2016). Cell Death Induced by Endoplasmic Reticulum Stress. *FEBS J.* 283, 2640–2652. doi:10.1111/febs.13598

Jones, S. A., and Jenkins, B. J. (2018). Recent Insights into Targeting the IL-6 Cytokine Family in Inflammatory Diseases and Cancer. *Nat. Rev. Immunol.* 18, 773–789. doi:10.1038/s41577-018-0066-7

Kouhestani, S., Jafari, A., and Babaei, P. (2018). Kaempferol Attenuates Cognitive Deficit via Regulating Oxidative Stress and Neuroinflammation in an Ovariectomized Rat Model of Sporadic Dementia. *Neural Regen. Res.* 13, 1827–1832. doi:10.4103/1673-5374.238714

Lebeaupin, C., Vallée, D., Rousseau, D., Patouraux, S., Bonnafous, S., Adam, G., et al. (2018). Bax Inhibitor-1 Protects from Nonalcoholic Steatohepatitis by Limiting Inositol-Requiring Enzyme 1 Alpha Signaling in Mice. *Hepatology* 68, 515–532. doi:10.1002/hep.29847

Lee, B., Kwon, M., Choi, J. S., Jeong, H. O., Chung, H. Y., and Kim, H. R. (2015a). Kaempferol Isolated from *Nelumbo nucifera* Inhibits Lipid Accumulation and Increases Fatty Acid Oxidation Signaling in Adipocytes. *J. Med. Food* 18, 1363–1370. doi:10.1089/jmf.2015.3457

Lee, Y.-J., Choi, H.-S., Seo, M.-J., Jeon, H.-J., Kim, K.-J., and Lee, B.-Y. (2015b). Kaempferol Suppresses Lipid Accumulation by Inhibiting Early Adipogenesis in 3T3-L1 Cells and Zebrafish. *Food Funct.* 6, 2824–2833. doi:10.1039/c5fo00481k

Li, B.-H., He, F.-P., Yang, X., Chen, Y.-W., and Fan, J.-G. (2017a). Steatosis Induced CCL5 Contributes to Early-Stage Liver Fibrosis in Nonalcoholic Fatty Liver Disease Progress. *Translational Res. : J. Lab. Clin. Med.* 180. doi:10.1016/j.trsl.2016.08.006

Li, F., Yang, Y., Yang, L., Wang, K., Zhang, X., Zong, Y., et al. (2017b). Resveratrol Alleviates FFA and CCl4 Induced Apoptosis in HepG2 Cells via Restoring Endoplasmic Reticulum Stress. *Oncotarget* 8, 43799–43809. doi:10.18632/oncotarget.16460

Li, S., and Pu, X.-P. (2011). Neuroprotective Effect of Kaempferol against a 1-Methyl-4-Phenyl-1,2,3,6-Tetrahydropyridine-Induced Mouse Model of Parkinson's Disease. *Biol. Pharm. Bull.* 34, 1291–1296. doi:10.1248/bpb.34.1291

Liu, J., Lin, B., Chen, Z., Deng, M., Wang, Y., Wang, J., et al. (2020). Identification of Key Pathways and Genes in Nonalcoholic Fatty Liver Disease Using Bioinformatics Analysis. *Arch. Med. Sci.* 16, 374–385. doi:10.5114/aoms.2020.93343

Liu, W., Qin, L., Yu, H., Lv, F., and Wang, Y. (2014). Apolipoprotein A-I and Adenosine Triphosphate-Binding Cassette Transporter A1 Expression Alleviates Lipid Accumulation in Hepatocytes. *J. Gastroenterol. Hepatol.* 29, 614–622. doi:10.1111/jgh.12430

Lu, Y., Shao, M., Xiang, H., Zheng, P., Wu, T., and Ji, G. (2020). Integrative Transcriptomics and Metabolomics Explore the Mechanism of Kaempferol on Improving Nonalcoholic Steatohepatitis. *Food Funct.* 11, 10058–10069. doi:10.1039/d0fo02123g

Luhr, M., Torgersen, M. L., Szalai, P., Hashim, A., Brech, A., Staerk, J., et al. (2019). The Kinase PERK and the Transcription Factor ATF4 Play Distinct and Essential Roles in Autophagy Resulting from Tunicamycin-Induced ER Stress. *J. Biol. Chem.* 294, 8197–8217. doi:10.1074/jbc.RA118.002829

Malaviya, R., Laskin, J. D., and Laskin, D. L. (2017). Anti-Tnfα Therapy in Inflammatory Lung Diseases. *Pharmacol. Ther.* 180, 90–98. doi:10.1016/j.pharmthera.2017.06.008

Malhi, H., and Kaufman, R. J. (2011). Endoplasmic Reticulum Stress in Liver Disease. *J. Hepatol.* 54, 795–809. doi:10.1016/j.jhep.2010.11.005

Marciniak, S. J., Yun, C. Y., Oyadomari, S., Novoa, I., Zhang, Y., Jungreis, R., et al. (2004). CHOP Induces Death by Promoting Protein Synthesis and Oxidation in the Stressed Endoplasmic Reticulum. *Genes Dev.* 18, 3066–3077. doi:10.1101/gad.1250704

Marra, F., and Tacke, F. (2014). Roles for Chemokines in Liver Disease. *Gastroenterology* 147, 577–e1. doi:10.1053/j.gastro.2014.06.043

Montagner, A., Polizzi, A., Fouché, E., Ducheix, S., Lippi, Y., Lasserre, F., et al. (2016a). Liver PPARα Is Crucial for Whole-Body Fatty Acid Homeostasis and Is Protective against NAFLD. *Gut* 65, 1202–1214. doi:10.1136/gutjnl-2015-310798

Nakagawa, H., Umemura, A., Taniguchi, K., Font-Burgada, J., Dhar, D., Ogata, H., et al. (2014). ER Stress Cooperates with Hypernutrition to Trigger TNF-dependent Spontaneous HCC Development. *Cancer cell* 26, 331–343. doi:10.1016/j.ccr.2014.07.001

Nobili, V., Alisi, A., Valenti, L., Miele, L., Feldstein, A. E., and Alkhouri, N. (2019). NAFLD in Children: New Genes, New Diagnostic Modalities and New Drugs. *Nat. Rev. Gastroenterol. Hepatol.* 16, 517–530. doi:10.1038/s41575-019-0169-z

Ozcan, L., and Tabas, I. (2012). Role of Endoplasmic Reticulum Stress in Metabolic Disease and Other Disorders. *Annu. Rev. Med.* 63, 317–328. doi:10.1146/annurev-med-043010-144749

Pandolfi, F., Franza, L., Carusi, V., Altamura, S., Andriollo, G., and Nucera, E. (2020). Interleukin-6 in Rheumatoid Arthritis. *Int. J. Mol. Sci.* 21. doi:10.3390/ijms21155238

Pawlak, M., Lefebvre, P., and Staels, B. (2015). Molecular Mechanism of PPARα Action and its Impact on Lipid Metabolism, Inflammation and Fibrosis in Non-alcoholic Fatty Liver Disease. *J. Hepatol.* 62, 720–733. doi:10.1016/j.jhep.2014.10.039

Phillips, M. C. (2018). Is ABCA1 a Lipid Transfer Protein? *J. Lipid Res.* 59, 749–763. doi:10.1194/jlr.R082313

Ren, J., Lu, Y., Qian, Y., Chen, B., Wu, T., and Ji, G. (2019). Recent Progress Regarding Kaempferol for the Treatment of Various Diseases. *Exp. Ther. Med.* 18, 2759–2776. doi:10.3892/etm.2019.7886

Rong, X., Albert, C. J., Hong, C., Duerr, M. A., Chamberlain, B. T., Tarling, E. J., et al. (2013). LXRs Regulate ER Stress and Inflammation through Dynamic Modulation of Membrane Phospholipid Composition. *Cell Metab* 18, 685–697. doi:10.1016/j.cmet.2013.10.002

Sheka, A. C., Adeyi, O., Thompson, J., Hameed, B., Crawford, P. A., and Ikramuddin, S. (2020). Nonalcoholic Steatohepatitis: A Review. *JAMA* 323, 1175–1183. doi:10.1001/jama.2020.2298

Shen, X., Guo, H., Xu, J., and Wang, J. (2019). Inhibition of lncRNA HULC Improves Hepatic Fibrosis and Hepatocyte Apoptosis by Inhibiting the MAPK Signaling Pathway in Rats with Nonalcoholic Fatty Liver Disease. *J. Cel Physiol* 234, 18169–18179. doi:10.1002/jcp.28450

Singh, A. B., and Liu, J. (2017a). Identification of Hepatic Lysophosphatidylcholine Acyltransferase 3 as a Novel Target Gene Regulated by Peroxisome Proliferator-Activated Receptor δ. *J. Biol. Chem.* 292, 884–897. doi:10.1074/jbc.M116.743575

Suchal, K., Malik, S., Khan, S. I., Malhotra, R. K., Goyal, S. N., Bhatia, J., et al. (2017). Molecular Pathways Involved in the Amelioration of Myocardial Injury in Diabetic Rats by Kaempferol. *Int. J. Mol. Sci.* 18. doi:10.3390/ijms18051001

Takahashi, Y., and Fukusato, T. (2014). Histopathology of Nonalcoholic Fatty Liver Disease/nonalcoholic Steatohepatitis. *World J. Gastroenterol.* 20, 15539–15548. doi:10.3748/wjg.v20.i42.15539

Tomita, K., Teratani, T., Suzuki, T., Oshikawa, T., Yokoyama, H., Shimamura, K., et al. (2012). p53/p66Shc-mediated Signaling Contributes to the Progression of Non-alcoholic Steatohepatitis in Humans and Mice. *J. Hepatol.* 57, 837–843. doi:10.1016/j.jhep.2012.05.013

Van Schouwenburg, P. A., Rispens, T., and Wolbink, G. J. (2013). Immunogenicity of Anti-TNF Biologic Therapies for Rheumatoid Arthritis. *Nat. Rev. Rheumatol.* 9, 164–172. doi:10.1038/nrrheum.2013.4

Vance, J. E. (2015). *Phospholipid Synthesis and Transport in Mammalian Cells.* Copenhagen, Denmark: Traffic, 16.

Walter, F., O'brien, A., Concannon, C. G., Düssmann, H., and Prehn, J. H. M. (2018). ER Stress Signaling Has an Activating Transcription Factor 6α (ATF6)-dependent "Off-Switch". *J. Biol. Chem.* 293, 18270–18284. doi:10.1074/jbc.RA118.002121

Wang, B., Rong, X., Duerr, M. A., Hermanson, D. J., Hedde, P. N., Wong, J. S., et al. (2016). Intestinal Phospholipid Remodeling Is Required for Dietary-Lipid Uptake and Survival on a High-Fat Diet. *Cel Metab* 23, 492–504. doi:10.1016/j.cmet.2016.01.001

Wang, H., Chen, L., Zhang, X., Xu, L., Xie, B., Shi, H., et al. (2019). Kaempferol Protects Mice from D-GalN/LPS-Induced Acute Liver Failure by Regulating the ER Stress-Grp78-CHOP Signaling Pathway. *Biomed. Pharmacother.* 111, 468–475. doi:10.1016/j.biopha.2018.12.105

Wang, M., and Kaufman, R. J. (2016). Protein Misfolding in the Endoplasmic Reticulum as a Conduit to Human Disease. *Nature* 529, 326–335. doi:10.1038/nature17041

Wang, M., Sun, S., Wu, T., Zhang, L., Song, H., Hao, W., et al. (2013). Inhibition of LXRα/SREBP-1c-Mediated Hepatic Steatosis by Jiang-Zhi Granule. *Evid. Based Complement. Alternat Med.* 2013, 584634. doi:10.1155/2013/584634

Yang, Y., Jiang, Y., Wang, Y., and An, W. (2010). Suppression of ABCA1 by Unsaturated Fatty Acids Leads to Lipid Accumulation in HepG2 Cells. *Biochimie* 92, 958–963. doi:10.1016/j.biochi.2010.04.002

Yoshida, H., Matsui, T., Yamamoto, A., Okada, T., and Mori, K. (2001). XBP1 mRNA Is Induced by ATF6 and Spliced by IRE1 in Response to ER Stress to Produce a Highly Active Transcription Factor. *Cell* 107, 881–891. doi:10.1016/s0092-8674(01)00611-0

Younossi, Z., Anstee, Q. M., Marietti, M., Hardy, T., Henry, L., Eslam, M., et al. (2018). Global burden of NAFLD and NASH: Trends, Predictions, Risk Factors and Prevention. *Nat. Rev. Gastroenterol. Hepatol.* 15, 11–20. doi:10.1038/nrgastro.2017.109

Zhang, C., Chen, X., Zhu, R. M., Zhang, Y., Yu, T., Wang, H., et al. (2012). Endoplasmic Reticulum Stress Is Involved in Hepatic SREBP-1c Activation and Lipid Accumulation in Fructose-Fed Mice. *Toxicol. Lett.* 212, 229–240. doi:10.1016/j.toxlet.2012.06.002

Zhang, X., Lin, Y., Lin, S., Li, C., Gao, J., Feng, Z., et al. (2020). Silencing of Functional P53 Attenuates NAFLD by Promoting HMGB1-Related Autophagy Induction. *Hepatol. Int.* 14, 828–841. doi:10.1007/s12072-020-10068-4

14

Bicyclol Alleviates Signs of BDL-Induced Cholestasis by Regulating Bile Acids and Autophagy-Mediated HMGB1/p62/Nrf2 Pathway

Jingwen Zhao[1†], Maojuan Ran[1,2†], Ting Yang[1,3†], Liwei Chen[1], Peixu Ji[1], Xiuxiu Xu[1], Lu Zhang[1], Siyuan Sun[1], Xin Liu[1], Simin Zhou[1], Lu Zhou[1*] and Jie Zhang[1*]*

[1]*Department of Gastroenterology and Hepatology, Tianjin Medical University General Hospital, Tianjin Institute of Digestive Disease, Tianjin Key Laboratory of Digestive Diseases, Tianjin, China,* [2]*Department of Gastroenterology and Hepatology, Chengdu Second People's Hospital, Chengdu, China,* [3]*Department of Gastroenterology, Shanxi Provincial People's Hospital, Taiyuan, China*

Correspondence:
Jingwen Zhao
jingwenzhao@tmu.edu.cn
Lu Zhou
zhou_lu@126.com
Jie Zhang
zhangjiezhj@163.com

†*These authors have contributed equally to this work and share first authorship*

Cholestasis is a liver disease characterized by the accumulation of toxic bile salts, bilirubin, and cholesterol, resulting in hepatocellular damage. Recent findings have revealed several key steps of cholestasis liver injury including the toxicity of bile acids and accumulation of proinflammatory mediator. In this study, we investigated the protective effect of bicyclol in cholestasis caused by bile duct ligation (BDL), as well as relevant mechanisms. Bicyclol attenuated liver damage in BDL mice by increasing the levels of hydrophilic bile acid such as α-MCA and β-MCA, regulating bile acid-related pathways and improving histopathological indexes. High-mobility group box 1 (HMGB1) is an extracellular damage-associated molecular pattern molecule which can be used as biomarkers of cells and host defense. Bicyclol treatment decreased extracellular release of HMGB1. In addition, HMGB1 is also involved in regulating autophagy in response to oxidative stress. Bicyclol promoted the lipidation of LC3 (microtubule-associated protein 1 light chain 3)-II to activate autophagy. The nuclear factor, E2-related factor 2 (Nrf2) and its antioxidant downstream genes were also activated. Our results indicate that bicyclol is a promising therapeutic strategy for cholestasis by regulating the bile acids and autophagy-mediated HMGB1/p62/Nrf2 pathway.

Keywords: liver injury, cholestasis, BDL, high mobility group box 1, autophagy, Nrf2, bicyclol

INTRODUCTION

Cholestasis is a pathological condition caused by obstruction or cessation of bile flow resulting in intrahepatic cholestasis and accompanied by cell injury, inflammatory infiltration, cell apoptosis, liver fibrosis, and even cirrhosis (Yokoda and Carey, 2019). Currently, the main drug treatment for chronic cholestatic liver injury is ursodeoxycholic acid (UDCA). However, some patients do not respond to this treatment (Wagner and Fickert, 2020). Hence, novel treatment approaches, which could be based on a comprehensive understanding of the mechanisms of the different stages of disease progression, are urgently needed.

A previous study found that primary bile acids conjugated with glycine or taurine were significantly increased in serum of patients with cholestasis liver injury (Woolbright et al., 2015). Bile acids (BAs), such as taurocholic acid (TCA), glycocholic acid (GCA), glycochenodeoxycholic acid (GCDCA), and glycodeoxycholic acid (GDCA), can be used as biomarkers of liver injury or as indicators of drug-induced liver injury (DILI) (Yang et al., 2019). The hydrophobicity of bile acids was affected by the number and orientation of the hydrophilic region, where lithocholic acid (LCA) was the most hydrophobic while cholic acid (CA) was less hydrophobic (Ashby et al., 2018). On the other hand, the conjugated groups also affected the hydrophobicity of bile acids, where unconjugated was the most hydrophobic and glycine conjugated was more hydrophobic than taurine or sulphate conjugated (Ashby et al., 2018). The toxicity of bile acids is mostly dependent on its hydrophobicity. According to previous studies, TCA, the major endogenous BAs in rodents, significantly increases the mRNA level of inflammatory cytokines monocyte chemotactic protein 1 (Ccl2) and macrophage inflammatory protein 2α (cxcl2) (Cai et al., 2017). The toxicity of BAs during obstructive cholestatic liver injury likely occurs because of biliary BAs leakage. Previous studies proved that biliary BAs at 0.5x dose resulted in significant hepatocyte necrosis (Woolbright et al., 2015).

High-mobility group box-1 (HMGB1) protein, a member of the high-mobility group 1 (HMG-1) family, modulates cell death in acute liver injury by NF-κB signal pathway activated by advanced glycan end products (RAGE) and toll-like receptor 4 (TLR4) (Eguchi et al., 2014). HMGB1 is involved in many liver diseases. Previous studies have found that the level of liver HMGB1 protein was correlated with alcoholic steatohepatitis (ASH) and primary biliary cirrhosis (PBC) in patients with chronic Hepatitis C virus (HCV), as well as in chronic carbon tetrachloride (CCl4) treated mice (Ge et al., 2018). HMGB1 levels also increased in BDL induced cholestatic mice (Woolbright et al., 2013; Dondorf et al., 2017), while carnosic acid provided protection against BDL induced fibrosis by inhibiting HMGB1 expression (Zhang et al., 2017a). HMGB1 is a proinflammatory cytokine released by injured cells and the innate immune system, which alerts other cells that infection or sterile injury has occurred (Andersson and Tracey, 2011). Neutrophils and Cxcl2, Ccl2 mRNA levels were significantly decreased in mice with hepatocyte-specific Hmgb1 knockout (Huebener et al., 2019).

Autophagy deficiency leads to the rise of HMGB1 levels and promotes ductular reaction and tumorigenesis *via* its receptor RAGE (Khambu et al., 2018). HMGB1 regulates autophagy under the circumstances of oxidative stress (Kang et al., 2011). The oxidation HMGB1 binding to Beclin1 causes the dissociation of Bcl-2 from Beclin1, leading to the induction of autophagy (Tang et al., 2010). So, autophagy and HMGB1 are closely connected. Autophagy includes five processes: initiation, elongation, closure, maturation, and degradation. LC3B and p62 are the most commonly used markers of autophagy. The carboxyl terminus of the LC3 protein is specifically cleaved to form LC3-I with the exposed carboxyl-terminal glycine, which is combined with phosphatidylethanolamine to form LC3-II (Kuma et al., 2017). LC3-II targets the inner and outer membranes of autophagosomes to participate in the elongation step of autophagy (Kuma et al., 2017; Qian et al., 2017). P62 as a receptor for ubiquitinated proteins and organelles is selectively transported into the autophagosomes, after which it is degraded by autophagy (Ichimura and Komatsu, 2010).

The high levels of p62 associated with the suppression of autophagy competitively interacts with Kelch-like ECH-associated protein-1 (Keap1), the nuclear factor Nrf2-binding site, resulting in activation of Nrf2 and its target genes (Komatsu et al., 2010; Jiang et al., 2015). The activation of Nrf2 protects from various liver diseases through different molecular mechanisms (Xu et al., 2018). After activation, Nrf2 is translocated to the nucleus to activate heme oxygenase-1 (HO-1), NADPH quinone oxidoreductase-1 (NQO1), glutamate cysteine ligase (GCLC), and other genes to resist damage caused by oxidative stress (Galicia-Moreno et al., 2020). Nrf2-knockout mice are more susceptible to hepatic injury after BDL, as vitamin A activates Nrf2 to protect liver function in BDL rats, thus proving that Nrf2 activation is beneficial in cholestatic liver injury (Weerachayaphorn et al., 2012; Shin et al., 2013; Wang et al., 2014).

Bicyclol (4,4′-dimethoxy-5,6,5′,6′-bis (methylenedioxy)-2-hydroxymethyl-2′-methoxycarbonyl biphenyl) is a synthetic drug widely used to treat HCV (Li et al., 2018; Huang et al., 2019). Bicyclol has been proven to induce autophagy and inhibit cell proliferation through PI3K/AKT and MEK/ERK pathways (Wang et al., 2016b). Previous studies in our laboratory have shown that bicyclol can activate Nrf2 to act against CCl_4 induced hepatotoxicity (Zhao et al., 2020). What's more, Zhen, Yong-Zhan et al. have found that BDL-induced liver fibrosis can be significantly attenuated by bicyclol through reversing fibrogenic gene expression (Zhen et al., 2015). Nonetheless, there are still few studies on the mechanism of the protective effect of bicyclol in BDL-induced liver damage.

In this study, we aimed to explore the protective effect of bicyclol in BDL induced liver injury. Our research was mainly based on two aspects: the synthesis, excretion, and composition of bile acid, and the pathway associated with autophagy-mediated by HMGB1.

MATERIALS AND METHODS

Animals

Eleven-weeks old male (22–23 g) c57BL/6 mice were purchased from Beijing HFK Bioscience CO., LTD. All mice were housed in the SPF animal room with a constant temperature (22°C), and a 12/12 h light/dark cycles and were given free access to water and food. Before the experiment, mice were allowed to adapt to the environment for 1 week. All animal studies (including the mice euthanasia procedure) were done in compliance with the regulations and guidelines of the Animal Ethical and Welfare Committee (AEWC) at the Institute of Radiation Medicine

Chinese Academy of Medical Sciences and conducted according to the AAALAC and the IACUC guidelines.

The mice were randomly divided into three groups: Sham group (n = 8), BDL group (n = 6), and BDL + Bicyclol group (n = 6); the different numbers in different groups are due to the injury following BDL surgery. BDL was employed to induce cholestatic liver injury as described in a previous study (Fickert et al., 2002). Briefly, after anesthesia with isoflurane, the bile duct was separated from the portal vein and hepatic artery, then ligated using a 6–0 suture. The sham group underwent similar laparotomy without BDL. BDL + Bicyclol group was orally administered with bicyclol at a dose of 100 mg/kg (Hu and Liu, 2006; Zhen et al., 2015) body weight daily for 14 days, while sham and BDL group were treated with volume-matched 0.5% carboxymethylcellulose sodium (CMC-Na). Bicyclol was a kind gift from the Beijing Union Pharmaceutical Company (Beijing, China) with a purity of over 99%. Animals were sacrificed on days 14 after the operation, after which the blood and liver were collected and stored at −80°C for further research.

Serum Biochemical Analysis

The serum levels of aspartate transaminase (AST), alanine transaminase (ALT), alkaline phosphatase (ALP), γ-glutamyl transpeptadase (GGT), serum bile acid (TBA), and total cholesterol (TC) were measured by the automated chemistry analyzer (AU5800, Beckman Coulter, United States) of the clinical laboratory (Tianjin medical university general hospital).

Histology

Liver tissue was fixed in 4% paraformaldehyde at room temperature and blocked with paraffin wax, after which they were sectioned into 4 um thick slices and stained with hematoxylin and eosin (H&E) according to the standard H&E protocol. The inflammatory cell infiltration and necrosis were assessed by two experienced pathologists according to Ishak scoring criteria, including piece-meal necrosis, fusion necrosis, lytic necrosis, and portal inflammation (Ishak et al., 1995). Images were taken by Leica microscope (Leica DM5000B; Germany) at 200X magnification.

Measurement of Gallbladder Bile Acids Composition

Gallbladder bile was collected, and its composition was measured with liquid chromatography-tandem mass spectrometry (LC-MS/MS) (Yang et al., 2017). Briefly, standard samples were added into 50 ul bile samples, the supernatant was extracted after oscillation and centrifuged at 12,000 rpm for 10 min and then further concentrated on the concentrator. The concentrate was reconstituted in 100 uL of methyl/water (50/50) and analyzed by the LC-MS/MS system. The chromatographic separation was performed on the ACQUITY UPLC HSS T3 column (2.1*100 mm, 1.8 um). Data acquisition systems mainly included Ultra Performance Liquid Chromatography (Shim-pack UFLC SHIMADZU CBM30A) and Tandem mass spectrometry (Applied Biosystems 6500 QTRAP).

Immunofluorescence

The slides with liver samples were dewaxed with xylene and various ethanol concentrations and blocked with 5% bovine serum albumin (BSA) for 30 min. After that, the slides were incubated with primary antibodies against p62/SQSTM1 (no. NBP1-48320SS; Novus) at 4°C overnight. After being washed with PBS, the sections were incubated with secondary antibodies at 37°C for 1 h. The nuclei were stained with 4′-6′-diamino-2-phenylindole dihydrochloride (DAPI), and then sealed with resins. The sections were observed under a fluorescence microscope (Leica DM5000B; Germany).

Cell Culture and Treatment

Alpha mouse liver 12 cell line AML12 were purchased from the Chinese Academy of Sciences Cell Bank (Shanghai, China) and cultured in Dulbecco's Modified Eagle Media: Nutrient Mixture F-12 (DMEM—F12) (#119435; Gibco) supplemented with 10% fetal bovine serum (Gibco), 1% Insulin—Transferrin-Selenium (ITS) (#41400045; Gibco),40 ng/ml dexamethasone. Cells were grown in a humidified atmosphere with 5% CO_2 at 37°C. Once the cells reached confluency near 80%, they were digested with 0.125% trypsin-EDTA and seeded into 6-well plates. For analysis of protein and mRNA levels, cells were stimulated for 24 h with 100 uM TCA and/or 500 uM bicyclol. Taurocholic acid (TCA) was purchased from Sigma-Aldrich.

Western Blot

Liver tissues and cells were homogenized in RIPA buffer (Solarbio, China) that contained PMSF (Solarbio, China) and phosphatase inhibitors on ice. The homogenates were centrifuged, and supernatants were extracted, after which 1/3 volume of loading buffer was added and stored at −80°C for further study. The protein was quantified by a BCA protein assay kit (Solarbio, China). Equal amounts of proteins were separated by SDS-PAGE gels and transferred to nitrocellulose membranes. After blocking with 5% non-fat milk, membranes were incubated with primary antibodies overnight at 4°C. The primary anti-CYP7A1 (#sc-518007, Santa Cruz), anti-BSEP (#sc-74500, Santa Cruz), anti-FXR (#ab235094, Abcam), anti- SQSTM1/p62 (#39749, Cell Signaling Technology), anti-LC3A/B (D11) (#3868, Cell Signaling Technology), anti-Beclin-1 (#3495, Cell Signaling Technology), anti-HMGB1 (#6893, Cell Signaling Technology), anti-RAGE (ab216329, Abcam, Cambridge, MA, United States), anti-TLR4 (#A17436, ABclonal Technology), anti-NRF2 (#12721, Cell Signaling Technology), anti-Keap1 (#A17061, ABclonal Technology) and anti-β-actin (#3700, Cell Signaling Technology) were used. The secondary horseradish peroxidase-conjugated goat anti-rabbit or anti-mouse IgG antibodies (Zhongshan Golden Bridge Biotechnology, Beijing, China) were incubated at room temperature for 1 h. After fully washing, the ECL Reagent (Solarbio, China) and Image Lab (Bio-Rad, America) were used to analyze the bands.

TABLE 1 | Specific qPCR primers used in this study.

Gene name	Forward primer (5'-3')	Reverse primer (5'-3')
Gapdh	GGAGAAACCTGCCAAGTATG	TGGGAGTTGCTGTTGAAGTC
Cyp7a1	AACAACCTGCCAGTACTAGATAG	GTGTAGAGTGAAGTCCTCCTTAGC
Fxr	GGCCTCTGGGTACCACTACA	TGTACACGGCGTTCTTGGTA
Bsep	CTGCCAAGGATGCTAATGCA	CGATGGCTACCCTTTGCTTCT
Tnf-α	GGTGCCATGTCTCAGCCTCTT	GCCATAGAACTGATGAGAGGGAG
IL-1β	GCCATAGAACTGATGAGAGGGAG	GCCATAGAACTGATGAGAGGGAG
Nrf2	CTTTAGTCAGCGACAGAAGGAC	AGGCATCTTGTTTGGGAATGTG
Nqo1	AGGATGGGAGGTACTCGAATC	TGCTAGAGATGACTCGGAAGG
Hmox1	GATAGAGCGCAACAAGCAGAA	CAGTGAGGCCCATACCAGAAG

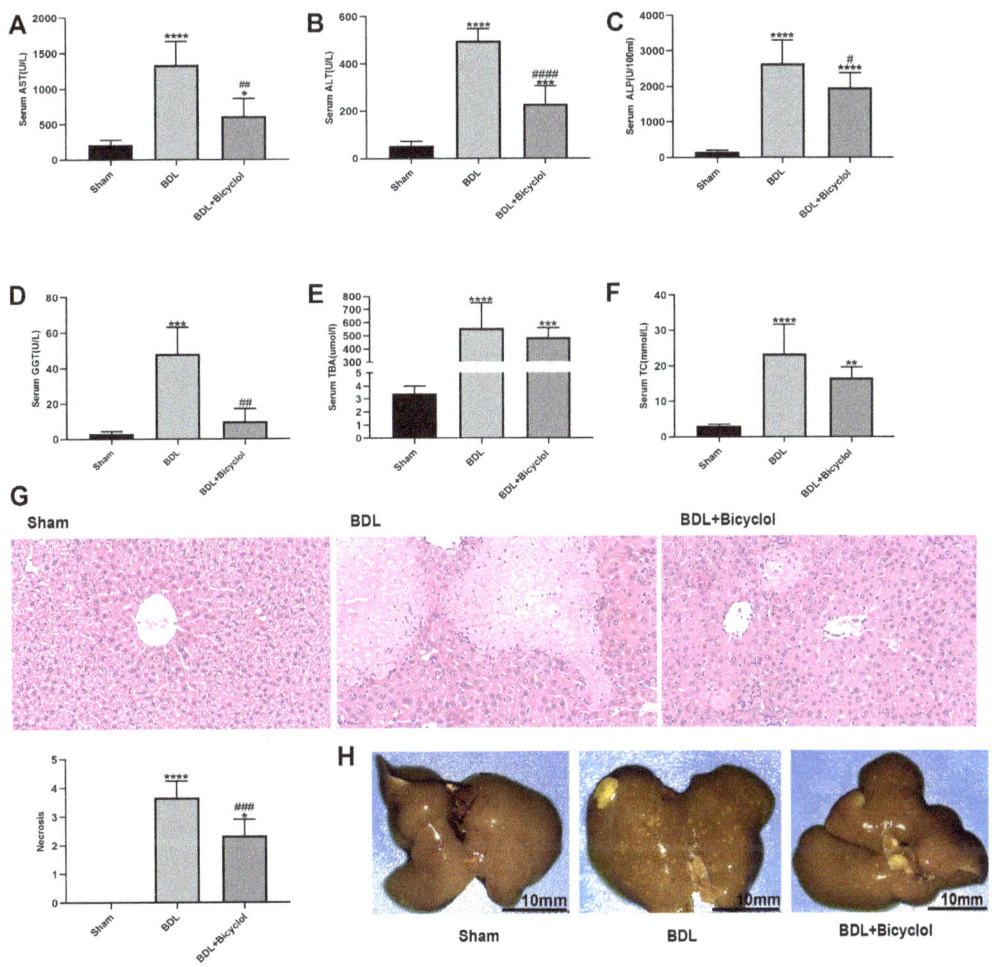

FIGURE 1 | Bicyclol markedly improved the liver enzyme, histology, and liver gross appearance in BDL mice. **(A–F)** Serum biochemistry including AST, ALT, ALP, GGT, TBA, and TC. **(G)** H&E stain liver histology (Scale bar, 100 um). **(H)** Gross liver appearance (Scale bar, 10 mm). AST, aspartate aminotransferase; ALT, alanine aminotransferase; ALP, alkaline phosphatase; GGT, γ-glutamyl transpeptidase; TBA, total bile acid; TC, total cholesterol. $^{*}p < 0.05$, $^{**}p < 0.01$, $^{***}p < 0.001$, $^{****}p < 0.0001$ vs. sham; $^{\#}p < 0.05$, $^{\#\#}p < 0.01$, $^{\#\#\#}p < 0.001$, $^{\#\#\#\#}p < 0.0001$ vs. BDL.

Real-Time RT-PCR

Total RNA was extracted from liver tissues, and AML12 cells using Trizol reagent and the concentration was determined by an enzyme-labeled instrument. The RNA was reverse-transcribed into cDNA using SuperScript III First-Strand Synthesis System (Invitrogen, Carlsbad, CA, United States). The reaction mix was performed as follows: 50°C (2 min); 95°C (5 min); followed by 50 cycles of 95°C (15 s) and 60°C (30 s).

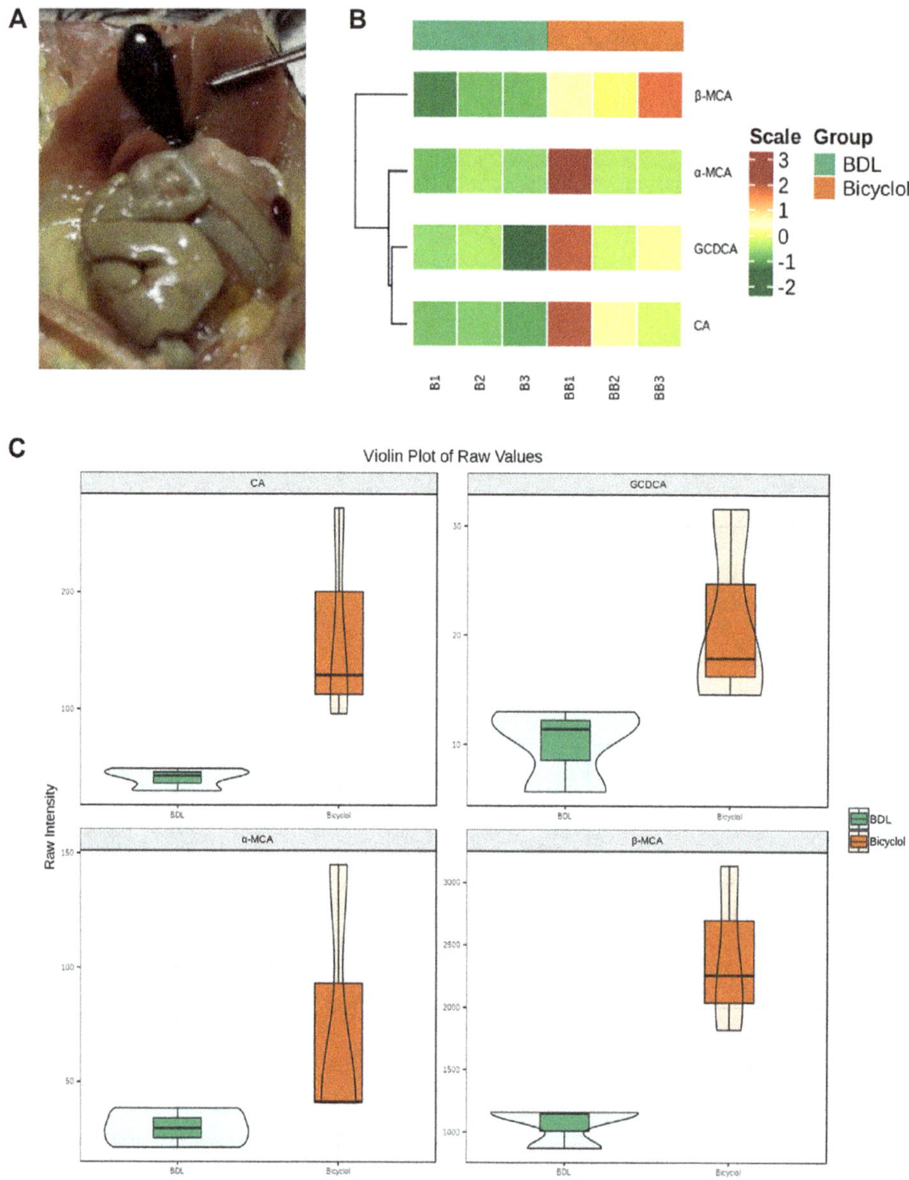

FIGURE 2 | Bile acid composition in the gallbladder. **(A)** The gallbladder of BDL mice. **(B)** Heatmap of differential bile acids of gallbladder bile samples. Rows represent different bile acids, while columns represent different samples. Colors from green to red indicate increasing levels from low to high. **(C)** Violin plot analysis comparing the levels of CA, GCDCA, α-MCA, β-MCA in the BDL and Bicyclol groups. Green represents the BDL group, whereas orange represents the Bicyclol group.

Relative expression of target genes was calculated by the $2^{-\Delta\Delta Ct}$ method and normalized to GAPDH. The primer sequences are shown in **Table 1**.

Statistical Analysis

Data are expressed as mean ± SEM and analyzed with GraphPad Prism 8.0.1 (GraphPad Software, United States). One-way ANOVA followed by Tukey's multiple comparisons test was used to calculate the statistical significance. A p-value of <0.05 was considered statistically significant.

RESULTS

Protective Effects of Bicyclol on Liver Injury in Bile Duct Ligation Mice

To explore the effects of bicyclol on BDL induced mice liver injury, we tested liver enzymes including AST, ALT, ALP, GGT, TBA, and TC, and liver pathology. The serum AST, ALT, ALP, GGT, TBA, and TC levels increased in BDL compared with the sham group (**Figures 1A–F**). Bicyclol significantly decreased the AST, ALT, ALP, and GGT levels. However, the TBA and TC levels were comparable between

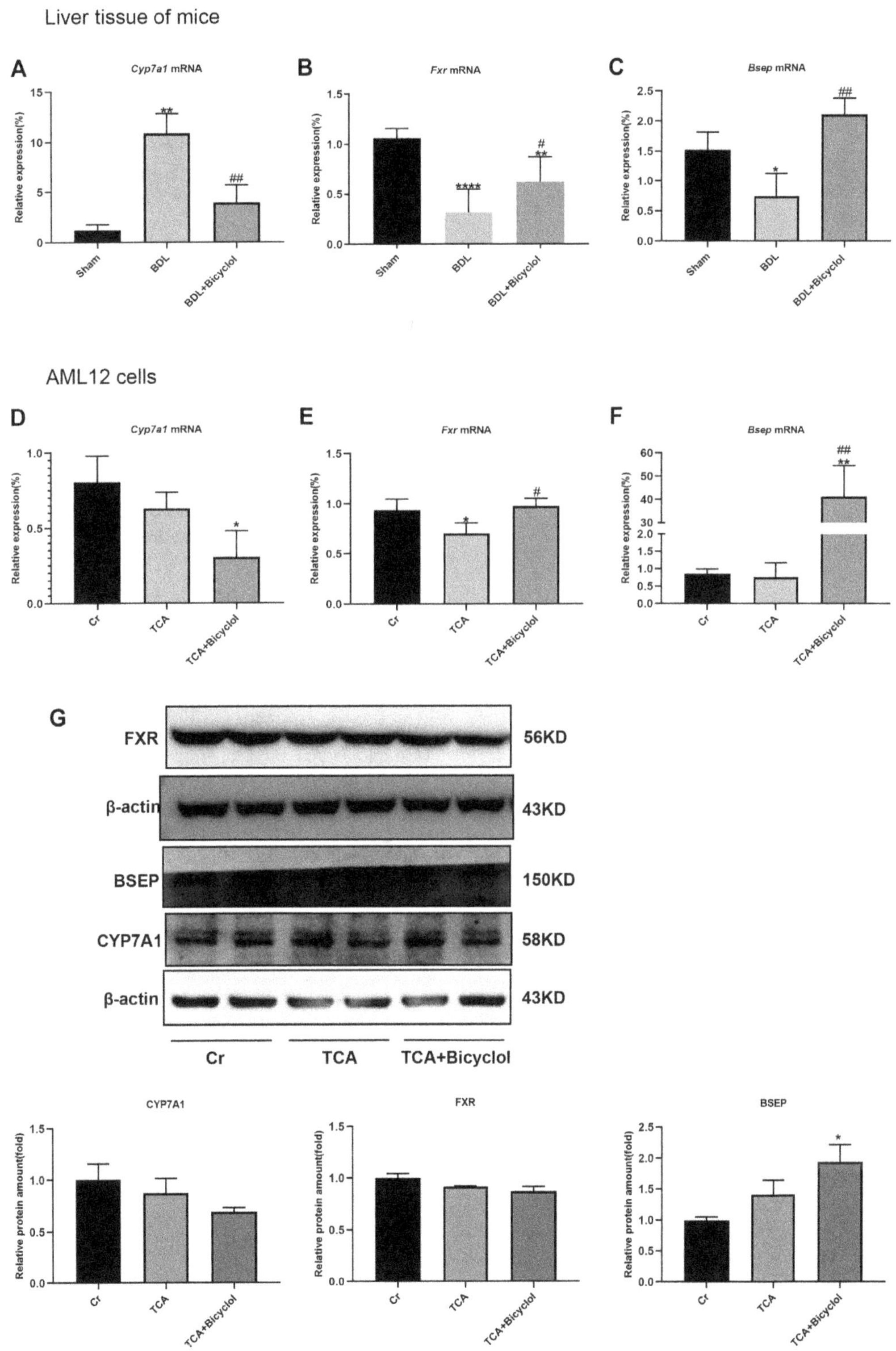

FIGURE 3 | Effects of bicyclol on genes related to bile metabolism. **(A–C)** The mRNA levels of bile metabolism-related genes (Fxr, Cyp7a1, Bsep) in BDL and bicyclol treatment mice. The mRNA levels **(D–F)** and protein levels **(G)** of bile metabolism-related genes (Fxr, Cyp7a1, Bsep) in AML12 cells after TCA and bicyclol exposure. Cr represents control group without special treatment, TCA means cells were stimulated with 100 uM TCA for 24 h, TCA + Bicyclol means cells were pretreated with 500 uM bicyclol for 2 h, then stimulated with 100 uM TCA for 24 h. Data are expressed as mean ± SD. *$p < 0.05$, **$p < 0.01$, ***$p < 0.001$, ****$p < 0.0001$ vs. sham or Cr; #$p < 0.05$, ##$p < 0.01$ vs. BDL or TCA.

BDL and BDL + Bicyclol groups. As indicated by H&E staining, BDL induced inflammatory cell infiltration and hepatic necrosis in mice liver, the effects of which were then ameliorated by bicyclol (**Figure 1G**). The beneficial effects were also proved by liver appearance, where livers from BDL mice had many yellow-white granules on the surface. In contrast, yellow-white granules of the liver were significantly improved in the bicyclol treatment group (**Figure 1H**). These results revealed that bicyclol could relieve BDL induced liver injury.

Bicyclol Treatment Changed Bile Acid Composition

In those mice with bile duct ligation, the gallbladder volume significantly increased, and the bile was stagnant (**Figure 2A**); thus, we collected the bile in the gallbladder and analyzed the composition. In total, we tested 25 different kinds of bile acids, finding four BAs CA, GCDCA, α-muricholic acid (α-MCA), β-muricholic acid (β-MCA) levels that differed between BDL and bicyclol groups (**Figure 2**). A heatmap was plotted to show the levels of four bile acids (**Figure 2B**). CA, GCDCA, α-MCA, β-MCA in three samples of the bicyclol group were higher than that in the BDL group. In addition, violin plot analysis showed that the levels of bile acids, including CA, GCDCA, α-MCA, and β-MCA were higher in the bicyclol group than in the BDL group (**Figure 2C**). Previous studies have found that cholate and β-muricholate were the main components of mouse bile acid pool (Kerr et al., 2002), with the following order from hydrophobic to hydrophilic: LCA > deoxycholic acid (DCA) > chenodeoxycholic acid (CDCA) > CA > UDCA > MCA (de Aguiar Vallim et al., 2013). Our results showed that bicyclol could increase hydrophilic bile acid, mainly the α-MCA, β-MCA levels.

Bicyclol Prevented Liver Injury by Preventing Hepatic Bile Acid Synthesis and Promoting Bile Acid Excretion

Cyp7a1 is the key enzyme in the classic bile acid synthesis pathway (Chiang and Ferrell, 2019). *Fxr* is a nuclear receptor that suppresses *Cyp7a1* expression (Xu et al., 2016). In our study, liver *Cyp7a1* mRNA expression level was elevated by BDL and significantly reduced post bicyclol treatment (**Figure 3A**). BDL significantly reduced *Fxr* expression at the mRNA level, which was then reversed by bicyclol (**Figure 3B**). *Bsep* expression at the mRNA level was also decreased in the BDL group and increased in BDL + Bicyclol group (**Figure 3C**). TCA resulted in the most abundant BAs in blood, which was significantly increased in cirrhosis and hepatocellular carcinoma (HCC) patients, and induced inflammatory gene expression in liver cells. Consequently, we treated TCA cells to mimic the cell damage caused by bile (Chen et al., 2011; Wang et al., 2016a). TCA caused a down-regulation of *Fxr* [F (2,7) = 7.736], which was reversed by bicyclol. *Fxr* further caused a decrease of *Cyp7a1* and an increase of *Bsep* (**Figures 3D–F**). At the same time, bicyclol significantly up-regulated the protein expression of BSEP and inhibited the protein level of CYP7A1 although there was no significant difference, even if the FXR protein expression was not changed by bicyclol (**Figure 3G**). These results suggested that bicyclol could activate *Fxr* to suppress *Cyp7a1* expression, which led to a reduction of BA synthesis and acceleration of BA excretion.

Bicyclol Ameliorates Bile Duct Ligation-Induced Liver Injury by Down-Regulation of High-Mobility Group Box-1

Inflammatory factors, including tumor necrosis factor-α (TNF-α), interleukin-1 β (IL-1β), interleukin- 6 (IL-6), transforming growth factor-β (TGF-β), are involved in drug-induced liver injury, cholestasis, alcoholic and non-alcoholic fatty liver diseases, and other chronic liver disease processes (Szabo and Csak, 2012). Severe bile duct damage often triggers inflammation. To further verify the liver damage caused by BDL and the effect of bicyclol, we tested the mRNA levels of *TNF-α* and *IL-1β*. The results showed that bicyclol recovered the BDL-induced *IL-1β*, *TNF-α* mRNA higher expression (**Figures 4A,B**). HMGB1, as a member of damage-associated molecular patterns (DAMPs) and its receptor RAGE, promote neutrophil infiltration in necrotic tissue, thus aggravating necrosis (Huebener et al., 2015). So, we also measured the protein expression changes of HMGB1 in the liver and AML12 cells. The HMGB1 expression levels were upregulated in the BDL or TCA groups, and this upregulation was offset by bicyclol (**Figures 4C,E**). Similarly, BDL and TCA also caused the up-regulation of RAGE protein and was also reversed by bicyclol (**Figures 4D,F**). TLR4 can be activated by HMGB1, the expression of TLR4 was upregulated at TCA and TCA + Bicyclol groups compare to Cr group (**Figure 4G**).

Bicyclol Stimulated Autophagy in Mice and Alpha Mouse Liver 12 Cells

To analyze the effect of bicyclol on autophagy, two important markers of autophagy were detected. The conversion from LC3-I (soluble form) to LC3-II (lapidated form) and p62 protein are autophagy activation indicators. Western blot showed that the expression of LC3-II levels was increased, and p62 was decreased in the BDL group. Also, bicyclol treatment further upregulated the LC3-II., but the p62 levels were also increased by bicyclol (**Figure 5A**). *In vitro*, bicyclol enhanced the TCA induced accumulation of LC3-II and p62 (**Figure 5C**). We also observed the expression of p62 in the liver by immunofluorescence (**Figure 5B**). The results showed that the nucleus of the cholestasis site was broken and dissolved, there was no normal structure, and the fluorescence of p62 was significantly reduced. Bicyclol significantly improved cell necrosis with p62 fluorescence increased dramatically (**Figure 5B**). These results were consistent with the western blot findings. Besides these, the expression levels of pro-autophagy protein Beclin-1 were upregulated by TCA, even though there was no significant difference (**Figure 5D**).

Bicyclol Regulated Nuclear Factor, E2-Related Factor 2 Mediated Antioxidant Response

Cholestasis is related to oxidative stress. Under basal conditions, Nrf2 binds to Keap1 in the cytoplasm; under oxidative stress,

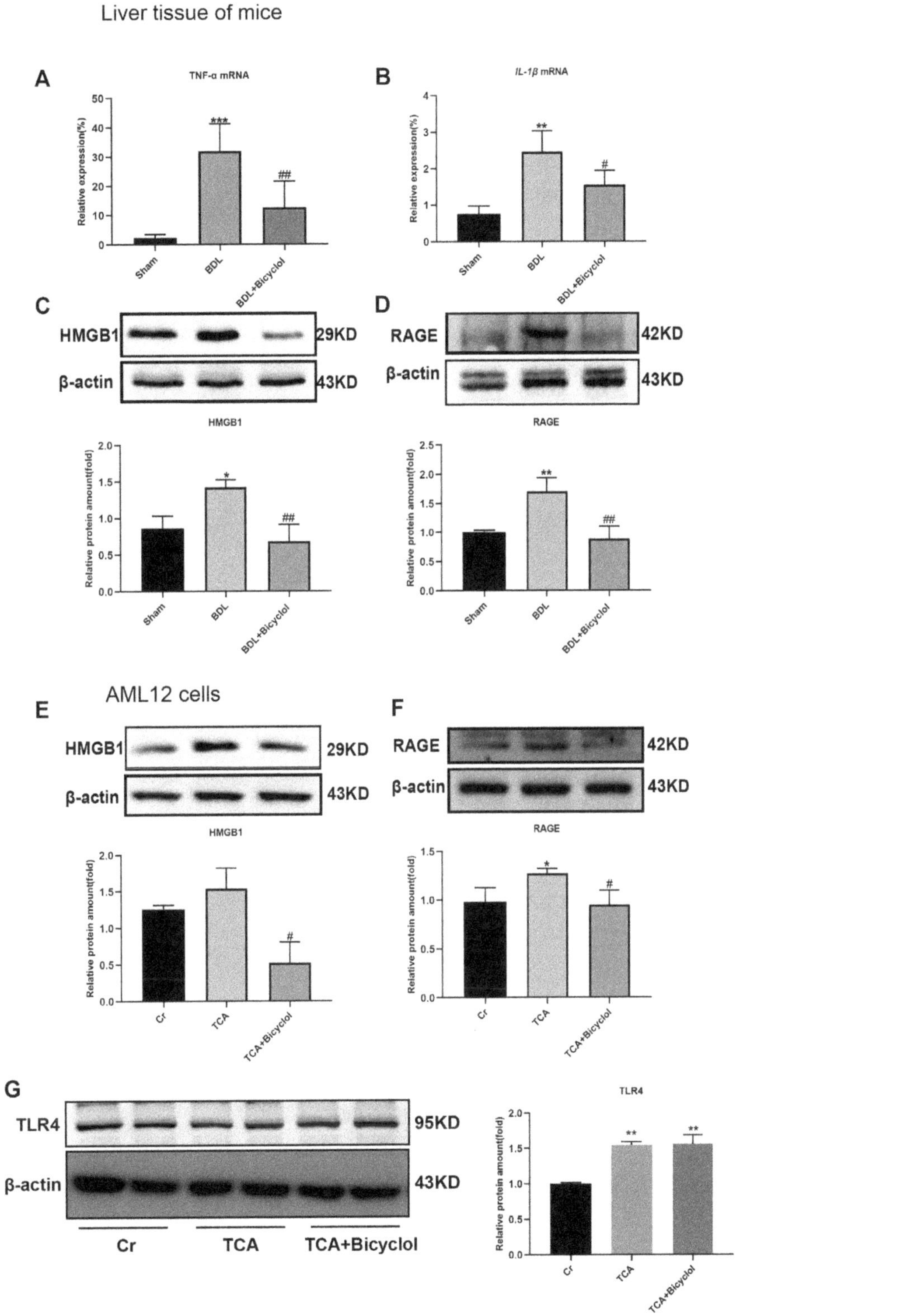

FIGURE 4 | Effect of bicyclol on inflammatory cytokines, HMGB1, and its receptor RAGE and TLR4. The mRNA level of Tnf-α **(A)** and IL-1β **(B)** in mouse liver tissue. **(C,D)** Immunoblots for HMGB1 and RAGE in mouse liver. **(E,F)** Immunoblots for HMGB1 and RAGE in AML12 cells. **(G)** Immunoblots for TLR4 in AML12 cells. $^{*}p < 0.05$, $^{**}p < 0.01$, $^{***}p < 0.001$ vs. sham or Cr; $^{\#}p < 0.05$, $^{\#\#}p < 0.01$ vs. BDL or TCA. Protein levels were normalized to levels of β-actin.

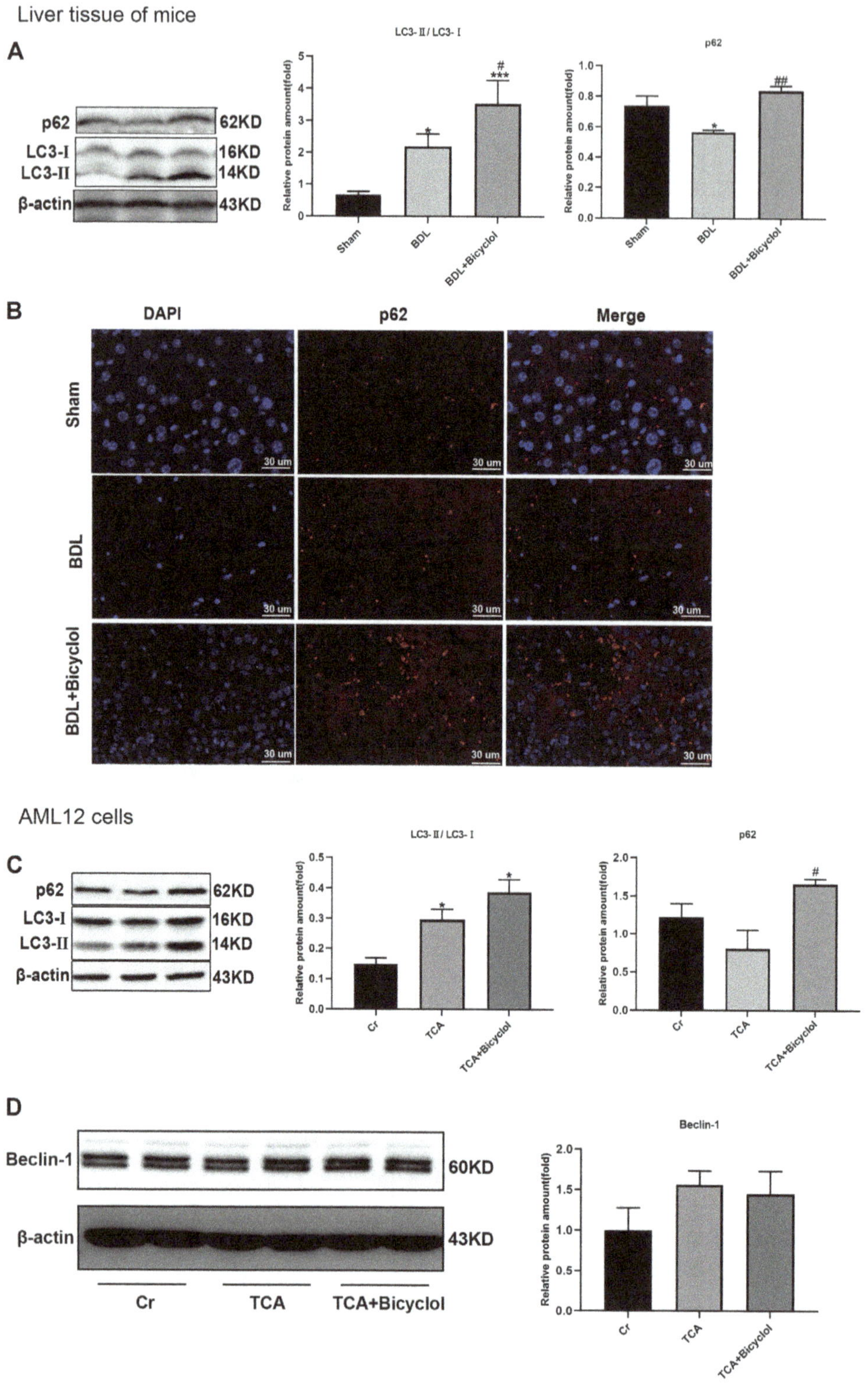

FIGURE 5 | Effect of bicyclol on autophagy. **(A)** P62 and LC3-II protein levels in mice were detected by western blot. **(B)** Paraffin sections of liver tissue were stained with p62 (red) and counterstained with DAPI to visualize nuclei (blue) by immunofluorescence. Scale bar, 30 um. **(C)** Immunoblots for p62 and LC3-II in AML12 cells. **(D)** Immunoblots for Beclin-1 in AML12 cells. $^{*}p < 0.05$ vs. sham or Cr; $^{\#}p < 0.05$, $^{\#\#}p < 0.01$, $^{\#\#\#}p < 0.001$ vs. BDL or TCA. Protein levels were normalized to levels of β-actin.

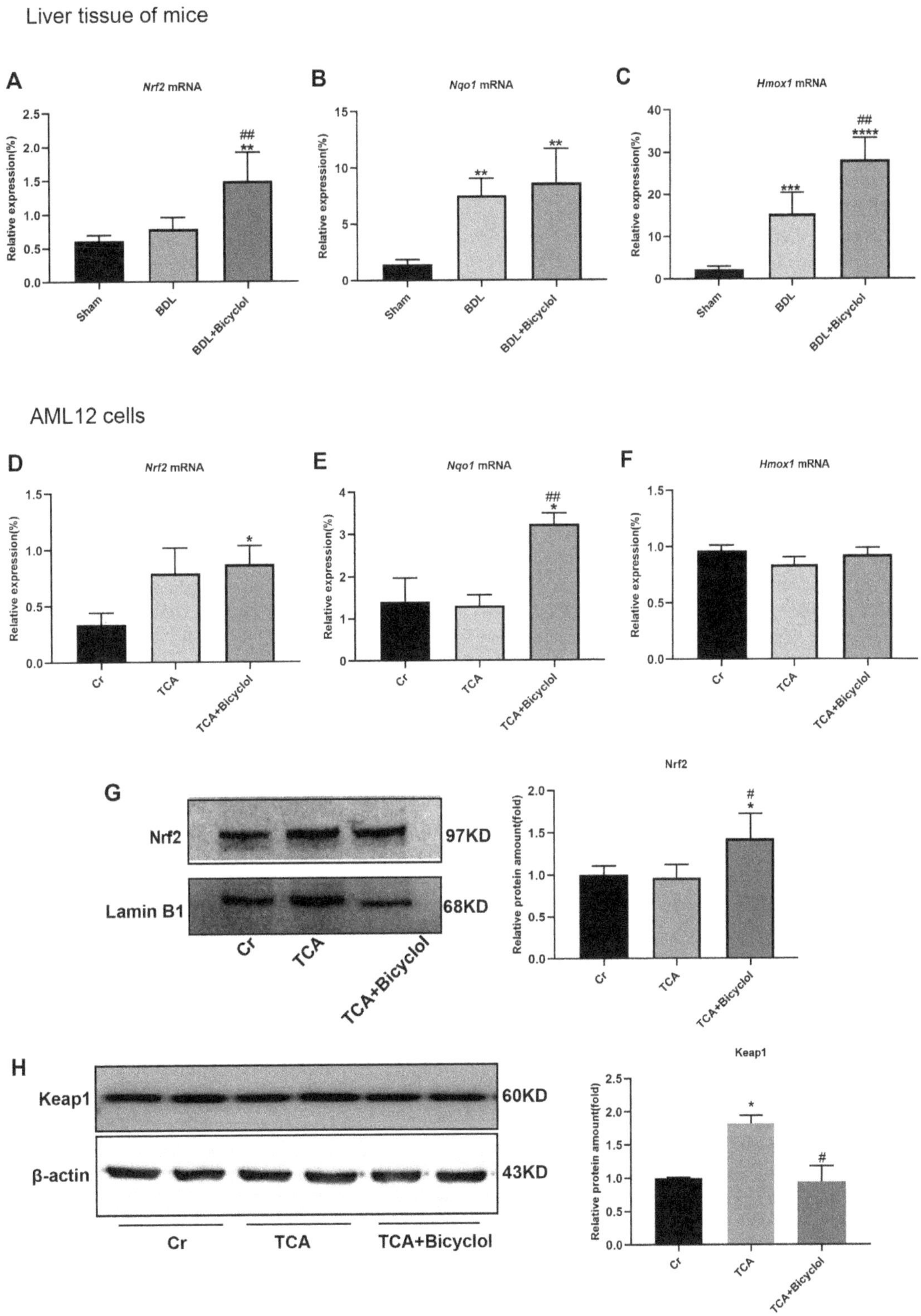

FIGURE 6 | Effects of bicyclol on Nrf2 and its target genes. **(A–C)** The mRNA levels of Nrf2, Nqo1, Hmox1 in BDL and bicyclol treatment mice. **(D–F)** The mRNA levels of Nrf2, Nqo1, Hmox1; The protein levels of Nrf2 **(G)** and Keap1 **(H)** in AML12 cells after TCA and bicyclol exposure. Dates are expressed as mean ± SD. $^{*}p < 0.05$, $^{**}p < 0.01$, $^{***}p < 0.001$, $^{****}p < 0.0001$ vs. sham or Cr; $^{\#}p < 0.05$, $^{\#\#}p < 0.01$ vs. BDL or TCA.

Nrf2 dissociates from the Nrf2/Keap1 complex and translocate to the nucleus, thereby initiating the transcription of anti-oxidative stress genes. As shown in **Figure 6A** *Nrf2* mRNA level was significantly increased in BDL + Bicyclol group compared with the Sham and BDL groups. In addition, the downstream target genes, including NADPH: quinone oxidoreductase 1 (*Nqo1*) and heme oxygenase-1 (*Hmox1*), were also determined. The results showed that *Nqo1* and *Hmox1* were upregulated in BDL and BDL + Bicyclol groups compared with the Sham group (**Figures 6B,C**). The level of *Hmox1* was further upregulated by bicyclol. The *Nrf2* and *Nqo1* mRNA levels were increased in bicyclol-treated AML12 cells; however, there were no significant differences in TCA-treated AML12 cells (**Figures 6D,E**). In addition, the protein level of Nrf2 also increased by bicyclol (**Figure 6G**). The expression level of Keap1 was significant increased after TCA exposure, while pretreatment with bicyclol reversed the upregulation (**Figure 6H**).

DISCUSSION

Cholestasis is a liver disease characterized by the accumulation of toxic bile salts, bilirubin, and cholesterol, resulting in hepatocellular injury, which eventually develop into fibrosis and cirrhosis. UDCA, as an exogenous hydrophilic bile acid that replaces endogenous hydrophobic bile acids and obeticholic acid as FXR agonists, have been used to treat PBC (Gulamhusein and Hirschfield, 2020). Besides UDCA and obeticholic acid, 24-norursodeoxycholic acid (norUDCA) is also used to treat PSC and cholestasis liver diseases with favorable outcomes (Fickert et al., 2013; Fickert et al., 2017). Unfortunately, 40% of patients do not have a satisfactory response to UDCA and are at risk of cirrhosis or non-neoplastic complications (Leung et al., 2020; Wagner and Fickert, 2020). The results of the present study demonstrated that BDL could lead to the accumulation of serum TBA and TC which induce a significant liver injury, as evidenced by the increasing of serum ALT, AST, ALP, GGT and hepatic necrosis. Bicyclol treatment exhibited significant protection against BDL induced liver injury by reducing the elevated serum ALT, AST, ALP, GGT levels and hepatic necrosis. Bicyclol also improved bile stasis in the liver as evidenced by the liver gross appearance that yellow-white granules were significantly decreased by bicyclol. These results are consistent with a previous study that bicyclol treatment ameliorated liver condition in BDL rats (Zhen et al., 2015). In addition, our research supplements the potential mechanisms that may be involved.

The composition of bile acids in different species is different. In the human body, CA and CDCA are the main components, while CA and muricholic acid (MCA) are the main bile acid components in mice (de Aguiar Vallim et al., 2013). Due to the presence or absence of hydroxyl groups in the corresponding position and direction on the molecular skeleton, bile acids' hydrophilicity is different. The order from hydrophilic to hydrophobic reads as follows: MCA > UDCA > CA > CDCA > DCA > LCA (de Aguiar Vallim et al., 2013). The previous study has shown that colesevelam can improve cholestatic liver and biliary tract damage by changing biliary BA composition, mainly by causing hydrophilization of BAs (up-regulating liver and biliary α-MCA, β-MCA and ω-MCA levels) (Fuchs et al., 2018). Another study found that the FXR agonist obeticholic acid increased the levels of α/β MCA from 11.3 to 29.4% and reduced the absorption of cholesterol (Xu et al., 2016). Our experiments revealed that the levels of hydrophilic bile acids such as α-MCA and β-MCA were significantly up-regulated after bicyclol treatment compared to the BDL group. It seems that bicyclol treatment promoted the excretion of the bile acids from the body through the circulation, thus reducing the toxic damage of bile acids. Clinical trials have also found that the bile acid composition in PBC patients treated with UDCA was also changed as the bile was enriched with UDCA, while CA and CDCA were significantly down-regulated, and endogenous bile acids combined with glycine were also increased (Combes et al., 1999). Yet, in our study, we found a different result, i.e., bicyclol treatment increased the levels of CA and GCDCA. Our explanation is that while bicyclol improves the laboratory indicators of BDL accompanied by ongoing liver damage, but GCDCA accumulation can cause liver cell damage because of its hydrophobicity.

BAs are synthesized from cholesterol in the liver through classical and alternative pathways that involve 14 enzymes. Among them, the classical pathway is catalyzed by *Cyp7a1* to synthesize primary bile acids CA and CDCA (Russell, 2003). Cyp7a1 overexpressed mice have increased bile acid pool and a higher level of hepatic cholesterol (Li et al., 2011). Nuclear receptors are also involved in BAs balance. *Fxr* regulates most of the bile acid formation processes, including transport and detoxification, and limits the overload of bile acids in liver cells (Wagner et al., 2011). *Fxr* participates in BAs balance through a variety of ways, including inhibiting liver *Cyp7a1* transcription, inducing intestinal *Fgf-15* to activate liver FGF receptor 4 (FGFR-4), repressing Na/taurocholate cotransporter (NTCP), activating the bile salt export pump *Bsep* and similar (Wagner et al., 2011). The Fxr agonist obeticholic acid (OCA) inhibits the expression of *Cyp7a1* by activating liver *Fxr* and *Shp* expression and changes the bile acid pool size and composition to inhibit intestinal cholesterol absorption (Xu et al., 2016). Our results showed that treatment with bicyclol in BDL mice up-regulated *Fxr* transcription while down-regulating *Cyp7a1* and up-regulating the expression of *Bsep*. Many previous studies have proven that gut microbes are involved in the synthesis and excretion of bile acids and the conversion of components, such as VSL#3 probiotics (including eight different probiotic strains) (Degirolamo et al., 2014) and probiotic *Lactobacillus rhamnosus* GG (LGG) (Liu et al., 2020), while bile acids can also affect bacterial structure *in vitro* and *in vivo* (Tian et al., 2020). Besides affecting the growth of intestinal bacteria, bile also participates in anti-adhesion and neutralizing endotoxins (Wiest et al., 2014). The lack of intestinal bile leads to bacterial translocation and intestinal inflammation, which promotes the progression and development of colorectal cancer (Jia et al., 2018). Therefore, intestinal bacteria and pathological changes after BDL should also be investigated due to the lack of bile in the intestinal.

HMGB1 can have both favorable and unfavorable consequences. On the one hand, hepatocyte-specific HMGB1 knockout mice suffer from increased mitochondrial damage and cell death during liver ischemia/reperfusion (Huang et al., 2014). On the other hand, hepatocyte HMGB1 is involved in the pathogenesis of ALD (Ge et al., 2014). Zhang *et al* found that NF-KBp65 was significantly up-regulated after treatment with FXR siRNA or inhibitor, accompanied by the up-regulation of IL-1β and TNF-α (Zhang et al., 2017b). In the present study, we found that bicyclol increased the FXR expression while it decreased the mRNA levels of inflammatory factors TNFα and IL-1β and the protein level of HMGB1 in the liver. Autophagy, which maintains liver homeostasis by eliminating toxic substances in the liver, is involved in accumulation disorders, non-alcoholic fatty liver disease, fibrosis, hepatocellular carcinoma, hyperammonaemia, viral infections and other liver diseases (Hazari et al., 2020). HMGB1 can stimulate autophagy in a variety of ways, including BECN1 in the cytoplasm, HSPB1 in the nucleus, and RAGE outside the cell. Previous studies have also shown that HMGB1 deficiency has no adverse impact on liver function, nor does it affect mitochondrial quality and autophagy (Huebener et al., 2014; Sun and Tang, 2014). We detected LC3-II/I and p62, which are two markers of autophagy. The results showed that BDL resulted in the up-regulation of LC3-II/I ratio and the degradation of p62 to activate autophagy and protect the liver from cholestasis damage. Bicyclol further increased the LC3-II/I ratio, but caused the accumulation of p62, which in turn activated autophagy to provide protection. Although our experiment did not find that bicyclol could change the expression of pro-autophagy protein Beclin-1, previous study has reported that Beclin-1 and Atg7 were up-regulated by bicyclol (Zhao et al., 2020). All these demonstrate that bicyclol can resist the progression of cholestasis liver injury through autophagy.

The p62-Keap1-Nrf2 pathway is part of the cellular antioxidant defense mechanism, in which p62 accumulates and competitively combines with Keap1 to activate Nrf2 (Komatsu et al., 2010). A recent study showed that activation of the p62-Keap1-Nrf2 pathway protects the ferroptosis in hepatocellular carcinoma cells (Sun et al., 2016). In our study, we found that the decrease of p62 led to the upregulation of Keap1, and Nrf2 was no significant changes. The accumulation of p62 caused by bicyclol treatment resulted in the degradation of Keap1 and activation of Nrf2. Nrf2 is one of the nuclear transcription factors, which provide protection against oxidative stress by regulating the expression of endogenous antioxidants. Genes regulated by Nrf2 are involved in the synthesis and regeneration of GSH, the expression of GST and GPx, the production of NADPH, and the expression of genes encoding iron chelation (Battino et al., 2018). In this study, we detected the mRNA levels of *Nrf2* and its downstream target genes *Nqo1*, *Hmox1*, and *Gclc*. Our results demonstrate that *Gclc* was not significantly different in animal experiments or cell experiments (data not shown). Heping *et al* reported that the mRNA and protein levels of GCLC, GCLM, and NRF2 all temporarily increased during BDL and then fell to baseline or below. These results suggested that either ursodeoxycholic acid or S-adenosylmethionine therapy alone can prevent the down-regulation of GCLC, GCLM, and NRF2 protein levels, while the combination of the two can increase these levels even higher (Yang et al., 2009). Other studies have shown that BDL leads to increased nuclear migration of NRF2, the expression of downstream target genes *Nqo1*, *Hmox1*, and *Gclm* is also up-regulated, and Vitamin A or baicalin intervention further increases the above performance (Wang et al., 2014; Shen et al., 2017). In our study, the mRNA level of *Nrf2* was not significantly up-regulated in the BDL group, while the levels of *Nqo1* and *Hmox1* were substantially up-regulated. Bicyclol not only up-regulated the mRNA level of *Nqo1* and *Hmox1*, but it also up-regulated the level of *Nrf2*. *In vitro* cell experiments, TCA only up-regulated the level of *Nrf2* mRNA without significant difference, while bicyclol up-regulated the mRNA and protein levels of *Nrf2* and *Nqo1*. So, bicyclol also improved liver damage caused by BDL by activating *Nrf2* and its downstream targets *Nqo1* and *Hmox1*, which is consistent with previous studies (Zhang et al., 2014; Zhao et al., 2020).

CONCLUSION

These results indicate that bicyclol can improve liver damage caused by BDL in obstructive cholestasis. The bicyclol treatment promotes hydrophilization of bile acids, inhibits bile acid synthesis through Fxr/Cyp7a1, and promotes the excretion of bile acids through the Fxr/Bsep pathway. In addition, the fact that bicyclol treatment exerts its therapeutic effect through p62-Nrf2 anti-inflammatory and antioxidant pathways further the research on cholestasis liver injury.

Institutional Review Board Statement: The study was conducted according to the guidelines of the Declaration of Helsinki, and approved by the Institutional Review Board (or Ethics Committee) of Radiation Medicine Chinese Academy of Medical Sciences (IRM-DWLL-2018104, November 20, 2018).

ETHICS STATEMENT

The animal study was reviewed and approved by the Institutional Review Board (or Ethics Committee) of Radiation Medicine Chinese Academy of Medical Sciences.

AUTHOR CONTRIBUTIONS

JWZ, JZ, and LZ designed the research; MR, TY, XX, PJ, and LZ performed the experiments; MR, LC, SS, XL, and SZ analyzed data; MR, JWZ, and LC wrote the paper; JWZ, JZ, and LZ read and revised the manuscript.

REFERENCES

Andersson, U., and Tracey, K. J. (2011). HMGB1 Is a Therapeutic Target for Sterile Inflammation and Infection. *Annu. Rev. Immunol.* 29, 139–162. doi:10.1146/annurev-immunol-030409-101323

Ashby, K., Navarro Almario, E. E., Tong, W., Borlak, J., Mehta, R., and Chen, M. (2018). Review Article: Therapeutic Bile Acids and the Risks for Hepatotoxicity. *Aliment. Pharmacol. Ther.* 47 (12), 1623 1638. doi:10.1111/apt.14678

Battino, M., Giampieri, F., Pistollato, F., Sureda, A., de Oliveira, M. R., Pittalà, V., et al. (2018). Nrf2 as Regulator of Innate Immunity: A Molecular Swiss Army Knife!. *Biotechnol. Adv.* 36 (2), 358–370. doi:10.1016/j.biotechadv.2017.12.012

Cai, S.-Y., Ouyang, X., Chen, Y., Soroka, C. J., Wang, J., Mennone, A., et al. (2017). Bile Acids Initiate Cholestatic Liver Injury by Triggering a Hepatocyte-specific Inflammatory Response. *JCI insight* 2 (5), e90780. doi:10.1172/jci.insight.90780

Chen, T., Xie, G., Wang, X., Fan, J., Qiu, Y., Zheng, X., et al. (2011). Serum and Urine Metabolite Profiling Reveals Potential Biomarkers of Human Hepatocellular Carcinoma. *Mol. Cell Proteomics* 10 (7), M110004945. doi:10.1074/mcp.M110.004945

Chiang, J. Y. L., and Ferrell, J. M. (2019). Bile Acids as Metabolic Regulators and Nutrient Sensors. *Annu. Rev. Nutr.* 39, 175–200. doi:10.1146/annurev-nutr-082018-124344

Combes, B., Carithers, R. L., Maddrey, W. C., Munoz, S., Garcia-Tsao, G., Bonner, G. F., et al. (1999). Biliary Bile Acids in Primary Biliary Cirrhosis: Effect of Ursodeoxycholic Acid. *Hepatology* 29 (6), 1649–1654. doi:10.1002/hep.510290618

de Aguiar Vallim, T. Q., Tarling, E. J., and Edwards, P. A. (2013). Pleiotropic Roles of Bile Acids in Metabolism. *Cell Metab* 17 (5), 657–669. doi:10.1016/j.cmet.2013.03.013

Degirolamo, C., Rainaldi, S., Bovenga, F., Murzilli, S., and Moschetta, A. (2014). Microbiota Modification with Probiotics Induces Hepatic Bile Acid Synthesis via Downregulation of the Fxr-Fgf15 axis in Mice. *Cel Rep.* 7 (1), 12–18. doi:10.1016/j.celrep.2014.02.032

Dondorf, F., Fahrner, R., Ardelt, M., Patsenker, E., Stickel, F., Dahmen, U., et al. (2017). Induction of Chronic Cholestasis without Liver Cirrhosis - Creation of an Animal Model. *Wjg* 23 (23), 4191–4199. doi:10.3748/wjg.v23.i23.4191

Eguchi, A., Wree, A., and Feldstein, A. E. (2014). Biomarkers of Liver Cell Death. *J. Hepatol.* 60 (5), 1063–1074. doi:10.1016/j.jhep.2013.12.026

Fickert, P., Hirschfield, G. M., Denk, G., Marschall, H.-U., Altorjay, I., Färkkilä, M., et al. (2017). norUrsodeoxycholic Acid Improves Cholestasis in Primary Sclerosing Cholangitis. *J. Hepatol.* 67 (3), 549–558. doi:10.1016/j.jhep.2017.05.009

Fickert, P., Pollheimer, M. J., Silbert, D., Moustafa, T., Halilbasic, E., Krones, E., et al. (2013). Differential Effects of norUDCA and UDCA in Obstructive Cholestasis in Mice. *J. Hepatol.* 58 (6), 1201–1208. doi:10.1016/j.jhep.2013.01.026

Fickert, P., Zollner, G., Fuchsbichler, A., Stumptner, C., Weiglein, A. H., Lammert, F., et al. (2002). Ursodeoxycholic Acid Aggravates Bile Infarcts in Bile Duct-Ligated and Mdr2 Knockout Mice via Disruption of Cholangioles. *Gastroenterology* 123 (4), 1238–1251. doi:10.1053/gast.2002.35948

Fuchs, C. D., Paumgartner, G., Mlitz, V., Kunczer, V., Halilbasic, E., Leditznig, N., et al. (2018). Colesevelam Attenuates Cholestatic Liver and Bile Duct Injury in Mdr2−/− Mice by Modulating Composition, Signalling and Excretion of Faecal Bile Acids. *Gut* 67 (9), 1683–1691. doi:10.1136/gutjnl-2017-314553

Galicia-Moreno, M., Lucano-Landeros, S., Monroy-Ramirez, H. C., Silva-Gomez, J., Gutierrez-Cuevas, J., Santos, A., et al. (2020). Roles of Nrf2 in Liver Diseases: Molecular, Pharmacological, and Epigenetic Aspects. *Antioxidants* 9 (10), 980. doi:10.3390/antiox9100980

Ge, X., Antoine, D. J., Lu, Y., Arriazu, E., Leung, T.-M., Klepper, A. L., et al. (2014). High Mobility Group Box-1 (HMGB1) Participates in the Pathogenesis of Alcoholic Liver Disease (ALD). *J. Biol. Chem.* 289 (33), 22672–22691. doi:10.1074/jbc.M114.552141

Ge, X., Arriazu, E., Magdaleno, F., Antoine, D. J., Dela Cruz, R., Theise, N., et al. (2018). High Mobility Group Box-1 Drives Fibrosis Progression Signaling via the Receptor for Advanced Glycation End Products in Mice. *Hepatology* 68 (6), 2380–2404. doi:10.1002/hep.30093

Gulamhusein, A. F., and Hirschfield, G. M. (2020). Primary Biliary Cholangitis: Pathogenesis and Therapeutic Opportunities. *Nat. Rev. Gastroenterol. Hepatolgastroenterology Hepatology* 17 (2), 93–110. doi:10.1038/s41575-019-0226-7

Hazari, Y., Bravo-San Pedro, J. M., Hetz, C., Galluzzi, L., and Kroemer, G. (2020). Autophagy in Hepatic Adaptation to Stress. *J. Hepatol.* 72 (1), 183–196. doi:10.1016/j.jhep.2019.08.026

Hu, Q.-W., and Liu, G.-T. (2006). Effects of Bicyclol on Dimethylnitrosamine-Induced Liver Fibrosis in Mice and its Mechanism of Action. *Life Sci.* 79 (6), 606–612. doi:10.1016/j.lfs.2006.02.025

Huang, H., Nace, G. W., McDonald, K.-A., Tai, S., Klune, J. R., Rosborough, B. R., et al. (2014). Hepatocyte-specific High-Mobility Group Box 1 Deletion Worsens the Injury in Liver Ischemia/reperfusion: a Role for Intracellular High-Mobility Group Box 1 in Cellular protection. *Hepatology* 59 (5), 1984–1997. doi:10.1002/hep.26976

Huang, M.-H., Li, H., Xue, R., Li, J., Wang, L., Cheng, J., et al. (2019). Up-regulation of Glycolipid Transfer Protein by Bicyclol Causes Spontaneous Restriction of Hepatitis C Virus Replication. *Acta Pharmaceutica Sinica. B* 9 (4), 769–781. doi:10.1016/j.apsb.2019.01.013

Huebener, P., Gwak, G.-Y., Pradere, J.-P., Quinzii, C. M., Friedman, R., Lin, C.-S., et al. (2014). High-mobility Group Box 1 Is Dispensable for Autophagy, Mitochondrial Quality Control, and Organ Function *In Vivo*. *Cel Metab.* 19 (3), 539–547. doi:10.1016/j.cmet.2014.01.014

Huebener, P., Pradere, J.-P., Hernandez, C., Gwak, G.-Y., Caviglia, J. M., Mu, X., et al. (2015). The HMGB1/RAGE axis Triggers Neutrophil-Mediated Injury Amplification Following Necrosis. *J. Clin. Invest.* 125 (2), 539–550. doi:10.1172/JCI76887

Huebener, P., Pradere, J.-P., Hernandez, C., Gwak, G.-Y., Caviglia, J. M., Mu, X., et al. (2019). The HMGB1/RAGE axis Triggers Neutrophil-Mediated Injury Amplification Following Necrosis. *J. Clin. Invest.* 129, 1802. doi:10.1172/JCI12697510.1172/jci126976

Ichimura, Y., and Komatsu, M. (2010). Selective Degradation of P62 by Autophagy. *Semin. Immunopathol* 32 (4), 431–436. doi:10.1007/s00281-010-0220-1

Ishak, K., Baptista, A., Bianchi, L., Callea, F., De Groote, J., Gudat, F., et al. (1995). Histological Grading and Staging of Chronic Hepatitis. *J. Hepatol.* 22 (6), 696–699. doi:10.1016/0168-8278(95)80226-6

Jia, W., Xie, G., and Jia, W. (2018). Bile Acid-Microbiota Crosstalk in Gastrointestinal Inflammation and Carcinogenesis. *Nat. Rev. Gastroenterol. Hepatol.* 15 (2), 111–128. doi:10.1038/nrgastro.2017.119

Jiang, T., Harder, B., Rojo de la Vega, M., Wong, P. K., Chapman, E., and Zhang, D. D. (2015). p62 Links Autophagy and Nrf2 Signaling. *Free Radic. Biol. Med.* 88 (Pt B), 199–204. doi:10.1016/j.freeradbiomed.2015.06.014

Kang, R., Livesey, K. M., Zeh, III, H. J., Lotze, M. T., and Tang, D. (2011). HMGB1 as an Autophagy Sensor in Oxidative Stress. *Autophagy* 7 (8), 904–906. doi:10.4161/auto.7.8.15704

Kerr, T. A., Saeki, S., Schneider, M., Schaefer, K., Berdy, S., Redder, T., et al. (2002). Loss of Nuclear Receptor SHP Impairs but Does Not Eliminate Negative Feedback Regulation of Bile Acid Synthesis. *Developmental Cel.* 2 (6), 713–720. doi:10.1016/s1534-5807(02)00154-5

Khambu, B., Huda, N., Chen, X., Antoine, D. J., Li, Y., Dai, G., et al. (2018). HMGB1 Promotes Ductular Reaction and Tumorigenesis in Autophagy-Deficient Livers. *J. Clin. Invest.* 128 (6), 2419–2435. doi:10.1172/JCI91814

Komatsu, M., Kurokawa, H., Waguri, S., Taguchi, K., Kobayashi, A., Ichimura, Y., et al. (2010). The Selective Autophagy Substrate P62 Activates the Stress Responsive Transcription Factor Nrf2 through Inactivation of Keap1. *Nat. Cel Biol.* 12 (3), 213–223. doi:10.1038/ncb2021

Kuma, A., Komatsu, M., and Mizushima, N. (2017). Autophagy-monitoring and Autophagy-Deficient Mice. *Autophagy* 13 (10), 1619–1628. doi:10.1080/15548627.2017.1343770

Leung, K. K., Deeb, M., and Hirschfield, G. M. (2020). Review Article: Pathophysiology and Management of Primary Biliary Cholangitis. *Aliment. Pharmacol. Ther.* 52 (7), 1150–1164. doi:10.1111/apt.16023

Li, H., Li, J.-R., Huang, M.-H., Chen, J.-H., Lv, X.-Q., Zou, L.-L., et al. (2018). Bicyclol Attenuates Liver Inflammation Induced by Infection of Hepatitis C Virus via Repressing ROS-Mediated Activation of MAPK/NF-κB Signaling Pathway. *Front. Pharmacol.* 9, 1438. doi:10.3389/fphar.2018.01438

Li, T., Matozel, M., Boehme, S., Kong, B., Nilsson, L.-M., Guo, G., et al. (2011). Overexpression of Cholesterol 7α-Hydroxylase Promotes Hepatic Bile Acid Synthesis and Secretion and Maintains Cholesterol Homeostasis. *Hepatology* 53 (3), 996–1006. doi:10.1002/hep.24107

Liu, Y., Chen, K., Li, F., Gu, Z., Liu, Q., He, L., et al. (2020). Probiotic Lactobacillus Rhamnosus GG Prevents Liver Fibrosis through Inhibiting Hepatic Bile Acid Synthesis and Enhancing Bile Acid Excretion in Mice. *Hepatology* 71 (6), 2050–2066. doi:10.1002/hep.30975

Qian, M., Fang, X., and Wang, X. (2017). Autophagy and Inflammation. *Clin. translational Med.* 6 (1), 24. doi:10.1186/s40169-017-0154-5

Russell, D. W. (2003). The Enzymes, Regulation, and Genetics of Bile Acid Synthesis. *Annu. Rev. Biochem.* 72, 137–174. doi:10.1146/annurev.biochem.72.121801.161712

Shen, K., Feng, X., Pan, H., Zhang, F., Xie, H., and Zheng, S. (2017). Baicalin Ameliorates Experimental Liver Cholestasis in Mice by Modulation of

Oxidative Stress, Inflammation, and NRF2 Transcription Factor. *Oxidative Med. Cell. longevity* 2017, 1–11. doi:10.1155/2017/6169128
Shin, S. M., Yang, J. H., and Ki, S. H. (2013). Role of the Nrf2-ARE Pathway in Liver Diseases. *Oxidative Med. Cell. longevity* 2013, 1–9. doi:10.1155/2013/763257
Sun, X., Ou, Z., Chen, R., Niu, X., Chen, D., Kang, R., et al. (2016). Activation of the P62-Keap1-NRF2 Pathway Protects against Ferroptosis in Hepatocellular Carcinoma Cells. *Hepatology* 63 (1), 173–184. doi:10.1002/hep.28251
Sun, X., and Tang, D. (2014). HMGB1-dependent and -independent Autophagy. *Autophagy* 10 (10), 1873–1876. doi:10.4161/auto.32184
Szabo, G., and Csak, T. (2012). Inflammasomes in Liver Diseases. *J. Hepatol.* 57 (3), 642–654. doi:10.1016/j.jhep.2012.03.035
Tang, D., Kang, R., Livesey, K. M., Cheh, C.-W., Farkas, A., Loughran, P., et al. (2010). Endogenous HMGB1 Regulates Autophagy. *J. Cel. Biol.* 190 (5), 881–892. doi:10.1083/jcb.200911078
Tian, Y., Gui, W., Koo, I., Smith, P. B., Allman, E. L., Nichols, R. G., et al. (2020). The Microbiome Modulating Activity of Bile Acids. *Gut microbes* 11 (4), 979–996. doi:10.1080/19490976.2020.1732268
Wagner, M., and Fickert, P. (2020). Drug Therapies for Chronic Cholestatic Liver Diseases. *Annu. Rev. Pharmacol. Toxicol.* 60, 503–527. doi:10.1146/annurev-pharmtox-010818-021059
Wagner, M., Zollner, G., and Trauner, M. (2011). Nuclear Receptors in Liver Disease. *Hepatology* 53 (3), 1023–1034. doi:10.1002/hep.24148
Wang, G., Xiu, P., Li, F., Xin, C., and Li, K. (2014). Vitamin A Supplementation Alleviates Extrahepatic Cholestasis Liver Injury through Nrf2 Activation. *Oxidative Med. Cell. longevity* 2014, 1–10. doi:10.1155/2014/273692
Wang, X., Xie, G., Zhao, A., Zheng, X., Huang, F., Wang, Y., et al. (2016a). Serum Bile Acids Are Associated with Pathological Progression of Hepatitis B-Induced Cirrhosis. *J. Proteome Res.* 15 (4), 1126–1134. doi:10.1021/acs.jproteome.5b00217
Wang, Y., Nie, H., Zhao, X., Qin, Y., and Gong, X. (2016b). Bicyclol Induces Cell Cycle Arrest and Autophagy in HepG2 Human Hepatocellular Carcinoma Cells through the PI3K/AKT and Ras/Raf/MEK/ERK Pathways. *BMC cancer* 16 (1), 742. doi:10.1186/s12885-016-2767-2
Weerachayaphorn, J., Mennone, A., Soroka, C. J., Harry, K., Hagey, L. R., Kensler, T. W., et al. (2012). Nuclear Factor-E2-Related Factor 2 Is a Major Determinant of Bile Acid Homeostasis in the Liver and Intestine. *Am. J. Physiology-Gastrointestinal Liver Physiol.* 302 (9), G925–G936. doi:10.1152/ajpgi.00263.2011
Wiest, R., Lawson, M., and Geuking, M. (2014). Pathological Bacterial Translocation in Liver Cirrhosis. *J. Hepatol.* 60 (1), 197–209. doi:10.1016/j.jhep.2013.07.044
Woolbright, B. L., Antoine, D. J., Jenkins, R. E., Bajt, M. L., Park, B. K., and Jaeschke, H. (2013). Plasma Biomarkers of Liver Injury and Inflammation Demonstrate a Lack of Apoptosis during Obstructive Cholestasis in Mice. *Toxicol. Appl. Pharmacol.* 273 (3), 524–531. doi:10.1016/j.taap.2013.09.023
Woolbright, B. L., Dorko, K., Antoine, D. J., Clarke, J. I., Gholami, P., Li, F., et al. (2015). Bile Acid-Induced Necrosis in Primary Human Hepatocytes and in Patients with Obstructive Cholestasis. *Toxicol. Appl. Pharmacol.* 283 (3), 168–177. doi:10.1016/j.taap.2015.01.015
Xu, D., Xu, M., Jeong, S., Qian, Y., Wu, H., Xia, Q., et al. (2018). The Role of Nrf2 in Liver Disease: Novel Molecular Mechanisms and Therapeutic Approaches. *Front. Pharmacol.* 9, 1428. doi:10.3389/fphar.2018.01428
Xu, Y., Li, F., Zalzala, M., Xu, J., Gonzalez, F. J., Adorini, L., et al. (2016). Farnesoid X Receptor Activation Increases Reverse Cholesterol Transport by Modulating Bile Acid Composition and Cholesterol Absorption in Mice. *Hepatology* 64 (4), 1072–1085. doi:10.1002/hep.28712
Yang, H., Ramani, K., Xia, M., Ko, K. S., Li, T. W. H., Oh, P., et al. (2009). Dysregulation of Glutathione Synthesis during Cholestasis in Mice: Molecular Mechanisms and Therapeutic Implications. *Hepatology* 49 (6), 1982–1991. doi:10.1002/hep.22908
Yang, T., Khan, G. J., Wu, Z., Wang, X., Zhang, L., and Jiang, Z. (2019). Bile Acid Homeostasis Paradigm and its Connotation with Cholestatic Liver Diseases. *Drug Discov. Today* 24 (1), 112–128. doi:10.1016/j.drudis.2018.09.007
Yang, T., Shu, T., Liu, G., Mei, H., Zhu, X., Huang, X., et al. (2017). Quantitative Profiling of 19 Bile Acids in Rat Plasma, Liver, Bile and Different Intestinal Section Contents to Investigate Bile Acid Homeostasis and the Application of Temporal Variation of Endogenous Bile Acids. *J. Steroid Biochem. Mol. Biol.* 172, 69–78. doi:10.1016/j.jsbmb.2017.05.015
Yokoda, R. T., and Carey, E. J. (2019). Primary Biliary Cholangitis and Primary Sclerosing Cholangitis. *Am. J. Gastroenterol.* 114 (10), 1593–1605. doi:10.14309/ajg.0000000000000268
Zhang, J., Fu, B., Zhang, X., Zhang, L., Bai, X., Zhao, X., et al. (2014). Bicyclol Upregulates Transcription Factor Nrf2, HO-1 Expression and Protects Rat Brains against Focal Ischemia. *Brain Res. Bull.* 100, 38–43. doi:10.1016/j.brainresbull.2013.11.001
Zhang, S., Wang, Z., Zhu, J., Xu, T., Zhao, Y., Zhao, H., et al. (2017a). Carnosic Acid Alleviates BDL-Induced Liver Fibrosis through miR-29b-3p-Mediated Inhibition of the High-Mobility Group Box 1/Toll-like Receptor 4 Signaling Pathway in Rats. *Front. Pharmacol.* 8, 976. doi:10.3389/fphar.2017.00976
Zhang, Y., Xu, Y., Qi, Y., Xu, L., Song, S., Yin, L., et al. (2017b). Protective Effects of Dioscin against Doxorubicin-Induced Nephrotoxicity via Adjusting FXR-Mediated Oxidative Stress and Inflammation. *Toxicology* 378, 53–64. doi:10.1016/j.tox.2017.01.007
Zhao, T.-M., Wang, Y., Deng, Y., Fan, X.-F., Cao, X.-C., Hou, L.-J., et al. (2020). Bicyclol Attenuates Acute Liver Injury by Activating Autophagy, Anti-oxidative and Anti-inflammatory Capabilities in Mice. *Front. Pharmacol.* 11, 463. doi:10.3389/fphar.2020.00463
Zhen, Y.-Z., Li, N.-R., He, H.-W., Zhao, S.-S., Zhang, G.-L., Hao, X.-F., et al. (2015). Protective Effect of Bicyclol against Bile Duct Ligation-Induced Hepatic Fibrosis in Rats. *Wjg* 21 (23), 7155–7164. doi:10.3748/wjg.v21.i23.7155

15

Metformin Exerts Anti-Inflammatory and Mucus Barrier Protective Effects by Enriching Akkermansia muciniphila in Mice with Ulcerative Colitis

Haoran Ke[1†], *Fang Li*[1,2†], *Wenlin Deng*[1,3†], *Zitong Li*[1†], *Siqi Wang*[1], *Pinjing Lv*[1] *and Ye Chen*[1*]

[1]*Department of Gastroenterology, State Key Laboratory of Organ Failure Research, Guangdong Provincial Key Laboratory of Gastroenterology, Nanfang Hospital, Southern Medical University, Guangzhou, China,* [2]*Hainan General Hospital, Haikou, China,* [3]*Department of Pediatrics, The Sixth Affiliated Hospital of Sun Yat-sen University, Guangzhou, China*

Correspondence:
Ye Chen
yechen@smu.edu.cn

[†]*These authors have contributed equally to this work and share first authorship*

The present study aimed to determine if metformin exerts anti-inflammatory and mucus-protective effects *via* the gut microbiota. Metformin has extensive benefits including anti-inflammatory effects. Previous studies showed that metformin changed the gut microbiota composition and increases the number of goblet cells. Intestinal dysbiosis and goblet cell depletion are important features of ulcerative colitis (UC). The underlying mechanism and whether metformin can improve the mucus barrier in UC remain unclear. Metformin (400 mg/kg/day) was administered to mice with dextran sulfate sodium (DSS)-induced UC for 2 wk to investigate the effects of metformin on the intestinal mucus barrier. The gut microbiota was depleted, using antibiotics, to explore its role in the mucus-protecting effects of metformin. *Akkermansia muciniphila (A. muciniphila)*, which was enriched in metformin-treated mice, was administered to mice to investigate the effects of the bacteria on UC and the mucus barrier. Metformin attenuated DSS-induced UC in mice, as evidenced by the alleviation of diarrhea, hematochezia, and the decrease in body weight. The expression of mucin2, a prominent mucus barrier protein, was increased in the metformin-treated group compared to the DSS-treated group. Furthermore, fecal 16S rRNA analysis showed that metformin treatment changed the gut microbiota composition by increasing the relative abundance of *Lactobacillus* and *Akkermansia* species while decreasing *Erysipelatoclostridium* at the genus level. Antibiotic treatment partly abolished the anti-inflammatory and mucus-protecting effects of metformin. Administration of *A. muciniphila* alleviated the colonic inflammation and mucus barrier disruption. Metformin alleviated DSS-induced UC in mice and protected against cell damage *via* affecting the gut microbiota, thereby providing a new mechanism for the therapeutic effect of metformin in patients with UC. This study also provides evidence that *A. muciniphila* as a probiotic has potential benefits for UC.

Keywords: intestinal barrier, inflammatory bowel diseases, probiotics, gut microbiota, mucin2

INTRODUCTION

Ulcerative colitis (UC), characterized by chronic and relapsing inflammation in the colon, is becoming a global disease (M'Koma, 2013). However, the underlying pathogenesis of UC is incompletely understood. It is thought to involve genetic factors, abnormal immune responses, environmental factors, intestinal barrier dysfunction, and dysbiosis (Zhang and Li, 2014; Testa et al., 2017; Ungaro et al., 2017). Goblet cell depletion and gut dysbiosis are important features of UC (Strugala et al., 2008; Gersemann et al., 2009; Johansson et al., 2014).

Mucus barrier dysfunction plays a significant role in the pathogenesis of UC. The mucus barrier, organized by the Mucin2 (Muc2) mucin, is a gel that covers the intestinal epithelium (Johansson and Hansson, 2011; Kühn and Klar, 2015). Several studies have shown that the thickness of the mucus is decreased in wild-type mice with DSS-induced UC, while Muc2-deficient mice developed spontaneous UC and were more susceptible to DSS-induced colitis (Van der Sluis et al., 2006; Heazlewood et al., 2008; Petersson et al., 2010). The mucus barrier is also impaired in patients with UC (Shen et al., 2018) (Van der Post et al., 2019).

The gut microbiota plays an important role in the pathogenesis of UC. The composition, diversity and richness of the gut microbiota are altered in patients with inflammatory bowel disease (IBD) (Knox et al., 2019) and are related to disease severity as well as treatment efficacy (Zhou et al., 2018). Furthermore, in animal models, the absence of gut microbiota reduces inflammation in the mouse colon (Hernández-Chirlaque et al., 2016). The manipulation of the microbiota by fecal microbiota transplantation (FMT) or administration of probiotics may have potential benefits in the treatment of IBD (Shen et al., 2014; Paramsothy et al., 2017).

Metformin, with a relatively low cost and a superior safety profile, is the first-line treatment for type 2 diabetes (McCreight et al., 2016). Recent studies have demonstrated that metformin has extensive benefits, besides its anti-diabetic effects, including anticancer effects (Leone et al., 2014), cardiovascular benefits (Rena and Lang, 2018; Van der Post et al., 2019), anti-aging effects (Anisimov, 2013), and anti-inflammatory effects (Saisho, 2015; Cameron Amy et al., 2016). In particular, metformin treatment increases the number of goblet cells in the intestine (Shin et al., 2014; Xue et al., 2016), indicating that metformin may have mucus protective effects. Several studies have established that metformin can attenuate colitis in mice by suppressing nuclear factor kappa-light-chain-enhancer of activated B cells (NF-kB) (Koh et al., 2014), Phosphorylated-Signal transducer and activator of transcription 3 (pSTAT3) (Lee et al., 2015), Jun N-terminal kinases (JNK) (Deng et al., 2018) and p38 mitogen-activated protein kinase (MAPK) activation (Di Fusco et al., 2018). However, most of these studies focus on the mechanisms involved in the host factor and the influence of gut microbiota on the therapeutic effects of metformin in colitis the is not fully understood.

Metformin can alter the gut microbiota by increasing the abundance of *Akkermansia muciniphila (A. muciniphila)* and *Lactobacillus* (Hur and Lee, 2015; Bauer et al., 2018; Zhang, 2019), both of which have an anti-inflammatory profile. Emerging evidence shows that *A. muciniphila* is decreased in inflammatory bowel diseases, which is negatively associated with inflammation scores (Png et al., 2010; Rajilić-Stojanović et al., 2013; Earley et al., 2019). *Lactobacillus* also shows potential benefits for IBD, as it has anti-inflammatory and gut barrier-protective effects (Vich Vila et al., 2018). The gut microbiota also has significant impacts on the mucus barrier: gut microbiota and their bacterial products regulate Muc2 secretion by goblet cells, and, hence, the properties of the mucus barrier (Petersson et al., 2010; Jakobsson et al., 2015; Birchenough et al., 2016). These studies suggest that gut microbiota altered by metformin may play a critical role in its anti-inflammatory effects. However, whether metformin exerts its anti-inflammatory and mucus barrier protective effects in UC *via* affecting the gut microbiota has not been determined.

Here, the present study proved that metformin exerted its anti-inflammatory and mucus-protective effects *via* affecting the gut microbiota, particularly, *via* enriching *A. muciniphila*.

METHODS

Animal Model

All animal studies were carried out in specific pathogen-free (SPF) laboratory of the Department of Laboratory Animal, Southern Medical University, in accordance with the guidelines of the Southern Medical University Committee for Experimental Animals. And the protocols were approved by the Animal Experimental Ethics Committee of the Southern Medical University, China (**L2018225**). Wild-type male C57BL/6 mice (6–8-wk-old) ranging from 20 to 25 g in weight were purchased from the Animal Center of the Southern Medical University in China. The animals were housed at 22–24°C with an artificial 12 h/12 h day/night cycle in SPF conditions. Mice (6–8-wk-old) were treated with metformin (400 mg/kg/d), administered *via* oral gavage, 7 days before dextran sulfate sodium salt (DSS) treatment, and then in parallel with DSS treatment. Colitis in mice was induced as previously described (Chassaing et al., 2014). To be brief, DSS (MPbio, Solon, OH, United States) (2% w/v), with a molecular weight of 36,000–50,000 Da, was added to drinking water and administered to the mice for 6 days, followed by 1 day of regular water administration. The disease activity index (DAI) was evaluated after DSS administration as previously described (Wang et al., 2015). Fecal samples were collected on day 6 following DSS treatment. The mice were anesthetized by 100 mg/kg pentobarbital sodium (provide by the Department of Laboratory Animal, Nanfang Hospital) and euthanized by using cervical dislocation on day 7 after DSS treatment and the colons were removed.

Depletion of the Gut Microbiota Using Antibiotics

The gut microbiota of mice was depleted according to a method described previously (Chen et al., 2020) with minor adjustments.

Mice were administered with an antibiotic cocktail consisting of vancomycin 100 mg/kg/day, metronidazole 200 mg/kg/day, gentamicin 40 mg/kg/day, and ampicillin 200 mg/kg/day. The antibiotic cocktail was administered to the mice by oral gavage for 5 days prior to metformin treatment and the induction of experimental colitis described above. The fecal substance was collected on day 5 to evaluate the effect of the antibiotic treatment on the gut microbiota by using gel electrophoresis.

Bacterial Culture and Animal Treatment

Akkermansia muciniphila bacteria (ATTC BAA-835), purchased from ATCC (Manassas, VA, United States), were cultured anaerobically (80% N2, 10% CO2, and 10% H2) at 37°C in brain heart infusion (BHI) medium (Zhai et al., 2019) with an AnoxomatTM MarkII anaerobic system (Mart Microbiology). Bacteria used for oral gavage were washed once using 5 ml of anaerobic phosphate-buffered saline (PBS, pH = 7.4) after centrifugation, and then resuspended in anaerobic PBS. The mice were orally gavaged with 1.50×10^{11} CFU bacterial cells per kilogram of body weight per day for 7 days prior to DSS treatment and 6 days parallel with DSS treatment. All the experiments were performed according to the General Requirements for Biosafety (GB 19489-2008).

Histological Analysis

Tissues were embedded in paraffin and were cut into 4-μm sections and stained with hematoxylin and eosin (HE). The scores were assessed by two blinded investigators from the aspects of inflammation level, inflammation extent, crypt damage and involvement percentage according to the protocols devised by Deng et al. (Deng et al., 2018). Briefly, the level of inflammation was graded as (0) none; (1) slight; (2) moderate; (3) severe. The inflammation extent was graded as: (0) none; (1) mucosa; (2) mucosa and submucosa; (3) transmural. The crypt damage was graded on a scale from 0 to 4: (0) none; (1) basal 1/3 damaged; (2) basal 2/3 damaged; (3) only surface epithelium intact; (4) entire crypt and epithelium lost. These changes were quantified based on the percentage of disease process involvement as follows: (1) 1–25%; (2) 26–50%; (3) 51–75%; (4) 76–100% (**Supplementary Table S1**).

Immunofluorescence

Immunofluorescence staining was performed as previously described with minor modifications (Robertson et al., 2008). Sections were deparaffinized in xylene three times for 10 min, and their endogenous peroxidase was quenched for 15 min using 3% hydrogen peroxide in methanol. Subsequently, the sections were rehydrated using a graded ethanol series and antigen retrieval was performed using a sodium citrate buffer at a sub-boiling temperature for 10 min. The slides were then cooled at the bench-top and washed with PBS three times for 5 min, blocked with 10% BSA for 1 h, and incubated overnight at 4°C with the following primary antibodies: anti-MUC2 (1:200, #MA5-12345; Invitrogen), anti-Kruppel-like factor 4 (KLF4) (1:100, #ab129473; Abcam), anti-mouse atonal homolog 1 (MATH1) (1:300, #PA5-29392; Abcam), anti-hairy and enhancer of split type-1 (Hes1) (1:200, #ab71559; Abcam), anti-SAM pointed domain-containing ETS transcription factor (SPDEF) (1:100, #LS-C749124; LSBIO). After washing three times for 5 min with PBS, the slides were incubated with the appropriate secondary antibodies conjugated with a fluorescent label for 1 h at room temperature in the dark. The sections were washed three times for 5 min in PBS and incubated with 4′,6-diamidino-2-phenylindole (DAPI) for 3 min at room temperature followed by PBS washing for another three times. Finally, the slides were mounted and investigated under a fluorescence microscope (BX53F; Olympus, Tokyo, Japan) using cellSens Dimension software.

Alcian Blue-periodic Acid-Shiff (AB-PAS) Staining and Goblet Cell Counting

AB-PAS staining was performed using commercial kits (DG0007100; Solarbio, Beijing, China) according to the manufacturer's manual. The number of goblet cells was determined by counting the Alcian Blue positive vacuoles (Becker et al., 2013).

RNA Extraction

The total RNA from colon tissue was isolated using the Trizol method (Rio et al., 2010). Briefly, the colon samples were homogenized using 1 ml Trizol reagent per 80 mg of tissue. The homogenized samples were incubated for 10 min at room temperature. A total of 0.2 ml chloroform per 1 ml homogenized sample was used and the mixture was vortexed vigorously for 15 s. Then, the samples were incubated for 10 min at room temperature and centrifuged at 12,000 g for 10 min at 4°C. After centrifugation, the upper layer was transferred into a fresh tube. Then, 0.5 ml isopropyl alcohol was added to each tube and the samples were incubated for 10 min at room temperature. Next, the samples were centrifuged at 12,000 g for 10 min at 4°C and the supernatant was completely removed. A total of 1 ml of 75% ethanol was added per tube and the tube was washed gently. The samples were incubated for 10 min at room temperature and then centrifuged at 12,000 g for 10 min at 4°C. All the remaining ethanol was removed, the samples were air-dried and 20 μl diethylpyrocarbonate (DEPC) water was added per tube to dissolve the RNA.

Real-time Quantitative PCR (RT-qPCR)

First-strand cDNA was synthesized using the PrimeScript RT Master Mix (Takara) according to the manufacturer's manual, and RT-qPCR was performed using the Roche LightCycler 480II with the SYBR Premix Ex Taq. The primer sequences are provided in **Supplementary Table S2**. The $2^{\Delta\Delta CT}$ method was used to calculate the expression of the detected mRNA using β-actin as the reference gene (Deng et al., 2018).

DNA Extraction

DNA was extracted from fecal samples by using the TIANamp Stool DNA Kit (#DP328; TIANGEN Biotech) according to the manufacturer's instructions (Shao et al., 2017). The DNA was diluted to 1 ng/μl.

PCR Amplification

Fecal DNA was amplified using the TIANGEN 2× Taq PCR MasterMix (KT201), according to the manufacturer's manual

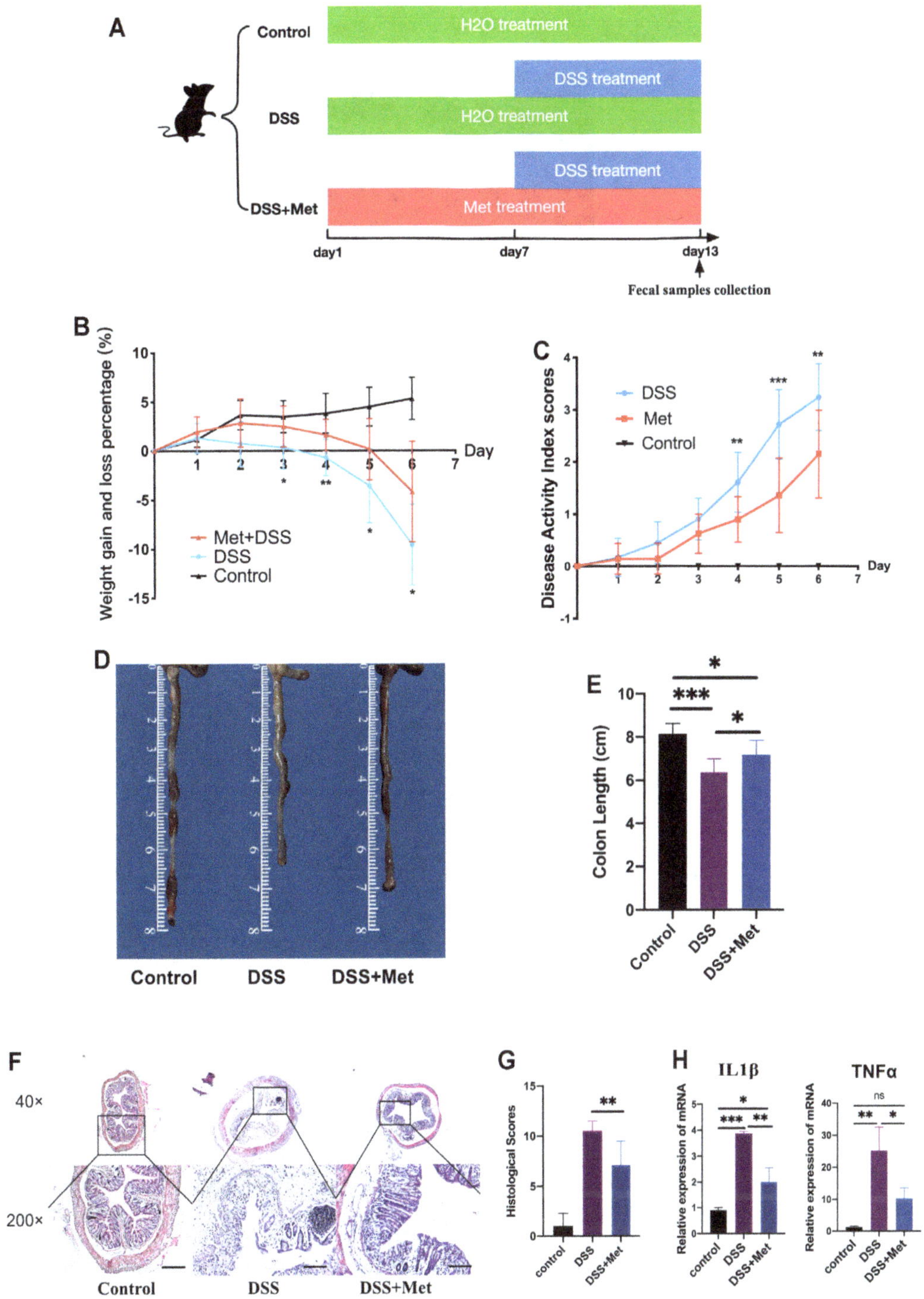

FIGURE 1 | Metformin alleviates dextran sulfate sodium (DSS)-induced ulcerative colitis (UC) in mice. Flow chart of animal treatment (n = 6–10) **(A)**, weight loss and gain (n = 6–10) **(B)**, disease activity index (DAI) scores (n = 6–10) **(C)**, representative pictures of the mouse colon (n = 6–10) **(D)**, colon length (n = 6–10) **(E)**, hematoxylin and eosin (HE) staining (scale bars, 400 μm) (n = 6–10) **(F)**, and histological scores (n = 6–10) **(G)**. RT-qPCR assay of tumor necrosis factor-α (TNF-α) and interleukin 1β (IL1β) in colon tissue (n = 3) **(H)** and statistical comparison was made using an ANOVA test followed by Tukey-Kramer *post-hoc* tests. $^{*}p < 0.05$, $^{**}p < 0.01$, $^{***}p < 0.001$.

and the V4 primers 514F (5′-GTGCCAGCMGCCGCGGTAA-3′) and 805R (5′-GGACTACHVGGGTWTCTAAT-3′) (Yin et al., 2015).

16S rRNA Sequencing

16S rRNA sequencing was performed as previously described (Janda and Abbott, 2007). Briefly, fecal DNA amplification

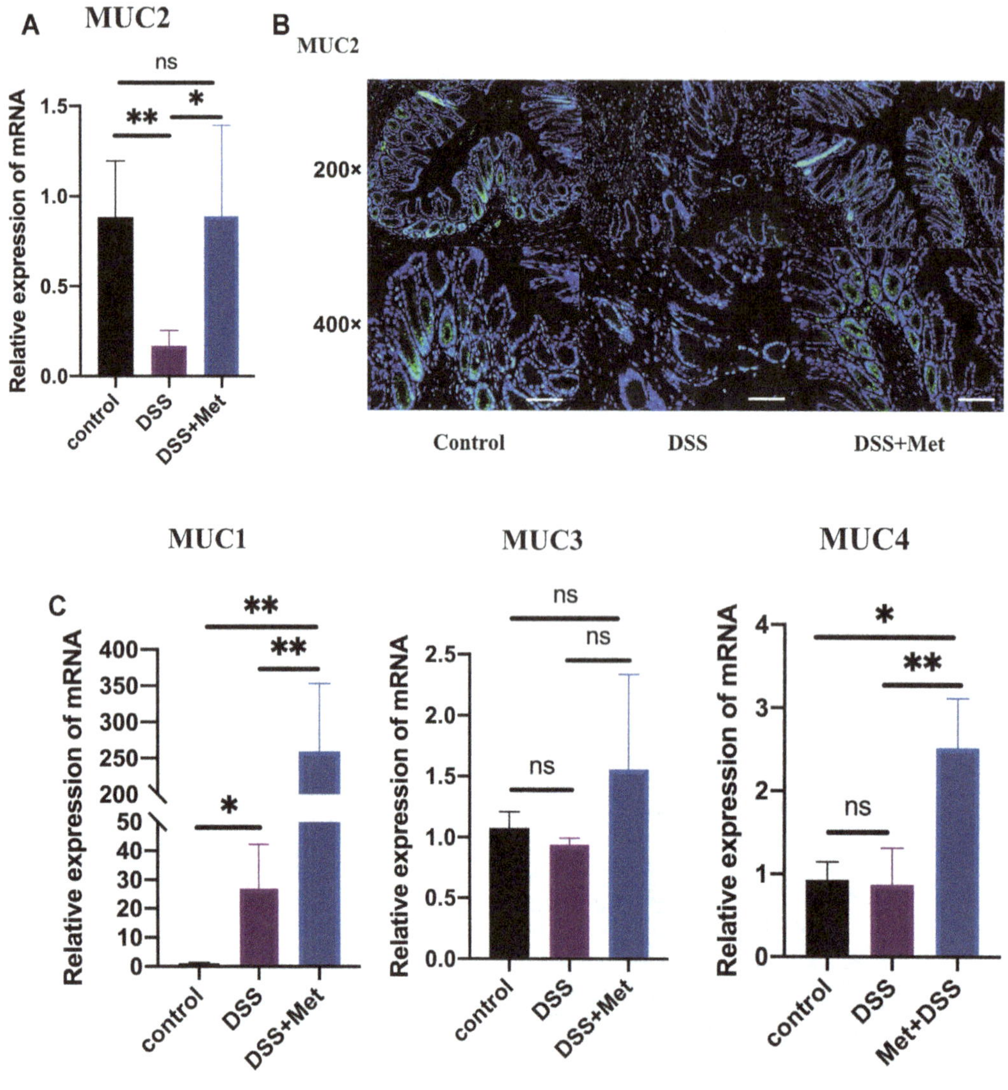

FIGURE 2 | Metformin protects the mucus barrier by increasing the expression of mucins in ulcerative colitis (UC). RT-qPCR assay of mucin 2 (MUC2) expression of colon tissue (n = 3–4) **(A)**, immunofluorescence assay showing the expression of mucin2 protein in colon tissue (scale bars, 200 μm) (n = 4) **(B)**, and RT-qPCR assay (n = 3–6) of the relative expression levels of MUC1, MUC3, and MUC4 in colon tissue at mRNA level **(C)** and statistical comparison was made using an ANOVA test followed by Tukey-Kramer *post-hoc* tests. $^{*}p < 0.05$, $^{**}p < 0.01$, $^{***}p < 0.001$, ns, no significance.

was performed using the TIANGEN 2× Taq PCR MasterMix (KT201), according to the manufacturer's manual. Amplification of the 16S/18S rRNA genes was performed using the specific primers with the barcodes: 16S V4: 515F-806R; 18S V4: 528F-706R; 18S V9: 1380F-1510R; ITS1: ITS5-1737F, ITS2-2043R; ITS2: ITS3-2024F, ITS4-2409R. Then, the PCR products were sequenced using the Illumina GAII (Illumina, San Diego, CA, United States) at the Beijing Genomic Institute (Shenzhen, China) and the data were clustered using the Illumina paired barcoded-sequencing (end) (BIPES) (PE) process for preliminary analysis. The rest of the sequences were screened by UCHIME and the suspected chimeric sequences were removed. All the reads were sorted into different samples according to their barcodes.

Statistical Analysis

All the data from at least three independent experiments were displayed as the mean ± standard deviation (SD). The student's t-test and/or one-way analysis of variance (ANOVA) with a proper post hoc Tukey-Kramer test comparison was carried out to determine if the differences were statistically significant. A p value of less than 0.05 was considered statistically significant.

RESULTS

Metformin Alleviated DSS-induced UC in Mice

To determine if metformin can attenuate colitis, mice were first treated with 2% DSS to induce colitis and then treated with

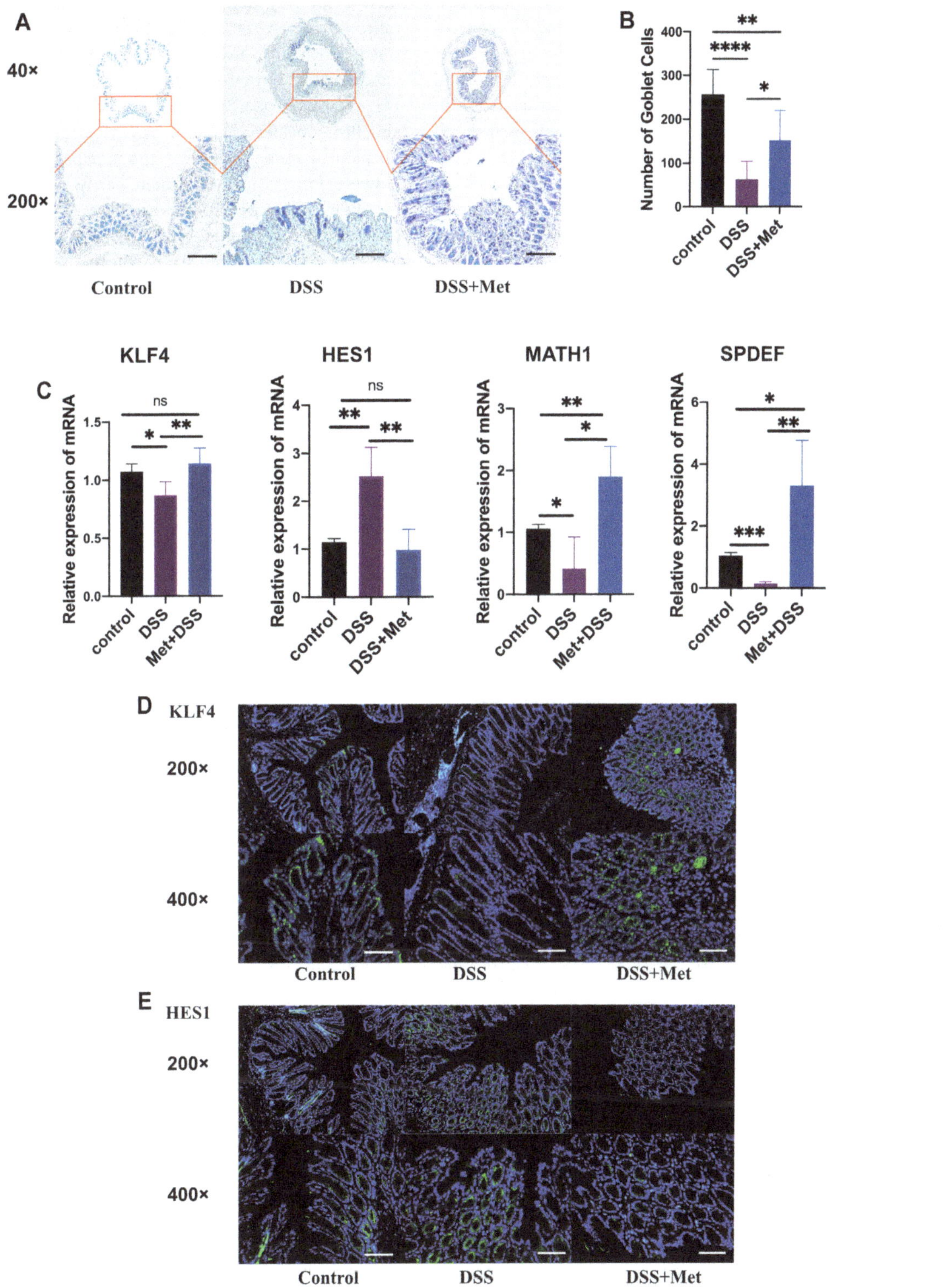

FIGURE 3 | Metformin positively regulates the differentiation of goblet cells. Alcian blue-periodic acid-Shiff (AB-PAS) staining of colon tissue (scale bars, 400 μm) (n = 4–7) **(A)** and count of goblet cells (n = 4–7) **(B)**, RT-qPCR assay (n = 3–6) of Kruppel-like factor 4 (KLF4), hairy and enhancer of split type-1 (HES1), MATH1 and SAM pointed domain containing ETS transcription factor (SPDEF) at the mRNA level **(C)**, immunofluorescence assay of Klf4 (scale bars, 200 m) (n = 4) **(D)** and Hes1 (scale bars, 200 μm) (n = 4) **(E)** protein detection in the mouse colon and statistical comparison was made using an ANOVA test followed by Tukey-Kramer *post-hoc* tests. $^{*}p < 0.05$, $^{**}p < 0.01$, $^{***}p < 0.001$.

400 mg/kg/day metformin or PBS solution (**Figure 1A**). Metformin reduced the severity of UC in mice as manifested by the reduced weight loss and less severe DAI scores (**Figures 1B,C**). Next, the colon length of mice was measured, and less colon length shortening was found in metformin-treated mice compared to mice treated with PBS (**Figures 1D,E**). Colon histology showed that metformin alleviated the damage and inflammation caused by DSS and reduced the histological scores (**Figures 1F,G**). The expression of pro-inflammatory cytokines interleukin 1β (IL1β) and tumor necrosis factor-α (TNF-α) in the colon were assessed. Consistent with previous results, metformin significantly reduced the level of IL1β and TNF-α (**Figure 1H**). These indicated that metformin had an anti-inflammatory effect.

Metformin Protected Against Mucus Barrier Dysfunction in DSS-induced UC

Mucus barrier dysfunction plays an important role in the pathogenesis of UC. The present study has shown that metformin can attenuate UC in mice. We explored the effects of metformin on the mucus barrier of the mouse colon. The expression of MUC2, the major component of the mucus barrier, was increased in DSS-induced colitis at the mRNA level (**Figure 2A**). Additionally, immunofluorescence assays were performed to assess the expression level of mucin2 protein. Metformin treatment also increased mucin2 expression at the protein level (**Figure 2B**). Mucin1 (Muc1), mucin3 (Muc3), and mucin4 (Muc4) are critical components of the colon mucus barrier. Metformin treatment significantly increased the expression of Mucl and Muc4 (**Figure 2C**). These results suggested that metformin can protect against mucus barrier dysfunction by increasing the expression of mucins, particularly that of mucin2, in the colon and thus contributed to its anti-inflammatory effect.

Metformin Positively Regulated the Differentiation of Goblet Cells

Mucin2 is synthesized and secreted by goblet cells. To explore the effects of metformin on goblet cells, the numbers of goblet cells in the colon were measured. Metformin treatment significantly increased the number of goblet cells (**Figures 3A,B**). KLF4, MATH1, SPDEF and HES1 play an important role in regulating the differentiation of goblet cells: KLF4, MATH1 and SPDEF can promote the differentiation of goblet cells while HES1 has an opposite effect. The expressions of them were assessed by RT-qPCR assays. Mice treated with metformin had a higher expression of KLF4, MATH1 and SPDEF and a lower expression of HES1 (**Figure 3C**). Furthermore, immunofluorescence assays showed that metformin treatment increased the expression of Klf4 and decreased that of Hes1 in colon tissue (**Figures 3D,E**), which suggested that metformin increased the number of goblet cells by promoting its differentiation.

Metformin Changed the Structure of the Gut Microbiota in DSS-induced UC in Mice

Previous studies have shown that metformin altered the structure of the gut microbiota of mice on a high-fat diet (Shin et al., 2014), which may play an important role in the anti-inflammatory and mucus-protective effects of metformin. 16S rRNA sequencing was performed to investigate the influence of metformin on the gut microbiota in DSS-induced UC in mice. At the phylum level, DSS treatment decreased the relative abundance of Bacteroidetes and Proteobacteria while it increased the relative abundance of Firmicutes compared with the normal control (**Figure 4A**). However, metformin treatment partly restored the structure of the gut microbiota in DSS-induced UC. The relative abundance of the phylum Bacteroidetes in the metformin group was increased, while the relative abundance of the phylum Firmicutes was decreased compared with the DSS group (**Figure 4A**). Furthermore, the relative abundance of the phylum Verrucomicrobia was increased after metformin treatment compared with the DSS and control groups (**Figure 4A**). At the genus level, metformin increased the abundance of *Bacteroides* and *Lactobacillus* compared with the DSS group. Metformin also increased the abundance of the genus *Akkermansia* compared with the DSS and control groups (**Figure 4B**). Increased or decreased Firmicutes/Bacteroidetes (F/B) ratio is regard as dysbiosis (Mariat et al., 2009). The F/B ratio increased by DSS treatment was lowered by metformin (**Figure 4C**), indicating that metformin reversed the dysbiosis in colitis mice. Importantly, the relative abundance of the genus *Akkermansia* was enriched in the metformin group (**Figure 4D**). These results showed that metformin can partly restore the structure of gut microbiota impaired by DSS treatment and enrich *Akkermansia* at the same time.

Antibiotic Treatment Abolished the Anti-inflammatory Effects of Metformin

To further investigate the effects of the gut microbiota on the anti-inflammatory beneficence of metformin, mice were treated with an antibiotic cocktail to deplete the gut microbiota (**Figure 5A**). The microbiota was depleted effectively after a 5-day antibiotic cocktail treatment (**Supplementary Figure S1**). There was no significant difference between the DSS and the antibiotics + DSS + metformin (abx + DSS + Met) group in weight loss and DAI (**Figures 5B,C**), which indicated that antibiotic treatment abolished the protective effects of metformin in DSS-induced UC. Mice in the abx + DSS + Met group also experienced more severe colon shortening compared with mice in the DSS + metformin (DSS + Met) group (**Figures 5D,E**). Histological analysis of colon tissue was performed for further verification. Although metformin inhibited the damage of colon tissue in DSS-induced UC, antibiotic treatment abolished these protective effects (**Figures 5F,G**), which suggested that gut microbiota is of great significance in the anti-inflammatory effects of metformin.

Antibiotic Treatment Abolished the Mucus-protective Effects of Metformin

Furthermore, the effects of the depletion of the gut microbiota on the mucus-protective effects of metformin were investigated by

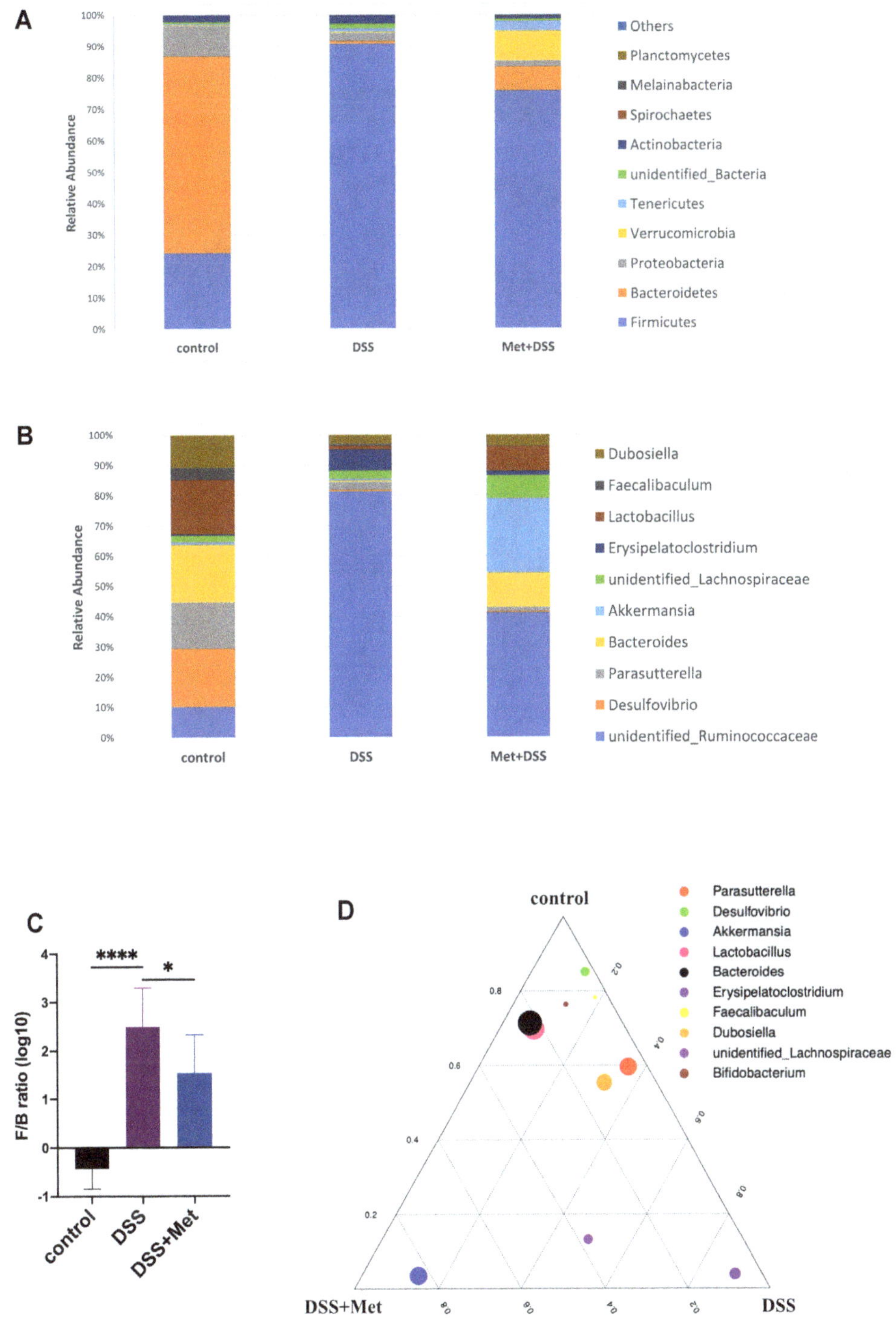

FIGURE 4 | Metformin changes the structure of the gut microbiota (*n* = 4–10). Fecal 16S rRNA sequencing of gut microbiota of the metformin, dextran sulfate sodium (DSS) and control group. Relative abundance (% of the total community) of 10 most abundant phyla **(A)** and 10 most abundant genera **(B)**, Firmicutes/Bacteroidetes (F/B) ratio (log10 transformation) **(C)** and ternary plot indicating the fraction of 10 most abundant genera in the metformin group (bottom left corner), dextran sulfate sodium (DSS) group (bottom right corner) and control group (top corner) with the size of each dot representing the relative abundance **(D)**.

assessing the number of goblet cells and the expression of mucin2 at the mRNA and protein levels. The number of goblet cells in the DSS + Met group was increased compared with that of the DSS group while antibiotics treatment abolished such effects (**Figures 6A,B**). Antibiotics also inhibited the metformin-induced expression of MUC2 at the mRNA level and of mucin2 at the

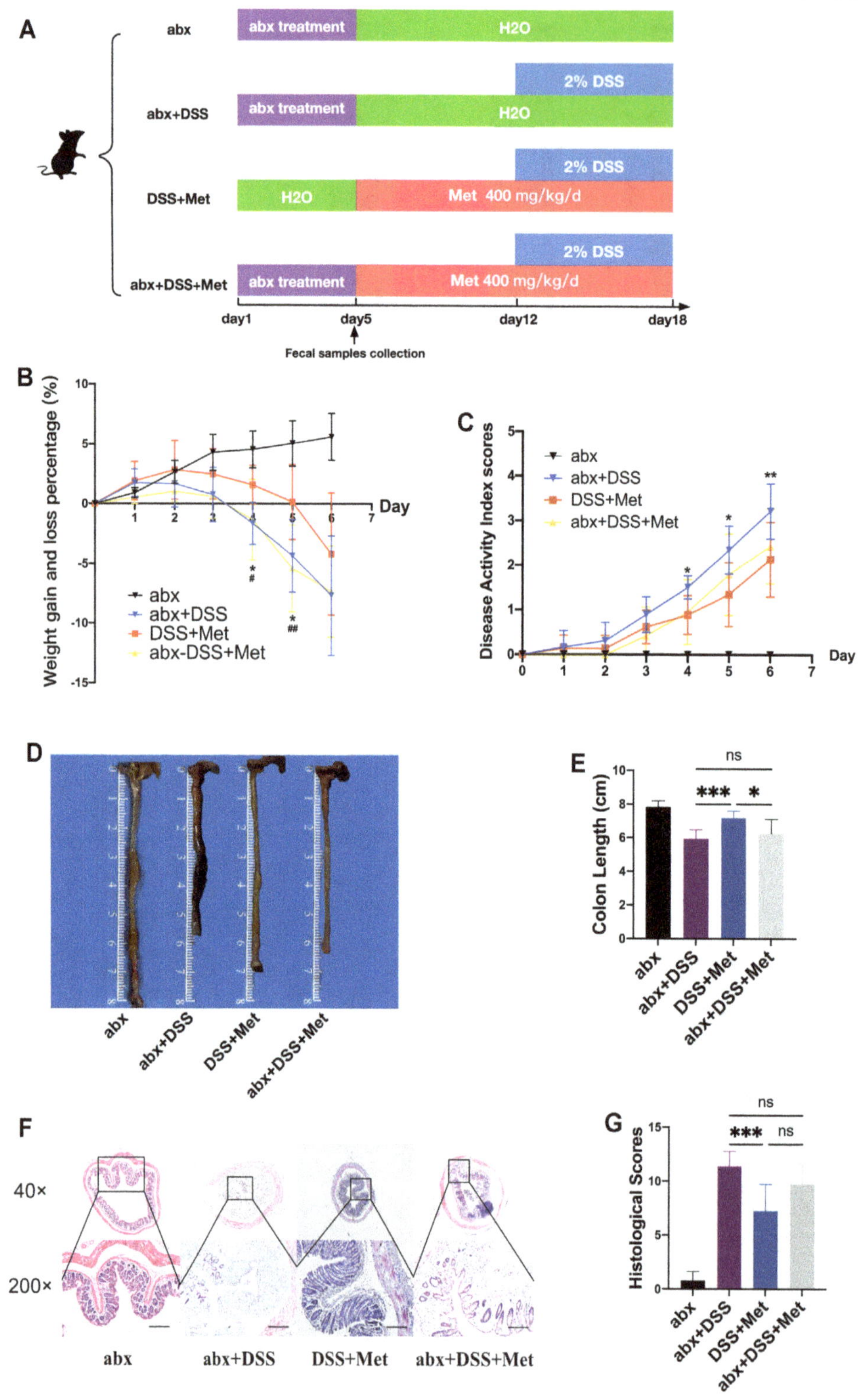

FIGURE 5 | Antibiotics abolish the anti-inflammatory effects of metformin. Flow chart of animal treatment **(A)**, weight loss and gain (n = 6–10) **(B)**, disease activity index (DAI) scores (n = 6–10) **(C)**, representative pictures of the mouse colon (n = 6–10) **(D)**, colon length (n = 6–10) **(E)**, hematoxylin and eosin (HE) staining (scale bars, 400 μm) **(F)**, histological scores (n = 5–8) **(G)** $^*p < 0.05$ (DSS+Met vs abx+DSS) and statistical comparison was made using an ANOVA test followed by Dunnett's *post-hoc* tests. $^{**}p < 0.01$, $^{***}p < 0.00$, $^{\#}p < 0.05$ (DSS+Met vs abx+DSS+Met), $^{\#\#}p < 0.01$.

protein level (**Figures 6C,D**). The mucus-protective effect of metformin was also influenced by gut microbiota.

A. muciniphila Exerted Anti-inflammatory and Mucus-protective Effects Similar to Those of Metformin

To explore whether *A. muciniphila* (akk)—which was enriched in the metformin group-exerts anti-inflammatory and mucus-barrier-protective effects like metformin, mice were administered with *A. muciniphila via* oral gavage (**Figure 7A**). *A. muciniphila* reduced weight loss (**Figures 7B,C**) and DAI scores (**Figure 7D**) in mice treated with DSS. Significant differences were found between the akk + DSS and DSS groups in colon length (**Figures 7E,F**) and histological scores (**Figures 7G,H**). Administration of *A. muciniphila* reduced the expression of TNF-α and IL1β, which were induced by DSS treatment (**Figure 7I**). In addition, *A. muciniphila* increased the number of goblet cells (**Figures 8A,B**) and the expression of mucin2 mucins (**Figures 8C,D**) compared with the DSS group, demonstrating that *A. muciniphila* has similar anti-inflammatory and mucus-protective effects.

DISCUSSION

The present study shows that metformin reduced colonic inflammation and protected against mucus barrier disruption along with an alteration of the gut microbiota during UC. Importantly, depletion of the gut microbiota partly abolished the anti-inflammatory and mucus-protective effects of metformin, indicating that metformin exerts its effects *via* the gut microbiota. Furthermore, administration of *A. muciniphila* alone, which was enriched in the metformin-treated group, to mice with DSS-induced UC mimicked the anti-inflammatory and mucus-protective effects of metformin. Based on these results the current study provides a critical understanding of the role of the gut microbiota in the anti-inflammatory and mucus-protective effects of metformin.

The results show that metformin mitigates the severity of mouse UC. Consistently, there is evidence showing that metformin exerts anti-inflammatory effects in mouse colitis: Di Fusco et al. reported that metformin reduced colonic inflammation by activating the AMP-activated protein kinase (AMPK) signaling pathway (Di Fusco et al., 2018); Lee et al. showed that metformin ameliorated colitis by suppressing STAT3 signaling *via* activating the AMPK signaling pathway (Lee et al., 2015). Deng et al. also has proved that metformin protected against intestinal barrier dysfunction *via* AMPKa1-dependent inhibition of JNK signaling activation and, thus, attenuated mouse colitis (Deng et al., 2018).

Accompanied by reduced colonic inflammation, metformin also restored the DSS-induced mucus barrier destruction by increasing the expression of mucin2, mucin1, mucin3, mucin4 and the number of goblet cells. Mucin1, mucin3 and mucin4 are transmembrane mucins. Their highly glycosylated extracellular domains can form a tight mesh structure and exert a barrier function. And their intracellular domains are involved in signaling pathways that regulate inflammation and cell differentiation (Putten and Strijbis, 2017). Mucin1 is upregulated in inflammation (Paone and Cani, 2020) which is consistent with the results of the present study. Mucin1 serves as a negative regulator of inflammation by suppressing the T helper 17-cell response (Nishida et al., 2012), toll-like receptor pathway and NLRP3 inflammasome complex activation (Dhar and McAuley, 2019), which may contribute to the anti-inflammatory effects of metformin in the current research. On the contrary, mucin3 and mucin4 are decreased during inflammation (Lindén et al., 2008). Mucin3 is negatively correlated with inflammation and dysbiosis levels (Algieri et al., 2021) *in vivo*, and can inhibit bacteria adherence *in vitro* (Pan et al., 2013). Kim et al. showed that mucin4 expression was decreased during DSS-induced colitis (Kim et al., 2019). However, contrary to Kim's and results of the present research, Song et al. found that mucin3 was increased in the azoxymethane (AOM)/DSS colon cancer mouse model (Song et al., 2018). These may be due to the different experimental models that were used. Consistently, Xue et al. showed that metformin treatment increased the number of goblet cells by promoting secretory cell lineage differentiation, and reduced colonic inflammation *via* AMPK activation in IL10-knockout mice (Xue et al., 2016). Shin et al. also found that metformin treatment increased the number of goblet cells in mice fed a high-fat diet (Shin et al., 2014). In the clinic, goblet cell depletion and mucus barrier disruption were common in UC patients (Swidsinski et al., 2007; Strugala et al., 2008; Van der Post et al., 2019). Furthermore, the abnormality of the mucus barrier plays an important role in the pathogenesis of UC. Previous studies have shown that the aberrant mucus barrier structure caused by Muc2 deficiency led to a more severe colonic inflammation in a mouse colitis model (Van der Sluis et al., 2006; Heazlewood et al., 2008; Petersson et al., 2010). In this study metformin also promoted the differentiation of goblet cells by increasing the expression of KLF4, MATH1 and SPDEF and decreasing that of HES1. Wnt and Notch signaling play a central role in the regulation of intestinal epithelium differentiation (van der Flier and Clevers, 2009). More specifically, Wnt signaling promotes secretory cells differentiation (i.e., goblet, Paneth and enteroendocrine cells) and Notch signaling is required for enterocyte development. KLF4, MATH1 and SPDEF, which are stimulated by the Wnt pathway and inhibited by the Notch pathway, are critical for goblet cells formation (Gregorieff et al., 2009; van der Flier and Clevers, 2009). HES1, on the contrary, is promoted by Notch signaling and inhibits goblet cells development by decreasing the expression of MATH1 (van der Flier and Clevers, 2009). These findings indicate that the mucus barrier may have a critical protective effect against UC and metformin exerts a mucus-protective effect in DSS-induced colitis. Thus, we conclude that the mucus-barrier-protective effects of metformin may be attributed to its anti-inflammatory effects in the colon.

Metformin is a widely used anti-diabetic treatment. The interaction between metformin and the gut microbiota has been reported in previous studies. The concentrations of

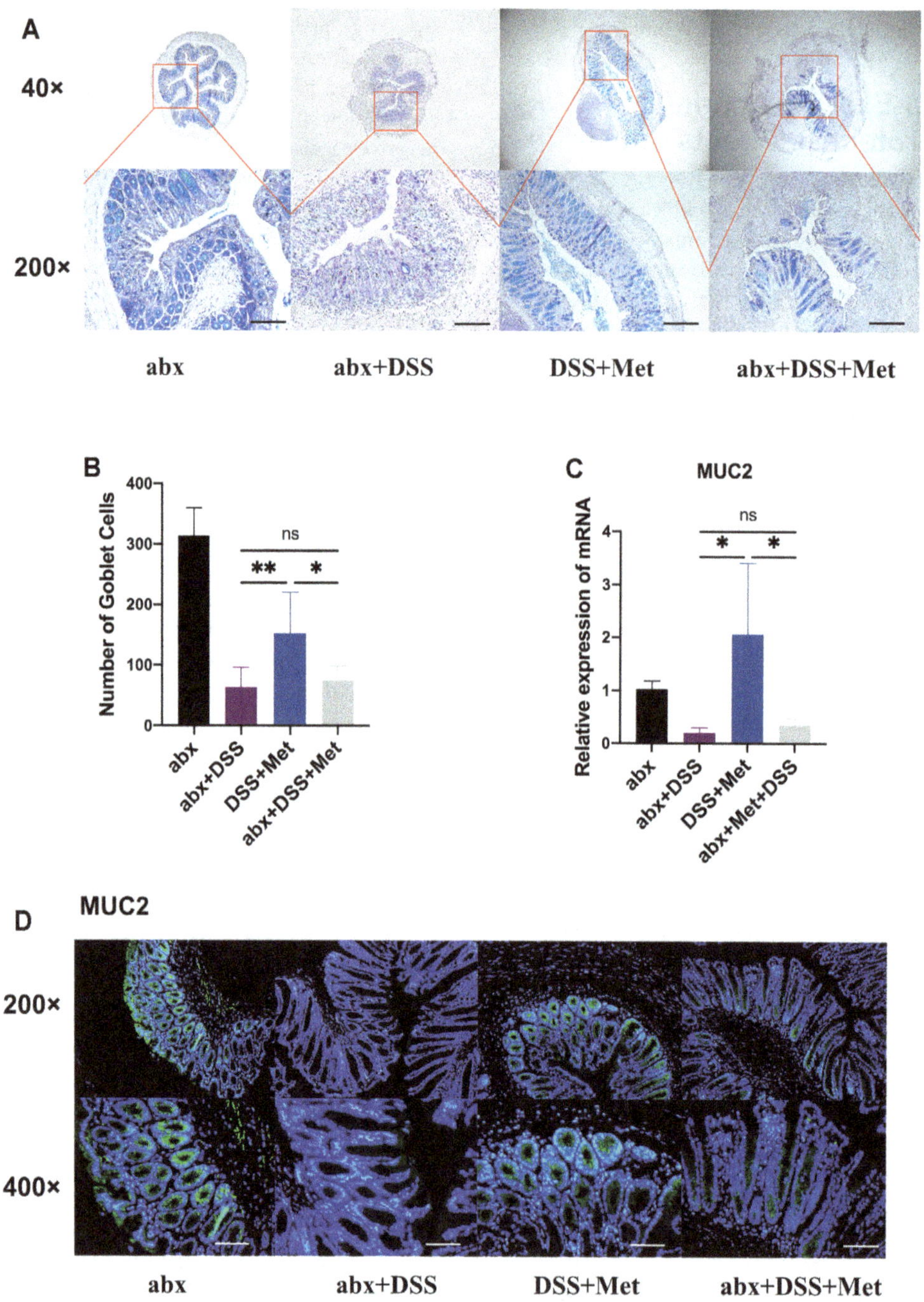

FIGURE 6 | Antibiotics abolish the mucus-protective effects of metformin. Alcian blue-periodic acid-Shiff (AB-PAS) staining (scale bars, 400 μm) (n = 5–7) **(A)** and count of goblet cells (n = 5–7) **(B)**, relative expression levels of mucin 2 (MUC2) (n = 3–4) **(C)**, and immunofluorescence assay of mucin2 protein in the mouse colon (scale bars, 200 μm) (n = 3) **(D)** and statistical comparison was made using an ANOVA test followed by Dunnett's *post-hoc* tests. $^*p < 0.05$, $^{**}p < 0.01$, $^{***}p < 0.001$.

metformin in the intestine are much higher than those in the plasma (Bailey et al., 2008). Shin et al. showed that metformin exerted its pharmacological effects by modulating the gut microbiota in a diet-induced diabetes mouse model (Shin et al., 2014). Similar results have been reported by Bauer et al. (Bauer et al., 2018). However, most of these studies focus on diabetes mellitus. Although the gut microbiota plays a critical role in the pathogenesis of UC (Zhang and Li, 2014; Testa et al., 2017; Ungaro et al., 2017), its role in the pharmacological effects of metformin on UC remains unclear. In the current study, we showed that metformin changed the structure of the gut microbiota. At the phylum level, the alteration of the gut microbiota in IBD remains controversial. Santoru et al. showed that the levels of Firmicutes and Proteobacteria were increased in IBD, whereas those of Bacteroidetes were decreased (Santoru et al., 2017). In contrast, Frank et al. reported that the

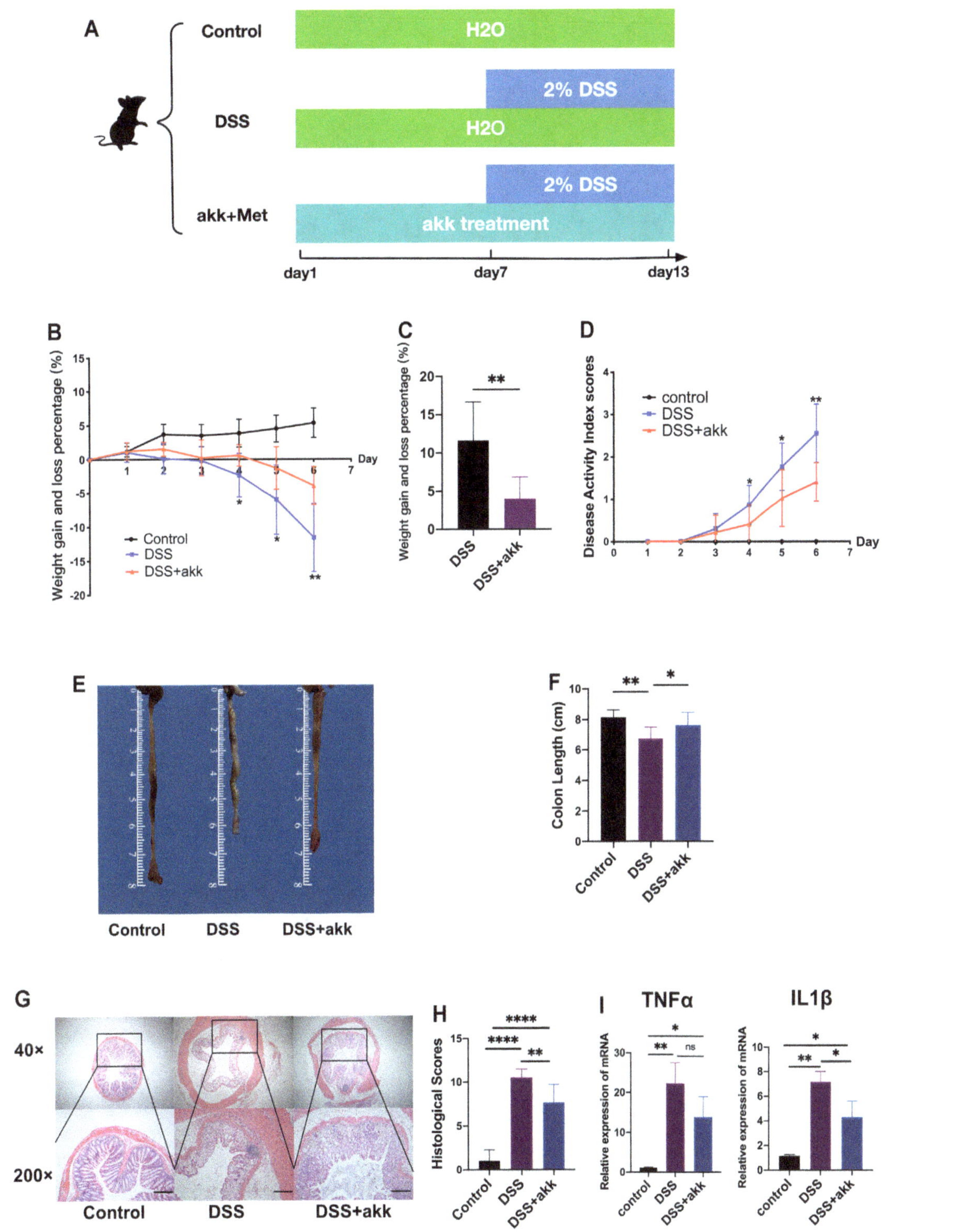

FIGURE 7 | *Akkermansia muciniphila* alleviates dextran sulfate sodium (DSS)-induced ulcerative colitis (UC) in mice. Flow chart of animal treatment **(A)**, weight loss and gain during DSS treatment (n = 6–14) **(B)** and weight loss percentage at day 6 (n = 6–14) **(C)**, disease activity index (DAI) scores (n = 6–14) **(D)**, representative pictures of the mouse colon (n = 6–14) **(E)**, colon length (n = 6–14) **(F)**, hematoxylin and eosin (HE) staining of colon tissue (scale bars, 400 μm) (n = 6–10) **(G)**, colon histological scores (n = 6–10) **(H)**, and RT-qPCR assay of tumor necrosis factor-α (TNF-α) and interleukin 1β (IL1β) in colon tissue (n = 2–6) **(I)** and statistical comparison was made using an ANOVA test followed by Tukey-Kramer *post-hoc* tests. *$p < 0.05$, **$p < 0.01$, ***$p < 0.001$.

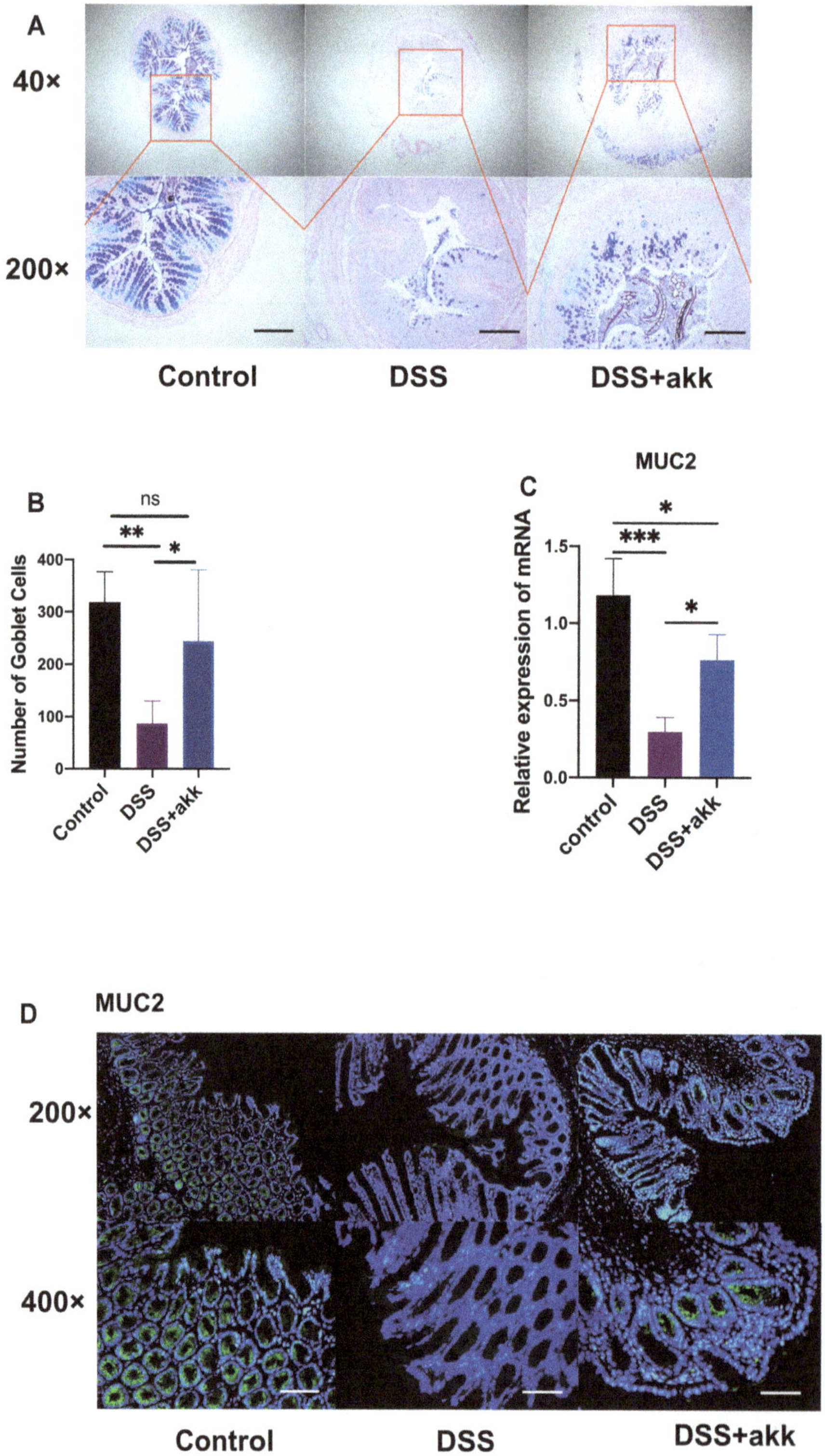

FIGURE 8 | *Akkermansia muciniphila* protects the mucus barrier in ulcerative colitis (UC). Alcian blue-periodic acid-Shiff (AB-PAS) staining of colon tissue (scale bars, 400 μm) (n = 6–7) **(A)** and count of goblet cells (n = 6–7) **(B)**, RT-qPCR assay of mucin 2 (MUC2) (n = 3–4) **(C)**, and immunofluorescence assay of mucin2 protein detection in colon tissue (scale bars, 200 μm) (n = 4) **(D)** and statistical comparison was made using an ANOVA test followed by Tukey-Kramer *post-hoc* tests. *$p < 0.05$, **$p < 0.01$, ***$p < 0.001$, ns, no significance.

levels of Firmicutes and Bacteroidetes were decreased in IBD (Frank et al., 2007). Furthermore, Walker et al. showed that Firmicutes levels were decreased while those of Bacteroidetes were increased in IBD (Walker et al., 2011). Although the results of these studies are contradictory, they are to a certain extent consistent with our results. Importantly, metformin treatment partly restored the structure of the gut microbiota which was altered by DSS treatment at the phylum level. Furthermore, similar results were found at the genus level. Moreover, metformin treatment increased the relative abundance of the genera *Bacteroides*, *Lactobacillus* and *Akkermansia*, which are considered to be potential probiotics (Shin et al., 2014; Bauer et al., 2018; Tan et al., 2019). Accordingly, the F/B ratio increased by DSS treatment was restored by metformin. F/B ratio is widely accepted as a significant marker for intestinal homeostasis-increased or decreased F/B ratio is regarded as dysbiosis (Mariat et al., 2009). Previous studies have shown that the F/B ratio was increased in the DSS model and decreased when colitis was alleviated (Rodríguez-Nogales et al., 2018; Yeo et al., 2020). Taken together, these findings suggest that metformin may exert its anti-inflammatory and mucus-protective effects *via* modulating the gut microbiota. To confirm the hypothesis, we administered an antibiotic cocktail to mice *via* oral gavage to deplete the gut microbiota and the anti-inflammatory and mucus-protective effects of metformin were partly abrogated. The gut microbiota also has an important role in shaping the mucus barrier (Jakobsson et al., 2015). In germ-free rats, the structure of mucus in the colon is impaired and the thickness is reduced (Schroeder, 2019). Bergström et al. reported that compared with germ-free mice, the presence of the microbiota increased the expression level of Muc2 (Bergström et al., 2012). Moreover, Troll et al. reported that the microbiota promoted the differentiation of goblet cells by activating the Notch signaling pathway (Troll et al., 2018).

Notably, in the current study, *A. muciniphila* was enriched only in the metformin-treated group. *A. muciniphila* is a gram-negative, anaerobic bacterium (Derrien, 2004) which has been reported to be decreased in patients with UC (Earley et al., 2019). Shin et al. have shown that metformin increased the levels of *A. muciniphila* in mice on a high-fat diet, improved glucose homeostasis, and, interestingly, increased the number of goblet cells (Shin et al., 2014). The present study found that administration of *A. muciniphila* reduced the colonic inflammation and protected the mucus barrier disruption in UC. Bian et al. reported that the severity of DSS-induced colitis in mice was relieved upon administration of A. muciniphila (Bian et al., 2019), whereas Kang et al. reported that extracellular vesicles derived from A. muciniphila protected against DSS-induced colitis (Kang et al., 2013). These results further confirmed that metformin exerted its therapeutic effects on UC *via* modulating the gut microbiota and increasing the levels of potential probiotics (e.g. *A. muciniphila*).

The doses of metformin that used in this study are similar to those in patients receiving metformin treatment. In clinical practice, patients typically receive 500–2000 mg metformin per day (Scarpello and Howlett, 2008). According to a method based on body surface area normalization (Nair and Jacob, 2016), the human equivalent dose of 400 mg/kg/d in mice is 32.43 mg/kg/day or 1946 mg per day for a 60 kg adult, which is within the recommended range. Although lower doses of metformin may have fewer side effects, DSS-treated mice receiving 100 mg/kg/day metformin (equivalent to 486 mg per day for human) or 200 mg/kg/day metformin (equivalent to 972 mg per day for human) had more weight loss and more severe DAI scores compared to those treated with DSS and 400 mg/kg/day metformin (**Supplementary Figure S2**) in the current experimental settings. The current study chose the dose of metformin at 400 mg/kg/day. However, further study may be needed to investigate the effects of lower doses of metformin especially from the aspects of adverse events.

The limitations of the present study should be also mentioned. First, instead of germ-free mice, which are inaccessible to our facility, antibiotic-treated mice were used to explore the role of the gut microbiota in the effects of metformin on UC. Compared with germ-free mice, which is considered to be the golden standard for the study of microbiota, antibiotic-treated models may be more inconsistent. However, an antibiotic-treated mouse model is a less expensive and more accessible alternative that has been widely used by many researchers for the study of microbiota (Kennedy et al., 2018). Second, although significant differences were not observed between conventional mice and antibiotic-treated mice in the DSS-induced colitis model (data not shown), other potential unknown effects of antibiotic treatment on DSS-induced colitis were not taken into account in the present study. DSS-induced colitis model is very popular in IBD research because of its rapidity, reproducibility and similarities to human IBD (Solomon et al., 2010; Chassaing et al., 2014). But the exact mechanism through which DSS initiates colitis is unknown (Solomon et al., 2010). Previous studies have successfully developed DSS-induced colitis in germ-free and antibiotic-treated “pseudo-germ-free” mice (Hudcovic et al., 2001; Hernández-Chirlaque et al., 2016; Gancarcikova et al., 2020), indicating that gut microbiota may not be indispensable for the initiation of DSS-induced colitis. In addition, the manifestations of DSS-induced colitis in antibiotic-treated “pseudo-germ-free” mice are similar to those in conventional mice. Hernández-Chirlaque et al. showed that antibiotic-treated “pseudo-germ-free” mice had similar manifestations of DSS-induced colitis in aspects of weight loss, colonic inflammation and mucosal barrier function (Hernández-Chirlaque et al., 2016). Accordingly, Gancarcikova et al. revealed that antibiotic-treated “pseudo-germ-free” mice did not have changes that could influence the initiation or development of DSS-induced colitis, and the inflammatory process developed during DSS treatment was mostly due to the exposure to DSS and its toxic action on compactness and integrity of mucosal barrier (Gancarcikova et al., 2020). So, it is a feasible solution to use the antibiotic cocktail to explore the role of gut microbiota in the therapeutic effects of metformin in the DSS model. Third, except for *A. muciniphila*, the roles of other bacteria were not investigated, which may influence the pharmacological effects of metformin on colonic inflammation and the mucus barrier. The current study focused on the effects of *A. muciniphila* as it was enriched only in the metformin-treated group. However, these topics will be further investigated.

In summary, the results suggest that metformin alters the composition of the gut microbiota by increasing the levels of potential probiotics (e.g. *A. muciniphila*) and restoring the dysbiosis in mice with DSS-induced UC, which play a critical role in its anti-inflammatory and mucus-protective effects. The novelty of the current study is offering new insights into the role of the gut microbiota in the mucus-barrier-protective and anti-inflammatory effects of metformin, which indicates that metformin has the potential as a supplement or alternative to existing treatment for UC. It also provides evidence that A. muciniphila as a probiotic has potential benefits for the treatment of UC.

ETHICS STATEMENT

All animal studies were carried out in accordance with the guidelines of the Southern Medical University Committee for Experimental Animals. And the protocols were approved by the Animal Experimental Ethics Committee of the Southern Medical University, China (L2018225).

AUTHOR CONTRIBUTIONS

All authors contributed to the study's conception and design. YC, HK, FL, WD, and ZL were involved in the study design. Material preparation, data collection, and analysis were performed by HK, FL, WD, ZL, SW, and PL. The first draft of the manuscript was written by HK and FL. All authors commented on previous versions of the manuscript. All authors read and approved the final manuscript.

ACKNOWLEDGMENTS

The authors thank Xia Chen, Yuyan Xu, Qin Liu, Zhanjun Chen, Zhigang Hu, Yanfei Gao, and Qingmao Zhang for their general support.

REFERENCES

Algieri, F., Garrido-Mesa, J., Vezza, T., Rodríguez-Sojo, M. J., Rodríguez-Cabezas, M. E., Olivares, M., et al. (2021). Intestinal Anti-inflammatory Effects of Probiotics in DNBS-Colitis via Modulation of Gut Microbiota and microRNAs. *Eur. J. Nutr.* 60, 2537–2551. doi:10.1007/s00394-020-02441-8

Anisimov, V. N. (2013). Metformin: Do We Finally Have an Anti-aging Drug. *Cell Cycle* 12, 3483–3489. doi:10.4161/cc.26928

Bailey, C. J., Wilcock, C., and Scarpello, J. H. (2008). Metformin and the Intestine. *Diabetologia* 51, 1552–1553. doi:10.1007/s00125-008-1053-5

Bauer, P. V., Duca, F. A., Waise, T. M. Z., Rasmussen, B. A., Abraham, M. A., Dranse, H. J., et al. (2018). Metformin Alters Upper Small Intestinal Microbiota that Impact a Glucose-SGLT1-Sensing Glucoregulatory Pathway. *Cell Metab* 27, 101–117.e5. doi:10.1016/j.cmet.2017.09.019

Becker, S., Oelschlaeger, T. A., Wullaert, A., Vlantis, K., Pasparakis, M., Wehkamp, J., et al. (2013). Bacteria Regulate Intestinal Epithelial Cell Differentiation Factors Both In Vitro and In Vivo. *PLOS ONE* 8, e55620. doi:10.1371/journal.pone.0055620

Bergström, A., Kristensen, M. B., Bahl, M. I., Metzdorff, S. B., Fink, L. N., Frøkiaer, H., et al. (2012). Nature of Bacterial Colonization Influences Transcription of Mucin Genes in Mice during the First Week of Life. *BMC Res. Notes* 5, 402. doi:10.1186/1756-0500-5-402

Birchenough, G. M., Nyström, E. E., Johansson, M. E., and Hansson, G. C. (2016). A Sentinel Goblet Cell Guards the Colonic Crypt by Triggering Nlrp6-dependent Muc2 Secretion. *Science* 352, 1535–1542. doi:10.1126/science.aaf7419

Cameron, A. R., Morrison, V. L., Levin, D., Mohan, M., Forteath, C., Beall, C., et al. (2016). Anti-Inflammatory Effects of Metformin Irrespective of Diabetes Status. *Circ. Res.* 119, 652–665. doi:10.1161/CIRCRESAHA.116.308445

Chassaing, B., Aitken, J. D., Malleshappa, M., and Vijay-Kumar, M. (2014). Dextran Sulfate Sodium (DSS)-Induced Colitis in Mice. *Curr. Protoc. Immunol.* 104, 15–1415. doi:10.1002/0471142735.im1525s104

Chen, X., Li, P., Liu, M., Zheng, H., He, Y., Chen, M. X., et al. (2020). Gut Dysbiosis Induces the Development of Pre-eclampsia Through Bacterial Translocation. *Gut* 69, 513–522. doi:10.1136/gutjnl-2019-319101

Deng, J., Zeng, L., Lai, X., Li, J., Liu, L., Lin, Q., et al. (2018). Metformin Protects Against Intestinal Barrier Dysfunction via AMPKα1-dependent Inhibition of JNK Signalling Activation. *J. Cel. Mol. Med.* 22, 546–557. doi:10.1111/jcmm.13342

Derrien, M., Vaughan, E. E., Plugge, C. M., and de Vos, W. M. (2004). Akkermansia Muciniphila Gen. nov., Sp. nov., a Human Intestinal Mucin-Degrading Bacterium. *Int. J. Syst. Evol. Microbiol.* 54, 1469–1476. doi:10.1099/ijs.0.02873-0

Dhar, P., and McAuley, J. (2019). The Role of the Cell Surface Mucin MUC1 as a Barrier to Infection and Regulator of Inflammation. *Front. Cel. Infect. Microbiol.* 9, 117. doi:10.3389/fcimb.2019.00117

Di Fusco, D., Dinallo, V., Monteleone, I., Laudisi, F., Marafini, I., Franzè, E., et al. (2018). Metformin Inhibits Inflammatory Signals in the Gut by Controlling AMPK and P38 MAP Kinase Activation. *Clin. Sci. (Lond)* 132, 1155–1168. doi:10.1042/CS20180167

Earley, H., Lennon, G., Balfe, Á., Coffey, J. C., Winter, D. C., and O'Connell, P. R. (2019). The Abundance of Akkermansia Muciniphila and its Relationship with Sulphated Colonic Mucins in Health and Ulcerative Colitis. *Sci. Rep.* 9, 15683–15689. doi:10.1038/s41598-019-51878-3

Frank, D. N., St Amand, A. L., Feldman, R. A., Boedeker, E. C., Harpaz, N., and Pace, N. R. (2007). Molecular-phylogenetic Characterization of Microbial Community Imbalances in Human Inflammatory Bowel Diseases. *Proc. Natl. Acad. Sci. U S A.* 104, 13780–13785. doi:10.1073/pnas.0706625104

Gancarcikova, S., Lauko, S., Hrckova, G., Andrejcakova, Z., Hajduckova, V., Madar, M., et al. (2020). Innovative Animal Model of DSS-Induced Ulcerative Colitis in Pseudo Germ-free Mice. *Cells* 9, 2571. doi:10.3390/cells9122571

Gersemann, M., Becker, S., Kübler, I., Koslowski, M., Wang, G., Herrlinger, K. R., et al. (2009). Differences in Goblet Cell Differentiation Between Crohn's Disease and Ulcerative Colitis. *Differentiation* 77, 84–94. doi:10.1016/j.diff.2008.09.008

Gregorieff, A., Stange, D. E., Kujala, P., Begthel, H., van den Born, M., Korving, J., et al. (2009). The Ets-Domain Transcription Factor Spdef Promotes Maturation of Goblet and Paneth Cells in the Intestinal Epithelium. *Gastroenterology* 137, 1333–1345.e1-e3. doi:10.1053/j.gastro.2009.06.044

Heazlewood, C. K., Cook, M. C., Eri, R., Price, G. R., Tauro, S. B., Taupin, D., et al. (2008). Aberrant Mucin Assembly in Mice Causes Endoplasmic Reticulum Stress and Spontaneous Inflammation Resembling Ulcerative Colitis. *Plos Med.* 5, e54. doi:10.1371/journal.pmed.0050054

Hernández-Chirlaque, C., Aranda, C. J., Ocón, B., Capitán-Cañadas, F., Ortega-González, M., Carrero, J. J., et al. (2016). Germ-free and Antibiotic-Treated Mice Are Highly Susceptible to Epithelial Injury in DSS Colitis. *J. Crohns Colitis* 10, 1324–1335. doi:10.1093/ecco-jcc/jjw096

Hudcovic, T., Stěpánková, R., Cebra, J., and Tlaskalová-Hogenová, H. (2001). The Role of Microflora in the Development of Intestinal Inflammation: Acute and Chronic Colitis Induced by Dextran Sulfate in Germ-free and Conventionally Reared Immunocompetent and Immunodeficient Mice. *Folia Microbiol. (Praha)* 46, 565–572. doi:10.1007/BF02818004

Hur, K. Y., and Lee, M. S. (2015). New Mechanisms of Metformin Action: Focusing on Mitochondria and the Gut. *J. Diabetes Investig.* 6, 600–609. doi:10.1111/jdi.12328

Jakobsson, H. E., Rodríguez-Piñeiro, A. M., Schütte, A., Ermund, A., Boysen, P., Bemark, M., et al. (2015). The Composition of the Gut Microbiota Shapes the Colon Mucus Barrier. *EMBO Rep.* 16, 164–177. doi:10.15252/embr.201439263

Janda, J. M., and Abbott, S. L. (2007). 16S rRNA Gene Sequencing for Bacterial Identification in the Diagnostic Laboratory: Pluses, Perils, and Pitfalls. *J. Clin. Microbiol.* 45, 2761–2764. doi:10.1128/JCM.01228-07

Johansson, M. E., Gustafsson, J. K., Holmén-Larsson, J., Jabbar, K. S., Xia, L., Xu, H., et al. (2014). Bacteria Penetrate the Normally Impenetrable Inner Colon Mucus Layer in Both Murine Colitis Models and Patients with Ulcerative Colitis. *Gut* 63, 281–291. doi:10.1136/gutjnl-2012-303207

Johansson, M. E., and Hansson, G. C. (2011). Microbiology. Keeping Bacteria at a Distance. *Science* 334, 182–183. doi:10.1126/science.1213909

Kennedy, E. A., King, K. Y., and Baldridge, M. T. (2018). Mouse Microbiota Models: Comparing Germ-free Mice and Antibiotics Treatment as Tools for Modifying Gut Bacteria. *Front. Physiol.* 9, 1534. doi:10.3389/fphys.2018.01534

Kim, W.-K., Jang, Y. J., Seo, B., Han, D. H., Park, S., and Ko, G. (2019). Administration of Lactobacillus Paracasei Strains Improves Immunomodulation and Changes the Composition of Gut Microbiota Leading to Improvement of Colitis in Mice. *J. Funct. Foods* 52, 565–575. doi:10.1016/j.jff.2018.11.035

Knox, N. C., Forbes, J. D., Van Domselaar, G., and Bernstein, C. N. (2019). The Gut Microbiome as a Target for IBD Treatment: Are We There yet. *Curr. Treat. Options. Gastroenterol.* 17, 115–126. doi:10.1007/s11938-019-00221-w

Koh, S. J., Kim, J. M., Kim, I. K., Ko, S. H., and Kim, J. S. (2014). Anti-inflammatory Mechanism of Metformin and its Effects in Intestinal Inflammation and Colitis-Associated Colon Cancer. *J. Gastroenterol. Hepatol.* 29, 502–510. doi:10.1111/jgh.12435

Kühn, F., and Klar, E. (2015). Surgical Principles in the Treatment of Ulcerative Colitis. *Viszeralmedizin* 31, 246–250. doi:10.1159/000438894

Lee, S. Y., Lee, S. H., Yang, E. J., Kim, E. K., Kim, J. K., Shin, D. Y., et al. (2015). Metformin Ameliorates Inflammatory Bowel Disease by Suppression of the STAT3 Signaling Pathway and Regulation of the Between Th17/Treg Balance. *PLOS ONE* 10, e0135858. doi:10.1371/journal.pone.0135858

Leone, A., Di Gennaro, E., Bruzzese, F., Avallone, A., and Budillon, A. (2014). "New Perspective for an Old Antidiabetic Drug: Metformin as Anticancer Agent," in *Advances In Nutrition And Cancer Treatment and Research*. Editors V. Zappia, S. Panico, G. L. Russo, A. Budillon, and F. Della Ragione (Berlin, Heidelberg: Springer), 355–376. doi:10.1007/978-3-642-38007-5_21

Lindén, S. K., Florin, T. H. J., and McGuckin, M. A. (2008). Mucin Dynamics in Intestinal Bacterial Infection. *PLOS ONE* 3, e3952. doi:10.1371/journal.pone.0003952

M'koma, A. E. (2013). Inflammatory Bowel Disease: An Expanding Global Health Problem. *Clin. Med. Insights Gastroenterol.* 6, 33–47. doi:10.4137/CGast.S12731

Mariat, D., Firmesse, O., Levenez, F., Guimarães, V., Sokol, H., Doré, J., et al. (2009). The Firmicutes/Bacteroidetes Ratio of the Human Microbiota Changes with Age. *BMC Microbiol.* 9, 123–126. doi:10.1186/1471-2180-9-123

McCreight, L. J., Bailey, C. J., and Pearson, E. R. (2016). Metformin and the Gastrointestinal Tract. *Diabetologia* 59, 426–435. doi:10.1007/s00125-015-3844-9

Nair, A. B., and Jacob, S. (2016). A Simple Practice Guide for Dose Conversion Between Animals and Human. *J. Basic Clin. Pharm.* 7, 27–31. doi:10.4103/0976-0105.177703

Nishida, A., Lau, C. W., Zhang, M., Andoh, A., Shi, H. N., Mizoguchi, E., et al. (2012). The Membrane-Bound Mucin Muc1 Regulates T Helper 17-Cell Responses and Colitis in Mice. *Gastroenterology* 142, 865–874.e2. doi:10.1053/j.gastro.2011.12.036

Pan, Q., Tian, Y., Li, X., Ye, J., Liu, Y., Song, L., et al. (2013). Enhanced Membrane-Tethered Mucin 3 (MUC3) Expression by a Tetrameric Branched Peptide with a Conserved TFLK Motif Inhibits Bacteria Adherence. *J. Biol. Chem.* 288, 5407–5416. doi:10.1074/jbc.M112.408245

Paone, P., and Cani, P. D. (2020). Mucus Barrier, Mucins and Gut Microbiota: The Expected Slimy Partners. *Gut* 69, 2232–2243. doi:10.1136/gutjnl-2020-322260

Paramsothy, S., Kamm, M. A., Kaakoush, N. O., Walsh, A. J., van den Bogaerde, J., Samuel, D., et al. (2017). Multidonor Intensive Faecal Microbiota Transplantation for Active Ulcerative Colitis: A Randomised Placebo-Controlled Trial. *Lancet* 389, 1218–1228. doi:10.1016/S0140-6736(17)30182-4

Petersson, J., Schreiber, O., Hansson, G. C., Gendler, S. J., Velcich, A., Lundberg, J. O., et al. (2010). Importance and Regulation of the Colonic Mucus Barrier in a Mouse Model of Colitis. *Am. J. Physiol. Gastrointest. Liver Physiol.* 300, G327–G333. doi:10.1152/ajpgi.00422.2010

Png, C. W., Lindén, S. K., Gilshenan, K. S., Zoetendal, E. G., McSweeney, C. S., Sly, L. I., et al. (2010). Mucolytic Bacteria with Increased Prevalence in IBD Mucosa Augment In Vitro Utilization of Mucin by Other Bacteria. *Am. J. Gastroenterol.* 105, 2420–2428. doi:10.1038/ajg.2010.281

Rajilić-Stojanović, M., Shanahan, F., Guarner, F., and de Vos, W. M. (2013). Phylogenetic Analysis of Dysbiosis in Ulcerative Colitis During Remission. *Inflamm. Bowel Dis.* 19, 481–488. doi:10.1097/MIB.0b013e31827fec6d

Rena, G., and Lang, C. C. (2018). Repurposing Metformin for Cardiovascular Disease. *Circulation* 137, 422–424. doi:10.1161/CIRCULATIONAHA.117.031735

Rio, D. C., Ares, M., Hannon, G. J., and Nilsen, T. W. (2010). Purification of RNA Using TRIzol (TRI Reagent). *Cold Spring Harb. Protoc.* 2010, 5439. doi:10.1101/pdb.prot5439

Robertson, D., Savage, K., Reis-Filho, J. S., and Isacke, C. M. (2008). Multiple Immunofluorescence Labelling of Formalin-Fixed Paraffin-Embedded (FFPE) Tissue. *BMC Cel Biol* 9, 13. doi:10.1186/1471-2121-9-13

Rodríguez-Nogales, A., Algieri, F., Garrido-Mesa, J., Vezza, T., Utrilla, M. P., Chueca, N., et al. (2018). The Administration of *Escherichia coli* Nissle 1917 Ameliorates Development of DSS-Induced Colitis in Mice. *Front. Pharmacol.* 9, 468. doi:10.3389/fphar.2018.00468

Saisho, Y. (2015). Metformin and Inflammation: Its Potential beyond Glucose-Lowering Effect. *Endocr. Metab. Immune Disord. Drug Targets* 15, 196–205. doi:10.2174/1871530315666150316124019

Santoru, M. L., Piras, C., Murgia, A., Palmas, V., Camboni, T., Liggi, S., et al. (2017). Cross Sectional Evaluation of the Gut-Microbiome Metabolome Axis in an Italian Cohort of IBD Patients. *Sci. Rep.* 7, 9523. doi:10.1038/s41598-017-10034-5

Scarpello, J. H., and Howlett, H. C. (2008). Metformin Therapy and Clinical Uses. *Diab. Vasc. Dis. Res.* 5, 157–167. doi:10.3132/dvdr.2008.027

Schroeder, B. O. (2019). Fight Them or Feed Them: How the Intestinal Mucus Layer Manages the Gut Microbiota. *Gastroenterol. Rep. (Oxf)* 7, 3–12. doi:10.1093/gastro/goy052

Shao, Y., Ding, R., Xu, B., Hua, R., Shen, Q., He, K., et al. (2017). Alterations of Gut Microbiota After Roux-En-Y Gastric Bypass and Sleeve Gastrectomy in Sprague-Dawley Rats. *Obes. Surg.* 27, 295–302. doi:10.1007/s11695-016-2297-7

Shen, J., Zuo, Z. X., and Mao, A. P. (2014). Effect of Probiotics on Inducing Remission and Maintaining Therapy in Ulcerative Colitis, Crohn's Disease, and Pouchitis: Meta-Analysis of Randomized Controlled Trials. *Inflamm. Bowel Dis.* 20, 21–35. doi:10.1097/01.MIB.0000437495.30052.be

Shen, Z. H., Zhu, C. X., Quan, Y. S., Yang, Z. Y., Wu, S., Luo, W. W., et al. (2018). Relationship Between Intestinal Microbiota and Ulcerative Colitis: Mechanisms and Clinical Application of Probiotics and Fecal Microbiota Transplantation. *World J. Gastroenterol.* 24, 5–14. doi:10.3748/wjg.v24.i1.5

Shin, N. R., Lee, J. C., Lee, H. Y., Kim, M. S., Whon, T. W., Lee, M. S., et al. (2014). An Increase in the Akkermansia Spp. Population Induced by Metformin Treatment Improves Glucose Homeostasis in Diet-Induced Obese Mice. *Gut* 63, 727–735. doi:10.1136/gutjnl-2012-303839

Solomon, L., Mansor, S., Mallon, P., Donnelly, E., Hoper, M., Loughrey, M., et al. (2010). The Dextran Sulphate Sodium (DSS) Model of Colitis: An Overview. *Comp. Clin. Pathol.* 19, 235 239. doi:10.1007/s00580-010-0979-4

Song, C. H., Kim, N., Sohn, S. H., Lee, S. M., Nam, R. H., Na, H. Y., et al. (2018). Effects of 17β-Estradiol on Colonic Permeability and Inflammation in an Azoxymethane/Dextran Sulfate Sodium-Induced Colitis Mouse Model. *Gut Liver* 12, 682–693. doi:10.5009/gnl18221

Strugala, V., Dettmar, P. W., and Pearson, J. P. (2008). Thickness and Continuity of the Adherent Colonic Mucus Barrier in Active and Quiescent Ulcerative Colitis and Crohn's Disease. *Int. J. Clin. Pract.* 62, 762–769. doi:10.1111/j.1742-1241.2007.01665.x

Swidsinski, A., Loening-Baucke, V., Theissig, F., Engelhardt, H., Bengmark, S., Koch, S., et al. (2007). Comparative Study of the Intestinal Mucus Barrier in Normal and Inflamed Colon. *Gut* 56, 343–350. doi:10.1136/gut.2006.098160

Tan, H., Zhai, Q., and Chen, W. (2019). Investigations of Bacteroides Spp. Towards Next-Generation Probiotics. *Food Res. Int.* 116, 637–644. doi:10.1016/j.foodres.2018.08.088

Testa, A., Castiglione, F., Nardone, O. M., and Colombo, G. L. (2017). Adherence in Ulcerative Colitis: An Overview. *Patient Prefer Adherence* 11, 297–303. doi:10.2147/PPA.S127039

Troll, J. V., Hamilton, M. K., Abel, M. L., Ganz, J., Bates, J. M., Stephens, W. Z., et al. (2018). Microbiota Promote Secretory Cell Determination in the Intestinal Epithelium by Modulating Host Notch Signaling. *Development* 145, dev155317. doi:10.1242/dev.155317

Ungaro, R., Mehandru, S., Allen, P. B., Peyrin-Biroulet, L., and Colombel, J. F. (2017). Ulcerative Colitis. *Lancet* 389, 1756–1770. doi:10.1016/S0140-6736(16)32126-2

van der Flier, L. G., and Clevers, H. (2009). Stem Cells, Self-Renewal, and Differentiation in the Intestinal Epithelium. *Annu. Rev. Physiol.* 71, 241–260. doi:10.1146/annurev.physiol.010908.163145

van der Post, S., Jabbar, K. S., Birchenough, G., Arike, L., Akhtar, N., Sjovall, H., et al. (2019). Structural Weakening of the Colonic Mucus Barrier Is an Early Event in Ulcerative Colitis Pathogenesis. *Gut* 68, 2142–2151. doi:10.1136/gutjnl-2018-317571

Van der Sluis, M., De Koning, B. A., De Bruijn, A. C., Velcich, A., Meijerink, J. P., Van Goudoever, J. B., et al. (2006). Muc2-Deficient Mice Spontaneously Develop Colitis, Indicating that MUC2 Is Critical for Colonic Protection. *Gastroenterology* 131, 117–129. doi:10.1053/j.gastro.2006.04.020

van Putten, J. P. M., and Strijbis, K. (2017). Transmembrane Mucins: Signaling Receptors at the Intersection of Inflammation and Cancer. *J. Innate Immun.* 9, 281–299. doi:10.1159/000453594

Vich Vila, A., Imhann, F., Collij, V., Jankipersadsing, S. A., Gurry, T., Mujagic, Z., et al. (2018). Gut Microbiota Composition and Functional Changes in Inflammatory Bowel Disease and Irritable Bowel Syndrome. *Sci. Transl. Med.* 10, eaap8914. doi:10.1126/scitranslmed.aap8914

Walker, A. W., Sanderson, J. D., Churcher, C., Parkes, G. C., Hudspith, B. N., Rayment, N., et al. (2011). High-throughput Clone Library Analysis of the Mucosa-Associated Microbiota Reveals Dysbiosis and Differences Between Inflamed and Non-inflamed Regions of the Intestine in Inflammatory Bowel Disease. *BMC Microbiol.* 11, 7. doi:10.1186/1471-2180-11-7

Wang, Z., Li, R., Tan, J., Peng, L., Wang, P., Liu, J., et al. (2015). Syndecan-1 Acts in Synergy with Tight Junction Through Stat3 Signaling to Maintain Intestinal Mucosal Barrier and Prevent Bacterial Translocation. *Inflamm. Bowel Dis.* 21, 1894–1907. doi:10.1097/MIB.0000000000000421

Xue, Y., Zhang, H., Sun, X., and Zhu, M.-J. (2016). Metformin Improves Ileal Epithelial Barrier Function in Interleukin-10 Deficient Mice. *PLoS ONE* 11, e0168670. doi:10.1371/journal.pone.0168670

Yeo, S., Park, H., Seo, E., Kim, J., Kim, B. K., Choi, I. S., et al. (2020). Anti-Inflammatory and Gut Microbiota Modulatory Effect of Lactobacillus Rhamnosus Strain LDTM 7511 in a Dextran Sulfate Sodium-Induced Colitis Murine Model. *Microorganisms* 8, 845. doi:10.3390/microorganisms8060845

Yin, J., Liao, S. X., He, Y., Wang, S., Xia, G. H., Liu, F. T., et al. (2015). Dysbiosis of Gut Microbiota with Reduced Trimethylamine-N-Oxide Level in Patients with Large-Artery Atherosclerotic Stroke or Transient Ischemic Attack. *J. Am. Heart Assoc.* 4, e002699. doi:10.1161/JAHA.115.002699

Zhai, R., Xue, X., Zhang, L., Yang, X., Zhao, L., and Zhang, C. (2019). Strain-Specific Anti-inflammatory Properties of Two Akkermansia Muciniphila Strains on Chronic Colitis in Mice. *Front. Cel. Infect. Microbiol.* 9, 239. doi:10.3389/fcimb.2019.00239

Zhang, M. (2019). Tu1852 – Metformin Ameliorated Inflammatory Bowel Disease by Enhancing Akkermansia Muciniphila. *Gastroenterology* 156, S1148. doi:10.1016/S0016-5085(19)39838-5

Zhang, Y. Z., and Li, Y. Y. (2014). Inflammatory Bowel Disease: Pathogenesis. *World J. Gastroenterol.* 20, 91–99. doi:10.3748/wjg.v20.i1.91

Zhou, Y., Xu, Z. Z., He, Y., Yang, Y., Liu, L., Lin, Q., et al. (2018). Gut Microbiota Offers Universal Biomarkers Across Ethnicity in Inflammatory Bowel Disease Diagnosis and Infliximab Response Prediction. *mSystems* 3, 1–14. doi:10.1128/mSystems.00188-17

16

An Update for Pharmacologists on New Treatment Options for Inflammatory Bowel Disease: The Clinicians' Perspective

Carsten Schmidt[1], *Philip C. Grunert*[2] *and Andreas Stallmach*[2]*

[1]*Medizinische Klinik II, Klinikum Fulda AG, Universitätsmedizin Marburg - Campus Fulda, Fulda, Germany,* [2]*Klinik für Innere Medizin IV, Universitätsklinikum Jena, Friedrich-Schiller Universität Jena, Jena, Germany*

***Correspondence:**
Andreas Stallmach,
andreas.stallmach@med.uni-jena.de

The introduction of anti-tumor necrosis factor antibodies resulted in a considerable expansion of the options available for the treatment of inflammatory bowel disease. Unfortunately, approximately one third of treated patients do not respond to these modalities, and drug efficacy may be lost over time. These drugs are also associated with contraindications, adverse events, and intolerance. As such, there is an ongoing need for new therapeutic strategies. Despite several recent advances, including antibodies against pro-inflammatory cytokines and cell adhesion molecules, Janus kinase inhibitors, and modulators of sphingosine-1-phosphate receptors, not all problems associated with IBD have been solved. In this manuscript, we review the current state of development of several new treatment options. Ongoing evaluation will require specific proof of efficacy as well as direct comparisons with established treatments. Results from head-to-head comparisons are needed to provide clinicians with critical information on how to formulate effective therapeutic approaches for each patient.

Keywords: interleukin-23, anti-integrin drugs, sphingosine-1-phosphate receptor modulator, JAK inhibitor, fecal microbiota transplantation, biologics, small molecule

INTRODUCTION

Patients diagnosed with inflammatory bowel disease (IBD), including those with Crohn´s disease (CD) and ulcerative colitis (UC), can be difficult to manage clinically given the broad spectrum of disease, including both intestinal and extraintestinal manifestations. IBD is an immunologically-mediated disease with increasing prevalence across Western Europe, North America, and Australia, as well as in newly-industrialized areas of Asia and South America. The prevalence of IBD has been estimated at 0.3–0.5% in Western Europe, including at least 420,000 patients in Germany alone. Similarly, population-based data from Canada predict that the prevalence of IBD, estimated at 725 patients per 100,000 (0.73%) in 2018 will increase to as many as 981 patients per 100,000 (0.98%) in 2030 (Coward et al., 2019). If we apply this calculation to the current patient population in Germany, we might anticipate an increase to 0.67% in 2030, representing >560,000 patients.

While the physiologic mechanisms contributing to the development of IBD have not been fully clarified, current research suggests that genetically-susceptible individuals respond to routine environmental factors with alterations at the gastrointestinal barrier and exaggerated (or poorly-suppressed) innate and adaptive immune responses. These findings have provided a theoretical and practical basis for the development of new therapies. Indeed, the introduction of the anti-tumor

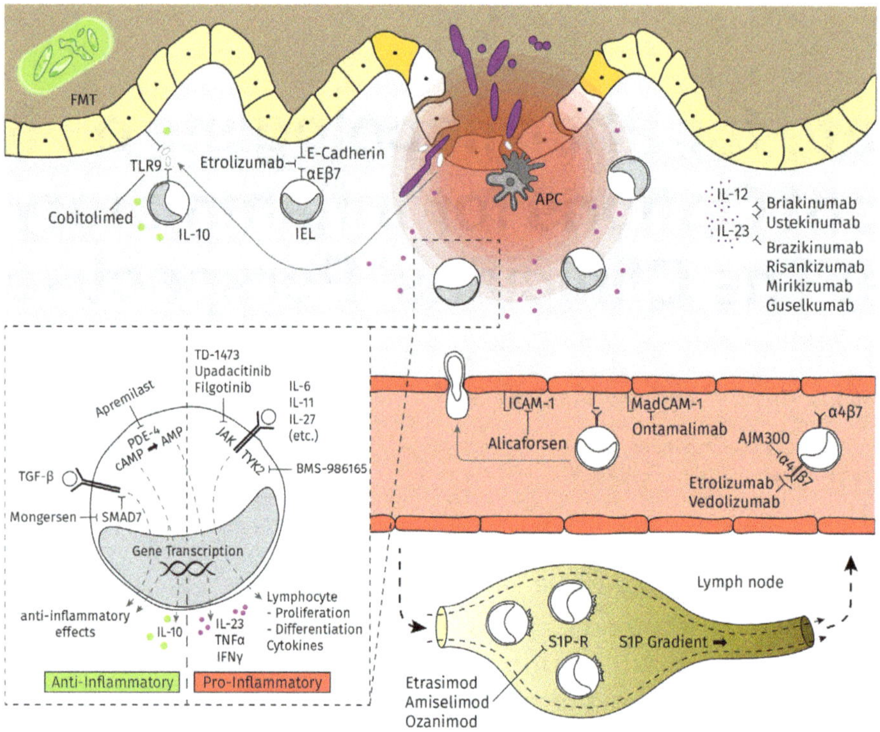

FIGURE 1 | Mechanisms of action of several of the new therapeutic agents used to treat IBD.

necrosis factor (TNF) antibody, infliximab, first for CD (in 1999) and later for UC (in 2006), revolutionized the treatment of these conditions. Other anti-TNF antibodies (all under the broad category known as "biologics"), including adalimumab, golimumab, or certolizumab pegol [certolizumab pegol is not approved by the European Medicines Agency (EMA)] were developed shortly thereafter. With the availability of biosimilars for infliximab and adalimumab and the approval of both ustekinumab, a monoclonal antibody (mAb) that antagonizes the actions of proinflammatory cytokines IL-12 and IL-23, and vedolizumab, a mAb that specifically targets $\alpha_4\beta_7$-integrin, physicians now have access to a broad range of unique biologics that can be used to manage intestinal inflammation. This armamentarium also includes tofacitinib, which is a small-molecule inhibitor of Janus kinases (JAKs) that can be used to treat patients diagnosed with UC. Unfortunately, not all patients respond to these new therapies (known as "primary non-responders"). Depending on the respective phase III study, the proportion of primary non-responders may be as high as 30–50%. Other patients may experience secondary loss of response due to the development of neutralizing antibodies or *via* other, as yet not well-understood mechanisms (e.g., as observed in patients treated with tofacitinib). The comparatively high incidence of adverse events also limits the use of these new therapeutic options. As such, additional research is needed that focuses on approaches that can be used to achieve long-lasting, steroid-free remission without adverse effects in all patients diagnosed with IBD.

The mechanisms of action of the new therapeutic agents used to treat IBD are summarized in **Figure 1**. It is critical to understand that the published studies focused on each of these agents feature different patient populations and have different inclusion and exclusion criteria; among these are differences in disease duration and activity, previous experience with anti-IBD therapies, duration of induction therapy, primary endpoints, and design of maintenance protocols (i.e., "treat-through" vs. "randomized responder"). As such, significant caution must be exercised when comparing the results of different studies.

Due to the multitude of new as well as already established modes of action and specific substances for the treatment of IBD a targeted selection of a medication for an individual patient is of utmost importance. Therefore, several biomarkers (e.g., fecal calprotectin, CRP, serological and genetic parameters, histological findings and microbiota) have been and are currently being evaluated with regard to the prediction of treatment response. At present, however, biomarkers of this type are not yet established for daily clinical practice. Further, from a clinical point of view improvement of disease activity and patient related outcome parameters are more important than changes in biomarkers. For these reasons, we aimed not to discuss such parameters in this overview on the effectiveness and safety of new therapeutics.

An electronic database search using PubMed, spanning up to November 2020, was conducted. Abstracts were also reviewed from Digestive Diseases Week, European Crohn's and Colitis Organization congress, and United European Gastroenterology Week 2019 and 2020, respectively.

ANTI-INTEGRIN ANTIBODIES

Integrins are cell adhesion molecules that form transmembrane dimers consisting of α- and β-chains. The goal of an anti-integrin strategy is to block the actions of adhesion molecules on circulating immune cells and/or those of their receptors on endothelial cells. For example, $\alpha_4\beta_7$-integrin on the surface of $CD4^+$ T lymphocytes binds specifically to MadCAM-1 (mucosal addressin cell adhesion molecule-1) on endothelial cells in the gastrointestinal tract and thereby mediates "gut-selective" lymphocyte migration into the gastrointestinal mucosa. **Vedolizumab** is a humanized mAb that targets $\alpha_4\beta_7$-integrin and was first approved for the treatment of CD and UC in 2014 with a favorable safety profile in clinical trials. This assessment was reinforced with the first direct, head-to-head comparison of biologic therapies for IBD carried out in 2019 as the VARSITY study. The results of this study revealed that vedolizumab had a more favorable therapeutic impact on inducing clinical remission compared to results obtained using adalimumab (Sands et al., 2019a).

Given the overall efficacy and "gut-selective" effects of vedolizumab, it is not surprising that cell adhesion molecules are among the most prominent targets of new therapeutics under development. Various inhibitors of the integrin β_7-subunit and its endothelial ligand, MadCAM-1, are currently undergoing evaluation in numerous studies. For example, in one phase II study, Vermeire and colleagues (Vermeire et al., 2014) found that the anti-β_7 antibody, **etrolizumab**, was more effective than placebo at inducing remission in patients with symptomatic UC. One important aspect of etrolizumab is the fact that it targets not only $\alpha_4\beta_7$-integrin (similar to vedolizumab) but also can inhibit $\alpha_E\beta_7$-integrin-mediated interactions between intraepithelial lymphocytes and E-cadherin expressed by enterocytes, thereby reducing the extent of lymphocyte accumulation at this site. This is a critical finding, as the probability of remission correlated strongly with mucosal expression of the α_E-subunit, which was also identified as the first established predictor of the response to mAb therapy. These results were followed by eight randomized-controlled and open-label studies of this modality for the treatment of CD and UC. More than 3,000 UC and CD patients were enrolled in two open-label and safety studies as well as in six phase III trials, including comparative studies against both adalimumab and infliximab (Sandborn et al., 2020e). However, in August 2020, Roche investigators reported mixed results from their studies and announced that the study program for patients diagnosed with UC was to be halted, while studies focused on CD were to be continued. The favorable safety profile for etrolizumab was consistent with the results of previous studies, although the results of the various treatment studies for UC were not as convincing. In the "Hibiscus-I" induction study, the primary endpoint of clinical remission at week 10 was achieved in response to etrolizumab among patients who had not undergone prior treatment with anti-TNF mAbs (19.4 vs. 6.9%; p = 0.0173). By contrast, in the "*Hibiscus* II" induction study (which also included anti-TNF-naïve patients) the same primary endpoint was not met (18.2 vs. 11.1%; p = 0.1729) (Dotan et al., 2020). In the "Hickory" study, the primary endpoint of induction (clinical remission at week 14: 18.5 vs. 6.3%; p = 0.0033), but not maintenance of remission (among clinical responders at week 14) was achieved in response to etrolizumab among patients with a history of previous anti-TNF treatment (24.1 vs. 20.2% at week 66; p = 0.4956) (Peyrin-Biroulet et al., 2020a). Finally, in the "Laurel" maintenance study, the primary endpoint of clinical remission at week 62 among responders at week 10 was not achieved in patients with no history of anti-TNF treatment (29.6 vs. 20.6%; p = 0.1942) (Vermeire et al., 2020). The consequences of these results and their impact on the further development of etrolizumab remain to be determined.

AJM300 is a small molecule administered orally that blocks the α_4-integrin subunit that has been investigated in patients with moderately-active UC. In one phase II study, 102 patients were treated with 960 mg AJM300 or placebo three times a day for 8 weeks. 62.7% of the patients in the treatment (AJM300) group exhibited a clinical response (a decrease in the Mayo Score by >3 points or at least 30% with a reduction in the rectal bleeding subscore by >1 point) compared to only 25.5% of the patients in the placebo group (p = 0.002). Furthermore, clinical remission was observed in 23.5% vs. 3.9% of patients (p = 0.01) (Yoshimura et al., 2015); This drug is currently undergoing evaluation in a phase III study involving patients with UC.

Ontamalimab (PF-00547659) is a mAb that targets MadCAM-1. A phase II study in patients with UC documented the superiority of this drug in inducing clinical remission compared to placebo (16.7% vs. 2.7% at week 12; p = 0.01). Patients who responded to therapy were treated for up to 72 weeks in an open-label extension study; in this study, positive effects on the maintenance of remission were more pronounced in patients that received higher drug doses. By contrast, no differences were observed in a comparison between PF-00547659 and placebo in patients with moderate-to-severe CD, despite the observed decreases in the concentration of circulating MAdCAM-1 and a dose-dependent increase in $\beta7^+$ memory T-cells, which are both findings that document the pharmacologic efficacy of the drug (Sandborn et al., 2018). Takeda (who acquired ontamalimab through the acquisition of Shire in 2018) announced the end of the study program in May 2020.

The results of six studies focused on achieving clinical remission in both CD and UC using anti-integrin strategies are summarized in **Table 1**.

COMMENT

Given the well-characterized positive responses to treatment with vedolizumab, the largely negative results of studies focused on etrolizumab for the treatment of UC are somewhat surprising. The full publications may ultimately provide more information to explain the underlying issues. Given the well-established favorable safety profile for vedolizumab, therapeutic agents directed against integrin-mediated interactions might be suitable for use as combination therapy with drugs that have

TABLE 1 | Frequency of achieving clinical remission in anti-integrin directed studies of patients with CD (a) and UC (b).

Drug	Study phase	Induction treatment				Study type	Maintenance treatment				References
		Week	Study drug	Placebo	*p*		Week	Study drug	Placebo	*p*	
a) CD											
Vedolizumab[a]	III	6	14.5	6.8%	0.02	rr	85	39.0	21.6%	<0.001	Sandborn et al. (2013)
Ontamalimab	II	8	29.1	16.7%	n.s						Sandborn et al. (2018)

Drug	Study phase	Induction treatment				Study type	Maintenance treatment				References
		Week	Study drug	Placebo	*p*		Week	Study drug	Placebo	*p*	
b) UC											
Vedolizumab[a]	III	6	16.9	5.4%	<0.001	rr	52	44.8	15.9%	<0.001	Feagan et al. (2013)
Etrolizumab	III	10	19.4	6.9%	0.0173	rr	62	29.6	20.6%	0,194	Dotan et al. (2020)
	III	10	18.2	11.1%	0.1729						Vermeire et al. (2020)
Etrolizumab	III	14	18.5	6.3%	0.0033	rr	66	24.1	20.2%	0,4956	Peyrin-Biroulet et al. (2020a)
Ontamalimab	II	12	16.7	2.7%	0.01	OLE	40–72	22.8	nd	Na	Vermeire et al. (2017a), Danese et al. (2019)
AJM300	II	8	23.5	3.9%	0.01						Yoshimura et al. (2015)

NB: In studies that feature different dosages or intervals, the most effective treatment has been presented.

[a]currently licensed for use as therapy in CD and UC; OLE, open-label extension; tt, treat-through; r, continuation of assigned treatment in responders; r 26, remission at week 26; rr, randomized responder; nd, not done; na, not applicable.

different mechanisms of action. Results of phase III studies of etrolizumab combined with other therapies may provide further insight into this possibility.

BLOCKADE OF INTERLEUKIN-23

Interleukin-12 (IL-12) and interleukin-23 (IL-23) are heterodimeric cytokines that share a common p40 subunit; this subunit has been identified as an effective target for mAbs designed to inhibit the actions of both pro-inflammatory mediators. By contrast, mAbs that target the second subunit of IL-23 (p19) alone promote selective inhibition of this cytokine. The anti-p40 mAb, **ustekinumab,** was approved for use in 2016, has proven effectiveness and a good safety profile when used to treat patients with CD and UC (Feagan et al., 2016; Sands et al., 2019b).

Briakinumab is another anti-p40 mAb that is currently under study for the treatment of psoriasis. Although higher response and remission rates were observed at weeks 6, 12, and 24 in a phase IIb study of patients with CD, the primary endpoint of the study, clinical remission at week 6, was not achieved (13,7 vs. 8.7%; p = 0.157) (Panaccione et al., 2015).

The potential use of **brazikumab (MEDI2070)**, a selective anti-p19mAb, was evaluated in a phase IIa study. In this trial, 119 patients with CD who had failed previous treatment with anti-TNF antibodies achieved a clinical response to brazikumab after 8 weeks, at a significantly higher rate than was observed for patients in the placebo-control group (49.2 vs. 26.7%; p = 0.01). Interestingly, higher serum concentrations of interleukin 22 (a "downstream" mediator in the IL-23 signaling pathway) were positively associated with treatment response; as such, IL-22 levels may be a predictor of treatment response (Sands et al., 2017).

Similarly, results of a phase II trial involving **risankizumab**, another anti-p19 mAb, revealed clinical remission at 12 weeks in 121 patients with CD significantly more frequently than in those receiving placebo (36.6 vs. 15.4%; p = 0.0252) (Feagan et al., 2017). When therapy was continued in the subset of patients who had achieved remission at week 26, clinical and endoscopic remission was achieved in 71 and 55% of the patients examined at week 52, respectively (Feagan et al., 2018).

In a phase II study of the anti-p19 mAb, **mirikizumab**, in 168 patients with UC, clinical remission was observed significantly more frequently in patients who received the study drug than in those receiving placebo (22.6 vs. 4.8%; p = 0.004), In this study, clinical responses were observed after intravenous induction therapy at a dose of 200 mg at weeks 0, 4 and 8; however, as insufficient responses were observed to doses of 50 or 600 mg, the primary endpoint of the study was not met. Nonetheless, it is important to note that clinical responses to therapy were observed more frequently among those who received one of the two higher doses (60 and 49% to 200 and 600 mg, respectively) than those in the placebo group (21%). Upon continuation of therapy, clinical remission was maintained up to week 52 in 37–47% of patients, depending on the dosage interval. As such, any future studies must first address the issue of the optimal dosage for induction therapy (Sandborn et al., 2020b).

In another phase II study featuring mirikizumab carried out in 191 CD patients, an endoscopic response (primary endpoint) was achieved significantly more frequently with induction doses of 600 mg (37.5%; p = 0.03) or 1,000 mg (43.8%; p < 0.001) than with placebo (10.9%). The rate of clinical response and clinical remission [600 mg: 40.6% (p < 0.001), 1,000 mg: 26.6% (p = 0.013) vs. placebo (9.4%), respectively] was also achieved significantly more frequently with mirikizumab (Sands et al., 2019). Findings in a recently published abstract reported that maintenance therapy after successful induction of an endoscopic response was successful in 59% of patients up to week 52, while

TABLE 2 | Frequency of achieving clinical remission in anti-IL-23 (±anti-IL-12) directed studies of patients with CD (a) or UC (b).

Drug	Study phase	Induction treatment				Study type	Maintenance treatment				References
		Week	Study drug	Placebo	*p*		Week	Study drug	Placebo	*p*	
a) CD											
Ustekinumab[a]	III	8	29.8	13.0%	<0.001	rr	52	53.1	35.9%	0.005	Feagan et al. (2016)
Briakinumab	II	6	17.3	8.7%	0.157						Panaccione et al. (2015)
Risankizumab	II	12	36.6	15.4%	0.0252	r 26	52	71.0	nd	Na	Feagan et al. (2017), Feagan et al. (2018)
Mirikizumab	II	12	40.6	9.4%	<0.001	rr	52	56.5	nd	Na	Sands et al. (2019), Sands et al. (2020b)
Brazikumab	II	8	27.1	15.0%	0.1						Sands et al. (2017)
Guselkumab	II	12	56.0	15.7%	0.001						(Sandborn et al., 2020)

Drug	Study phase	Induction treatment				Study type	Maintenance treatment				References
		Week	Study drug	Placebo	*p*		Week	Study drug	Placebo	*p*	
b) UC											
Ustekinumab[a]	III	8	15.5	5.3%	<0.001	rr	52	43.8	24.0%	<0.001	Sands et al. (2019b)
Mirikizumab	II	12	22.6	4.8%	0.004						Sandborn et al. (2020b)

NB: In studies that feature different dosages or intervals, the most effective treatment has been presented.
[a]currently licensed for use as therapy in CD and UC; OLE, open-label extension; tt, treat-through; r, continuation of assigned treatment in responders; r 26, remission at week 26; rr, randomized responder; nd, not done; na, not applicable.

clinical remission was achieved in 46% of patients (Sands et al., 2020a). A phase III study program (VIVID) aimed at evaluating the clinical efficacy of mirikizumab for the treatment of patients with CD is currently underway.

At United European Gastroenterology (UEG) Week 2020, data from the GALAXI 1 study that featured the treatment of CD patients with the anti-p19 mAb, **guselkumab,** were presented. Similar to risankizumab, this drug has already been approved for the treatment of plaque psoriasis. In this phase II study, the effectiveness of intravenous induction therapy with guselkumab was compared to placebo and induction with ustekinumab in 250 patients. Clinical remission was observed in 50–56% of patients at week 12 (and in 16 and 45% to placebo and ustekinumab, respectively). Other endpoints, including clinical, biochemical, and endoscopic responses were also achieved significantly more frequently with guselkumab than with placebo, although no dose-dependency was observed (Sandborn et al., 2020).

The results of eight studies focused on achieving clinical remission in both CD and UC using anti-IL-23 strategies are summarized in **Table 2**.

COMMENT

Taken together, results from the aforementioned studies suggest that combined inhibition of both IL-12 and IL-23 (as achieved with ustekinumab and possibly briakinumab) as well as selective inhibition of IL-23 alone (with brazikumab, risankizumab, mirikizumab, and guselkumab) are all effective therapies for patients with CD, and probably also for those with UC. It is not yet clear whether inhibition of one vs. two of the target cytokines offers advantages with regard to effectiveness and/or safety. In particular, ustekinumab, which has been approved for use as a treatment for both CD and UC, has a documented favorable safety profile based on the results of individual studies of patients who received this therapy for more than 5 years. We can assume that this good safety profile will most likely apply to the other, related drugs considered here, although their individual adverse event profiles require specific evaluation in future studies.

JAK INHIBITORS

The therapeutic modalities considered above were designed to interact with extracellular targets, including pro-inflammatory cytokines or cell-adhesion molecules. Another concept under development involves the blockade of intracellular signaling using inhibitors of tyrosine kinases. While more than 80 tyrosine kinases have been characterized, the Janus kinases (JAKs) have been identified as critical targets. Tofacitinib is a small-molecule inhibitor of JAK1 and JAK3 that has already been approved for the treatment of UC. A clinically relevant advantage of this class of medications is that unlike biologics, they are largely non-immunogenic. This is an important attribute, given that neutralizing immune responses are often the cause of secondary loss of response to biologics [see Overview (Vulliemoz et al., 2020)].

However, one notable disadvantage of tofacitinib is the increased risk for primary infection or reactivation of herpes zoster, as well as deep vein thrombosis and pulmonary embolism, especially in elder patients. **Upadacitinib**, a selective JAK1 inhibitor, has already been approved for the treatment of refractory rheumatoid arthritis and is currently under evaluation as induction and maintenance therapy for moderate to severe CD and UC. Clinical and endoscopic remissions after 16 weeks were defined as primary clinical end-points in these studies. The current results reveal endoscopic improvement and

TABLE 3 | Frequency of achieving clinical remission in studies featuring JAK inhibitors in patients with CD (a) or UC (b).

Drug	Study phase	Induction treatment				Study type	Maintenance treatment				Ref
		Week	Study drug	Placebo	*p*		Week	Study drug	Placebo	*p*	
a) CD											
Tofacitinib[a]	II	8	43.5	36.7%	0.325	rr	26	55.8	38.1%	0.13	Panés et al. (2017)
Upadacitinib	II	16	27.0	11.0%	<0.1	rr	52	41.0	32.0%	n.s	Sandborn et al. (2020c)
Filgotinib	II	10	47.0	23.0%	0.008						Vermeire et al. (2017b)

Drug	Study phase	Induction treatment				Study type	Maintenance treatment				Ref
		Week	Study drug	Placebo	*p*		Week	Study drug	Placebo	*p*	
b) UC											
Tofacitinib[a]	III	8	17.6	6.0%	<0.001	rr	52	40.6	11.0%	<0.001	Sandborn et al. (2017)
Upadacitinib	II	8	19.6	0.0%	0.002						Sandborn et al. (2020c)
Filgotinib	II/III	10	18.2	9.7%	0.001	rr	58	37.2	11.2%	<0.001	Feagan et al. (2020b), pooled data, Peyrin-Biroulet et al. (2020b)

NB: In studies that feature different dosages or intervals, the most effective treatment has been presented.
[a]currently licensed for use as therapy in CD and UC; OLE, open-label extension; tt, treat-through, r, continuation of assigned treatment in responders; r 26, remission at week 26; rr, randomized responder; nd, not done, na, not applicable.

clinical responses to induction therapy at daily doses of 6 and 7.5 mg, respectively. Of significant clinical relevance, the results of this study revealed that extraintestinal manifestations improved more frequently in response to upadacitinib compared to placebo in patients with CD (Peyrin-Biroulet et al., 2019).

Interestingly, more infections and more serious infections occurred in patients with CD in the upadacitinib treatment group than were reported in the group receiving placebo. While this was largely expected, this was not observed in studies involving the treatment of patients with UC (Sandborn et al., 2020a; Sandborn et al., 2020c).

Filgotinib is a selective JAK1 inhibitor that has recently been approved in Europe for the treatment of rheumatoid arthritis (September 2020); it has also been evaluated in patients with CD in the FITZROY phase II trial. Clinical remission was observed after 10 weeks in 47% of the patients receiving the study drug, compared to 23% in the placebo group ($p = 0.008$) (Vermeire et al., 2017b). A phase III trial in patients with CD is currently ongoing, together with additional phase II trials that feature subgroups of CD patients, including those with perianal fistulas or primarily small bowel disease. The recently closed phase IIb/III SELECTION study examined 1,348 patients with moderate to severe UC. Although the full publication remains pending, preliminary data reveal a significantly higher rate of clinical remission after 10 and 58 weeks among patients treated with 200 mg of filgotinib compared to placebo.

The results of six studies focused on achieving clinical remission in both CD and UC using JAK inhibitors are summarized in **Table 3**.

In addition to the previously characterized JAK inhibitors, other innovative approaches are currently under evaluation in clinical trials. For example, another potential therapeutic target is tyrosine kinase 2 (TYK2); this kinase is involved in the signal transduction mediated by the IBD-associated cytokines IL-12, IL-13, and the interferons. The TYK2 inhibitor, BMS-986165, is currently under evaluation for induction and maintenance of remission in a phase II trial in patients with CD.

Local/topical administration of JAK inhibitors is an important approach that is currently under consideration in an effort to reduce the frequency of treatment-associated infections. Toward this end, TD 1473 is a high-affinity JAK1-, JAK2-, JAK3- and TYK2-inhibitor that cannot be resorbed; this property results in high levels of drug within the inflamed gut mucosa with only minimal systemic exposure. Results of phase I trials indicated low plasma levels of this drug despite high concentrations in the colon. Data obtained in trials that included healthy subjects and also patients with UC revealed that a single dose of up to 1,000 mg or 14 days of a 300 mg daily dose appear to be safe and well-tolerated. As such, this might prove to be a promising approach for the treatment of UC.

COMMENT

In the coming years, additional tyrosine kinase inhibitors will be available for the treatment of IBD. Before treatment, the risk of herpes zoster reactivation and postherpetic neuralgia should be assessed and susceptible patients should be vaccinated. Likewise, there is an urgent need for direct head-to-head studies that compare the therapeutic potential of JAK inhibitors with previously-approved biological therapies. Due to the complexity of the JAK-mediated intracellular signaling pathways, it will be necessary to establish intensive long-term monitoring of patients who participated in registry studies to identify any long-term sequelae, including the potential for malignancies.

MODULATION OF SPHINGOSINE-1-PHOSPHATE RECEPTORS

Naïve lymphocytes reach the lymph nodes via afferent lymphatic vessels and ultimately enter the systemic circulation in response to an S1P gradient. Ligand-mediated activation leads to S1P-receptor (S1PR) internalization and therefore to a functional blockade of lymphocyte migration.

Fingolimod is an S1PR1 modulator that has already been approved for the treatment of multiple sclerosis. However, the use of this medication is associated with severe adverse effects, including cardiac sequelae, varicella zoster-encephalitis, hepatopathies, macular edema, and progressive multifocal leukoencephalopathy. A recent "Direct Health Care Professional Communication" issued by the EMA focused on fingolimod-induced liver injury, which can progress to acute liver failure requiring a liver transplant.

The TOUCHSTONE study featured responses of patients with UC to 32 weeks of therapy with the S1PR1/R5-modulator, **ozanimod**. The results of this study revealed a higher rate of clinical remission among those treated with the higher dose (1 mg/day) but not the lower dose (0.5 mg/day) of drug vs. those receiving placebo; this response was accompanied by a higher rate of mucosal healing (Sandborn et al., 2016). Data from the prolonged follow-up study (currently available as an abstract only) suggest that long-term control of inflammation can be achieved for up to 200 weeks.

An abstract of the results of the phase III study (TRUE NORTH) was presented at UEG Week 2020. In this study, 645 patients with UC were randomized 2:1 to receive treatment with 1 mg ozanimod (1 mg/day vs. placebo). After 10 weeks of therapy, clinical remission was achieved in 18.4 vs. 6.0% ($p = 0.001$) of the study participants, respectively; clinical remission was associated with a higher rate of mucosal healing. In the maintenance study that followed, 37% of the patients, that initially responded to the induction therapy reached a clinical remission after 52 weeks, compared to only 18.5% of those receiving placebo ($p < 0.001$) (Danese et al., 2020b; Sandborn et al., 2020f).

Preliminary data indicate that ozanimod is also effective in patients with CD. Sixty-nine patients were treated with ozanimod in the open STEPSTONE trial; after 12 weeks, 56.5% had a clinical response, 39.1% experienced clinical remission, and 23.2% had an endoscopic response (Feagan et al., 2020a). A placebo-controlled, phase III trial has been initiated.

A phase II study of the efficacy of **etrasimod**, an S1PR1/R4/R5 receptor modulator, in patients with UC indicated that treatment with this drug resulted in a marked improvement in the modified Mayo Scores when compared to placebo; this was especially notable in response to the higher dose (2 mg/day). Furthermore, a larger proportion of patients who achieved in clinical remission (33.0 vs. 8.1%; $p < 0.001$) and endoscopic improvement (41.8 vs. 17.8%; $p = 0.003$) could be identified after 12 weeks (Sandborn et al., 2020d).

Moreover, data from CD patients are available from a proof-of-concept-study that featured the S1PR1-modulator, **amiselimod**, although no clinical responses or biochemical improvement of disease activity was observed in comparison to placebo.

The results of four studies focused on achieving clinical remission in both CD and UC using S1PR modulators are summarized in **Table 4**.

COMMENT

As the modulation of the S1PRs is a novel therapeutic approach, its overall efficacy specifically for the treatment of patients with IBD requires further examination. Initial findings suggest no essential advantages when compared to previously established therapeutic regimens. Furthermore, it is unclear as to what might happen when the drug is discontinued. Of concern is the possibility of excessive rebound inflammation due to sudden removal of the blockade to lymphocyte migration.

PHOSPHODIESTERASE INHIBITORS

Apremilast is an inhibitor of the intracellular enzyme, phosphodiesterase 4. Blockade of this signaling pathway results in increased concentrations of intracellular cyclic AMP (cAMP); this leads to the inhibition of TNF-α–release and an increase in the level of the anti-inflammatory cytokine, IL-10. Apremilast has already been approved for the treatment of psoriasis. Although higher rates of clinical remission were observed at week 12 in comparison to placebo (30 mg: 31.6% and 40 mg 21.8 vs. Placebo: 12.1%; $p = 0.269$ and $p = 0.01$, resp.) in a current phase II study with 170 UC patients, these results did not achieve statistical significance (hierarchical, stepdown testing procedure), and as such, the primary endpoint of the study was not reached. However, remission was maintained in up to 40% of the patients that remained on the medication at week 52 (Danese et al., 2020b).

COMMENT

Inhibition of TNF-α *via* a mechanism that is unlikely to be vulnerable to immune-mediated loss of response is an interesting new therapeutic approach. However, the efficacy of this modality remains to be verified in future studies.

OLIGONUCLEOTIDE-BASED THERAPEUTICS

Specific inactivation of genes known to be involved in disease pathogenesis might constitute an effective therapeutic modality with fewer adverse effects. Clinical experience with this type of therapy is currently very limited. The phase III study featuring administration of **mongersen**, an antisense oligonucleotide inhibitor of Smad7, which is a critical regulator of TGF-ß mediated down-regulation of pro-inflammatory cytokines, did not fulfill the high expectations from the phase II study for patients with CD. The study was terminated early due to insufficient efficacy (Sands et al., 2020a).

The anti-sense oligonucleotide therapeutic, **alicaforsen,** leads to down-regulation of intercellular adhesion molecule-1 (ICAM-1). Although this agent had some impact on disease activity, no convincing efficacy was demonstrated in a phase II trial with patients diagnosed with IBD. There is an ongoing phase III trial in which this agent is administered *via* an enema preparation

TABLE 4 | Frequency of achieving clinical remission in studies featuring S1P-receptor modulators to treat patients with CD (a) or UC (b).

Drug	Study phase	Induction treatment				Study type	Maintenance treatment				Ref
		Week	Study drug (%)	Placebo	p		Week	Study drug	Placebo	p	
a) CD											
Ozanimod	II	12	39.1	nd	Na						Feagan et al. (2020a)
Amiselimod	II	12	28.2	40.5%	ns						D'Haens et al. (2019)

Drug	Study phase	Induction treatment				Study type	Maintenance treatment				Ref
		Week	Study drug	Placebo	p		Week	Study drug (%)	Placebo	p	
b) UC											
Ozanimod	III	10	18.4	6.0%	<0.001	rr	52	37.0	18.5%	<0.001	Danese et al. (2020a), Sandborn et al. (2020)
Etrasimod	II	12	33.0	8.1%	<0.001	tt	46	39.3	nd	Na	Vermeire et al. (2019), Sandborn et al. (2020d)

OLE, open-label extension; tt, treat-through; r, continuation of assigned treatment in responders; r 26, remission at week 26; rr, randomized responder; nd, not done; na, not applicable; ns not significant. NB: In studies that feature different dosages or intervals, the most effective treatment has been presented.

specifically in patients with pouchitis. At UEG Week 2020, the first findings released from a phase IIb study with **cobitolimod** used to treat patients with left-sided ulcerative colitis were presented. This oligonucleotide TLR 9-agonist induces the expression of both IL-10 and type I-interferon. Two topical administrations of 250 mg were well tolerated by 42 of the total 213 patients participating in the study. The initial findings also suggest superiority regarding clinical remission after 6 weeks. No long-term data are currently available, but a phase III study is planned.

COMMENT

The Mongersen study is an impressive example of the fact that positive results from phase II trials, notably those that mainly rely on subjective criteria such as the Clinical disease Activity Index (CDAI) as endpoints, may ultimately fail to be reproduced in larger phase III studies that apply objective criteria (e.g., luminal inflammation markers, such as fecal calprotectin, and/or endoscopic changes.) Likewise, although the study examining the rectal administration of cobitolimod provided useful proof of efficacy, this route is not suitable for long-term therapy of chronic diseases. Other modes of application will need to be developed.

FECAL MICROBIOTA TRANSPLANTATION: READY FOR PRIME TIME?

An inappropriate immunologic response to the gastrointestinal microbiota is thought to be of great importance in the pathogenesis of IBD. Numerous clinical observations suggest a close connection between pathologic gastrointestinal microbiota and the manifestation of disease in patients with IBD. However, considering that genetic factors and inflammatory reactions can change the composition of the gastrointestinal microbiota, it is not clear whether changes in the gut microbiome are the causes or consequences of the disease process. While FMT may be among the more drastic of the interventions used to influence the gastrointestinal microbiome, this modality is now an accepted regimen for the treatment of recurrent *Clostridium difficile* infection (Khoruts et al., 2020).

Multiple case studies and several randomized trials have explored this concept in patients with IBD. While most randomized studies involving patients with UC revealed that FMT had a significant impact on induction of remission (Stallmach et al., 2019; Tan et al., 2020), its efficacy has not been verified for patients with CD. Placebo-controlled trials involving patients with UC revealed that, although one out of every 3 to 4 patients achieved remission after FMT, one-time or short-term FMT leads to clinical failure over time. To address this problem, repeat colonoscopic FMT was performed once every 8 weeks in patients with UC; this led to the maintenance of both endoscopic and histologic remission. The role of FMT for the treatment of CD has been explored in case series and a single randomized study (Tan et al., 2020). Despite the very heterogeneous approaches, including different applications, target criteria, and patient groups (children, teenagers, or adults with CD), the data suggest an ~30% probability (76/255 patients) of remission in response to FMT. However, in the first and thus far only published controlled study, Sokol et al. (Sokol et al., 2020) reported no difference in the remission rates maintained at 24 weeks between the FMT and sham-control group (4/8 vs. 3/9). As such, proof of the efficacy of FMT in patients with CD remains pending.

COMMENT

To induce long-term and sustainable changes in microbiota, repetitive FMT applications are required. Our data in patients with UC have revealed that the diversity of gastrointestinal microbiota increases significantly and remains stable in response to the daily application of FMT-capsules over a 3 month period. Before the therapeutic concept of FMT can be established as a routine treatment for UC, several critical questions remain to be answered:

- Are certain donors more likely to be effective than others? Are there patient-specific factors that might be used to inform donor selection?
- When should FMT be performed in patients diagnosed with IBD? At an early stage of the disease or after exhaustion of all other established treatments?
- What is the influence of emerging infectious disease challenges (e.g., the COVID-19 pandemic) on the long-term success of an FMT protocol?

Of course, identification of the therapeutically active substance or substances in fecal microbiota presents the possibility that they might be produced exogenously and provided by more routine therapeutic routes. Nevertheless, FMT is an extremely interesting therapeutic concept that merits further consideration. However, due to multiple limitations and many as-yet unanswered, this procedure should not be performed outside of clinical trials.

CONCLUSION

This review covers the current status of seven different new therapeutic approaches that may be on the horizon for the treatment of IBD. The modalities shown to be effective in phase II studies of course require confirmation in larger phase III studies; in most cases, these trials are already underway. The approval of several new therapeutic agents is anticipated in the near future, including many with unique pharmacological mechanisms of action. By their nature, these novel therapeutics will enhance and broaden the scope of our currently available drug treatments for IBD. This of course leads to further questions as clinicians attempt to determine which therapeutic approach is the best option for each patient. Given the broad scope of disease manifestations, it is unlikely that all patients will benefit equally from each new drug or drug class. One important focus of future studies will be the identification of biomarkers that can be used to predict individual responses to therapy. Until such predictors are available, the responsible clinician focusing on personalized therapy will have the option to select a given therapy based on individual disease characteristics, treatment targets, and published literature.

AUTHOR CONTRIBUTIONS

CS and AS wrote the first draft of the article, PCG prepared figure and tables. All authors reviewed and edited the article. All authors read and approved the final article. AS had the final responsibility for the decision to submit for publication.

REFERENCES

Coward, S., Clement, F., Benchimol, E. I., Bernstein, C. N., Avina-Zubieta, J. A., Bitton, A., et al. (2019). Past and future burden of inflammatory bowel diseases based on modeling of population-based data. *Gastroenterology* 156 (5), 1345–1353. doi:10.1053/j.gastro.2019.01.002e1344

Danese, S., Feagan, B. G., Wolf, D. C., Hanauer, S. B., Jovanovic, I., Ghosh, S., et al. (2020a). "Ozanimod as maintenance therapy in patients with moderate-to-severe ulcerative colitis: results from the phase 3, randomized, double-blind," in *Placebo-controlled true north study* (Vienna, Austria: United European Gastroenterology Week), LB10.

Danese, S., Neurath, M. F., Kopoń, A., Zakko, S. F., Simmons, T. C., Fogel, R., et al. (2020b). Effects of apremilast, an oral inhibitor of phosphodiesterase 4, in a randomized trial of patients with active ulcerative colitis. *Clin. Gastroenterol. Hepatol.* 18 (11), 2526–2534. doi:10.1016/j.cgh.2019.12.032

Danese, S., Sandborn, W. J., Reinisch, W., Hébuterne, X., Kłopocka, M., Tarabar, D., et al. (2019). Long-term mucosal healing, clinical response and clinical remission in patients with ulcerative colitis treated with the anti-mucosal addressin cell adhesion molecule-1 (MAdCAM-1) antibody ontamalimab (SHP647): results from the open-label extension study TURANDOT II. *United European Gastroenterol. J.* 7 (8 Suppl. l), 84. doi:10.14309/01.ajg.0000592624.44779.ee

Dotan, I. P. J., Duvall, A., Bouhnik, Y., Radford-Smith, G., Higgins, P. D. R., Mishkin, D. S., et al. (2020). *Etrolizumab compared with adalimumab or placebo as induction therapy for ulcerative colitis: results from the randomized, phase 3* Hibiscus *I & ii trials*, LB09. Vienna, Austria: United European Gastroenterology Week.

D'Haens, G., D. S., Davies, M., Watanabe, M., and Hibi, T. (2019). Amiselimod, a selective S1P receptor modulator in Crohn's disease patients: a proof-of-concept study. *J. Crohns Colitis* 13 (S1), S055–S056. doi:10.1093/ecco-jcc/jjy222.082

Feagan, B. G., Loftus, E. V., Jr., Danese, S., Vermeire, S., Sandborn, W. J., Ritter, T., et al. (2020a). *Efficacy and safety of filgotinib as induction therapy for patients with moderately to severely active ulcerative colitis: results from the phase 2b/3 selection study.* Vienna, Austria: United European Gastroenterology Week, LB19

Feagan, B. G., Panés, J., Ferrante, M., Kaser, A., D'Haens, G. R., Sandborn, W. J., et al. (2018). Risankizumab in patients with moderate to severe Crohn's disease: an open-label extension study. *Lancet Gastroenterol. Hepatol.* 3 (10), 671–680. doi:10.1016/s2468-1253(18)30233-4

Feagan, B. G., Rutgeerts, P., Sands, B. E., Hanauer, S., Colombel, J.-F., Sandborn, W. J., et al. (2013). Vedolizumab as induction and maintenance therapy for ulcerative colitis. *N. Engl. J. Med.* 369 (8), 699–710. doi:10.1056/NEJMoa1215734

Feagan, B. G., Sandborn, W. J., D'Haens, G., Panés, J., Kaser, A., Ferrante, M., et al. (2017). Induction therapy with the selective interleukin-23 inhibitor risankizumab in patients with moderate-to-severe Crohn's disease: a randomised, double-blind, placebo-controlled phase 2 study. *The Lancet* 389 (10080), 1699–1709. doi:10.1016/s0140-6736(17)30570-6

Feagan, B. G., Sandborn, W. J., Danese, S., Wolf, D. C., Liu, W. J., Hua, S. Y., et al. (2020b). Ozanimod induction therapy for patients with moderate to severe Crohn's disease: a single-arm, phase 2, prospective observer-blinded endpoint study. *Lancet Gastroenterol. Hepatol.* 5 (9), 819–828. doi:10.1016/s2468-1253(20)30188-6

Feagan, B. G., Sandborn, W. J., Gasink, C., Jacobstein, D., Lang, Y., Friedman, J. R., et al. (2016). Ustekinumab as induction and maintenance therapy for crohn's disease. *N. Engl. J. Med.* 375 (20), 1946–1960. doi:10.1056/NEJMoa1602773

Khoruts, A., Staley, C., and Sadowsky, M. J. (2020). Faecal microbiota transplantation for Clostridioides *difficile*: mechanisms and pharmacology. *Nat. Rev. Gastroenterol. Hepatol.* 18, 67. doi:10.1038/s41575-020-0350-4

Panaccione, R., Sandborn, W. J., Gordon, G. L., Lee, S. D., Safdi, A., Sedghi, S., et al. (2015). Briakinumab for treatment of Crohn's disease. *Inflamm. Bowel Dis.* 21 (6), 1–1340. doi:10.1097/MIB.0000000000000366

Panés, J., Sandborn, W. J., Schreiber, S., Sands, B. E., Vermeire, S., D'Haens, G., et al. (2017). Tofacitinib for induction and maintenance therapy of Crohn's disease: results of two phase IIb randomised placebo-controlled trials. *Gut* 66 (6), 1049–1059. doi:10.1136/gutjnl-2016-312735

Peyrin-Biroulet, L., Danese, S., Louis, E., Higgins, P. D. R., Dubinsky, M., Cataldi, F., et al. (2019). DOP50 Effect of upadacitinib on extra-intestinal manifestations in patients with moderate to severe Crohn's disease: data from the CELEST study. *J. Crohns Colitis* 13 (S1), S057. doi:10.1093/ecco-jcc/jjy222.084

Peyrin-Biroulet, L., Hassan, A. L., Bossuyt, P., Long, M., Allez, M., Juillerat, P., et al. (2020a). "Etrolizumab as induction and maintenance therapy in patients with ulcerative colitis previously exposed to anti-tumor necrosis factor Agent: the randomized," in *Phase 3 hickory trial*, LB08.

Peyrin-Biroulet, L., Loftus, E. V., Jr, Danese, S., Vermeire, S., Sandborn, W. J., Fogel, R., et al. (2020b). *Efficacy and safety of filgotinib as maintenance therapy for patients with moderately to severely active ulcerative colitis: results from the phase 2b/3 selection study.* Vienna, Austria: United European Gastroenterology Week, LB20.

Sandborn, W. J., D'Haens, G. R., Wolf, D. C., Hanauer, S. B., Jovanovic, I., Ghosh, S., et al. (2020). "Ozanimod as induction therapy," in *Moderate-to severe ulcerative colitis: results from the phase 3, randomized, double-blind, placebo-controlled true North study* (Vienna, Austria: United European Gastroenterology Week), LB02. doi:10.1177/2050640620968709

Sandborn, W. J., Feagan, B. G., Loftus, E. V., Jr., Peyrin-Biroulet, L., Van Assche, G., D'Haens, G., et al. (2020b). Efficacy and safety of upadacitinib in a randomized trial of patients with crohn's disease. *Gastroenterology* 158 (8), 2123–2138. doi:10.1053/j.gastro.2020.01.047

Sandborn, W. J., Feagan, B. G., Rutgeerts, P., Hanauer, S., Colombel, J.-F., Sands, B. E., et al. (2013). Vedolizumab as induction and maintenance therapy for Crohn's disease. *N. Engl. J. Med.* 369 (8), 711–721. doi:10.1056/NEJMoa1215739

Sandborn, W. J., Feagan, B. G., Wolf, D. C., D'Haens, G., Vermeire, S., Hanauer, S. B., et al. (2016). Ozanimod induction and maintenance treatment for ulcerative colitis. *N. Engl. J. Med.* 374 (18), 1754–1762. doi:10.1056/NEJMoa1513248

Sandborn, W. J., Ferrante, M., Bhandari, B. R., Berliba, E., Feagan, B. G., Hibi, T., et al. (2020c). Efficacy and safety of mirikizumab in a randomized phase 2 study of patients with ulcerative colitis. *Gastroenterology* 158 (3), 537–549. doi:10.1053/j.gastro.2019.08.043e510

Sandborn, W. J., Ghosh, S., Panes, J., Schreiber, S., D'Haens, G., Tanida, S., et al. (2020d). Efficacy of upadacitinib in a randomized trial of patients with active ulcerative colitis. *Gastroenterology* 158 (8), 2139–2149. doi:10.1053/j.gastro.2020.02.030e2114

Sandborn, W. J., Lee, S. D., Tarabar, D., Louis, E., Klopocka, M., Klaus, J., et al. (2018). Phase II evaluation of anti-MAdCAM antibody PF-00547659 in the treatment of Crohn's disease: report of the OPERA study. *Gut* 67 (10), 1824–1835. doi:10.1136/gutjnl-2016-313457

Sandborn, W. J., Peyrin-Biroulet, L., Zhang, J., Chiorean, M., Vermeire, S., Lee, S. D., et al. (2020e). Efficacy and safety of etrasimod in a phase 2 randomized trial of patients with ulcerative colitis. *Gastroenterology* 158 (3), 550–561. doi:10.1053/j.gastro.2019.10.035

Sandborn, W. J., Su, C., Sands, B. E., D'Haens, G. R., Vermeire, S., Schreiber, S., et al. (2017). Tofacitinib as induction and maintenance therapy for ulcerative colitis. *N. Engl. J. Med.* 376 (18), 1723–1736. doi:10.1056/NEJMoa1606910

Sandborn, W. J., Vermeire, S., Vermeire, S., Tyrrell, H., Hassanali, A., Lacey, S., et al. (2020f). Etrolizumab for the treatment of ulcerative colitis and crohn's disease: an overview of the phase 3 clinical program. *Adv. Ther.* 37 (7), 3417–3431. doi:10.1007/s12325-020-01366-2

Sandborn, W. J., Wolf, C. D., Johanns, J., Lang, G., Adedokun, O. J., Afzali, A., et al. (2020a). The efficacy and safety of guselkumab induction therapy in patients with moderately to severely active Crohn's disease: week 12 interim analyses from the phase 2 galaxi 1 study. *United Eur. Gastroenterol J* 8 (8 Suppl. l), 64.

Sands, B., S. W., Peyrin-Biroulet, L., Higgins, P., Hirai, F., Belin, R., Gomez Valderas, E., et al. (2019). Efficacy and safety of mirikizumab (LY3074828) in a phase 2 study of patients with Crohn's disease. *United Eur. Gastroenterol J* 7 (8 Suppl. l), 92. doi:10.1177/2050640619854670

Sands, B. E., Chen, J., Feagan, B. G., Penney, M., Rees, W. A., Danese, S., et al. (2017). Efficacy and safety of MEDI2070, an antibody against interleukin 23, in patients with moderate to severe crohn's disease: a phase 2a study. *Gastroenterology* 153 (1), 77–86. doi:10.1053/j.gastro.2017.03.049

Sands, B. E., Feagan, B. G., Sandborn, W. J., Schreiber, S., Peyrin-Biroulet, L., Frédéric Colombel, J., et al. (2020b). Mongersen (GED-0301) for active crohn's disease: results of a phase 3 study. *Am. J. Gastroenterol.* 115 (5), 738–745. doi:10.14309/ajg.0000000000000493

Sands, B. E., Peyrin-Biroulet, L., Loftus, E. V., Jr., Danese, S., Colombel, J.-F., Törüner, M., et al. (2019a). Vedolizumab versus adalimumab for moderate-to-severe ulcerative colitis. *N. Engl. J. Med.* 381 (13), 1215–1226. doi:10.1056/NEJMoa1905725

Sands, B. E., Sandborn, W. J., Panaccione, R., O'Brien, C. D., Zhang, H., Johanns, J., et al. (2019b). Ustekinumab as induction and maintenance therapy for ulcerative colitis. *N. Engl. J. Med.* 381 (13), 1201–1214. doi:10.1056/NEJMoa1900750

Sands, B. E., Scully, S. W. J., Peyrin-Biroulet, L., Higgins, P., Hirai, F., Jairath, V., et al. (2020a). Efficacy and safety of mirikizumab after 52-weeks maintenance treatment in patients with moderate-to-severe Crohn's disease. *United Eur. Gastroenterol J* 8 (8 Suppl. l), 75–76. doi:10.1177/2050640620927344

Sokol, H., Landman, C., Landman, C., Seksik, P., Berard, L., Montil, M., et al. (2020). Fecal microbiota transplantation to maintain remission in Crohn's disease: a pilot randomized controlled study. *Microbiome* 8 (1), 12. doi:10.1186/s40168-020-0792-5

Stallmach, A., Grunert, P., Pieper, D., and Steube, A. (2019). Colitis ulcerosa: kann eine Modulation der intestinalen Mikrobiota eine langfristige Remission bedingen? *Z. Gastroenterol.* 57 (7), 834–842. doi:10.1055/a-0874-6603

Tan, P., Li, X., Shen, J., and Feng, Q. (2020). Fecal microbiota transplantation for the treatment of inflammatory bowel disease: an update. *Front. Pharmacol.* 11, 574533. doi:10.3389/fphar.2020.574533

Vermeire, S., L, P. L., Ritter, T., Hanauer, S., Bressler, B., Khanna, R., et al. (2020). *Etrolizumab versus placebo in tumor necrosis factor Antagonist naive patients with ulcerative colitis: results from the randomized phase 3 laurel trial.* Vienna, Austria: United European Gastroenterology Week, LB18.

Vermeire, S., O'Byrne, S., Keir, M., Williams, M., Lu, T. T., Mansfield, J. C., et al. (2014). Etrolizumab as induction therapy for ulcerative colitis: a randomised, controlled, phase 2 trial. *The Lancet* 384 (9940), 309–318. doi:10.1016/S0140-6736(14)60661-9

Vermeire, S., Pulley, J., Chiorean, M., Peyrin-Biroulet, L., Zhang, J., Sands, B. E., et al. (2019). Long-term efficacy and safety of etrasimod for ulcerative colitis: results from the open-label extension of the OASIS study. *United Eur. Gastroenterol. J.* 7 (8 Suppl. l), 352. doi:10.1177/2050640619854670

Vermeire, S., Sandborn, W. J., Danese, S., Hébuterne, X., Salzberg, B. A., Klopocka, M., et al. (2017a). Anti-MAdCAM antibody (PF-00547659) for ulcerative colitis (TURANDOT): a phase 2, randomised, double-blind, placebo-controlled trial. *The Lancet* 390 (10090), 135–144. doi:10.1016/s0140-6736(17)30930-3

Vermeire, S., Schreiber, S., Petryka, R., Kuehbacher, T., Hebuterne, X., Roblin, X., et al. (2017b). Clinical remission in patients with moderate-to-severe Crohn's disease treated with filgotinib (the FITZROY study): results from a phase 2, double-blind, randomised, placebo-controlled trial. *The Lancet* 389 (10066), 266–275. doi:10.1016/S0140-6736(16)32537-5

Vulliemoz, M., Brand, S., Juillerat, P., Mottet, C., Ben-Horin, S., and Michetti, P. (2020). TNF-alpha blockers in inflammatory bowel diseases: practical recommendations and a user's guide: an update. *Digestion* 101 (Suppl. 1), 16–26. doi:10.1159/000506898

Yoshimura, N., Watanabe, M., Motoya, S., Tominaga, K., Matsuoka, K., Iwakiri, R., et al. (2015). Safety and efficacy of AJM300, an oral antagonist of α4 integrin, in induction therapy for patients with active ulcerative colitis. *Gastroenterology* 149 (7), 1775–1783. doi:10.1053/j.gastro.2015.08.044

17

The Effects of Vitamin D Supplementation on Anthropometric and Biochemical Indices in Patients with Non-alcoholic Fatty Liver Disease

Shahla Rezaei[1,2], *Reza Tabrizi*[3], *Peyman Nowrouzi-Sohrabi*[2,4], *Mohammad Jalali*[5], *Mojtaba Shabani-Borujeni*[6], *Shayan Modaresi*[2], *Maryam Gholamalizadeh*[7] *and Saeid Doaei*[8]*

[1]*Nutrition Research Center, School of Nutrition and Food Sciences, Shiraz University of Medical Sciences, Shiraz, Iran,* [2]*Student Research Committee, Shiraz University of Medical Sciences, Shiraz, Iran,* [3]*Non-Communicable Diseases Research Center, Fasa University of Medical Sciences, Fasa, Iran,* [4]*Department of Biochemistry, School of Medicine, Shiraz University of Medical Sciences, Shiraz, Iran,* [5]*Nutrition Research Center, Student Research Committee, Shiraz University of Medical Sciences, Shiraz, Iran,* [6]*Department of Clinical Pharmacy, Faculty of Pharmacy, Shiraz University of Medical Sciences, Shiraz, Iran,* [7]*Student Research Committee, Cancer Research Center, Shahid Beheshti University of Medical Sciences, Tehran, Iran,* [8]*Research Center of Health and Enviroment, School of Health, Guilan University of Medical Sciences, Rasht, Iran*

Correspondence:
Saeid Doaei
sdoaee@yahoo.com

Background: Vitamin D was reported to be associated with non-alcoholic fatty liver disease (NAFLD). This systematic review and meta-analysis aimed to investigate the effects of the vitamin D supplementation on anthropometric and biochemical indices in patient with NAFLD.

Methods: PubMed, Web of science, Scopus, and Embase databases were explored to identify all randomized controlled trial (RCT) investigating the effects of vitamin D supplementation on anthropometric and biochemical indices in patients with NAFLD. A random-effects model was used to pool weighted mean difference (WMD) and corresponding 95% confidence intervals (CIs). The statistical heterogeneity among the studies was assessed using I2 statistic (high ≥ 50%, low < 50%) and Cochran's Q-test.

Results: Sixteen RCTs were included in this meta-analysis. The results identified that high-density lipoprotein-cholesterol (HDL-C) level significantly increased following vitamin D supplementation ($P = 0.008$). Vitamin D reduced body weight ($P = 0.007$), body mass index ($P = 0.002$), waist circumstance (WC) ($P = 0.02$), serum alanine transaminase (ALT) ($P = 0.01$), fasting blood sugar (FBS) ($P = 0.01$), homeostatic model assessment for insulin resistance (HOMA-IR) ($P = 0.004$), and calcium ($P = 0.01$). No significant changes were found on body fat, triglyceride (TG), total cholesterol, low-density lipoprotein-cholesterol

---

Abbreviations: NAFLD, with non-alcoholic fatty liver disease; BMI, body mass index; WC, waist circumstance; ALT, alanine transaminase; FBS, fasting blood sugar; HOMA-IR, homeostatic model assessment for insulin resistance; TG: triglyceride.

(LDL–C), aspartate transaminase, alkaline phosphatase, gamma–glutamyl transferase, and adiponectin following vitamin D supplementation.

Conclusion: Vitamin D had significant effects on anthropometric and biochemical indices including HDL–C, body weight, BMI, WC, serum ALT, serum FBS, HOMA–IR, and calcium. Vitamin D supplementation can be considered as an effective strategy in management of patients with NAFLD.

Systematic Review Registration: [website], identifier [registration number]

Keywords: vitamin D, NAFLD, liver enzyme, anthropometry, biochemical indices

BACKGROUND

Non-alcoholic fatty liver disease (NAFLD) is considered to be the most common cause of chronic liver disorders (Younossi, 2019). NAFLD includes a wide range of liver diseases such as fibrosis, cirrhosis and non–alcoholic hepatitis (Petta et al., 2016; Morvaridzadeh et al., 2021). The prevalence of NAFLD is about 20% in general population and about 70–90% in patients with type 2 diabetes (Tolman et al., 2007; Chalasani et al., 2012). The main causes of NAFLD are obesity, excessive dietary fat intake, insulin resistance, and dyslipidemia (Ludwig et al., 1980). Over the past few decades, various pharmacological and nutritional interventions have been assessed to treat NAFLD, but none indicated significant improvements. Currently, no medically approved drugs are available for NAFLD (Del Ben et al., 2014). Weight loss and nutritional interventions are considered standard treatments for NAFLD. Insulin resistance increases the rate of adipose tissue lipolysis and the flow of free fatty acids to the liver cell. Hyperglycemia also causes lipid–related changes in the liver cells by increasing lipogenesis while blocking fatty acid oxidation (FAO) and lipid transport in the liver (Kleiner et al., 2005; Schwimmer et al., 2005).

Vitamin D plays an important role in reducing insulin resistance, obesity, cardiovascular risk, prediabetes, metabolic syndrome, cancer, and cardiovascular diseases (CVD_S) (Sepidarkish et al., 2019; Gholamalizadeh et al., 2020). Low serum level of 25-hydroxyvitamin D [25 (OH) D] is reported to be a risk factor for NAFLD disease (Forouhi et al., 2008; Sepidarkish et al., 2019). Vitamin D hypovitaminosis is associated with the severity and incidence of NAFLD in patients with normal liver enzymes. Vitamin D can affect the liver function through the vitamin D receptor (VDR). VDR is naturally present in the liver cells and its higher expression can reduce inflammation in chronic liver diseases (Benetti et al., 2018). Vitamin D also has anti–fibrotic, proliferative, and inflammatory effects on the liver. Some studies on the effects of vitamin D on anthropometric and biochemical indices reported that vitamin D was associated with body weight, fasting blood sugar (FBS), homeostatic model assessment for insulin resistance (HOMA–IR), glucose homeostasis, insulin resistance, high–density lipoprotein–cholesterol (HDL-C), low-density lipoprotein-cholesterol (LDL-C), triglycerides (TG), total cholesterol (TC), liver enzyme, and adiponectin (Sarathy et al., 2015; Foroughi et al., 2016; Doaei et al., 2019). A recent systematic review also reported that vitamin D improves the level of inflammatory mediators in patients with nonalcoholic fatty liver disease, but has no effect on anthropometric and glycemic indexes (Hariri and Zohdi, 2019; Mehrdad et al., 2020). However, the findings on the effects of vitamin D on NAFLD were contradictory (Sharifi et al., 2014; Sarathy et al., 2015). Therefore, this study aimed to investigate the effect of Vitamin D supplementation on anthropometric and biochemical indices in patient with NAFLD.

METHODS

Preferred reporting items for systematic reviews and meta–analyses (PRISMA) (Moher et al., 2009) was used to demonstrate the process of study selection (**Figure 1**).

Search Strategy

Two independent researchers performed the process of the systematic search using the online databases such as PubMed, embase, Scopus, Web of Science, and Cochrane Library for publications from 1980 up to 2021 on the effects of vitamin D supplementation on anthropometric and biochemical indices in patients with NAFLD, without considering any restriction on the language to detect the relevant citations. The PubMed search strategy was improved by consulting with an epidemiologist and was designed as a combination of the following search terms: "Vitamin D OR Cholecalciferol OR Calciol OR "Vitamin D 3" OR "Vitamin D3" OR Cholecalciferols OR Hydroxycholecalciferols OR "Hydroxyvitamins D″ OR Hydroxycholecalciferol OR Calcifediol OR "25–Hydroxyvitamin D 3" OR "25 Hydroxyvitamin D 3" OR "25–Hydroxycholecalciferol" OR Calcidiol OR Hydroxycholecalciferol OR Dedrogyl OR Hidroferol OR Calderol OR Dihydroxycholecalciferols OR "Dihydroxyvitamins D" OR "24,25–Dihydroxyvitamin D 3" OR Dihydroxyvitamin OR "24,25-Dihydroxyvitamin" OR "24,25-Dihydroxycholecalciferol" OR Dihydroxyvitamin OR Calcitriol OR "1 alpha,25-Dihydroxyvitamin" OR "1,25-Dihydroxyvitamin" OR "1,25-Dihydroxyvitamin" OR "1 alpha,25-Dihydroxycholecalciferol" OR "1,25–Dihydroxycholecalciferol" OR Dihydroxycholecalciferol OR Bocatriol OR Calcijex OR Decostriol OR MC1288 OR "MC–1288" OR "MC 1288" OR Osteotriol OR Renatriol OR Rocaltrol OR Silkis OR Sitriol OR Soltriol OR Tirocal" AND "Fatty Liver" OR

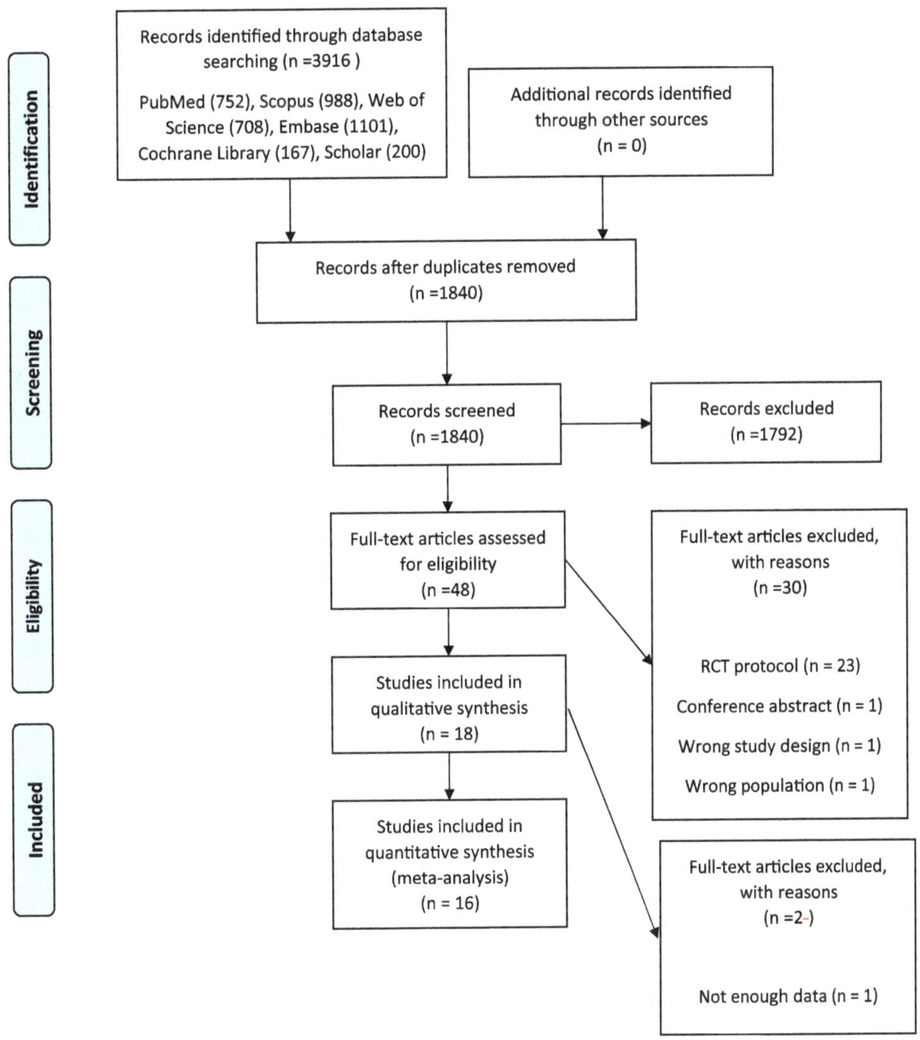

FIGURE 1 | Flow chart of the literature search strategy and study selection.

"Fatty Liver" OR Steatohepatitis OR Steatohepatitides OR "Steatosis of Liver" OR "Visceral Steatosis" OR Steatoses OR Steatosis OR "Visceral Steatoses" OR "Liver Steatosis" OR "Liver Steatoses" OR "Non–alcoholic Fatty Liver Disease" OR "Non–alcoholic Fatty Liver Disease" OR "Nonalcoholic Fatty Liver Disease" OR NAFLD OR "Nonalcoholic Fatty Liver Disease" OR Nonalcoholic OR "Nonalcoholic" OR "Nonalcoholic Fatty" OR "Non–alcoholic Fatty" OR "Nonalcoholic Fatty Liver" OR "Nonalcoholic Fatty Livers" OR NASH OR "Nonalcoholic Steatohepatitis" OR "Nonalcoholic Steatohepatitides" OR Steatohepatitis OR "liver cirrhosis" OR cirrhosis OR cirrhosis. To improve the search strategy, the wild–card term "*" was implicated and the reference lists of relevant articles were hand–scanned. Any doubts were resolved through discussing with the corresponding author.

Inclusion and Exclusion Criteria

Based on PICOS criteria, the aim of the present review study on patients with NAFLD (as population) was to evaluate the effect of vitamin D supplementation (as intervention) compared with placebo (as comparator) on anthropometric and biochemical outcomes (as outcome) in randomized interventional trials (as study design). Two independent reviewers initiated the assessment process of the collected papers and following inclusion criteria were considered (Younossi, 2019): randomized controlled trials (RCTs) with parallel design (Petta et al., 2016), studies that assessed the effects of vitamin D supplementation on patients with NAFLD. The exclusion criteria were (Younossi, 2019) being experimental study (Petta et al., 2016), lacking the essential data, for example, non–extractable or unconvertable data (Morvaridzadeh et al., 2021), studies without a suitable control group (Chalasani et al., 2012), trials with combined supplementation of nutrients or/and medicines besides vitamin D and also (Tolman et al., 2007) unpublished data, grey literature, conference abstracts, book chapters, and brief reports. The corresponding author was involved to solve disagreements.

Data Extraction

Following data were extracted from the included trials by two independent investigators: first authors' last name, publication date, country of study, study design, participants' characteristics, dosage of the supplement, intervention duration, quality of trials, mean changes and standard deviations (SDs) for each outcomes in pre–treatment and post–treatment. The third reviewer solved disagreements.

Risk of Bias Assessment

Two independent reviewers were assigned to qualify the included RCTs and explore the potential risk of bias for the following domains using the Cochrane Risk of Bias Tool: random sequence generation, allocation concealment, blinding of participants and personnel, blinding of outcome assessment, incomplete outcome data, and selective outcome reporting and other biases. "low", "high" or "unclear" terms were used to grade each item (Higgins et al., 2011).

Each question was answered as low risk of bias (score = 1), high risk of bias (score = −1), or unclear (score = 0). Disagreements was resolved by the third author. Scores were summed and studies with scores −6–0, 1–3 and 4–6 considered as low, medium and high quality, respectively (**Table 3**).

Statistical Analysis

A meta–analysis was performed using *STATA* software v13 (StataCorp, Texas) and a random–effects model was used to pool weighted mean difference (WMD) and corresponding 95% confidence intervals (CIs). The statistical heterogeneity among the studies was assessed using I^2 statistic (high ≥50%, low <50%) and Cochran's Q–test (Higgins et al., 2019). In presence of high inter–study heterogeneity, a random–effects meta–regression was performed to find its potential sources. Subgroup analysis was done based on country (Iran vs. other), duration of treatment (>12 weeks, ≤ 12 weeks), and dosage (>25,000 IU/day, ≤ 25,000 IU/day). Mean changes of the interested outcomes and the relevant SDs were obtained executing following formulas, respectively: (mean at post intervention–mean at baseline), SD = √([SD2–baseline + SD^2–post] − [2r × SD–baseline × SD–post]), assuming correlation coefficient (r) as 0.5 (Higgins et al., 2019). Sensitivity analysis was planned to assess the impact of each study on the pooled results by removing one study in a turn (Higgins et al., 2019). Potential publication bias was evaluated applying Egger regression and Begg's tests. If there was a significant publication bias, "trim and fills" analysis was done to check the possible change of the significance of the result (Duval and Tweedie, 2000). A P–value < 0.05 was considered as statistically significant.

RESULTS

Literature Search

A total of 3,916 potentially relevant articles were collected in the primary search (**Figure 1**). No additional article was detected via the hand searching. Among all of the references, 1840 were removed as duplicates. After title and abstract screening, 48 articles remained and after full-text review, 32 articles were excluded from the current study for different reasons. Thus, the final systematic review and meta-analysis was done on 16 papers (**Table 1**) (Sharifi et al., 2014; Foroughi et al., 2015; Barchetta et al., 2016; Foroughi et al., 2016; Nadjarzadeh et al., 2016; Sharifi et al., 2016; Lorvand Amiri et al., 2017; Sakpal et al., 2017; Dabbaghmanesh et al., 2018; Geier et al., 2018; Mansourian Hosseini et al., 2018; MOUODI et al., 2018; Hajiaghamohammadi et al., 2019; Hussain et al., 2019; Shidfar et al., 2019; Foroughi et al., 2014).

Meta–Analyses

Effect of Vitamin D on Lipid Profile

A significant improvement of serum HDL–C [WMD = 1.60, 95% CI = (0.41, 2.78), p = 0.008, I^2 = 0.0%] was found following vitamin D intake compared to the controls. Serum levels of TG [WMD = 0.65, 95% CI = (−12.60, 13.91), p = 0.92, I^2 = 40.9%], TC [WMD = 5.62, 95% CI = (−4.20, 15.45), p = 0.26, I^2 = 69.0%] and LDL–C [WMD = 3.53, 95% CI = (−0.91, 7.97), p = 0.11, I^2 = 12.8%] were not significantly affected in the group receiving vitamin D (**Figure 2**).

Effect of Vitamin D on Anthropometric Indices

Pooled results of the meta–analysis revealed a significant reduction in body weight [WMD = −0.88, 95% CI = (−1.52, −0.24), p = 0.007, I^2 = 29.7%], BMI [WMD = −0.33, 95% CI = (−0.54, −0.12), p = 0.002, I^2 = 21.5%], and WC [WMD = −1.04, 95% CI = (−1.97, −0.10), p = 0.02, I^2 = 64.0%] in the treatment groups compared with the controls. In contrast, body fat [WMD = 0.46, 95% CI = (−0.47, 1.40), p = 0.33, I^2 = 60.5%] was not changed following vitamin D supplementation (**Figure 3**).

Effect of Vitamin D on Liver Enzymes

Pooled estimate of 16 papers indicated a significant reduction of serum ALT [WMD = −4.03, 95% CI = (−7.41, −0.66), p = 0.01, I^2 = 78.5%] following vitamin D supplementation. However, serum AST [WMD = −1.05, 95% CI = (−3.50, 1.39), p = 0.39, I^2 = 78.2%], ALP [WMD = −5.43, 95% CI = (−18.08, 7.22), p = 0.40, I^2 = 62.4%], and GGT [WMD = −2.24, 95% CI = (−9.66, 5.18), p = 0.54, I^2 = 0.0%] were not affected by vitamin D supplementation (**Figure 4**).

Effect of Vitamin D on Glycemic Indices

As shown in **Figure 5**, receiving vitamin D significantly improved serum FBS [WMD = −5.02, 95% CI = (−8.95, −1.09), p = 0.01, I^2 = 81.6%] and HOMA–IR [WMD = −0.79, 95% CI = (−1.33, −0.25), p = 0.004, I^2 = 89.0%] compared with to the controls.

Effect of Vitamin D on Adiponectin and Calcium

As shown in **Figure 5**, serum calcium was significantly increased after vitamin D supplementation [WMD = 1.97, 95% CI = (0.38, 3.55), p = 0.01, I^2 = 99.3%]. Adiponectin was not significantly affected [WMD = 0.45, 95% CI = (−0.35, 1.24), p = 0.26, I^2 = 88.3%] by vitamin D supplementation.

Subgroup Analyses

As shown in **Table 2,** serum HDL–C was significantly affected by vitamin D supplementation when subgroup analysis conducted

TABLE 1 | Characteristics of the primary studies included in the meta-analysis.

Authors	Publication year	Country	Sample size case/ control	Dosage of vitamin D	Type of intervention in control group	Follow-up duration	Significant out comes
Foroughi et al. (Foroughi et al., 2015)	2015	Iran	30/30	50,000 IU/ week	Placebo	10 weeks	Vitamin D supplementation resulted in increased serum 25-hydroxy vitamin D concentration in the intervention group compared to the control group. Intake of vitamin D supplements led to a marginally significant decrease in fasting blood glucose in the intervention group compared to the control group. HOMA-IR decreased in the intervention group compared to the control group
Mansourian Hosseini et al. (Mansourian Hosseini et al., 2018)	2018	Iran	41/41	600,000 IU	Placebo	4 weeks	serum 25-hydroxyvitamin D significantly increased in the intervention group vs. the control. Total body fat decreased in the intervention group. while visceral fat was significantly different between the groups. Adiponectin, calcium, phosphors, and PTH levels increased, while liver enzymes, insulin, and HOMA-IR decreased in both. There were significant differences in mean changes of serum 25(OH) D, PTH, ALT, AST, ALP, and FBS between the groups after adjusting for baseline, TF and VF. Vitamin D injection did improve NAFLD severity
Hajiaghamoham madi et al. (Hajiaghamohammadi et al., 2019)	2019	Iran	40/40	50,000 IU/ week	Placebo	10 weeks	A significant reduction in the variables including AST, ALT, total cholesterol, and LDL-C in both groups ($p < 0.05$). As for the two indices of FBG and TG, the control group exhibited significantly less variations ($p < 0.05$)
Shidfar et al. (Shidfar et al., 2019)	2019	Iran	Group1: (n = 37), group2 (n = 37) group3 (n = 36)	Group1: (n = 37) 1000 IU vitamin D + Group2: (n = 37) 1000 IU vitamin D + 500 mg/d as calcium Group3: (n = 36), placebo	Placebo	12 weeks	Reduction in serum ALT, AST, LDL-C/ HDL-C, TC/HDL-C, and non-HDL C were significantly higher in the CaD compared with the P group
Geier et al. (Geier et al., 2018)	2018	Switzerland	30/30	2100 IU/daily	Placebo	18 weeks	Significant change was not observed in AST, AP, and GGT levels; significant change was observed in ALT
Dabbaghmanesh et al. (Dabbaghmanesh et al., 2018)	2018	Iran	Group1: 35, group2: 35, group3: 36	Group1:50,000 IU vitamin, Group2: 0.25 mg calcitriol, Group3: placebo	Placebo	12 weeks	serum alkaline phosphatase levels was significantly decreased from baseline levels in vitamin D3 group. Serum and gamma GGT level was also significantly decreased compared to the baseline levels in treatment group. There was no statistically significant difference between placebo and vitamin D3 group in terms of serum aminotransferase, ALP, serum GGT and lipid profile serum ALP levels was significantly decreased from baseline levels in calcitriol treated group. There was no statistically significant difference between placebo and calcitriol groups in terms of serum aminotransferase, ALP, serum GGT and lipid profile

(Continued on following page)

TABLE 1 | *(Continued)* Characteristics of the primary studies included in the meta-analysis.

Authors	Publication year	Country	Sample size case/ control	Dosage of vitamin D	Type of intervention in control group	Follow-up duration	Significant out comes
Hussain et al. (Hussain et al., 2019)	2019	Iran	55/54	50,000 IU vitamin	Placebo	12 weeks	A reduction in HOMA-IR, liver enzymes ALT, AST, serum CRP and increase in serum adiponectin as compared to placebo group. However no significant changes were observed in both groups in terms of body weight, BMI, and serum lipid profiles
Taghvaei et al. (MOUODI et al., 2018)	2018	Iran	20/20	50,000 IU vitamin	Placebo	12 weeks	Mean BMI and serum liver enzymes decreased significantly in two groups. A significant improvement was observed in steatosis in both groups. No significant differences were observed between the two groups in steatosis when measured by CAP parameter
Foroughi et al. (Foroughi et al., 2016)	2020	Iran	30/30	50,000 IU vitamin	Placebo	10 weeks	Vitamin D supplementation resulted in an increase of serum 25(OH) D concentrations in inter group and intra-group in intervention group. At the end of the study, in the intervention group, TG and CRP reduced significantly compare with baseline. A significant increase was seen in calcium serum in the intervention group in comparison with baseline and compared with the placebo group
Nadjarzadeh et al. (Nadjarzadeh et al., 2016)	2010	Iran	36/37	Group1: low calorie diet+ 50,000 IU vitamin D, Group2: low calorie diet + placebo	Placebo	12 weeks	Significant reduction was observed in ALT and AP Significant change was not observed in AST levels
Amiri et al. (Lorvand Amiri et al., 2017)	2016	Iran	37/36	1000 IU/day	Placebo	12 weeks	Significant reduction in FPG, insulin, insulin resistance (by HOMA-IR) and TG concentrations and an increase in HDL.C was seen over the 12 weeks of study in each group. Adjusting to the baseline measurements, there was significant difference in FPG, HOMA-IR, serum insulin, TG and HDL.C among the groups after 12 weeks of the study. The calcium plus calcitriol group showed a significant decrease in ALT and FPG and increase in HDL.C level compared with the calcitriol group, adjusted to the baseline measures
Sharifiet al. (Sharifi et al., 2016)	2016	Iran	27/26	50,000 IU vitamin D	Placebo	every 14 days for 4 months	In both genders, serum 25(OH) D3 increased significantly. This increase was accompanied by significant decrease in serum TC and LDL-C in women. However, in men, vitamin D supplementation increased the levels of serum TC with no significant effects on LDL-C. Moreover, vitamin D significantly reduced serum hs-CRP in women. The median daily calcium intake in both genders was well below the dietary reference intake for adults
Sharifi et al. (Sharifi et al., 2014)	2014	Iran	27/26	50,000 IU/ 2 weeks	Placebo	12 weeks	In vitamin D supplementation compared to the controls, the median of serum 25(OH)D3 significantly increased. This increase accompanied by significant decrease in serum MDA and near significant changes in serum hs-CRP. Other variables showed no significant changes

(Continued on following page)

TABLE 1 | *(Continued)* Characteristics of the primary studies included in the meta-analysis.

Authors	Publication year	Country	Sample size case/ control	Dosage of vitamin D	Type of intervention in control group	Follow-up duration	Significant out comes
Barchetta et al. (Barchetta et al., 2016)	2016	Italia	26/29	2000 IU/daily	Placebo	48 weeks	25(OH) vitamin D significantly increased in the treated group, no group differences were found in HFF, transaminases, CK18-M30, P3NP levels or FLI after 24 weeks. Vitamin D neither changed the metabolic profile nor the cardiovascular parameters
Foroughi et al. (Foroughi et al., 2016)	2014	Iran	30/30	50,000 IU vitamin D	Placebo	10 weeks	Vitamin D supplementation resulted in an increase of serum 25(OH) D concentrations in inter group and intra-group in intervention group. At the end of the study, in the intervention group, TG and CRP reduced significantly compare with baseline. A significant increase was seen in calcium serum in the intervention group in comparison with baseline and compared with the placebo group
Sakpal et al. (Sakpal et al., 2017)	2010	India	51/30	600,000 IU	Placebo	24 weeks	Significant improvement in serum ALT and serum adiponectin levels of intervention group

by country (Iran), duration (≤12 weeks), and dose (≤25,000 IU). BMI was changed in country (Iran), duration (>12 weeks), and dose (≤25,000 IU) subgroups. Body weight was changed in studies conducted in Iran and also when used >25,000 IU doses of when which interventions last >12 weeks, serum FBS was significantly affected when studies performed in Iran, last ≤12 weeks, and used doses more than 25,000 IU vitamin D. HOMA–IR was significantly improved all subgroups, except in trials last more than 12 weeks.

Meta–Regression and Sensitivity Analysis

The results of meta–regression and sensitivity analysis indicated that total sample size was regarded as a source of inter–study heterogeneity for AST [Coefficient: −0.19, 95% CI = (−0.29, −0.08), p = 0.001]. Sensitivity analyses showed that pooled results of interested outcomes are not sensitive to removing any of included trials.

Publication Bias

A significant publication bias was found for HOMA-IR, HDL-C and GGT. Hence, trim and fill analysis was done to detect the potential change of their results. Only the significance of HDL–C was changed and turned into non–significant.

DISCUSSION

To the best of the authors' knowledge, this is the first study to systematically review and meta analyze the findings of intervention studies on the effect of vitamin D on a wide range of anthropometric and biochemical indices in patient with NAFLD. The results of the present study indicated that vitamin D supplementation significantly improved the body weight, BMI, WC, HDL-C, ALT, FBS, and HOMA-IR in the intervention group compared to the control group. However, no significant differences were found on body fat, TG, LDL-C, AST, and GGT. Subgroup analyses also showed that the effect of vitamin D on most indices was affected by study location, duration of study and dose used for vitamin D.

Some studies investigated the association between vitamin D supplementation with lipid profile in NAFLD. In line with this study, Dabaghmanesh et al. indicated that 12 weeks of vitamin D supplementation significantly increased HDL-C (Dabbaghmanesh et al., 2018). Another study found that supplementation with calcium combined with vitamin D improved serum ALT and HDL-C levels (Lorvand Amiri et al., 2017).

However, the results regarding the effect of vitamin D on lipid profile have been contradictory. Sharifi et al. found that vitamin D intake supplementation for 4 months significantly decreed LDL-C and total cholesterol in woman (Sharifi et al., 2016). A meta-analysis indicated that supplementation with vitamin D significantly increased LDL-C and had not significant effect on TG and HDL-C in patients with CVDs (Wang et al., 2012). One study found that vitamin D supplementation reduced LDL-C but no significant change was found on HDL-C (Hajiaghamohammadi et al., 2019). In another study supplementation with vitamin D3 as 50,000 IU per week for 12 weeks in NAFLD had no significant effect on lipid profile and body composition (Hussain et al., 2019). The effect of vitamin D on lipid profile in people with NAFLD may be different from its effect in healthy people or in people with other chronic diseases.

Some effects of vitamin D are exerted through its effect on increasing calcium absorption. Therefore, dietary calcium intake can also affect the role of vitamin D in determining serum lipid profile. Shidfar et al. found that vitamin D combined with calcium

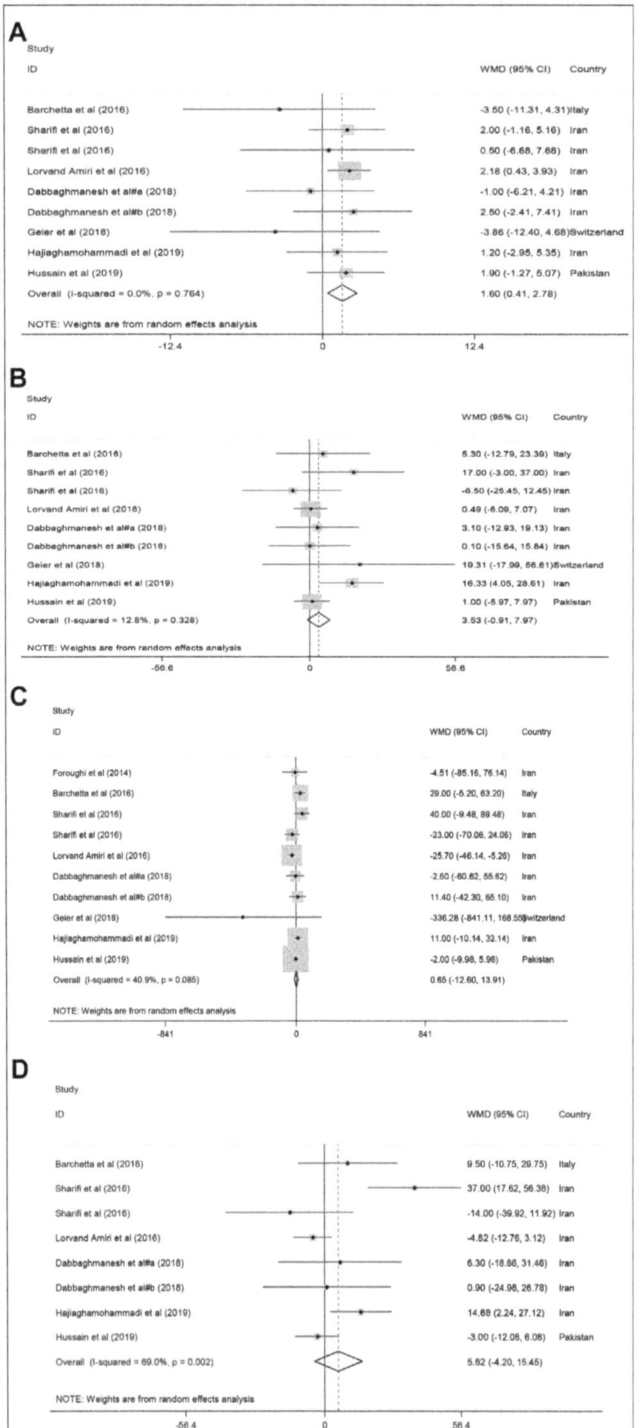

FIGURE 2 | The lipid profile standardized mean differences estimates for **(A)** HDL-C, **(B)** LDL-C, **(C)** TG and **(D)** TC between intervention group (receiving vitamin D supplementation) and placebo groups.

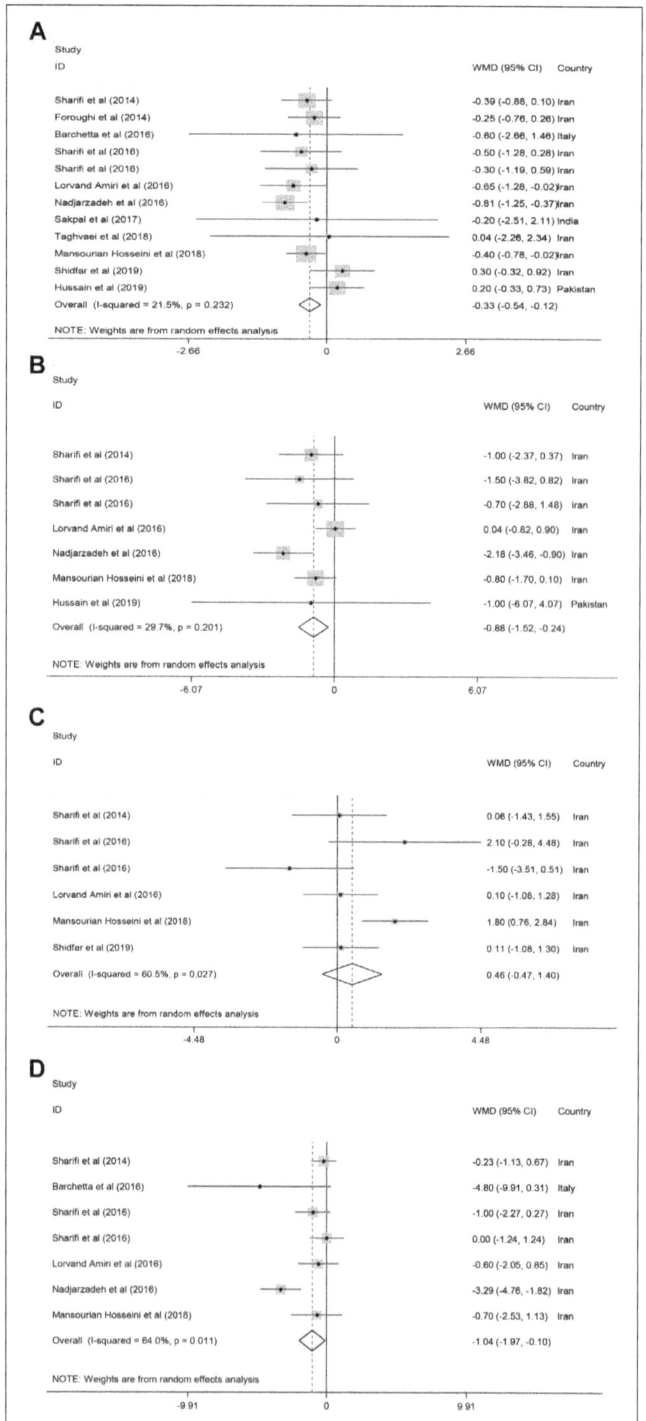

FIGURE 3 | The anthropometric parameters standardized mean differences estimates for **(A)** BMI, **(B)** weight, and **(C)** body fat and **(D)** WC between intervention group (receiving vitamin D supplementation) and placebo groups.

for 12 weeks reduced ALT, AST, LDL-C/HDL-C, TC/HDL-C, and increased non–HDL–C compared with group revived only vitamin D (Shidfar et al., 2019). Moreover, some studies suggested an inverse association between serum 25(OH)-D levels and TG (Chon et al., 2014). The underlying mechanisms of the effects of vitamin D on lipid profile has not been completely yet understood. The low levels of vitamin D can lead to hyperparathyroidism which can lower serum TG. On the other hand, lower vitamin D level can activate microsomal

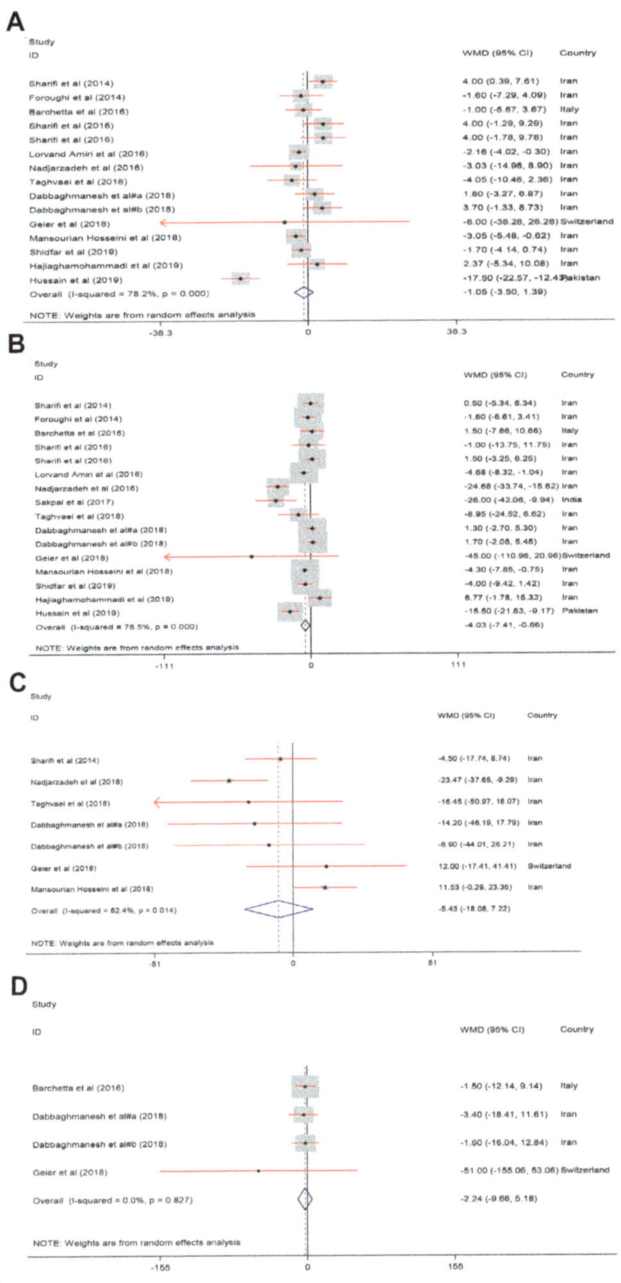

FIGURE 4 | The Liver enzymes standardized mean differences estimates for **(A)** AST **(B)** ALT, **(C)** ALP and **(D)** GGT between intervention group (receiving vitamin D supplementation) and placebo groups.

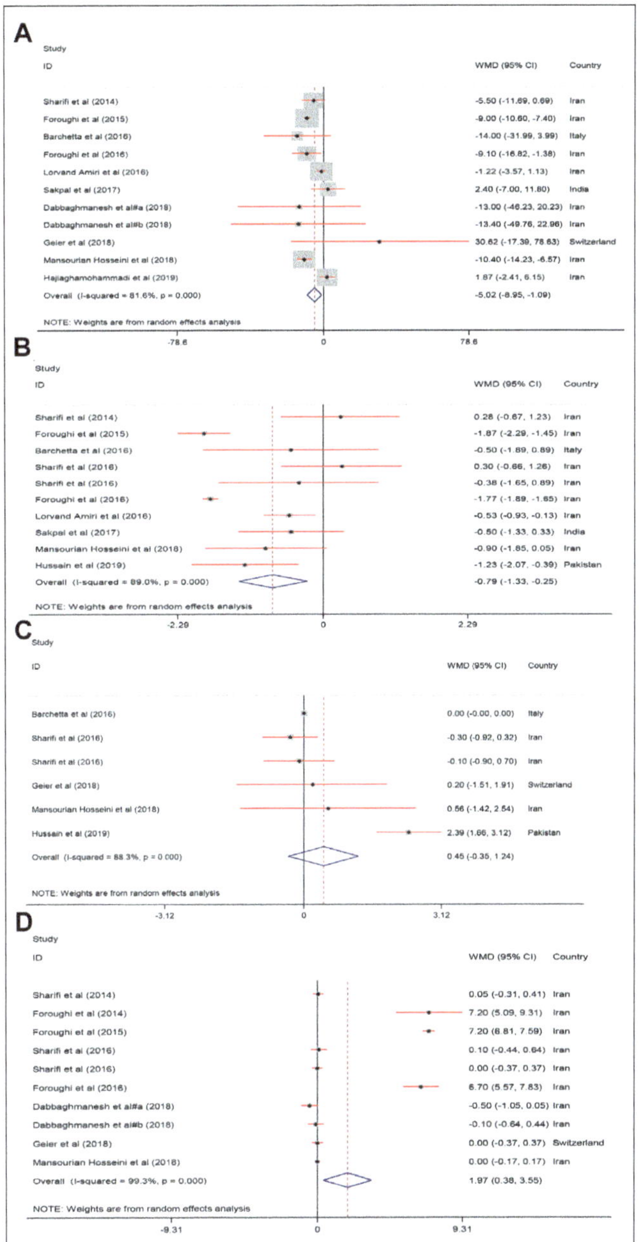

FIGURE 5 | The FBS, HOMA, Adiponectin and calcium mean differences estimates for **(A)** FBG, **(B)** HOMA–IR, **(C)** Adiponectin and **(D)** calcium FBS: fasting plasma glucose; homeostasis model assessment of insulin resistance; RCTs, randomized controlled trials.

TG-transfer protein, which leads to increased TG. Vitamin D also regulates macrophage function in reverse cholesterol transportation and reduces inflammation and insulin resistance (Shidfar et al., 2019).

Regarding to anthropometric measurements, this meta–analysis found that vitamin D reduced body weight, BMI, and WC but no significant change was found in body fat. Hussain et al. investigated the association between vitamin D intake and BMI, body fat, and WC in NAFLD and reported that 50,000 IU vitamin D for 12 weeks had no significant effect on anthropometric indices (Hussain et al., 2019). Another study found that the injection of cholecalciferol (600,000 IU) reduced weight, WC, and BMI (Mansourian Hosseini et al., 2018). Sharifi et al. reported that the intervention group with 50,000 IU vitamin D3 for 4 month had lower weight, WC, and BMI compared with the controls (Sharifi et al., 2016). The reason for these differences may be the differences in doses of vitamin D supplementation and also differences in seum level of vitamin D. Doaei et al. reported that the serum level of vitamin D is inversely associated

TABLE 2 | The results of subgroup analysis.

Subgroups		No. of study	WMD (95% CI)	p	Heterogeneity (I^2, P)
TG					
Country	Iran	7	−1.73 (−21.01, 17.55)	0.86	41.4%, 0.11
	Other	3	8.29 (−24.32, 40.90)	0.61	57.4%, 0.09
Duration	>12 weeks	4	14.03 (−25.09, 53.15)	0.48	49.7%, 0.11
	≤12 weeks	6	−3.87 (−15.21, 7.47)	0.50	26.0%, 0.23
Dosage	≤25,000 IU	5	1.31 (−34.31, 36.94)	0.94	69.2%, 0.01
	>25,000 IU	5	−0.23 (−7.53, 7.08)	0.95	0.0%, 0.83
TC					
Country	Iran	6	7.19 (−6.90, 21.27)	0.31	75.8%, 0.001
	Other	2	−0.16 (−10.43, 10.10)	0.97	17.9%, 0.27
Duration	>12 weeks	3	11.84 (−16.20, 39.89)	0.40	80.1%, 0.007
	≤12 weeks	5	1.39 (−6.58, 9.36)	0.73	46.1%, 0.11
Dosage	≤25,000 IU	4	7.02 −13.62, 27.66)	0.50	82.6%, 0.001
	>25,000 IU	4	4.45 (−5.80, 14.71)	0.39	0.16
HDL–C					
Country	Iran	6	1.82 (0.51, 3.13)	0.007	0.0%, 0.90
	Other	3	−0.22 (−4.17, 3.72)	0.91	27.3%, 0.25
Duration	>12 weeks	4	0.66 (−1.92, 3.25)	0.61	0.0%, 0.41
	≤12 weeks	5	1.84 (0.51, 3.18)	0.007	0.0%, 0.83
Dosage	≤25,000 IU	5	1.70 (0.25, 3.15)	0.02	0.0%, 0.43
	>25,000 IU	4	1.38 (−0.68, 3.44)	0.18	0.0%, 0.77
BMI					
Country	Iran	9	−0.40 (−0.61, −0.19)	<0.0001	15.1%, 0.30
	Other	3	0.13 (−0.37, 0.64)	0.60	0.0%, 0.73
Duration	>12 weeks	5	−0.40 (−0.77, −0.03)	0.03	0.0%, 0.99
	≤12 weeks	7	−0.29 (−0.61, 0.04)	0.08	56.2%, 0.03
Dosage	≤25,000 IU	7	−0.31 (−0.59, −0.02)	0.03	0.0%, 0.51
	>25,000 IU	5	−0.33 (−0.69, 0.03)	0.07	53.9%, 0.06
Body weight					
Country	Iran	6	−0.90 (−1.60, −0.20)	0.01	41.4%, 0.12
	Other	1	−1 (−6.07, 4.07)	–	–
Duration	>12 weeks	3	−1.03 (−2.07, 0.01)	0.05	0.0%, 0.88
	≤12 weeks	4	−0.89 (−1.94, 0.16)	0.09	62.6%, 0.04
Dosage	≤25,000 IU	4	−0.40 (−1.06, 0.27)	0.23	0.0%, 0.44
	>25,000 IU	3	−1.35 (−2.40, −0.31)	0.01	33.3%, 0.22
ALT					
Country	Iran	12	−2.37 (−5.46, 0.73)	0.13	74.0%, <0.0001
	Other	4	−13.61 (−27.33, 0.10)	0.05	77.6%, 0.004
Duration	>12 weeks	6	−2.41 (−8.67, 3.85)	0.45	59.6%, 0.03
	≤12 weeks	10	−4.69 (−8.79, −0.59)	0.02	83.6%, <0.0001
Dosage	≤25,000 IU	8	−2.72 (−6.67, 1.22)	0.17	56.3%, 0.02
	>25,000 IU	8	−4.98 (−10.41, 0.45)	0.07	87.0%, <0.0001
AST					
Country	Iran	12	0.10 (−1.70, 1.90)	0.91	54.9%, 0.01
	Other	3	−8.77 (−23.21, 5.67)	0.23	90.9%, <0.0001
Duration	>12 weeks	5	2.74 (0.44, 5.04)	0.02	0.0%, 0.46
	≤12 weeks	10	−2.59 (−5.45, 0.27)	0.07	79.9%, <0.0001
Dosage	≤25,000 IU	7	0.53 (−1.86, 2.91)	0.66	60.5%, 0.01
	>25,000 IU	8	−2.76 (−7.44, 1.91)	0.24	84.0%, <0.0001
ALP					
Country	Iran	6	−7.62 (−21.34, 6.09)	0.27	66.2%, 0.01
	Other	1	12.00 (−17.41, 41.41)	–	–
Duration	>12 weeks	2	−1.69 (−13.84, 10.46)	0.78	0.5%, 0.31
	≤12 weeks	5	−9.11 (−27.90, 9.67)	0.34	73.0%, 0.005
Dosage	≤25,000 IU	2	−1.69 (−13.84, 10.46)	0.78	0.5%, 0.31
	>25,000 IU	5	−9.11 (−27.90, 9.67)	0.34	73.0%, 0.005

(Continued on following page)

TABLE 2 | (*Continued*) The results of subgroup analysis.

Subgroups		No. of study	WMD (95% CI)	*p*	Heterogeneity (I^2, *P*)
FBS					
Country	Iran	8	−5.63 (−9.78, −1.48)	0.008	85.5%, <0.0001
	Other	3	−0.85 (−16.87, 15.17)	0.91	51.7%, 0.12
Duration	>12 weeks	4	−3.09 (−11.24, 5.07)	0.45	41.9%, 0.16
	≤12 weeks	7	−5.68 9—10.34, −1.01)	0.01	87.5%, <0.0001
Dosage	≤25,000 IU	5	−2.20 (−6.33, 1.93)	0.29	31.9%, 0.20
	>25,000 IU	6	−6.87 (−11.81, −1.94)	0.006	78.8%, <0.0001
HOMA–IR					
Country	Iran	7	−0.79 (−1.44, −0.14)	0.01	91.7%, <0.0001
	Other	3	−0.81 (−1.35, −0.26)	0.004	0.0%, 0.43
Duration	>12 weeks	5	−0.12 (−0.58, 0.34)	0.60	0.0%, 0.61
	≤12 weeks	5	−1.30 (−1.88, −0.73)	<0.0001	89.4%, <0.0001
Dosage	≤25,000 IU	6	−0.35 (−0.65, −0.05)	0.02	0.0%, 0.49
	>25,000 IU	4	−1.68 (−1.96, −1.40)	<0.0001	39.0%, 0.17

TABLE 3 | The results of risk of bias.

First author	Country	Random sequence generation (selection bias)	Alloation concealment (selection bias)	Blinding or participants and personnel (performance bias)	Blinding of outcome assessment (detection bias)	Incomplete outcome data addressed (attrition bias)	Selective reporting (reporting bias)	Other sources of bias (e.g. bias of study design, trial stopped early, extreme baseline imbalance and fraudulent)
Sharifi et al. (2014)	Iran	Unclear	Unclear	Low risk	Low risk	Low risk	Low risk	Low risk
Foroughi et al. (2014)	Iran	Unclear	Unclear	Low risk	Low risk	Low risk	High risk	Low risk
Foroughi et al. (2015)	Iran	Unclear	Unclear	Low risk	Low risk	Low risk	Low risk	Low risk
Barchetta et al. (2016)	Italy	Low risk	Low risk	Low risk	Low risk	High risk	Low risk	Low risk
Sharifi et al. (2016)	Iran	Unclear	Unclear	Low risk	Low risk	Low risk	Low risk	Low risk
Foroughi et al. (2016)	Iran	Low risk	Low risk	Low risk	Low risk	Low risk	Low risk	Low risk
Lorvandamiri et al. (2016)	Iran	Low risk	Low risk	Low risk	Low risk	Low risk	Low risk	Low risk
Nadjarzadeh et al. (2016)	Iran	Unclear	Unclear	Low risk	Low risk	Low risk	High risk	Low risk
Sakpal et al. (2017)	India	Unclear	Unclear	Unclear	Low risk	Unclear	Unclear	Low risk
Taghvaei et al. (2018)	Iran	Low risk	Low risk	Low risk	Low risk	Low risk	Low risk	Low risk
Dabbaghmanesh et al. (2018)	Iran	Low risk	Low risk	Low risk	Low risk	Low risk	Low risk	Low risk
Geier et al. (2018)	Switzerland	Unclear	Unclear	Low risk	Low risk	Low risk	Low risk	Low risk
Mansourian Hosseini et al. (2018)	Iran	Low risk	Low risk	Unclear	Low risk	High risk	Low risk	Low risk
Shidfar et al. (2019)	Iran	Low risk	Low risk	Low risk	Low risk	Unclear	High risk	Low risk
Hajiaghamohammadi et al. (2019)	Iran	Unclear	Unclear	Low risk	Low risk	Unclear	High risk	Low risk
Hussain et al. (2019)	Pakistan	Low risk	Low risk	Low risk	Low risk	Low risk	Unclear	Low risk

with obesity. However, short term changes of serum vitamin D was not related to changes in weight (Doaei et al., 2020).

The present study identified that ALT increased and some liver enzymes such as AST, ALP, GGT were not affected following vitamin D supplementation. Vitamin D receptor (VDR) is abundantly expressed on liver cells and this vitamin was reported to have an anti–inflammatory effect on liver (Bozic et al., 2016). One study found that 50,000 IU/wk vitamin D supplementation for 10 weeks reduced AST and ALT in the intervention group compared with the control group (Hajiaghamohammadi et al., 2019). The vitamin D supplementation for 48 weeks decreased liver enzyme in patients with NAFLD (Geier et al., 2018). The difference in the results of the effect of vitamin D on the serum level of liver enzymes may be due to the fact that the levels of liver enzymes is greatly affected by other lifestyle and dietary factors. Sakpal et al. indicated that vitamin D intake along with lifestyle modifications improved serum ALT levels (Jamali et al., 2013). Another placebo–controlled study found that 12–weeks hypocaloric diet combined with calcitriol improved ALT and AST in the intervention group compared with the control group (Amiri et al., 2016).

The levels of FBS and HOMA-IR were improved following vitamin D intake. In line with this study, one study indicated that calcitriol intake (25 mg) for 12 weeks improved HOMA–IR in patients with NAFLD (Amiri et al., 2016). A recent study reported that vitamin D intake increased insulin sensitivity (Inzucchi et al., 1998). Another study found a negative association between vitamin D supplementation and FBS (Pittas et al., 2007). In another study, calcitriol supplementation for a short term increased insulin sensitivity (Foroughi et al., 2016). One meta–analysis suggested that vitamin D administration could improve FBS and insulin resistance in patents with impaired glucose tolerance or HOMA–IR (George et al., 2012). However, the results regarding the effect of vitamin D on serum glucose indices were contradictory. One study reported that vitamin D had no association with FBS (Kitson and Roberts, 2012). Interestingly, Lind et al. found that long–term calcitriol supplementation for 2 years decreased HOMA–IR but had no effect on insulin (Lind et al., 1989). The short–term vitamin D intake was associated with lower FBS in renal disease patients while had no effect on fasting insulin levels (Sarathy et al., 2015). The underlying mechanism of the effect of vitamin D on blood glucose is not yet clear. Vitamin D deficiency increase serum parathyroid hormone levels (PTH) and the PTH plays an important role in NAFLD through increasing insulin resistance (IR) (Foss, 2009).

The results of the present study indicated that the level of adiponectin was not significantly affected by vitamin D supplementation. Some studies reported that patients with NAFLD had lower adiponectin concentration compared with the others and adiponectin can be considered as a predictor of the severity of hepatic steatosis (Targher et al., 2006; Nakano et al., 2011). In line with our study, two previous studies reported that vitamin D intake had no effect on serum adiponectin in people with type 2 diabetes and obese children (Patel et al., 2010; Belenchia et al., 2013). On the other hand, Nakano et al. reported that phototherapy and vitamin D increased adiponectin concentration in rats with NAFLD (Kitson and Roberts, 2012). Adiponectin is secreted from adipose tissue and could influence on metabolism of fat and glucose. Adiponectin increased liver insulin sensitivity and decreased glucose excretion from the liver which can lead to prevent of high blood sugar. It has been suggested that vitamin D regulates adiponectin gene expression in adipose tissue (Hajiaghamohammadi et al., 2019). It seems that many factors may influence the effects of vitamin D on serum adiponectin such as differences in doses of vitamin D supplementation, follow–up duration, and VDR gene polymorphisms. Moreover, the association between vitamin D intake and adiponectin may be influenced by other factors such as calcium intake and body weight. The results of a recent meta–analysis study indicated that vitamin D may promote secretion of adiponectin in subjects with diabetes and this effect may be potentiated if vitamin D intake is on daily basis and in combination with calcium but can be weakened by increasing BMI (Nikooyeh and Neyestani, 2021).

The present study found that vitamin D supplementation improved the level of serum calcium. In contrast with this result, Geier et al. found that adiponectin and calcium levels were not significantly different after vitamin D supplementation (Geier et al., 2018). Sharifi et al. showed that vitamin D supplementation has no effect on serum level of calcium (Sharifi et al., 2016). A recent study of more than 5,000 people found that taking a monthly vitamin D supplement did not alter serum calcium (Malihi et al., 2019). Serum calcium levels play an important role in the cardiovascular and muscular system and are maintained at a certain level by complex mechanisms (Fleet, 2017). Further studies on the effect of vitamin D on serum calcium levels and considering the interaction of various factors on serum calcium levels are needed.

CONCLUSION

The present study showed that Vitamin D supplementation had significant effect on HDL-C, body weight, BMI, WC, serum ALT, serum FBS, HOMA-IR, calcium and no effect on TG, TC, LDL-C, AST, ALP, GGT, and adiponectin. Further studies are needed to identify the underlying mechanisms of the effects of vitamin D supplementation on the anthropometric and biochemical indices in patient with NAFLD.

AUTHOR CONTRIBUTIONS

SR and RT designed the study, and were involved in the data collection, analysis, and drafting of the manuscript. SR, PN-S, MJ, MS-B, SM, SD, and MG were involved in the design of the study, analysis of the data, and critically reviewed the manuscript. All authors read and approved the final manuscript.

ACKNOWLEDGMENTS

This study was conducted at the school of Nutrition and Food Sciences and shahid beheshti University of Medical Sciences, Tehran, Iran.

REFERENCES

Amiri, H. L., Agah, S., Mousavi, S. N., Hosseini, A. F., and Shidfar, F. (2016). Regression of Non–alcoholic Fatty Liver by Vitamin D Supplement: a Double–Blind Randomized Controlled Clinical Trial. *Arch. Iranian Med.* 19 (9), 0.

Barchetta, I., Del Ben, M., Angelico, F., Di Martino, M., Fraioli, A., La Torre, G., et al. (2016). No Effects of Oral Vitamin D Supplementation on Non–alcoholic Fatty Liver Disease in Patients with Type 2 Diabetes: a Randomized, Double–Blind, Placebo–Controlled Trial. *BMC Med.* 14 (1), 92–10. doi:10.1186/s12916-016-0638-y

Belenchia, A. M., Tosh, A. K., Hillman, L. S., and Peterson, C. A. (2013). Correcting Vitamin D Insufficiency Improves Insulin Sensitivity in Obese Adolescents: a Randomized Controlled Trial. *Am. J. Clin. Nutr.* 97 (4), 774–781. doi:10.3945/ajcn.112.050013

Benetti, E., Mastrocola, R., Chiazza, F., Nigro, D., D'Antona, G., Bordano, V., et al. (2018). Effects of Vitamin D on Insulin Resistance and Myosteatosis in

Diet–Induced Obese Mice. *PLoS One* 13 (1), e0189707. doi:10.1371/journal.pone.0189707

Bozic, M., Guzmán, C., Benet, M., Sánchez–Campos, S., García–Monzón, C., Gari, E., et al. (2016). Hepatocyte Vitamin D Receptor Regulates Lipid Metabolism and Mediates Experimental Diet–Induced Steatosis. *J. Hepatol.* 65 (4), 748–757. doi:10.1016/j.jhep.2016.05.031

Chalasani, N., Younossi, Z., Lavine, J. E., Diehl, A. M., Brunt, E. M., Cusi, K., et al. (2012). The Diagnosis and Management of Non–alcoholic Fatty Liver Disease: Practice Guideline by the American Association for the Study of Liver Diseases, American College of Gastroenterology, and the American Gastroenterological Association. *Hepatology* 55 (6), 2005–2023. doi:10.1002/hep.25762

Chon, S. J., Yun, B. H., Jung, Y. S., Cho, S. H., Choi, Y. S., Kim, S. Y., et al. (2014). Association between Vitamin D Status and Risk of Metabolic Syndrome Among Korean Postmenopausal Women. *PloS one* 9 (2), e89721. doi:10.1371/journal.pone.0089721

Dabbaghmanesh, M. H., Danafar, F., Eshraghian, A., and Omrani, G. R. (2018). Vitamin D Supplementation for the Treatment of Non–alcoholic Fatty Liver Disease: A Randomized Double Blind Placebo Controlled Trial. *Diabetes Metab. Syndr.* 12 (4), 513–517. doi:10.1016/j.dsx.2018.03.006

Del Ben, M., Polimeni, L., Baratta, F., Pastori, D., Loffredo, L., and Angelico, F. (2014). Modern Approach to the Clinical Management of Non–alcoholic Fatty Liver Disease. *World J. Gastroenterol.* 20 (26), 8341–8350. doi:10.3748/wjg.v20.i26.8341

Doaei, S., Jarrahi, S., Torki, S., Haghshenas, R., Jamshidi, Z., Rezaei, S., et al. (2020). Serum Vitamin D Level May Be Associated with Body Weight and Body Composition in Male Adolescents; a Longitudinal Study. *Pediatr. Endocrinol. Diabetes Metab.* 26 (3), 125–131. doi:10.5114/pedm.2020.97466

Doaei, S., Kalantari, N., Izadi, P., Salonurmi, T., Mosavi Jarrahi, A., Rafieifar, S., et al. (2019). Changes in FTO and IRX3 Gene Expression in Obese and Overweight Male Adolescents Undergoing an Intensive Lifestyle Intervention and the Role of FTO Genotype in This Interaction. *J. Transl Med.* 17 (1), 176–178. doi:10.1186/s12967–019–1921–4

Duval, S., and Tweedie, R. (2000). Trim and Fill: A Simple Funnel–Plot–Based Method of Testing and Adjusting for Publication Bias in Meta–Analysis. *Biometrics* 56 (2), 455–463. doi:10.1111/j.0006–341x.2000.00455.x

Fleet, J. C. (2017). The Role of Vitamin D in the Endocrinology Controlling Calcium Homeostasis. *Mol. Cel Endocrinol* 453, 36–45. doi:10.1016/j.mce.2017.04.008

Foroughi, M., Maghsoudi, Z., and Askari, G. (2016). The Effect of Vitamin D Supplementation on Blood Sugar and Different Indices of Insulin Resistance in Patients with Non–alcoholic Fatty Liver Disease (NAFLD). *Iran J. Nurs. Midwifery Res.* 21 (1), 100–104. doi:10.4103/1735–9066.174759

Foroughi, M., Maghsoudi, Z., Ghiasvand, R., Iraj, B., and Askari, G. (2014). Effect of Vitamin D Supplementation on C–Reactive Protein in Patients with Nonalcoholic Fatty Liver. *Int. J. Prev. Med.* 5 (8), 969–975.

Foroughi, M., Maghsoudi, Z., Ghiasvand, R., Iraj, B., and Askari, G. (2015). The Effect of Vitamin D Supplementation on Insulin Resistance in Patients with Nonalcoholic Fatty Liver. *J. Isfahan Med. Sch.* 33 (342), 1076–1085.

Forouhi, N. G., Luan, J., Cooper, A., Boucher, B. J., and Wareham, N. J. (2008). Baseline Serum 25–hydroxy Vitamin D Is Predictive of Future Glycemic Status and Insulin Resistance: the Medical Research Council Ely Prospective Study 1990–2000. *Diabetes* 57 (10), 2619–2625. doi:10.2337/db08–0593

Foss, Y. J. (2009). Vitamin D Deficiency Is the Cause of Common Obesity. *Med. Hypotheses* 72 (3), 314–321. doi:10.1016/j.mehy.2008.10.005

Geier, A., Eichinger, M., Stirnimann, G., Semela, D., Tay, F., Seifert, B., et al. (2018). Treatment of Non–alcoholic Steatohepatitis Patients with Vitamin D: a Double–Blinded, Randomized, Placebo–Controlled Pilot Study. *Scand. J. Gastroenterol.* 53 (9), 1114–1120. doi:10.1080/00365521.2018.1501091

George, P. S., Pearson, E. R., and Witham, M. D. (2012). Effect of Vitamin D Supplementation on Glycaemic Control and Insulin Resistance: a Systematic Review and Meta–Analysis. *Diabet Med.* 29 (8), e142–50. doi:10.1111/j.1464–5491.2012.03672.x

Gholamalizadeh, M., Jarrahi, A. M., Akbari, M. E., Bourbour, F., Mokhtari, Z., Salahshoornezhad, S., et al. (2020). Association between FTO Gene Polymorphisms and Breast Cancer: the Role of Estrogen. *Expert Rev. Endocrinol. Metab.* 15 (2), 115–121. doi:10.1080/17446651.2020.1730176

Hajiaghamohammadi, A., Shafikhani, A. A., Akbar Shafikhani, A., Bastani, A., and Gaemi, N. (2019). Effect of Vitamin D Replacement on Liver Enzymes in Patients with Non–alcoholic Fatty Liver Disease. *J. Gastroenterol. Hepatol. Res.* 8 (3), 2907–2910. doi:10.17554/j.issn.2224–3992.2019.08.819

Hariri, M., and Zohdi, S. (2019). Effect of Vitamin D on Non–alcoholic Fatty Liver Disease: a Systematic Review of Randomized Controlled Clinical Trials. *Int. J. Prev. Med.* 10, 14. doi:10.4103/ijpvm.IJPVM_499_17

Higgins, J., Thomas, J., Chandler, J., Cumpston, M., Li, T., Page, M., et al. (2019). *Cochrane Handbook for Systematic Reviews of Interventions*. Wiley, NJ, USA, version 6.0(updated July 2019), .

Higgins, J. P., Altman, D. G., Gøtzsche, P. C., Jüni, P., Moher, D., Oxman, A. D., et al. (2011). The Cochrane Collaboration's Tool for Assessing Risk of Bias in Randomised Trials. *BMJ* 343, d5928. doi:10.1136/bmj.d5928

Hussain, M., Iqbal, J., Malik, S. A., Waheed, A., Shabnum, S., Akhtar, L., et al. (2019). Effect of Vitamin D Supplementation on Various Parameters in Non–alcoholic Fatty Liver Disease Patients. *Pak J. Pharm. Sci.* 32, 1343–1348.

Inzucchi, S. E., Maggs, D. G., Spollett, G. R., Page, S. L., Rife, F. S., Walton, V., et al. (1998). Efficacy and Metabolic Effects of Metformin and Troglitazone in Type II Diabetes Mellitus. *N. Engl. J. Med.* 338 (13), 867–872. doi:10.1056/NEJM199803263381303

Jamali, R., Mofid, A., Vahedi, H., Farzaneh, R., and Dowlatshahi, S. (2013). The Effect of helicobacter Pylori Eradication on Liver Fat Content in Subjects with Non–alcoholic Fatty Liver Disease: a Randomized Open–Label Clinical Trial. *Hepat. Mon* 13 (12), e14679. doi:10.5812/hepatmon.14679

Kitson, M. T., and Roberts, S. K. (2012). D–livering the Message: the Importance of Vitamin D Status in Chronic Liver Disease. *J. Hepatol.* 57 (4), 897–909. doi:10.1016/j.jhep.2012.04.033

Kleiner, D. E., Brunt, E. M., Van Natta, M., Behling, C., Contos, M. J., Cummings, O. W., et al. (2005). Design and Validation of a Histological Scoring System for Nonalcoholic Fatty Liver Disease. *Hepatology* 41 (6), 1313–1321. doi:10.1002/hep.20701

Lind, L., Pollare, T., Hvarfner, A., Lithell, H., Sørensen, O. H., and Ljunghall, S. (1989). Long–term Treatment with Active Vitamin D (Alphacalcidol) in Middle–Aged Men with Impaired Glucose Tolerance. Effects on Insulin Secretion and Sensitivity, Glucose Tolerance and Blood Pressure. *Diabetes Res.* 11 (3), 141–147.

Lorvand Amiri, H., Agah, S., Tolouei Azar, J., Hosseini, S., Shidfar, F., and Mousavi, S. N. (2017). Effect of Daily Calcitriol Supplementation with and without Calcium on Disease Regression in Non–alcoholic Fatty Liver Patients Following an Energy–Restricted Diet: Randomized, Controlled, Double–Blind Trial. *Clin. Nutr.* 36 (6), 1490–1497. doi:10.1016/j.clnu.2016.09.020

Ludwig, J., Viggiano, T R., Mcgill, D. B., and Oh, B. J. (1980). "Nonalcoholic Steatohepatitis: Mayo Clinic Experiences with a Hitherto Unnamed Disease," in *Mayo Clinic Proceedings*, 55, 7, 434–438, .

Malihi, Z., Lawes, C. M. M., Wu, Z., Huang, Y., Waayer, D., Toop, L., et al. (2019). Monthly High–Dose Vitamin D Supplementation Does Not Increase Kidney Stone Risk or Serum Calcium: Results from a Randomized Controlled Trial. *Am. J. Clin. Nutr.* 109 (6), 1578–1587. doi:10.1093/ajcn/nqy378

Mansourian, S. H., Aliashrafi, S., and Ebrahimi, M. M. (2018). The Effect of a Single Intramuscular Injection of Cholecalciferol on the Serum Levels of Vitamin D, Adiponectin, Insulin Resistance, and Liver Function in Women with Non–alcoholic Fatty Liver Disease (NAFLD): A Randomized, Controlled Clinical Trial. *Iranian Red Crescent Med. J.* 20 (10). doi:10.5812/ircmj.60746

Mehrdad, M., Doaei, S., Gholamalizadeh, M., Fardaei, M., Fararouei, M., and Eftekhari, M. H. (2020). Association of FTO Rs9939609 Polymorphism with Serum Leptin, Insulin, Adiponectin, and Lipid Profile in Overweight Adults. *Adipocyte* 9 (1), 51–56. doi:10.1080/21623945.2020.1722550

Moher, D., Liberati, A., Tetzlaff, J., and Altman, D. G. (2009). Preferred Reporting Items for Systematic Reviews and Meta–Analyses: the PRISMA Statement. *BMJ* 339 (4), b2535–9. doi:10.1136/bmj.b2535

Morvaridzadeh, M., Nachvak, S. M., Mohammadi, R., Moradi, S., Mostafai, R., Pizarro, A. B., et al. (2021). Probiotic Yogurt Fortified with Vitamin D Can Improve Glycemic Status in Non–alcoholic Fatty Liver Disease Patients: a Randomized Clinical Trial. *Clin. Nutr. Res.* 10 (1), 36–47. doi:10.7762/cnr.2021.10.1.36

Mouodi, M., Fakheri, H. T., Kashi, Z., Maleki, I., and Mohammadpour, R. (2018). Effects of Vitamin D Supplementation on Patients with Non–alcoholic Fatty Liver Disease (NAFLD). *Acta Med.* 34, 415.

Nadjarzadeh, A., Jani, N., Khoshnevisan, M., Molajaafari, A., Fallahzadeh, H., Khabiri, F., et al. (2016). Effects of Low Caloric Diet with and without Vitamin D Supplementation on Anthropometric Parameters in Patients with Non–alcoholic Fatty Liver. *Tolooebehdasht* 14 (6), 410–422.

Nakano, T., Cheng, Y. F., Lai, C. Y., Hsu, L. W., Chang, Y. C., Deng, J. Y., et al. (2011). Impact of Artificial Sunlight Therapy on the Progress of Non–alcoholic

Fatty Liver Disease in Rats. *J. Hepatol.* 55 (2), 415–425. doi:10.1016/j.jhep.2010.11.028

Nikooyeh, B., and Neyestani, T. R. (2021). Can Vitamin D Be Considered an Adiponectin Secretagogue? A Systematic Review and Meta–Analysis. *J. Steroid Biochem. Mol. Biol.* 212, 105925. doi:10.1016/j.jsbmb.2021.105925

Patel, P., Poretsky, L., and Liao, E. (2010). Lack of Effect of Subtherapeutic Vitamin D Treatment on Glycemic and Lipid Parameters in Type 2 Diabetes: a Pilot Prospective Randomized Trial. *J. Diabetes* 2 (1), 36–40. doi:10.1111/j.1753–0407.2009.00057.x

Petta, S., Gastaldelli, A., Rebelos, E., Bugianesi, E., Messa, P., Miele, L., et al. (2016). Pathophysiology of Non Alcoholic Fatty Liver Disease. *Int. J. Mol. Sci.* 17 (12), 2082. doi:10.3390/ijms17122082

Pittas, A. G., Harris, S. S., Stark, P. C., and Dawson, B. H. (2007). The Effects of Calcium and Vitamin D Supplementation on Blood Glucose and Markers of Inflammation in Nondiabetic Adults. *Diabetes care* 30 (4), 980–986. doi:10.2337/dc06–1994

Sakpal, M., Satsangi, S., Mehta, M., Duseja, A., Bhadada, S., Das, A., et al. (2017). Vitamin D Supplementation in Patients with Nonalcoholic Fatty Liver Disease: A Randomized Controlled Trial. *JGH Open* 1 (2), 62–67. doi:10.1002/jgh3.12010

Sarathy, H., Pramanik, V., Kahn, J., Abramowitz, M. K., Meier, K., Kishore, P., et al. (2015). The Effects of Short–Term Vitamin D Supplementation on Glucose Metabolism in Dialysis Patients: a Systematic Review and Meta–Analysis. *Int. Urol. Nephrol.* 47 (3), 537–549. doi:10.1007/s11255–015–0909–0

Schwimmer, J. B., Behling, C., Newbury, R., Deutsch, R., Nievergelt, C., Schork, N. J., et al. (2005). Histopathology of Pediatric Nonalcoholic Fatty Liver Disease. *Hepatology* 42 (3), 641–649. doi:10.1002/hep.20842

Sepidarkish, M., Farsi, F., Akbari, M. F., Namazi, N., Almasi, A. H., Maleki, A. H., et al. (2019). The Effect of Vitamin D Supplementation on Oxidative Stress Parameters: a Systematic Review and Meta–Analysis of Clinical Trials. *Pharmacol. Res.* 139, 141–152. doi:10.1016/j.phrs.2018.11.011

Sharifi, N., Amani, R., Hajiani, E., and Cheraghian, B. (2014). Does Vitamin D Improve Liver Enzymes, Oxidative Stress, and Inflammatory Biomarkers in Adults with Non–alcoholic Fatty Liver Disease? A Randomized Clinical Trial. *Endocrine* 47 (1), 70–80. doi:10.1007/s12020–014–0336–5

Sharifi, N., Amani, R., Hajiani, E., and Cheraghian, B. (2016). Women May Respond Different from Men to Vitamin D Supplementation Regarding Cardiometabolic Biomarkers. *Exp. Biol. Med. (Maywood)* 241 (8), 830–838. doi:10.1177/1535370216629009

Shidfar, F., Mousavi, S. N., Lorvand, H. A., Agah, S., Hoseini, S., and Hajimiresmail, S. J. (2019). Reduction of Some Atherogenic Indices in Patients with Non–alcoholic Fatty Liver by Vitamin D and Calcium Co–supplementation: a Double Blind Randomized Controlled Clinical Trial. *Iran J. Pharm. Res.* 18 (1), 496–505.

Targher, G., Bertolini, L., Rodella, S., Zoppini, G., Scala, L., Zenari, L., et al. (2006). Associations between Plasma Adiponectin Concentrations and Liver Histology in Patients with Nonalcoholic Fatty Liver Disease. *Clin. Endocrinol. (Oxf)* 64 (6), 679–683. doi:10.1111/j.1365–2265.2006.02527.x

Taghvaei, T., Akha, O., Mouodi, M., Fakheri, H. T., Kashi, Z., Maleki, I., Mohammadpour, R., et al. (2018). Effects of Vitamin D Supplementation on Patients with Non-Alcoholic Fatty Liver Disease (NAFLD). *Acta Medica.* 34 (415). doi:10.19193/0393-6384_2018_2_66

Tolman, K. G., Fonseca, V., Dalpiaz, A., and Tan, M. H. (2007). Spectrum of Liver Disease in Type 2 Diabetes and Management of Patients with Diabetes and Liver Disease. *Diabetes care* 30 (3), 734–743. doi:10.2337/dc06–1539

Wang, H., Xia, N., Yang, Y., and Peng, D. Q. (2012). Influence of Vitamin D Supplementation on Plasma Lipid Profiles: a Meta–Analysis of Randomized Controlled Trials. *Lipids Health Dis.* 11 (1), 42–49. doi:10.1186/1476–511X–11–42

Younossi, Z. M. (2019). Non–alcoholic Fatty Liver Disease – A Global Public Health Perspective. *J. Hepatol.* 70 (3), 531–544. doi:10.1016/j.jhep.2018.10.033

Permissions

All chapters in this book were first published by Frontiers; hereby published with permission under the Creative Commons Attribution License or equivalent. Every chapter published in this book has been scrutinized by our experts. Their significance has been extensively debated. The topics covered herein carry significant findings which will fuel the growth of the discipline. They may even be implemented as practical applications or may be referred to as a beginning point for another development.

The contributors of this book come from diverse backgrounds, making this book a truly international effort. This book will bring forth new frontiers with its revolutionizing research information and detailed analysis of the nascent developments around the world.

We would like to thank all the contributing authors for lending their expertise to make the book truly unique. They have played a crucial role in the development of this book. Without their invaluable contributions this book wouldn't have been possible. They have made vital efforts to compile up to date information on the varied aspects of this subject to make this book a valuable addition to the collection of many professionals and students.

This book was conceptualized with the vision of imparting up-to-date information and advanced data in this field. To ensure the same, a matchless editorial board was set up. Every individual on the board went through rigorous rounds of assessment to prove their worth. After which they invested a large part of their time researching and compiling the most relevant data for our readers.

The editorial board has been involved in producing this book since its inception. They have spent rigorous hours researching and exploring the diverse topics which have resulted in the successful publishing of this book. They have passed on their knowledge of decades through this book. To expedite this challenging task, the publisher supported the team at every step. A small team of assistant editors was also appointed to further simplify the editing procedure and attain best results for the readers.

Apart from the editorial board, the designing team has also invested a significant amount of their time in understanding the subject and creating the most relevant covers. They scrutinized every image to scout for the most suitable representation of the subject and create an appropriate cover for the book.

The publishing team has been an ardent support to the editorial, designing and production team. Their endless efforts to recruit the best for this project, has resulted in the accomplishment of this book. They are a veteran in the field of academics and their pool of knowledge is as vast as their experience in printing. Their expertise and guidance has proved useful at every step. Their uncompromising quality standards have made this book an exceptional effort. Their encouragement from time to time has been an inspiration for everyone.

The publisher and the editorial board hope that this book will prove to be a valuable piece of knowledge for researchers, students, practitioners and scholars across the globe.

List of Contributors

Su Yeon An and Anca D. Petrescu
Division of Pharmacology and Toxicology, College of Pharmacy, The University of Texas at Austin, Austin, TX, United States

Sharon De Morrow
Division of Pharmacology and Toxicology, College of Pharmacy, The University of Texas at Austin, Austin, TX, United States

Qiannan Ye and Changqing Zhao
Shuguang Hospital Affiliated to Shanghai University of Traditional Chinese Medicine, Shanghai, China
Institute of Liver Diseases, Shanghai University of Traditional Chinese Medicine, Shanghai, China

Yang Zhou
Yueyang Hospital Affiliated to Shanghai University of Traditional Chinese Medicine, Shanghai, China

Lieming Xu
Shuguang Hospital Affiliated to Shanghai University of Traditional Chinese Medicine, Shanghai, China
Institute of Liver Diseases, Shanghai University of Traditional Chinese Medicine, Shanghai, China
Shanghai Key Laboratory of Traditional Chinese Medicine, Shanghai, China
Key Laboratory of Liver and Kidney Diseases, Ministry of Education, Shanghai, China

Jian Ping
Shuguang Hospital Affiliated to Shanghai University of Traditional Chinese Medicine, Shanghai, China
Key Laboratory of Liver and Kidney Diseases, Ministry of Education, Shanghai, China

Kanchana K. Ayyar and Alan C. Moss
Division of Gastroenterology, Department of Medicine, Boston Medical Center, Boston, MA, United States

Francesca Ferretti, Rosanna Cannatelli, Sandro Ardizzone and Giovanni Maconi
Gastroenterology Unit—ASST Fatebenefratelli-Sacco, Department of Biomedical and Clinical Sciences (DIBIC) L. Sacco, Università degli Studi di Milano, Milan, Italy

Jeanette A. Maier
General Pathology—Department of Biomedical and Clinical Sciences (DIBIC) L. Sacco, Università degli Studi di Milano, Milan, Italy

Yanling Zhao
Department of Pharmacy, Fifth Medical Center of PLA General Hospital, Beijing, China

Xing Chen, Shihua Wu, Jianxia Wen, Tao Yang, Ying Wei, Sichen Ren and Yuling Tong
Department of Pharmacy, Fifth Medical Center of PLA General Hospital, Beijing, China
College of Pharmacy, Chengdu University of Traditional Chinese Medicine, Chengdu, China

Jianzhong Zhang
Center of Disease Control and Prevention, National Institute for Communicable Disease Control and Prevention, Beijing, China

Ruilin Wang and Honghong Liu
Integrative Medical Center, Fifth Medical Center of PLA General Hospital, Beijing, China

Chunmei Bao
Division of Clinical Microbiology, Fifth Medical Center of PLA General Hospital, Beijing, China

Badr Al-Bawardy and Deborah D. Proctor
Section of Digestive Diseases, Yale School of Medicine, New Haven, CT, United States

Raina Shivashankar
Division of Gastroenterology and Hepatology, Thomas Jefferson University, Philadelphia, PA, United States

Lijun Kong, Hewei Zhang, Hongjian Huang, Yushu Zheng, Yongqiang Wang and Hongwei Wang
Key Laboratory of Diagnosis and Treatment of Severe Hepato-Pancreatic Diseases of Zhejiang Province, The First Affiliated Hospital of Wenzhou Medical University, Wenzhou, China

Chaosheng Lu and Dan Wang
Department of Pediatrics, The First Affiliated Hospital of Wenzhou Medical University, Wenzhou, China

Keqing Shi
Translational Medicine Laboratory, The First Affiliated Hospital of Wenzhou Medical University, Wenzhou, China

Wei Huang
Department of Nutrition, The First Affiliated Hospital of Wenzhou Medical University, Wenzhou, China

Chang Han, Wen Chen, Jia Yao, Cong Li, Jinqiu Hou and Dongmei Qin
Key Laboratory of Xinjiang Phytomedicine Resource and Utilization, Ministry of Education, School of Pharmacy, Shihezi University, Shihezi, China

Xi Wu
Dongfang Hospital, Beijing University of Chinese Medicine, Beijing, China

Nan Zou and Jinqi Yuan
First Affiliated Hospital, School of Medicine, Shihezi University, Shihezi, China

Yuefeng Gao
State Key Laboratory of Animal Nutrition, College of Animal Science and Technology, China Agricultural University, Beijing, China

Yunsheng Zhang
Husbandry Research Institute, Xinjiang Academy of Animal Science, Urumqi, China

Bianca J. Parker and Pamela A. Wearsch
Department of Pathology, Case Western Reserve University School of Medicine, Cleveland, OH, United States

Alida C. M. Veloo
Department of Medical Microbiology, University Medical Centre Groningen, University of Groningen, Groningen, Netherlands

Alex Rodriguez-Palacios
Division of Gastroenterology and Liver Disease, Case Western Reserve University School of Medicine, Cleveland, OH, United States
Germ-Free and Gut Microbiome, Digestive Health Research Institute, Case Western Reserve University, Cleveland, OH, United States

Yang Yang
Department of Gastroenterology and the Center of Inflammatory Bowel Disease, West China Hospital, Sichuan University, Chengdu, China
Lab of Inflammatory Bowel Disease, Clinical Institute of Inflammation and Immunology, Frontiers Science Center for Disease-related Molecular Network, West China Hospital, Sichuan University, Chengdu, China
Department of Gastroenterology, Daping Hospital, Army Medical University, Chongqing, China

DongFeng Chen
Department of Gastroenterology, Daping Hospital, Army Medical University, Chongqing, China

Jian Zeng
Department of Gastroenterology, Chongqing Traditional Chinese Medicine Hospital, Chongqing, China

Jiao Nie
Lab of Inflammatory Bowel Disease, Clinical Instituteof Inflammation and Immunology, Frontiers Science Center for Disease-related Molecular Network, West China Hospital, Sichuan University, Chengdu, China
Department of Geriatrics and National Clinical Research Center for Geriatric, West China Hospital, Sichuan University, Chengdu, China

Hua-Tian Gan
Department of Gastroenterology and the Center of Inflammatory Bowel Disease, West China Hospital, Sichuan University, Chengdu, China
Lab of Inflammatory Bowel Disease, Clinical Institute of Inflammation and Immunology, Frontiers Science Center for Disease-related Molecular Network, West China Hospital, Sichuan University, Chengdu, China

Qi-Shan Zeng and Min Zou
Department of Gastroenterology and the Center of Inflammatory Bowel Disease, West China Hospital, Sichuan University, Chengdu, China
Lab of Inflammatory Bowel Disease, Clinical Institute of Inflammation and Immunology, Frontiers Science Center for Disease-related Molecular Network, West China Hospital, Sichuan University, Chengdu, China

Ryohtaroh Matsumoto and Daisuke Takahashi
Division of Biochemistry, Graduate School of Pharmaceutical Science and Faculty of Pharmacy, Keio University, Tokyo, Japan

Masaki Watanabe, Shunsuke Nakatani, Yuta Takamura, Yuji Kurosaki and Hiroki Kakuta
Division of Pharmaceutical Sciences, Graduate School of Medicine Dentistry and Pharmaceutical Sciences, Okayama University, Okayama, Japan

Koji Hase
Division of Biochemistry, Graduate School of Pharmaceutical Science and Faculty of Pharmacy, Keio University, Tokyo, Japan
International Research and Development Center for Mucosal Vaccines, The Institute of Medical Science, The University of Tokyo (IMSUT), Tokyo, Japan

Vu Q. Nguyen and Kristin K. Knight
IBD Center, Division of Gastroenterology, Virginia Tech Carilion School of Medicine, Roanoke, VA, United States

Holly A. Morrison, Megan B. Sammons and Siena Sorrentino
Department of Biomedical Sciences and Pathobiology, Virginia-Maryland College of Veterinary Medicine, Virginia Tech, Blacksburg, VA, United States

Kristin Eden
Department of Biomedical Sciences and Pathobiology, Virginia-Maryland College of Veterinary Medicine, Virginia Tech, Blacksburg, VA, United States
Department of Basic Science Education, Virginia Tech Carilion School of Medicine, Roanoke, VA, United States

Irving C. Allen
Department of Biomedical Sciences and Pathobiology, Virginia-Maryland College of Veterinary Medicine, Virginia Tech, Blacksburg, VA, United States
Department of Basic Science Education, Virginia Tech Carilion School of Medicine, Roanoke, VA, United States
Graduate Program in Translational Biology, Medicine and Health, Virginia Tech, Blacksburg, VA, United States

Rebecca M. Brock
Graduate Program in Translational Biology, Medicine and Health, Virginia Tech, Blacksburg, VA, United States

Douglas J. Grider
Department of Pathology, Virginia Tech Carilion School of Medicine, Roanoke, VA, United States

Dario Sorrentino
IBD Center, Division of Gastroenterology, Virginia Tech Carilion School of Medicine, Roanoke, VA, United States
Department of Clinical and Experimental Medical Sciences, University of Udine School of Medicine, Udine, Italy

Hongjiao Xiang, Mingmei Shao, Yifei Lu, Junmin Wang and Tao Wu
Institute of Interdisciplinary Integrative Medicine Research, Shanghai University of Traditional Chinese Medicine, Shanghai, China

Guang Ji
Institute of Digestive Disease, Longhua Hospital, Shanghai University of Traditional Chinese Medicine, Shanghai, China

Jingwen Zhao, Liwei Chen, Peixu Ji, Xiuxiu Xu, Lu Zhang, Siyuan Sun, Xin Liu, Simin Zhou, Lu Zhou and Jie Zhang
Department of Gastroenterology and Hepatology, Tianjin Medical University General Hospital, Tianjin Institute of Digestive Disease, Tianjin Key Laboratory of Digestive Diseases, Tianjin, China

Maojuan Ran
Department of Gastroenterology and Hepatology, Tianjin Medical University General Hospital, Tianjin Institute of Digestive Disease, Tianjin Key Laboratory of Digestive Diseases, Tianjin, China
Department of Gastroenterology and Hepatology, Chengdu Second People's Hospital, Chengdu, China

Ting Yang
Department of Gastroenterology and Hepatology, Tianjin Medical University General Hospital, Tianjin Institute of Digestive Disease, Tianjin Key Laboratory of Digestive Diseases, Tianjin, China
Department of Gastroenterology, Shanxi Provincial People's Hospital, Taiyuan, China

Haoran Ke, Zitong Li, Siqi Wang, Pinjing Lv and Ye Chen
Department of Gastroenterology, State Key Laboratory of Organ Failure Research, Guangdong Provincial Key Laboratory of Gastroenterology, Nanfang Hospital, Southern Medical University, Guangzhou, China

Fang Li
Department of Gastroenterology, State Key Laboratory of Organ Failure Research, Guangdong Provincial Key Laboratory of Gastroenterology, Nanfang Hospital, Southern Medical University, Guangzhou, China
Hainan General Hospital, Haikou, China

Wenlin Deng
Department of Gastroenterology, State Key Laboratory of Organ Failure Research, Guangdong Provincial Key Laboratory of Gastroenterology, Nanfang Hospital, Southern Medical University Guangzhou, China
Department of Pediatrics, The Sixth Affiliated Hospital of Sun Yat-sen University, Guangzhou, China

Carsten Schmidt
Medizinische Klinik II, Klinikum Fulda AG, Universitätsmedizin Marburg - Campus Fulda, Fulda, Germany

Philip C. Grunert and Andreas Stallmach
Klinik für Innere Medizin IV, Universitätsklinikum Jena, Friedrich-Schiller Universität Jena, Jena, Germany

Shahla Rezaei
Nutrition Research Center, School of Nutrition and Food Sciences, Shiraz University of Medical Sciences, Shiraz, Iran
Student Research Committee, Shiraz University of Medical Sciences, Shiraz, Iran

Shayan Modaresi
Student Research Committee, Shiraz University of Medical Sciences, Shiraz, Iran

Reza Tabrizi
Non-Communicable Diseases Research Center, Fasa University of Medical Sciences, Fasa, Iran

Peyman Nowrouzi-Sohrabi
Student Research Committee, Shiraz University of Medical Sciences, Shiraz, Iran
Department of Biochemistry, School of Medicine, Shiraz University of Medical Sciences, Shiraz, Iran

Mohammad Jalali
Nutrition Research Center, Student Research Committee, Shiraz University of Medical Sciences, Shiraz, Iran

Mojtaba Shabani-Borujeni
Department of Clinical Pharmacy, Faculty of Pharmacy, Shiraz University of Medical Sciences, Shiraz, Iran

Maryam Gholamalizadeh
Student Research Committee, Cancer Research Center, Shahid Beheshti University of Medical Sciences, Tehran, Iran

Saeid Doaei
Research Center of Health and Enviroment, School of Health, Guilan University of Medical Sciences, Rasht, Iran

Index

M

N

P

R

S

T

U

www.ingramcontent.com/pod-product-compliance
Lightning Source LLC
LaVergne TN
LVHW082141200926
848484LV00008B/2087
9798887401300